What People All Over the World Are Saying About Betty Kamen's Life-Changing Daily Health Hints

"I have practiced nutritional medicine for 25 years and have been privileged to collaborate with Betty Kamen on numerous articles and books. I was involved in early discussions about the creation of 'nutritional hints' several years ago. Little did I know what a stunning success these daily hints would become and the positive impact it would have on so many lives. Dr. Kamen wisely understood that we learn the most one small bite (or byte) at a time. *Betty Kamen's 1,001 Health Secrets* invites each of us to savor a sumptuous feast of nutritional aphorisms from a master nutritionist."

— Michael Rosenbaum, MD, Corte Madera, CA

"As a busy physician, I look forward to Betty Kamen's Table Talk for accurate, pertinent facts on health and medical issues. Cutting through the rhetoric, she gets to the meat of important issues with useful and easy-to-understand hints that I can pass on to my patients."

— Spencer Thornton, MD

"I can take a hint! *Every* day, thank you! I so enjoy the hints and am amazed at how timely they are. As a body worker and yoga teacher I come in contact with dozens of folks per week.... Referring clients and students to your Table Talk Hints has been a blessing for all concerned. Keep hinting. I can take it ... really!"

— Melinda Maxwell-Smith, RCST, MT

"Betty Kamen's organization of her Daily Health Hints is something I've always wanted but was too afraid to ask for! Thank heaven she has done it all for me."

— Patricia Humes, Schuyler, VA

"I have greatly appreciated receiving the daily hints. I like that they are easily accessible, no need to connect to a website unless I want more information, and backed up by sound science. I feel comfortable passing on the hints to my colleagues and patients because of this."

— Mary Larsen, RN, Decatur, GA

"*Love* getting these daily hints. I forward them all over the place — to my daughter — to my friends.... I am not in health care, but got interested in your website when my youngest daughter was fighting AML. Your information helped her so much with combating the effects of chemo and the debilitating effects of her treatment. I regret to say that my precious daughter lost her battle with leukemia, but I remain a staunch promoter of your philosophy of health care."

— Pat Wittig, Miami, FL

"I value the gift of my good health so I decided to become proactive in safeguarding it with preventive measures rather than wait for something to go wrong. I really appreciate access to the latest findings in health research from a source I trust.... The brevity and user-friendly language of the hints are conducive to reading them and adopting the recommendations. I feel that I am continuing my education in this essential arena of life."

— Sister Adelaide Williamson, CSJ, Baton Rouge, LA

"How do I appreciate Betty Kamen's health hints? Let me count the ways ... but the ways are so many that they're uncountable! I have found answers to questions I didn't know I had to ask to address my basic health problems (I have been diagnosed with multiple sclerosis). Both of my parents have chronic degenerative health problems and have greatly benefited from the material you've found and published. So have a number of my friends.... It's all straight common sense out of peer-reviewed medical journals. Trustworthy information that's been sifted and intelligently commented upon. What more could anyone ask?"

— Colleen Scot

"I find Betty Kamen's 'Hint of the Day' to be a very valuable adjunct to my practice (Holistic Dentistry and Nutritional Counseling) and to my personal life. I'm healthier, happier, more prosperous and more energetic, and have gained much of this from Betty's Hints."

— Thomas E. Baldwin, DDS, MAGD, F/AIAOMT, Towson, MD

"I have been a keen supporter of natural health for many years, and shortly I will qualify as a Clinical Nutritionist. For several years I have been receiving your daily Table Talk Health Hints, which in addition to ensuring my health knowledge remains current, are a valuable reference resource that I use often."

— Marilyn Timms, Noosa Heads, Queensland, Australia

"I am a college professor who teaches nursing. I find the hints a great reminder to get my own house in order, on a daily basis."

— Rachel B. Johnson, Covington, VA

"Your tips are fabulous! Solid science combined with great applicability makes every tip a pleasure to read. Keep up the great work, and thanks."

— Lynn Fraley, RN, DrPH

"Velvet antler, info'd from a Betty hint, has changed my life from dismal to delightful!"

— Kate Paine, Honolulu, HI

"I do appreciate Betty's hints, they are like little affirmations to start the day. Knowledge is a good thing but even smart people don't concern themselves with healthy living and the pursuit of it. So thank you Betty for caring enough to pursue the knowledge of good nutrition, especially for making it available to us."

— Rich de Fazio

"I especially like that most are simple natural remedies. Also your warnings about hormone replacement therapy were well in advance of the medical profession's recent warnings. Keep 'em coming."

Don Guely, Schenectady, NY

"I have been reading Betty's wisdom and insight for years, and I enjoy her Daily Health Hints email and often forward them to my patients.... Betty is a pioneer, a woman ahead of her time, and a leader in the health field. Keep up the great work, Betty!"

— Elena Michaels, PhD, Psychotherapist and Nutritionist

"I am a health professional who has been receiving your daily health hints for about three years. I am an RN of over 30 years, emergency and home health nursing being the majority of my nursing practice.... I appreciate your professional search of journals to highlight some of the best and newest research in the nutrition and health areas to share with your readers. Please continue the good work!"

— Karen White, RN, WCMT, Rhinelander, WI

"If you would like to know some of the best approaches to health care 10 years before everyone else does, read this book."

— Ana Vertel, L.Ac, Berkeley, CA

"A lot of research said in a little space each day! Info not found elsewhere. My clients are easily able to assimilate the short bottom lines then later read more about it. Thank you, Betty!"

— Claudia MacGruer, Wholistic Healer, Austerlitz, NY

"I have appreciated receiving your Health Hints every day. On several occasions, the timing of particular hints was perfect. I was able to share the information with others who were dealing with particular health problems and didn't know where to turn for help."

— Gayle Cranford (recovered cancer patient since 1984), Hermitage, PA

If you would like the free one-line Table Talk Hints emailed to you daily, email to betty@well.com and write: "Hint" in the subject line.

Betty Kamen's 1,001 HEALTH SECRETS

WHAT THE LATEST RESEARCH REVEALS ABOUT

LIVING LONGER

LIVING HEALTHIER

LIVING BETTER

"THE SKEPTIC'S GUIDE TO ALTERNATIVE HEALTH CARE"

BETTY KAMEN, PhD

N E

NUTRITION ENCOUNTER, NOVATO, CALIFORNIA
www.bettykamen.com

All of the facts in this book have been very carefully researched and have been drawn from the scientific literature. In no way, however, are any of the suggestions meant to take the place of advice given by physicians. Please consult a medical or health professional should the need for one be indicated.

2003

Nutrition Encounter
PO Box 5847
Novato, CA 94948-5847
(415) 883-5154

Website: www.bettykamen.com

Email: betty@well.com

Printed in the United States of America
First Printing 2003

ISBN 0-944501-17-6

DEDICATED

to

Rita Leonard

who, with deep knowledge, integrity, and creativity has dedicated her life to helping others – spiritually, emotionally, and nutritionally!

ABOUT BETTY KAMEN

Years ago, on her popular radio program in New York City, Betty Kamen alerted her listeners to dozens of newly available supplements and treatments. Her program quickly developed into a center for disseminating innovative research and discoveries, featuring interviews with prominent alternative health care pioneers from around the world. Betty has written many cutting-edge health books, including the bestselling *Hormone Replacement Therapy, Yes or No? How to Make an Informed Decision* and *New Facts About Fiber.*

She received her MA in psychology in 1949, an MA in nutrition education in 1979, and her PhD in nutrition education in 1982. Betty taught at Hofstra University, developed a nutrition workshop at Stanford University Continuing Education Program for Doctors and Nurses, and served as nutrition consultant on the Committee of the Accrediting Council for Continuing Education and Training, Washington, DC.

A columnist for many health publications over the years, Betty has had hundreds of nutrition reports published. Articles written by or about Betty have appeared in the *New York Times, Chicago Tribune, San Francisco Progress, Prevention Magazine, Baltimore Sun,* and many other local and national publications. A full page photo of Betty and one of her grandchildren appeared in the March 1998 issue of *Time Magazine.*

But never mind all the credentials. Betty says her children describe her most aptly when they say, "Mom? She's just the oldest health nut in the country" — to which Betty responds: "If you have to be the oldest anything, 'health nut' is not so bad."

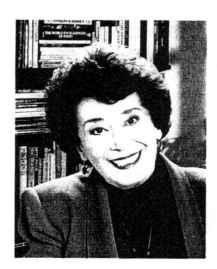

ACKNOWLEDGMENTS

Editing, Organization, & Guidance
David Hennessy

Co-author
Paul Kamen

Additional Assistance
Si Kamen
Kathi Kamen Goldmark
Tony Goldmark
Sam Barry

Cover Design
Raylene Buehler

...and the thousands of people receiving my daily nutrition hints who inspired me to categorize the research and publish this book!

Also From Betty Kamen
BOOKS

~ **Everything I Know About Nutrition I Learned from Barley**
   A Guide to Nutraceuticals and Functional Foods
~ **She's Gotta Have It!**
   The Essential Sex health Manual Every Woman Must Read!
~ **The Remarkable Healing Power of Velvet Antler**
~ **Hormone Replacement Therapy: Yes or No?**
   How to Make an Informed Decision
~ **Kamut**
   An Ancient Food for a Healthy Future
~ **Everything You Always Wanted to Know About Potassium But Were**
   Too Tired to Ask
~ **New Facts About Fiber**
   How Fiber Supplements Can Enhance Your Health
~ **The Chromium Connection**
   Diet & Supplement Strategy for Blood Sugar Control
~ **Startling New Facts About Osteoporosis**
   Why Calcium Alone Does Not Prevent Bone Disease
~ **Germanium**
   A New Approach to Immunity
~ **Siberian Ginseng**
   Up-to-Date Research on the Fabled Tonic Herb
~ **Sesame—The Superfood Seed**
   How It Can Add Vitality to Your Life
~ **Nutrition In Nursing — The New Approach**
   A Handbook of Nursing Science
~ **Osteoporosis**
   What It Is, How to Prevent It, How to Stop It
~ **In Pursuit of Youth**
   Everyday Nutrition for Everyone Over 35
~ **Kids Are What They Eat**
   What Every Parent Needs to Know About Nutrition
~ **Total Nutrition for Breast-Feeding Mothers**
~ **Total Nutrition During Pregnancy**
   How To Be Sure You and Your Baby Are Eating the Right Stuff

Also From Betty Kamen
TAPES

~ Table Talk Tapes: Lessons in Nutrition
   Six 1-hour Audio Cassette Tapes
     1. Supplements, 2. Food & Immunity, 3. Memory,
     4. Remedies, 5. Antioxidants (OPCs or Pycnogenol),
     6. Osteoporosis
~ Nutrition Breakthroughs
   Six 1-hour Audio Cassette Tapes
     1. Supplements, 2. Heart Health, 3. Scaling down,
     4. Immunity, 5. & 6. Common Problems
~ Individual Audio Tapes
   Locker Room Logic: For Men Only
   Things Your Mother Couldn't Tell You
   Hormonal Feedback
   Feminine and Afflicted
   Lactoferrin
      Helper Cells, Antioxidants, Immunity
   Cytolog
      Infopeptides and Cell Signaling
   Germanium
      Immunity, Alertness, Acuity

See www.bettykamen.com for details on all tapes and books, and for Betty Kamen's special reports on new products.

ONE-LINE ONLINE DAILY NUTRITION HINT

Betty's free Table Talk nutrition hint-of-the-day has been an overwhelming success. Betty emails a free online, brief, one-line daily Table Talk Nutrition Hint if you email a request to betty@well.com. Just write "hint" in the subject area.

The last ten hints, with expanded information and source references, are always available at the website.

CONTENTS

Part 1:
Health Challenges

Part 2:
HEALTHIER LIVING

AUTHOR'S NOTES

HOW THE HINTS STARTED

"I wish the vitamins were in the ice cream instead of the broccoli," said three-year-old Michael, our youngest son.

Paul, a little older, had questions about Butch, his friend down the street. "Butch says his parents would *never* allow him to have soda if it wasn't good for him! What do you say to that, Mom?"

At age six, our daughter Kathi had to cover up her embarrassment about not having sugar in the house when a sleep-over classmate asked for some for her breakfast cereal. Kathi thought for a long minute, then responded: "Sugar rots your brains. Didn't you know that?"

It wasn't easy for children to fully understand why our eating habits were so different from those of friends and neighbors in the 1950s and 60s.

As the children grew, I discovered that the best way to avoid their resistance was *not* to sermonize, *not* to offer long explanations – but to release small bits of information, just a little at a time. To accomplish this, I bought a few inexpensive paperback nutrition books (mostly by Carlton Fredericks, the lone voice of nutrition reason of that era), and cut the pages into meaningful little messages.

I inserted these brief snippets of nutrition wisdom into their lunch boxes, and later on, into their vitamin packs, camp letters and college correspondence. Although they moaned and groaned about those miserable "liver letters" (as Kathi dubbed them), I discovered that they not only read the short bulletins, but shared them with friends and classmates! (And at times, even with teachers, who had them read them aloud to the class.) My children eventually became the "mavens" as the nutrition movement began to surface and spread – easily answering friends' questions. More significant, *they couldn't help but notice that their health status was far superior to that of any of their peers.*

And so the "liver letters" laid the foundation for the Table Talk Hint-Of-The-Day.

THEY ARE NOT REALLY SECRETS

Slowly, my nutrition career began to unfold. Along the way I found myself in the spotlight – on the platform with doctors who were certain that supplements only enriched the vitamin manufacturer and the toilets. To give credence to my arguments (after all, I was *not* an MD), I knew I had to present nothing less than evidence-based information, preferably cross-over, double-blinded, placebo-controlled, and randomized. I began to spend every spare minute studying published medical research. Ten journal issues might yield one such nutrition disclosure – if it was a lucky day.

When I discussed the correlation between folic acid and birth anomalies more than twenty years ago, I was reprimanded by the AMA for daring to suggest that a nutrient deficiency could be responsible for such dire consequences. When I wrote an article about homocysteine and its relationship to atherosclerosis at least two decades ago, no one paid attention, except for Dr. Kilmer McKully, the first proponent of the concept. (No one was paying attention to him at that time, either, despite his Harvard degrees.) When the first edition of my book on hormone therapy was published, revealing the risks of cancer, I was labeled a scare-monger. "How come you know these secrets and no one else does?" asked the self-labeled quack busters.

Of course they weren't secrets – just as the information in *1,001 Health Secrets* are not really secrets! Anyone can go to the journals and be enlightened. But I refer to the "hints" as secrets because most people don't know how to go about doing the research, or just can't take the time. And it does require a bit of experience to separate the wheat from the chaff – to recognize how to tell a sincere study project from one sponsored by a company that has a financial interest in the outcome.

I dispense a "liver letter" almost every day now, and to a much wider audience than just my kids. Thanks to the Internet, "neither rain, nor snow, nor sleet, nor hail, nor gloom of night will stay me." If my telephone connection is disturbed, my broadband satellite system is at the ready. If there are no new medical reports of interest that day, I have a backlog of hints waiting in the memory wing of my computer.

WHAT THIS BOOK IS ABOUT

This book is not to be considered an encyclopedia of diseases. That is not its purpose. It is, rather, a compendium of *recent* research that demonstrates the importance of lifestyle change through exercise, diet improvements, and special supplementation. If a disease is not listed, it simply means that no new validated trials may have surfaced on that particular subject in the last few years – or nothing that I noticed in my extensive research. (Remember, I am looking for trustworthy studies.). That doesn't mean there are no natural ways to deal with the long list of health challenges that are *not* included here. Indeed, I believe there is rarely a health challenge that can't benefit from some general lifestyle shifts.

Please note: As you read through the text, you will notice that some information is inserted in brackets. That information is not part of the cited research, but my commentary.

IN SUMMARY

I don't know how else to sum up what I've learned in fifty years of nutrition research, except to say: *What you eat every day of your life affects the length and quality of your entire life.*

And, oh yes, there's our family crest:

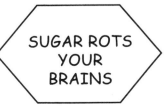

SUGAR ROTS
YOUR
BRAINS

INTRODUCTION

There was once a poor man who always prayed to God that he would win the lottery. Morning and night he lifted his gaze to the heavens and pleaded: "Dear God, please let me win the lottery! I have always been devout, followed your laws, and done what was right. I promise I will use my wealth wisely, and will give much to charity."

But the man's fortunes did not improve. Year after year he did not win the lottery, and he only became poorer and further in debt.

One day his prayers were particularly urgent. His meager business was failing, his family was coming apart, and he faced bankruptcy, eviction, rejection.

"This is my last chance on earth," he begged desperately from a hilltop. "I will be ruined, I will be disgraced. Just this once, please let me win the lottery."

To the man's astonishment, God answered. There was thunder and lightning, and the clouds parted above him. A ray of golden light beamed down upon him, and a majestic voice spoke from the sky: "Will you meet me halfway?" asked the voice of God.

"Yes, yes!" screamed the poor man. "I'll do anything to win the lottery!"

And God answered: "Then buy a ticket."

We are all playing a kind of lottery game with our health, and the prize is far more valuable than a million-dollar jackpot. But if we make the right choices in what we eat and how we live, the odds are very much in our favor.

The world of natural food, nutritional therapies, and alternative health care can be a jungle. There is a common perception that the health food industry has the moral high ground. We like to believe that health food stores are better than supermarkets, that vitamin companies have more integrity than drug manufacturers, and that alternative practitioners are of higher moral fiber than mainstream physicians.

As with most myths, there is a strong element of truth to these perceptions. But in general, the world of natural food and alternative health may sometimes be just as difficult to navigate as the industrialized food and drug industries.

Always be wary of claims that a single product has all the answers, or that one, and only one, regimen will cure every degenerative disease under the sun. Yes, it's true that some nutrients are very helpful for a wide range of disorders, but I can't think of anything that will turn your health status around all by itself.

So how do we tell the difference between good hype and good health? It is not really that hard, but you have to "buy a ticket." Which, in this context, means only one thing: READ.

The scientific standard of truth – or at least the closest approach possible in a relativistic world – is the peer-reviewed journal. All thousand and one hints in this book are supported by this kind of serious research.

Use this book to navigate the endless sea of claims and counter-claims. Also use it to track down the research that supports or refutes these claims. In so doing, you will almost certainly find conflicting data. Read more, and draw your own conclusions. There are many unresolved controversies, but there are also emerging areas of consensus that have not yet reached the popular consciousness (or the medical establishment, for that matter!).

Use this book to show your physician the research that he or she might not be aware of. Even traditional practitioners tend to be much more open to new ideas when they are supported by a peer-reviewed study in a respected medical journal. But ultimately we must all be our own doctors (or at the very least, our own dieticians and exercise coaches), and we must make our own choices.

Our good health and well-being are the grand prizes. The odds are good. Buy a ticket. Read.

Paul Kamen
Berkeley, CA

PART ONE:

HEALTH CHALLENGES

AGING

Most of us hope for a kinder, gentler aging process than that experienced by today's seniors. Is it possible to age without a health disorder? Is it possible to age without assisted care? While none of us can do anything about our chronological age, I believe that learning a few simple tactics can help us to grow older without disease, and to be able to live independently.

In the next decade the number of people over the age of 50 will increase by 48 percent, compared with 16 percent for the 13 to 24-year-old age group. With a continued increase in the overall age of the population, chronic problems such as heart disease, cancer, osteoporosis, Alzheimer's disease and age-related macular degeneration are inevitable {unless we learn the important tricks outlined in this book. (*Journal of Nutrition* **2002;132:3772-3781**)

IN THIS SECTION:
- BONE HEALTH & FALLS
- CONITIVE DECLINE
- CONSTIPATION
- DEPRESSION
- EYESIGHT
- EXERCISE THERAPY

- HYPERTENSION
- INCONTINENCE
- NUTRIENT ABSORPTION
- SLOWING THE AGING PROCESS
- VITAMINS & SUPPLEMENTS

AGING: BONE HEALTH & FALLS

1. HOW QUICKLY CAN YOU STAND UP?

Start measuring the time it takes you to get up out of a chair. When that time begins to increase, consider simple strength and resistance training to increase your sense of balance. Strength and resistance training can greatly reduce your risk of falling, an increasing problem among older people. Such training can improve lean body mass and bone mineral density, as well as general balance.

The time to start such training is middle age, so you can age *without* the symptoms experienced by those who are not in the best of health. After a few weeks of training, time yourself again – the difference may surprise you. [Weights are affordable and widely available in sporting goods stores. Or you might even consider joining the local gym.]

Source: *Journal of Aging Science* **1999;47:1208-1221.**
WANT TO KNOW MORE?
[To protect yourself from fractures, see the *Osteoporosis & Other Skeletal Problems* section for tips on how to improve your overall bone density and strength.]

2. PREDICT YOUR RISK OF FALLING

Try balancing on one leg, and see if you can hold this position for more than thirty seconds before switching to the other leg. If you can't, your risk of falling is high. Referred to as Unipedal Stance Time (UST), this quick and simple balance test can help predict future falls. Those with a history of falling have a significantly shorter average UST of 9.6 seconds, compared with 31.3 seconds in those who have not fallen. Age alone is a weak risk factor for falling. If you can't maintain 30 seconds balanced on one leg, then consider some of the following exercises to improve your balance:

~ Simple balance exercises: Standing, lift one knee and touch it with your opposite hand. Repeat on the other side. Continue this movement back and forth. You will find that you will gradually lift your knee higher and higher.

~ Tai Chi: Three months of 30-minute Tai Chi classes (twice a week) can bring about significant improvements in balance and functional mobility and reduce the fear of falling.

~ Dance aerobics: Dance-based aerobic exercise may reduce the risk of falling by improving balance and agility.

~ Resistance training: Compared with a flexibility exercise program, resistance training produces better gait and balance improvements in older people. Try this: Stand with your feet shoulder-length apart and press your hands hard against a wall. ·

Sources: *Archives of Physical and Medical Rehabilitation* **2000;81:587-591;** *Applied Nursing Research* **2002;15(4)235-242;** *Age Ageing* **2002;31(4):261-266;** *Australian Journal of Physiotherapy* **2002;48(3):215-219.**

3. KEEP "STEADY" WITH STEADY EXERCISE

Seniors who exercise at least twice a week can improve their sense of balance and protect themselves from falling. Both group exercise classes and exercise performed alone at home significantly reduce the incidence of falls among healthy, senior individuals living independently. At the end of 15 weeks, significant improvements in stability, balance, and leg strength are noted.

Sources: *British Medical Journal* **2002;325:128-131;** *American Journal of Medicine* **2002;112:733.**

WANT TO KNOW MORE?
Increased sense of balance offers more protection from falls at home than does reducing hazards. The evidence that exercise reduces the risk of falling is compelling. It can increase muscle strength even in octogenarians by 20 to 200 percent. (*Lakartidningen* [Sweden] **2002;99(35):3408-13**)

Falls are a major source of death and injury in older people. They cause 90 percent of hip fractures, costing the US about 10 billion dollars. (*Sports Medicine* **2001;31(6):427-38**)

4. WALK AWAY FROM RISK OF HIP FRACTURES

Walking and moderate levels of leisure-time physical activity protect against later hip fracture, while a decrease in physical activity over time increases this risk. Moderate levels of activity, including walking, are associated with substantially lower risk of hip fracture in postmenopausal women. Regular physical activity and maintenance of activity during the aging process should be an essential part of strategies aimed at controlling the alarming increase in hip fractures worldwide.

Sources: *Journal of the American Medical Association* 2002;288(18):2300-6; *American Journal of Epidemiology* 2001;154:60-68.

5. INCREASE BONE STRENGTH WITH WEIGHTS

A modest bi-weekly weight-lifting program helps improve bone mineral density and bone strength in older men and women. Lifting only 40 percent of your strength for 16 repetitions twice a week results in *significant* increases in bone mineral density. Starting a modest program of weight training can also produce big improvements in strength, such as the ability to lift a fair amount of weight. [As mentioned in Hint #1, weights are affordable and readily available in most sporting goods stores.] Keep in mind that older bones take longer to respond.

Sources: 24th Annual Meeting of the American Society of Bone and Mineral Research, San Antonio, TX, Sep 2002; American College of Sports Medicine meeting, Indianapolis, IN, Jun 2000; International Association for the Study of Pain, Seattle, WA, 2002.

6. VIGOROUS EXERCISE FOR BETTER BONES

Although mild exercise can reduce the risk of heart disease, only *vigorous* exercise will protect your bones and hold off or reduce age-related bone loss. Neither overall aerobic fitness nor participation in mild physical activity has a significant effect on bone-mineral density. But muscle strength, as well as abdominal obesity, *is* associated with denser bones. Having more body fat and stronger muscles (common in fatter people) has the most influence on bone.

Important note: Although being fat may be good for bone density, gaining weight is NOT the answer because of the harmful effects of obesity on many other aspects of your health. Try vigorous exercise instead. Stair climbing and brisk walking are associated with increased bone-mineral density at the hip and whole body in postmenopausal women.

Sources: *Journal of Internal Medicine* 2002;252; *International Journal of Epidemiology* 1999;28(2):241-246.

7. POTASSIUM CITRATE FOR HEALTHIER BONES

Supplements such as potassium citrate can help prevent normal age-related bone loss. Taking potassium citrate for 11 to 120 months can increase your bone density, which otherwise would normally decrease due to the aging process.

Source: *Journal of Urology* 2002;168:31-34.

WANT TO KNOW MORE?
[See my book, ***Everything You Always Wanted to Know About Potassium But Were Too Tired to Ask,*** in which I discuss the advantages of potassium citrate. Potassium deficiency is also the hidden side of chronic fatigue, high blood pressure, and headache, and, in fact, is an important contributor to all forms of degenerative disease. Also see the *Osteoporosis* section.]

AGING: COGNITIVE DECLINE

8. "DEMENTIA" MAY SIMPLY BE A SIDE EFFECT

If Grandma has memory loss, confusion or other symptoms of dementia, check the medications she's taking and investigate their side effects. Drugs widely used by older people have side effects that can be easily mistaken for dementia (often leading to the prescription of even *more* drugs). Older people tend to take more drugs and medications, and are therefore more at risk of symptoms such as confusion, memory loss, disorientation, glaucoma-like blurred vision, anxiety, and other symptoms associated with dementia.

Drugs used for Parkinson's disease, depression, allergies, migraine and irritable bowel syndrome may cause such side effects.

Over-the-counter drugs causing side effects include hay fever, cold and flu medicines, sleeping pills, and anti-diarrhea treatments.

Source: *Reuter's Health Report*, from the Medical University of South Carolina, Sep 2000.

WANT TO KNOW MORE?
In the US, people over 65 consume 30 percent of all prescriptions and 40 percent of over-the-counter remedies, despite making up only 13 percent of the population.

Other drug side effects are constipation, dry mouth, urinary problems, rapid shallow breathing, dizziness, the likelihood of falling, and irregular or rapid heartbeat.

9. EAT WELL TO THINK WELL

Nearly one-third of men and almost half of women over 70 have some cognitive deficit, but those who eat well reduce the risk of this decline. [Because the percentage of cognitive decline is too high for comfort, it should be the impetus to get us all to pay more attention to our diet. The good news is that we *can* influence our brain power!]

Source: *European Journal of Clinical Nutrition* 2001;55:1053-1058.

WANT TO KNOW MORE?
On average, female centenarians score lower than men in functional performance. However, these women are more able to endure diseases than men. Women tend to be more resilient. (**Annual Meeting of the Gerontological Society of America, Boston, MA, Nov 2002**)

10. UP YOUR Bs FOR A SHARPER MIND

Increasing B vitamins (folate and B12), which in turn decreases homocysteine, improves cognitive abilities as you age. [The best sources of folate (also known as folic acid) are green leafy vegetables such as spinach, kale, and beet greens, as well as beets, chard, asparagus, broccoli, bean sprouts (lentil, mung, and soy), and brewer's yeast.

B12 is found mainly in animal protein foods such as eggs, dairy products, organ meats, and seafood. It is also manufactured by bacteria in your intestines.

Laxatives and antacids can deplete your stores of B12.

Homocysteine is an amino acid produced naturally in your body, but even moderately high levels in your blood are associated with an increased risk of cardiovascular disease, among other health problems. Increasing your consumption of folate and B12 helps to regulate these levels, as does abstaining from filtered coffee.]

Source: *American Journal of Clinical Nutrition* 2002;75(5):908-913.

WANT TO KNOW MORE?
Low folate and vitamin B12 blood levels are associated with nerve and psychiatric disorders, but intervention with B vitamin supplements may reduce the severity of symptoms. Age-related changes may cause the accumulation of excess homocysteine.

High homocysteine concentrations are associated with impaired memory and lower total life quality in healthy seniors. Homocysteine is also reported to be elevated in patients with Alzheimer's disease.

11. UP YOUR Es WHILE YOU'RE AT IT

Foods and supplements containing vitamin E may help slow the decline in mental functioning that occurs with age. This translates to consumption of butter, egg yolk, liver, seeds, nuts, and tocotrienols. Vitamin E, an antioxidant, may counteract the damage done to brain cells by free radicals. [Vitamin E is a generic term for a group of naturally occurring tocopherol and tocotrienol derivatives.] Researchers studied more than 2,800 American men and women, aged 65 to 102. Those who had the highest intakes of vitamin E were found to have a 36 percent slower decline in mental function.

Source: *Archives of Neurology* **2002;59:1125-1132.**

WANT TO KNOW MORE?
[We consume very few foods today that contain vitamin E. An excellent vitamin E supplement is tocotrienol, found in palm oil, because it contains all the vitamin E complex forms in their natural context. Second best are formulas that contain the eight parts (or isomers) of vitamin E, or the d-mixed tocotrienols (not just the alpha-tocopherol varieties).

The amount of vitamin E in our diets has declined more than 90 percent in the last century, and very few people get all the E required from food alone.

Unfortunately, frying oils, processing and milling of foods, the bleaching of flours, cooking, and purifying vegetable oils are processes that remove most of the vitamin E from whole foods.]

High intake of vitamin E has also been linked to a 70 percent reduction in the risk of Alzheimer's disease when taken over a four-year period. For more information on the link between insufficient vitamin E and Alzheimer's disease, see the *Alzheimer* section.

12. ACTIVE WOMEN HAVE ACTIVE MINDS

In the latest study to link exercise with better health, researchers find that physically active older women are *significantly* less likely to suffer age-related mental decline. Women who exercise the most (through walking, gardening, or more rigorous activities) are less likely to suffer mental decline than those who exercise the least.

Other benefits of regular exercise include increased cerebral blood flow, reduced risk of cardiovascular disease in the body and brain, and stimulation of nerve-cell growth. Aerobic exercises protect against disability and early mortality, and are associated with the prolongation of a healthy, disease-free life.

Sources: *Archives of Internal Medicine* **2002;162:2285-2294.**

WANT TO KNOW MORE?
6,000 women 65 and older were studied for six to eight years. The group of women that exercised the most was 26 percent *less* likely to suffer mental decline than the group that exercised the least.

13. YOUR BRAIN: USE IT OR LOSE IT

Keep your brain active to keep it healthy, as a stimulating learning environment can encourage brain-cell growth as well as reduce brain-cell death. Read, do crossword puzzles, maybe even take a class – anything that stimulates your mind. "Use it or lose it" may be particularly true for brain cells. An enriched, more stimulating environment appears to protect against the brain-cell death that commonly accompanies aging. It is believed that the mechanisms involved in thought and mental activity cause the brain to become super-resistant to aging, to diseases such as Alzheimer's and Parkinson's, and to traumatic brain injury.

Source: *Nature Medicine* **1999;5:1113-6.**

AGING: CONSTIPATION
14. CONSTIPATION: A SIMPLE DIETARY SOLUTION

If you are a senior suffering from constipation, consuming oligosaccharides [from food or supplements] may help alleviate the problem. [Oligosaccharides are found in small quantities in foods such as wheat, onions, bananas, honey, garlic, leeks, and artichokes.] Adding oligosaccharides to your diet can effectively improve bowel movement, stool output, and health-promoting microbial fermentation in the colon, all without any adverse effects.

Constipation, a chronic problem among older people, is one of the most common disorders in the Western world. It can result in significant incidence of disease, especially among residents of nursing homes. The problem increases with age.

Ironically, habitual laxative use can cause chronic constipation.

Sources: *American College of Nutrition* **2001;20(1):44-49;** *Diseases of the Colon & Rectum* **2000;43(7):940-943;** *Nursing Times* **1997;93(4):35-36.**

WANT TO KNOW MORE?
Other factors associated with constipation are decreased fluid intake, pneumonia, Parkinson's disease, and allergies. [To learn more about oligosaccharides and how they can help, see my latest book, ***Everything I Know About Nutrition I Learned from Barley***. Also see the *Constipation* section here.

AGING: DEPRESSION

15. GET MOVIN' TO GET HAPPY

Physical activity can help to protect against age-related depression. Researchers studied a group of senior adults aged 50 to 94 over a five-year period. They found that physical activities such as walking, exercising, swimming, or playing sports are associated with a lower risk of depression.

One of the most common forms of physical activity is walking. It's simple, it does not involve costly equipment, and you already know how to do it.

Source: *American Journal of Epidemiology* **2002;156:328-334.**

WANT TO KNOW MORE?
Those who are physically active are more likely to shy away from smoking, overeating, not drinking to excess, and other less than beneficial activities.

AGING: EYESIGHT

16. KEEP YOUR EYES HEALTHY WITH VITAMIN E

Supplementing with vitamin E can help to protect your eyesight from degrading as you grow older. French clinicians report that vitamin E supplementation may help prevent age-related macular degeneration.

People with higher blood-plasma levels of alpha-tocopherol (one form of vitamin E) have an 82 percent decreased chance of developing this condition.

[Some good vitamin E-rich foods include dark green leafy vegetables, palm oil, legumes, nuts and seeds (purchased in their shells), whole grains, and eggs.

Brown rice and wheat germ are also high in vitamin E, but these foods rancidify very quickly because of their high oil content and lack of stability.]

Source: *Archives of Ophthalmology* **1999;117:1384-1390.**

AGING: EXERCISE

17. MEN OVER 45: EXERCISE NOW!

If you are a man over the age of 45, regular exercise can reduce your risk of sudden death associated with vigorous exertion. While physical activity [such as shoveling snow] can trigger sudden cardiac death, middle-aged men who engage in regular hearty exercise have a very low absolute risk of sudden death.

If you are going to start an exercise program, start it gradually and build up to levels of brisk exercise slowly.

Source: *New England Journal of Medicine* **2000;343:1355-1361,1409-1411.**

WANT TO KNOW MORE?
The risk of sudden death associated with vigorous exertion is higher in men who are sedentary or who exercise less than once a week, compared with those who exercise one or more times a week.

18. EXERCISE YOUR AGING HEART

As baby boomers grow older, entering the age when coronary artery disease becomes all too common, it is good to know that there is hope even for the older heart – provided one keeps physically active. A high level of physical activity continues to have a cardioprotective effect even in older adults. So staying in shape remains important at any age.

Source: *Journal of the American College of Cardiology* **2001;38:1357-1367.**

19. DON'T FORGET TO USE YOUR BODY!

There is no drug in current or prospective use that holds as much promise for sustained health as a lifetime program of physical exercise. There is a similarity between changes in the body seen during aging and changes seen during forced physical inactivity [because of a broken leg, for example]. Some changes are simply caused by disuse of the body. The good news is that these changes are subject to correction with an exercise program.

Sources: W. Bortz, *Living Longer for Dummies* (NY: Hungry Minds, 2001); *Journal of the American Geriatric Society* **1980;28(2):49-51;** *Journal of the American Medical Association* **1982;248(10):1203.**

20. WEIGHT TRAINING BENEFITS SENIORS

Since lifting weights increases muscle strength AND cardiovascular fitness, seniors are advised to add weight training to their daily walking exercise regimen. You are never too old to start. Improved aerobic power in healthy seniors can result from variable resistance training. Low- and high-intensity training three times a week can bring significant improvements in strength, endurance, and stair-climbing ability.

If you cannot get involved in a weight-training program, try adding wrist weights when you walk. Increase the weights as you see fit.

Sources: *Archives of Internal Medicine* 2002:162;673-678; *Journal of the American Geriatric Society* 2002;50:1100-1107.

WANT TO KNOW MORE?
Health benefits can be derived from a regimen that uses lighter weights and only takes 15 to 30 minutes, three times a week. You do not have to lift heavy weights that may cause injury, nor do you have to spend all day in the gym to improve your health.

21. SUPPLEMENTS + WEIGHTS = HEALTHY SENIORS

Nutritional supplements and resistance training for seniors help to maintain functionality, bone-mineral density, and cholesterol levels, as well as improved muscle strength. Body composition changes and loss of functionality in older people are related to substandard diets and a lack of physical activity.

Eighteen months of nutritional supplementation and resistance training can help maintain health benefits for those over 70. [Again – It's never too late to start.]

Source: *Journal of Nutrition* 2001;131:2441S-2446S

22. PROTEIN SOON AFTER TRAINING

Consumption of a protein supplement immediately after physical training is beneficial for counteracting age-related muscle loss. The findings confirm what body-builders, who routinely consume protein while they work out, know well.

Many older people could benefit tremendously from integrating a well-timed protein supplement with their training programs, helping them to gain both muscle mass and strength.

Men who drink 10 grams of liquid protein two hours after completing a weight-training program show no increase in muscle mass. But in men who drink the protein within minutes of the training session, a significant increase in muscle mass and strength is observed. [A scoop of whey dissolved in water would also work.]

Source: *Journal of Physiology* 2001;535:301-311.

23. DON'T WORRY ABOUT A LITTLE EXTRA WEIGHT

If you are older and *moderately* overweight, don't worry too much. Weight guidelines for seniors are changing, and new research shows that being moderately overweight is not a risk factor for increased illness or mortality. Current guidelines for ideal adult weight (defined as body mass index, regardless of age) may be "overly restrictive" for those 65 and older. Being mildly or moderately overweight is not a risk factor for any disease, including death from cardiovascular disease. [This does not mean, however, that you should stop exercising daily or start consuming junk foods.]

Source: *Archives of Internal Medicine* 2001;161:1194-1203.

AGING: HYPERTENSION

24. MEASURE YOUR SYSTOLIC PRESSURE ONLY

When having your blood pressure taken, diagnosis for seniors should be based on the *systolic* component of blood pressure only. New studies have found that the accuracy of diagnosis of hypertension in older people is more precise using systolic blood pressure alone rather than a combination of systolic and diastolic blood pressure.

By using this method, the risk for stroke, myocardial infarction [heart attack], heart failure, and kidney failure is much more accurate. Lowering systolic pressure markedly improves the health of older people.

Source: *Journal of Hypertension* 2000;2:132-133.

WANT TO KNOW MORE?
The combination of obesity with hypertension is a frequent finding. High blood pressure is directly connected with obesity in 70 percent of men and in 61 percent of women.

[For more information on how to combat these conditions, see the *Hypertension* and *Obesity* sections of this book.]

25. HYPERTENSION ALSO LEADS TO BONE LOSS

If you are a senior white woman with high blood pressure, don't neglect efforts to normalize your pressure, as you are also at risk for increased bone loss. One reason for this may be abnormal calcium metabolism that accompanies high blood pressure, resulting in the loss of bone-mineral density [leading to an increased risk of bone fractures and even osteoporosis].

The increased rate of bone loss associated with high blood pressure is not related to age, weight, weight changes over time, initial bone-mineral density, smoking, or use of hormone replacement therapy (HRT). Women with the highest systolic blood pressure lose bone at nearly *twice* the rate of those with the lowest.

Source: *Lancet* **1999;354:971-975.**

[For many helpful tips on how to treat hypertension, see the *Hypertension* section.]

AGING: INCONTINENCE

26. "KEGEL" AWAY INCONTINENCE

Learning "kegel" exercises and doing them about 200 times daily (this takes only about 10 minutes) can protect you from urinary incontinence. The earlier you start, the better. Kegeling involves a simple series of pelvic muscle contractions that you can do anytime, anywhere. The muscles involved are attached to the pelvic bone and act like a hammock, holding in your pelvic organs. So the first step is to locate where these pelvic floor muscles are:

Step 1: Sit forward on your chair and place your feet and knees wide apart. Place your elbows on your knees and lean forward. Your pelvic floor should now be touching the seat.

Step 2: Close your eyes and imagine that you want to stop yourself from passing wind.

Step 3: Squeeze the muscles tightly around your back and front passages and lift your pelvic floor up and away from the chair. See if you can hold each contraction for five seconds. Also, try "elevator" kegels, tightening the muscles in slow increments, like an elevator stopping on several floors.

You should NOT bear down (as during a contraction), hold your breath, or use stomach, thigh, or buttock muscles.

The overall rate for cure or significant improvement after exercising is about 60 percent. In addition, limit high fluid intake (keep to a quart a day), and treat any constipation. Diuretics such as caffeine should also be avoided.

Sources: *British Medical Journal* **2000;321:1326-1331;** *Current Opinions in Obstetrics and Gynecology* **1999;11(5):503-507; Boston Women's Health Book Collective,** *Our Bodies Ourselves* **(NY: Simon & Schuster, 1998).**

WANT TO KNOW MORE?
In a survey of over 10,000 adults aged 40 and older, the prevalence of incontinence in women was 20.2 percent. Kegeling is named after Dr. Arnold Kegel, who discovered it. These exercises have been used successfully since 1948. Kegeling is also known for:

~ making birth easier
~ helping prevent prolapses (displacements) of pelvic organs
~ preventing urine leakage during a sneeze or cough
~ enhancing sexual enjoyment.

[To learn about other advantages of kegeling, see my book, *She's Gotta Have It!*]

AGING:
NUTRIENT ABSORPTION
27. GET MORE BY EATING BETTER

Older people do not malabsorb nutrients (macronutrients or micronutrients) unless they are in poor health. Until a few years ago, we knew very little about nutrient absorption in older people.

We have now learned that those who do not absorb nutrients properly do so because of *disease*, not because of age.

[Unfortunately, what you have eaten every day of your life affects the length and quality of your entire life. But it's never too late to turn things around. Some of the best whole-food nutritional supplements include sprouted green grass powders, stabilized rice bran, brewer's yeast, probiotics such as *acidophilus* or viable yogurt, tocotrienols, and algae such as chlorella. These supplements not only provide nutrients, but may increase nutrient absorption from other foods you are consuming.]

Source: *Journal of Nutrition* **2001;131:1359S-1361S.**

[See the *Better Nutrition* and *Supplements* sections for helpful tips on improving your diet.]

SLOWING THE AGING PROCESS
28. LOW CALORIES, YOUNG HEARTS

Calorie restriction in middle age can have a profound slowing effect on the aging process. A low-calorie diet started at 14 months of age can lead to a 19 percent reduction in age-related changes. Caloric restriction reduces the normal progression of DNA damage, programmed cell death, and the normal progression of decreased immune activity. Caloric restriction has such a profound effect because it actually *reprograms* these age-related alterations in the body.

But it appears – again – that it's never too late! Since aging of the heart is associated with specific alterations, and since caloric restriction begun in middle age may retard heart aging, calorie restriction can extend your life.

[This is one reason I encourage the use of young barley green drinks; they provide nutrients and even a certain amount of satiety, but are low-cal!]

As the heart ages, there is a definite shift from fatty acid to carbohydrate metabolism. Older hearts utilize carbohydrates, which are faster burning but yield lower energy, leaving older hearts with less energy required to perform the same work.

Source: Proceedings of the National Academy of Sciences, 2002.

AGING:
VITAMINS & SUPPLEMENTS
29. OVER 60? INCREASE YOUR VITAMIN B12

If you are over 60 years of age, you should start taking supplemental vitamin B12. A deficiency in this vitamin is common among those in this age group, despite a lack of symptoms. One reason for this is related to the high prevalence of gastritis in older people, which in turn affects the absorption of vitamin B12 from food proteins. Bacterial overgrowth of the stomach and small intestine is also common, and these bacteria may bind passing vitamin B12 for their own use.

Researchers suggest that older people should try to obtain their vitamin B12 from supplemental sources to ensure adequate absorption from the gastrointestinal tract.

[One of the best supplemental sources of vitamin B12 is brewer's yeast. Another good source is the algae chlorella.]

Source: *Annual Review of Nutrition* 1999;19:357-377.

WANT TO KNOW MORE?
Because the American food supply is now being fortified with folic acid, concern is increasing about neurological problems in individuals with marginal vitamin B12 status and high-dose folate intake. [All the more reason to make sure your body is getting the vitamin B12 it needs.]

30. FOLATE AGAINST DISEASES OF OLD AGE

If you are older, increasing your consumption of folate can protect you from a large number of age-related diseases. [As mentioned in Hint #10, folate is a form of vitamin B. The best sources of folate (also known as folic acid) are green leafy vegetables such as spinach, kale, and beet greens, as well as beets, chard, asparagus, broccoli, bean sprouts (lentil, mung, and soy), and brewer's yeast.]

Recent findings have begun to reveal the cellular and molecular mechanisms whereby folate counteracts age-related disease.

Sources: *Journal of Nutrition* **2002;132:1361-1367;** *Aging Research Review* **2002;1(1):95-111.**

WANT TO KNOW MORE?
An increase in blood homocysteine levels is a major consequence of folate deficiency that may also have adverse effects on multiple organ systems. Homocysteine enhances accumulation of DNA damage, and in certain cells such DNA damage can lead to cancer, while in other cells (such as brain neurons) it promotes cell death.

The emerging data strongly suggest that elevated homocysteine levels increase the risk of multiple age-related diseases, and point to dietary supplementation with folate as a primary means of normalizing homocysteine levels and increasing your health.

You can significantly decrease homocysteine with only 0.8 milligrams of folic acid daily, reducing the risk of ischemic heart disease by 16 percent, deep-vein thrombosis by 25 percent, and stroke by 24 percent. (*British Medical Journal* **2002;325:1202**)

Coffee, but not caffeine, affects homocysteine metabolism within hours after intake, and the effect is still substantial after an overnight fast. (*American Journal of Clinical Nutrition* **2002;76(6):1244-1248**)

Regardless of your age, smoking, hypertension and cholesterol, and the number of fibrous plaques you have are associated with increased levels of homocysteine. Diabetes may also increase the association. (*Arteriosclerosis Thrombosis and Vascular Biology: Journal of the American Heart Association* **2002; 22:1936-1941**)

ALCOHOL
& YOUR HEALTH

Every time you take a drink you are putting your brain cells temporarily out of commission. Your perceptual and attentive mechanisms are affected after you have only *one* drink. Although your performance may not look any different, you have to work harder to keep your thoughts and actions together. (*How Much Is Too Much?*, L Gross (NY: Random House, 1983)

The effects of any given blood alcohol level vary greatly among people. Variety may occur on a personal level, too, because you can metabolize alcohol differently at different times of the day.

Total mortality increases remorselessly with intake above 12 to 16 grams of alcohol per day (12 to 16 grams equals about half an ounce), but even lesser amounts can result in very serious consequences. (*British Medical Journal* 2001;323:1439-1440) Little doubt exists that alcohol can change the effects of vitamins and other nutrients. And if there is any benefit to alcohol, that advantage is negated for anyone who is alcohol-dependent. (*Alcoholism, Clinical & Experimental Research* 2000;24:72-81)

Alcohol generally depresses the central nervous system and can also precipitate cardiac arrhythmia. Even modest concentrations may exert an inhibitory effect, turning an introvert into a garrulous exhibitionist. Most people retain some alcohol in their blood three to five hours after even moderate drinking. (*Journal of Nutrition* 2001;131:552S-561S)

For reasons not yet understood, binge drinking can cause a surge in blood pressure that does not occur with steady alcohol consumption. And we all know that higher concentrations can result in slurred speech, poor hand-eye coordination, and unsteadiness. (*Hypertension* 2001;38:1361-1366)

Chronic alcohol intake is associated with an increased incidence of a variety of cancers (including liver, oral cavity, esophagus, colorectal and breast). By impairing vitamin A metabolism, it promotes an environment for tumor formation. (*Journal of Nutrition* 2003;287S-290S)

As for breast cancer, moderate alcohol consumption increases the risk. Alcohol combined with estrogen replacement therapy makes the threat even worse! Alcohol as a breast cancer risk factor plays an important role not only in carcinogenesis, but also in promotion of cell invasion and migration. (*Cancer Research* 2000;60(20):5635-9; *Biochemical & Biophysical Research Communications* 2000; 273(2):448-53)

When it comes to hangovers, there's nothing new under the sun. Dietary exposure to alcohol via ingestion of fermenting fruit is theorized to have been around for about *40 million years!* (*Addiction* 2002;97(4):381-8)

IN THIS SECTION:
- HANGOVER CURES & TIPS
- RELATED DISEASES & CONDITIONS
- REVERSING DAMAGE

ALCOHOL: HANGOVER CURES & TIPS

31. HELPFUL HANGOVER HELPERS

To help avoid the hangover:

- Alcohol is very dehydrating, so drink about a quart of water before the party.
- Don't mix different types of alcoholic drinks.
- Don't drink on an empty stomach (food allows the alcohol to be absorbed more slowly into the bloodstream).
- Smoking intensifies the problems because of the additional toxins and further dehydration.
- Lack of sleep also increases susceptibility.

To help relieve the hangover:

- Continue to rehydrate by drinking lots of mineral water.
- Because alcohol also causes low blood sugar levels, consume a light meal to help relieve symptoms.
- Vitamin B6 is a great detoxifying nutrient that helps your body rid itself of the toxic acetaldehyde created by the alcohol. Nutritional yeasts are a good source of B vitamins (or consume any detoxifying mix you happen to have on hand).
- Vitamin C also reduces toxic effects. Take 1,000 mgs of C every hour for several hours, plus 250 mgs of magnesium hourly for three doses. (A morning-after cocktail of nutritional yeast, cayenne pepper, and orange juice can help.)
- Among helpful herbs are ginger (an anti-nausea substance that soothes the stomach). Stir into a glass of natural ginger ale and drink slowly. A combination of peppermint and fennel diluted in a cup of water also soothes the stomach. Other helpful herbs are sprouted green food mixes and Reishi mushrooms.
- Alternate hot and cold showers, with five minutes of hot water and a few seconds of cold.
- Beware analgesics! Aspirin can upset your stomach and intensify hangover symptoms.
- Caffeine can be a diuretic, but it can also assist with vessel constriction, impeding circulation.
- Go into a darkened, quiet room with an ice bag or cold compress on your forehead. The cold compress helps constrict the vessels in your head and reduce the hangover headache.

Sources: *Annals of Internal Medicine* **2000;132(11):897-902;** *Epidemiology* **1997;8(3):310-14.**

32. HANGOVERS NO LAUGHING MATTER

Since hangovers involve increased cardiac work (among other harmful heart actions), as well as increased levels of the anti-diuretic hormone (the hormone that controls water retention), intervention should include rehydration and vitamin B6. An alcohol hangover is characterized by headache, tremulousness, nausea, diarrhea, and fatigue, combined with decreased occupational, cognitive, and visual-spatial skill performance.

In summary, symptoms seem to be caused by dehydration, hormonal alterations, and toxic effects of the alcohol. Hangovers may pose substantial risk to you and to others – even if you have a normal blood-alcohol level. It can also be an independent risk factor for cardiac death.

Source: *Annals of Internal Medicine* 2000;132(11):897-902.

33. EAT AN EGG BEFORE THE PARTY

Before heading for a cocktail party or any event where you know you will be served alcohol, eat one egg and take some extra vitamin C, B6, and calcium. An egg provides quality protein and fat. Anything that delays gastric emptying will delay the absorption of alcohol into your bloodstream. The presence of foods rich in protein and fat initiate this delay. Russian politicians drink large amounts of milk before heading off to vodka-drenched banquets.

The additional nutrient supplements help to prevent the desperately hungry feeling that makes those drinks and hors d'oeuvres so irresistible. It may even give you enough resistance to nibble only on the crudités (raw vegetables) and avoid the more damaging snacks and beverages.

Chronic pretreatment with vitamin E helps to prevent alcohol-induced vascular injury and pathology in the brain. Interestingly, eggs contain vitamin E.

Sources: *Annals of Internal Medicine* 2000;132(11):897-902; *Alcohol* 1999;19(2):119-30.

WANT TO KNOW MORE?
Alcohol is associated with elevated sexual interest, an effect that may be due to known alcohol-caused testosterone elevations. (*Alcoholism, Clinical & Experimental Research* 1999;23(1):169-73) [It's amazing how the puzzle pieces fit together when we have enough information to understand *why* some of these physiological events occur.] But although interest is heightened, performance isn't.

See my book, *She's Gotta Have It!*, which discusses how alcohol causes sexual dysfunction, and why, contrary to the facts, women believe that alcohol enhances enjoyment and activity.]

The level of alcohol consumption associated with risk varies with age and sex. Any level of alcohol intake is associated with increased risk of mortality in men and women up to the age of 35. So abstinence in this age group increases survival. After age 65, however, the risk is lowered by drinking up to 27 grams of alcohol a week for women, and up to 72 grams a week for men. (*British Medical Journal* 2002;325:191-194.)

Approximately 59 percent of American women drink alcohol and six percent consume two or more drinks daily – an amount considered to be heavy drinking for women. The percentage of female college students who drink is now nearly equal to that of their male peers.

ALCOHOL-RELATED DISEASES
34. DRINKING CAN CAUSE BRAIN ATROPHY

Moderate alcohol consumption results in a higher prevalence of brain atrophy, which is associated with poorer neurological and cognitive function, as well as with a greater decline in cognitive function over time. These results are not influenced by gender, race, or cholesterol levels, nor does it matter whether the alcohol consumed comes from beer, wine, or liquor. Alcohol is alcohol, and its consumption negatively affects your brain.

Source: *Stroke* **2001;32:1939-1946**

WANT TO KNOW MORE?
Teenagers who drink heavily during early and middle adolescence are poorer at retrieving verbal and nonverbal information than are those with no history of alcohol abuse. (***Alcoholism, Clinical & Experimental Research* 2000;24)**

The good news is that long-term abstinence from alcohol reverses some of the structural changes in the brain associated with heavy consumption. (***Alcoholism, Clinical & Experimental Research* 2001; 25:1673-1682)**

35. ALCOHOL, COLON CANCER, & FOLIC ACID

Alcohol consumption has been related to an increased risk of colorectal cancer, but higher intakes of folic acid (either from dietary sources or from supplements) may lower your risk of this disease. Alcohol consumption has a strong anti-folic acid effect, and deficiency of this nutrient can lead to intestinal cancer. Dietary folic acid influences DNA manufacture and repair. An increasing number of studies indicate that higher intakes of folic acid may lower the risk of colorectal cancer. Dietary methionine may have a similar protective role.

[Folic acid (also known as folate) is very sensitive, and easily destroyed by light, heat, cooking method, storage, processing, or an acid pH below 4. The best sources are leafy greens, bean sprouts, and brewer's yeast.]

Methionine is generally low in the vegetarian diet, but can be found in significant quantities in eggs and fish. Methionine, by the way, also helps prevent problems of the skin and nails.]

Source: *Journal of Nutrition* **2002;132:2350S-2355S.**

36. NO BENEFITS TO ALCOHOL IN MODERATION

New findings bring into question the purported benefits of moderate alcohol consumption, and also show that heavy drinking may actually *double* your risk of stroke. There is no strong evidence that alcohol consumption reduces overall mortality for light and moderate drinkers. This conclusion was reached after examining the link between alcohol consumption and mortality in 5,766 working men, followed over 21 years. As alcohol consumption increases, so does the risk of mortality.

Daily consumption of 10 to 12 grams for women, and 20 to 24 grams for men is considered to be a moderate intake.

Sources: *British Medical Journal* 1999;318:1725-1729; *European Journal of Clinical Nutrition* 2002;56 Suppl 3:S50-3.

37. DON'T START NOW!

If you are a middle-aged male, do not start consuming alcohol regularly because it will increase your risk of mortality. Men who are regular drinkers or occasional drinkers have a slightly higher risk of death from causes other than heart disease. When compared with occasional drinkers, new drinkers do not have a reduction in death from coronary heart disease or cardiovascular mortality, and they have an increased risk of death from causes other than heart disease.

So the message is *don't start now*!

Source: *Heart* 2002;87:32-36.

WANT TO KNOW MORE?
Uric acid increases significantly after ingestion of red wine. And although red wine increases antioxidant compounds in your blood, the beneficial elixirs they offer never add up enough to influence oxidation of lipoproteins. So wine offers no benefit for your LDL, the bad variety of cholesterol. (***American Journal of Clinical Nutrition* 2002;71:67-74.**

Symptoms of insomnia occur frequently among those seeking treatment for alcohol dependence. In fact, if insomnia is present when alcoholic treatment is started, this is a good sign that there will be a subsequent relapse. (***American Journal of Psychiatry* 2001;158:399-404)**

Some Asian Americans, because of a genetic propensity, experience more severe hangovers – so bad, they are encouraged to abstain. So this unpleasant reaction may contribute, in part, to protection against the development of excessive or problematic drinking in this population. (***Journal of Alcoholic Studies* 2000;61(1):13-17)**

ALCOHOL: REVERSING DAMAGE

38. SAMe AGAINST ALCOHOLIC LIVER DAMAGE

Supplemental SAMe (S-adenosylmethionine) helps to stave off the liver-damaging effects of alcohol. In the past, alcoholic liver disease was attributed exclusively to dietary deficiencies, but studies have now established that alcohol, despite an adequate diet, can contribute to the entire spectrum of liver diseases, mainly by generating oxidative stress. It also interferes with nutrient activation, resulting in changes in nutritional requirements.

Supplemental SAMe has been shown to reduce lesions and mortality in test animals and patients suffering from cirrhosis. SAMe also replenishes stores of glutathione [a powerful antioxidant produced in the liver, and decreased in alcoholics].

Source: *Annual Review of Nutrition* **2000;20:395-430**.

39. FOLATE AGAINST ALCOHOLIC LIVER DAMAGE

Folate deficiency is present in most people with alcoholic liver disease, and abnormal methionine metabolism is exacerbated by folate deficiency. Actually, excessive alcohol ingestion disturbs the metabolism of most nutrients. It can lead to severe hypoglycemia, glucose intolerance, and altered lipid (fat) metabolism.

Alcoholics with a history of obesity have a two-to-three times higher risk of having alcoholic liver disease.

[Check out the *Liver Disease & Cirrhosis* section for more helpful information.]

Sources: *Transactions of the American Clinical & Climatological Association* **2002;113:151-62.**

WANT TO KNOW MORE?
Alcohol inhibits the function that builds your bones back, so it induces systemic bone loss and increases the risk of fracture.

Consider potassium, magnesium, and fruit and vegetable intakes because these are associated with greater bone-mineral density. (*Alcohol & Alcoholism* **2002;37(1):13-20;** *American Journal of Clinical Nutrition* **1999;69:727-736**)

ALLERGIES

Milk was responsible for my teenage acne. My friend Jane's pallor disappeared when she stopped drinking milk, although the doctors thought it was anemia. Dr. Lendon Smith (pediatrician of renown), told me that milk made him sneeze, and he was sure it was the cause of bed-wetting among his younger patients.

It's no surprise that milk is at the top of the allergic-foods list. But that list is long.

Chocolate causes my niece Alice to cough. My sister Trudy cannot wear cheap jewelry because of her sensitivity to nickel (the most common metal allergy in women). Tomatoes cause my cousin Gene to snort two or three times a minute. Corn makes my nephew John's ears itch deep inside. Sugar turns my grandson Tony's ears red.

Allergic reactions are usually, but not always, dose- and frequency-related.

Then there are the strange associations. For example, your risk of developing *atopy* by the age of 31 is increased by about 40 percent if your mother reached menarche (her first menstrual period) at a later age. (Atopy is an inherited allergic reaction such as hay fever, asthma, or eczema.) (***Thorax*** **2000;55:691-693**)

The many alternative physicians I interviewed over the years shared several allergy secrets with my radio and TV audiences. Of these, listeners reported that the following ideas worked best:

> ~ Consuming no more than two tablespoons of any food group every four hours (You could have several food groups at a meal, but no more than two tablespoons of each group within the four-hour period)
> ~ Eating only organic foods
> ~ Totally eliminating the seven or eight common food allergens (milk, wheat, peanuts, commercial eggs, soy, fish, shellfish, and other nuts) prevents allergy to *anything else*, including pollen, even if you don't appear to be allergic to these particular allergens
> ~ Taking huge amounts of friendly bacteria [such as acidophilus] after every meal
> ~ Adding enzymes also helps

And here's my discovery: When I handle too much paper from my computer printer or copy or fax machines, I go into a wild frenzy of sneezing. Dissolving a gram or two of vitamin C powder in a very small amount of liquid and placing the mix under my tongue works magic to *instantly* stop the sneezing spell. So we have our folklore and our clinical experience. In fact, some studies actually validate the suggestions I've just cited. Now let's see what this evidence-based research demonstrates.

IN THIS SECTION:
- DUST MITES & PET ALLERGENS
- FOOD ALLERGIES
- HAY FEVER
- PEANUT ALLERGIES
- WHEAT (GLUTEN) SENSITIVITY

DUST MITES & PET ALLERGENS

40. LOWER HUMIDITY AGAINST DUST MITES

Reducing indoor humidity to less than 51 percent is effective in reducing levels of house dust mites and their allergens. Houses wtih varying degrees of humidity were tested. Low-humidity homes began the study with 401 live mites and 17 micrograms of mite allergen per gram of dust. After 17 months of relative humidity below 51 percent, this fell to eight live mites and four micrograms of allergen per gram of dust.

In contrast, in other homes with higher humidity, live mites per gram of dust rose as high as 1,000 and allergen levels rose to as much as 70 micrograms. Allergen levels were more than 10 times lower in the low-humidity homes. This study shows that it is possible, practical, and effective to reduce indoor humidity to levels that will control dust-mite populations, thereby helping to reduce allergy incidence.

Source: *Journal of Allergy and Clinical Immunology* **2001;107:99-104.**

41. POLISH AWAY THOSE ALLERGENS

Using spray furniture polish dramatically reduces the amount of dust and allergens that become airborne, providing a less allergy-inducing home environment. A side-by-side comparison of spray furniture polish and dry dusting shows the superiority of the spray polish when comparing the amount of dust particles and house dust-mite and cat allergen released into the air while dusting.

Spray furniture polish can reduce airborne dust particles by 83.4 percent, dust mite allergen by 50.3 percent, and cat allergen by 57.4 percent. Spraying polish directly on the surface is even more effective in reducing airborne particles. Using this method, airborne dust particles are reduced by 92.9 percent, airborne dust-mite allergen by 95 percent or more, and cat allergen by 95 percent!

Source: *Journal of Allergy and Clinical Immunology* **2002;109:63-67.**

42. FEATHER PILLOWS BEST FOR THE ALLERGIC

Feather and down pillows contain much lower levels of pet allergens (even if you don't own pets!) and lower levels of dust-mite allergens than do synthetic pillows. Six to eight times as many pet allergens and five times as many dust mite allergens are found within synthetic pillows when compared with feather pillows. None of the pillows checked were from households that keep pets, but pet allergen float in the air and are carried by clothing. It is speculated that the more tightly woven covers required to keep feathers in the pillows are what prevent allergens from entering. [Feather bedding is also recommended for children with asthma.]

Source: Report presented at the American Academy of Allergy, Asthma and Immunology annual meeting in San Diego, CA, Mar 2000.

43. TRUCK EXHAUST CAN BE A TRIGGER

Exposure to particles in diesel exhaust, a major air pollutant from trucks, lowers your threshold for reactions, demonstrating how one allergen can trigger another. Diesel engines emit a mixture of gases and fine particles that contain some 40 chemicals, including benzene, dioxin, and mercury compounds – which exacerbate allergic response in adults with a history of allergic rhinitis and who respond to dust mites. (Rhinitis is an inflammation of the mucous membrane lining the nose, usually associated with nasal discharge.)

Only one-fifth of the amount of intranasal dust-mite allergen is required to induce symptoms, compared with the amount required *before* exposure to the diesel exhaust particles. (It is more than likely that other pollutants elicit the same response of lowered thresholds for allergic reactions, which explains why we are more sensitive at times.)

Unfortunately, levels of these particles are still on the rise. The Environmental Protection Agency released a report in September 2002 that concluded for the first time that diesel exhaust is a likely human carcinogen. Diesel fumes can also cause eye irritation, nausea, and respiratory problems.

Source: *Journal of Allergy and Clinical Immunology* 2000;106:1140-1146; *Reuter's Medical Health Report*, Dec 2002.

44. AVOID WOOL SWEATERS

Wearing wool sweaters can increase your exposure to cat allergens 11 times and to mite allergens 10 times. Clothing is a major source of both mite- and cat-allergen exposure, often transferring these allergens to cat-free environments.

Clothing that is not washed often can carry more of both allergens, in amounts that correspond to the amount of inhaled allergen.

By the end of the day, non-cat-owning workers working alongside cat owners can have a significant increase of mite and cat allergens on their own clothing.

Source: *Journal of Allergy and Clinical Immunology* 2000;106:874-879.

45. BLACK CATS *ARE* BAD LUCK AFTER ALL

If you suffer from allergies, black cats may indeed be bad luck! People with dark-haired cats experience more sneezing, runny nose, itchy and watery eyes, and swollen throat than do people with fairer felines. Those suffering the most are *six* times more likely to have a dark-haired cat than a light-haired one. Cat allergy is a common (and preventable) allergy, affecting five million sufferers in the US. It's not the animal's hair that causes the problem, but rather a protein in the saliva and dead skin flakes. Keeping your pet out of your bedroom is one helpful way of lessening the symptoms, as is covering mattresses and cushions with zippered, plastic casings to curtail the allergen build-up. If you have a choice, consider wood floors rather than carpeting, as carpets are notorious allergen collectors.

Sources: American Academy of Allergy, Asthma & Immunology Conference, Mar 2000.

WANT TO KNOW MORE?
There is no significant difference in symptom severity between those with no cats and those with light-colored cats. The hair of dark cats may contain higher concentrations of a cat antigen. [Antigens include toxins, bacteria, and foreign blood cells that stimulate the production of protective antibodies.]

ALLERGIES: FOOD

46. BOYS, MARGARINE & ALLERGIES

If you have a young boy at home, avoid giving him margarine as it appears to be associated with an increase in allergic sensitization and rhinitis symptoms in young boys. (Rhinitis is an inflammation of the mucous membranes of the nose.) The use of margarine, as compared with butter, is associated with a 30 percent increase in the risk of allergic sensitization and a more than 40 percent increase in rhinitis symptoms. For reasons not understood, further analysis revealed that this association is restricted to boys.

Source: *American Journal of Respiratory and Critical Care Medicine* 2001;163:277-279.

47. ENZYMES AGAINST FOOD ALLERGIES

If you have a food allergy, taking pancreatic enzymes at the same time as the allergenic food can reduce the severity of the allergic reaction. Ingesting pancreatic enzymes markedly reduces the severity of food-induced symptoms, perhaps because the enzymes improve digestion, thereby breaking down large, allergenic proteins into smaller, non-allergenic molecules. In addition, there is evidence that a proportion of orally administered enzymes can be absorbed intact into the bloodstream. Once inside the body, they are apparently capable of exerting an anti-inflammatory effect. The tablets used should be enteric-coated, so that your stomach's digestive juices do not destroy them.

Source: *Inflammation Research* 2002;51(Suppl 1):S13-14.

48. YOGURT AGAINST ALLERGIES

If you suffer from allergies, consumption of probiotic yogurt may help to relieve symptoms. [Probiotics are food supplements that promote the growth and proliferation of healthful bacteria in your body, such as the *Lactobacillus acidophilus* found in viable, cultured yogurt.] Live-culture yogurt consumption is associated with a decrease in allergic symptoms for all ages.

The microorganisms of the final product must be abundant and viable.

[Unfortunately, the majority of commercial yogurts in the marketplace do not meet this criterion. Look for yogurt in the refrigerated supplement section of your health food store.]

No adverse effects are associated with frequent consumption of yogurt.

Source: *Journal of Nutrition* 1999;129:1492S-1495S.

ALLERGIES: HAY FEVER
49. HOMEOPATHY FOR HAY FEVER

A homeopathic preparation for perennial allergic rhinitis [nasal inflammation associated with hay fever] appears to be effective. In a study of 50 patients with perennial allergic rhinitis, subjects were given either an oral 30c homeopathic preparation of their principal allergen, or a placebo. The homeopathy group had a significant improvement in nasal airflow compared with the placebo group.

The research group originally set out to show that homeopathy did *not* work, but the study failed to confirm the original hypothesis that homoeopathy is merely a placebo.

Source: *British Medical Journal* 2000;321:471-476.

WANT TO KNOW MORE?
Homeopathy in the US was in steep decline from the 1920s to the 1960s but has had a strong recovery since the 1970s. (*British Journal of Homeopathy* 2001;90(2):99-103)

Trials of homeopathy are difficult because there are no established animal models or examples of similar treatment for proved benefit. There is evidence, however, that homeopathic treatments are more effective than placebo. (*European Journal of Clinical Pharmacology* **2000;56(1):27-33**) In many countries, homeopathy has been integrated successfully for use by the modern physician. (*Medical Clinics of North American* **2002;86(1):47-62**)

50. HERBAL TREATMENT FOR HAY FEVER

If you are suffering from seasonal allergic rhinitis (hay fever), try taking butterbur, a well-tolerated herbal supplement that is just as successful as over-the-counter antihistamines – *without* **the side effects.** One tablet of butterbur taken four times daily for two consecutive weeks has the same effect as the antihistamine cetirizine. Over-the-counter medications may interact with alcohol, cause sedation, and hinder driving ability. Even though cetirizine is considered a non-sedating drug, two-thirds of those taking it report drowsiness and fatigue.

Butterbur has been used medicinally for centuries. During the Middle Ages it was used to treat plague and fever; in the 17th century for treating coughs, asthma, and skin wounds. Currently, its primary use is for migraines. Other common names for butterbur include pestwurz (German), blatterdock, bog rhubarb, and butter-dock.

Sources: *British Medical Journal* **2002;324:144**; *Alternative Medical Review* **2001;6(2):207-9**.

ALLERGIES: PEANUT ALLERGIES

51. STEALTH PEANUTS HIDING IN SNACK FOODS

Peanut allergy sufferers take note! Undisclosed traces of peanuts, which are highly allergenic, are found in 25 percent of snack foods tested, so don't trust the labels. Half the 30,000 annual emergency room admissions for food allergies are due to peanuts. About seven million Americans are estimated to have food allergies, and they rely on product labels to avoid ingredients that could trigger an anaphylactic reaction [a life-threatening allergic reaction]. But these food labels aren't always accurate.

Even trace amounts of allergens can provoke fatal reactions in susceptible individuals. Such trace amounts may even be due to cross-contamination, where utensils used in making one product are used in making another. Many airline companies have stopped supplying peanut snacks because of the prevalence of this allergy. Mothers who are breastfeeding should be aware that they could pass on the sensitivity through their milk.

Source: *British Medical Journal* **2001;322:883**.

52. MORE HIDDEN SOURCES OF PEANUT ALLERGY

Among peanut- and tree nut-allergic individuals who suffer reactions while eating out, commonly cited establishments are Asian restaurants (19 percent), ice cream shops (14 percent), and bakeries or doughnut shops (13 percent). So if you are allergic, be extra cautious when entering any of these restaurants. Symptoms may begin five minutes after ingestion. Desserts are a common cause (43 percent). In 50 percent of these incidents, the food item is "hidden" in sauces, dressings, egg rolls, etc. Reactions can occur from serving supplies, skin contact, inhalation (residual food on tables or peanut shells covering floors), or even being within two feet of the cooking of the food.

Source: *Journal of Allergy & Clinical Immunology* 2001;108(5 Part 1):867-870.

53. ROASTED PEANUTS MOST DANGEROUS

If you have a peanut allergy, be especially careful of roasted peanuts. You can reduce the allergy potency if the peanuts are fried or boiled, but roasting *increases* the reaction. Researchers roasted, boiled, and fried two types of peanuts grown in the US. The protein fractions of both varieties of peanuts are altered to a similar degree by frying or boiling, but differ when peanuts are roasted. Roasting uses higher temperatures that apparently increase the allergenic property of peanut proteins and may help explain the difference in the prevalence of peanut allergy. Some people may develop severe allergic reactions through skin contact or even by inhalation. Extremely sensitive people can have a reaction just from the peanut packets opened around them on an airplane.

Sources: *Journal of Allergy & Clinical Immunology* 2001;107:1077-1081; *Annals of Allergy & Asthma Immunology* 2001;86(5):583-586.

54. NUT ALLERGY? AVOID KISSING!

If you suffer from a nut allergy, be careful: you can have an anaphylactic reaction if you kiss someone who has recently eaten nuts to which you are allergic. (An anaphylactic reaction is a serious, often life-threatening allergic reaction characterized by low blood pressure, shock, and difficulty breathing.) People can have reactions up to six hours after the kisser has eaten nuts. In most cases, the kisser is a spouse, although some children have had a reaction after a kiss from a relative. One grandparent with a reaction was kissed by a grandchild who had eaten peanut butter. Brushing teeth and using mouthwash are ineffective measures for preventing this serious reaction.

Source: 59th Annual Meeting of the American College of Allergy, Asthma, & Immunology, Orlando, FL, Nov 2001.

55. BEWARE PEANUT OILS IN SKIN CREAMS

Watch out for skin creams containing arachis oil (peanut oil, ground nut oil) – a highly allergenic substance. Many of these creams are recommended for dry skin, cradle cap, eczema, diaper rash, or cracked nipples for nursing mothers. Arachis oil is also found in calamine lotion and zinc creams.

Source: *Lancet* 1996;348:759-760.

56. ECZEMA MEDICATION & PEANUT ALLERGIES

Topical drugs used to treat childhood eczema might be the cause of many cases of potentially life-threatening peanut allergy. Eczema creams containing peanut oil (as described in Hint #55 above) may sensitize children to these nuts. Eczema causes the skin barrier to break down, and immune cells in the skin could be exposed to substances that cause allergies.

Products containing peanuts or peanut oils may be responsible for starting these peanut allergies.

The problem of eczema among children is increasing, and peanut allergies are much more common than previously thought. Parents are warned to be careful about using these creams on children with rashes, especially if one or both parents have had eczema problems.

Source: Medical Research Council, London, reported in *Reuter's Medical Health Bulletin*.

WANT TO KNOW MORE?
For helpful tips on treating eczema, see the *Dermatological Problems* section.]

ALLERGIES: WHEAT (GLUTEN) SENSITIVITY

57. TEST YOURSELF FOR WHEAT SENSITIVITY

Try abstaining from all wheat products for three weeks, and there's a good chance you will feel better than you have in years. Celiac disease is much more prevalent in the US than previously believed. In this disease, the intestinal lining is inflamed in response to the ingestion of a protein known as gluten. Gluten is present in many grains including rye, oats, barley, and triticale, in addition to wheat. Gluten itself is even added to many prepared baked foods. It is now believed that the disease is rarely *diagnosed*, rather than rarely *occurring*.

Gluten-free diets are effective for those with small bowel mucosal problems, even if they appear to be minor. Dramatic clinical improvement in symptoms is noted in all those who are on a gluten-free diet, with symptoms virtually disappearing in everyone.

Among the symptoms of gluten sensitivity are diarrhea and unresponsive iron-deficiency anemia. It can also manifest itself in a form of dermatitis.

Source: Center for Celiac Research, University of Maryland, Baltimore, MD; *Journal of Clinical Gastroenterology* 2003;36(1):13-7; *Annals of Human Genetics* 2002;66(Pt6):387-92.

58. WHEAT: A WIDESPREAD PROBLEM

If you are really serious about optimum health, avoid anything made with wheat. Gluten is one of the most prevalent substances in foods, yet it contributes to illness for far too many people (even if consumed only occasionally). Many suffer for years before the diagnosis of wheat (gluten) intolerance is made. Eating foods containing wheat is so much a part of our lifestyle that giving it up can be very difficult. [Keep in mind that foods containing gluten are almost always highly processed, another contributing factor to illness.]

In addition to celiac disease, a widely prevalent autoimmune disease of the small intestine, long-term implications of gluten sensitivity include enhanced risk of malignancies (both cancer and lymphoma) of the small intestine, osteoporosis, abnormal small-intestinal structure, malabsorption, and many other disorders.

Sources: *Science* 2002;297(5590):2275-2279; *Gastroenterology* 2001;120:1526-1540.

WANT TO KNOW MORE?
Gluten intolerance was considered uncommon until recently, when the American Gastroenterological Association published an extensive technical review. Like other immune disorders such as type 1 diabetes, rheumatoid arthritis, or multiple sclerosis, environmental factors play a role in its onset.

Why wheat has become such a problem in our modern diets is explained in detail in my newest book, *Everything I Know About Nutrition I Learned from Barley*.]

59. WHEAT SENSITIVITY & PREGNANCY

If you are a woman of childbearing age, make sure to be tested for wheat (gluten) sensitivity. Those who are sensitive and don't change their diets reduce their reproductive capabilities. Undiagnosed celiac disease is not uncommon and can be a cause of unexplained infertility. A gluten-free diet may result in conception and favorable outcome of pregnancy. Celiac women who are on regular diets are more likely to experience miscarriage, have low-birth-weight babies, and short durations of breastfeeding.

Sources: Ginekologia Polska 2001;72(3):173-9; *Minerva Gynecology* 2002;54(2):151-9; *Hormone Research* 2002;57 Suppl 2:63-5; *Journal of Family Health Care* 2002;12(4):94-7.

WANT TO KNOW MORE?
Celiac disease also correlates strongly with a history of cigarette smoking. For more information on celiac disease and its effects on reproduction, see the *Pregnancy & Childbirth* section.

60. OATS IN SMALL AMOUNTS MAY BE OKAY

If you are wheat-sensitive, consuming oats in *small* amounts may not produce problems. Oats in the wheat-sensitive diet has been debated, but we now know that small amounts of oats are not usually problematical, but rye and barley in any quantity have an adverse effect on the intestinal mucosa of wheat-sensitive people. Adults with wheat sensitivity can consume moderate amounts of oats without too much risk. No research has been done yet on the effects of larger amounts. Maize (corn) and rice are also harmless.

Source: *Gut* 2000;46:327-331.

61. STARCH ENEMY!

If you are wheat sensitive, watch out for processed foods that contain modified starch, frequently used as a thickener or emulsifier, because this means gluten content. (Even yogurts can contain gluten.) You already know about abstaining from wheat, and, for many, the verboten list also includes rye, barley, and sometimes oats. Some exquisitely sensitive people cannot even eat butter if someone else has dipped into it with a crumb-coated knife.

If you generally feel run down, you might have your doctor check you out for wheat sensitivity. You will be amazed how your energy can soar when you are strict about eliminating gluten. (And since almost all gluten is found in less-than-healthful processed foods, eliminating these from your diet may also have a large impact on your improved sense of well-being.)

Source: *British Medical Journal* 2000;321(7269):1165.

WANT TO KNOW MORE?
Fewer test animals pretreated with a combination of vitamins E and C have reactions to allergy-triggering foods. The protective effect of antioxidants could be of practical therapeutic value in treating allergy. *(British Journal of Dermatology* 2002;146:649-656)

Children exposed to many other children in childhood appear to have a decreased risk of developing hay fever but an increased risk of developing asthma in adulthood. The risk of hay fever in adulthood decreases as the number of children a child is exposed to during childhood increases. But this inverse association only applies to those children who have parental allergy. *(Thorax* 2002;57:945-950)

Nine states, including New York and Wyoming, have introduced legislation in Congress that would require food companies to warn consumers that their products may contain food allergens.

62. GLUTEN-FREE DIET REDUCES DIABETES RISK

Six months of a gluten-free diet improves insulin secretion in those who are at high risk for type 1 diabetes. Removal of gluten from the diet reduces the incidence of diabetes. A trial consisting of six months of a gluten-free diet followed by another six months of a normal gluten-containing diet was performed in a group of first-degree relatives who were at high risk for diabetes. Insulin sensitivity improved after the gluten-free diet and subsequently returned after six months of the normal diet - demonstrating the beneficial effect of removing gluten for those at risk for type 1 diabetes.

Source: *Journal of Clinical Endocrinology Metabolism* **2003;88(1):162-5.**

WANT TO KNOW MORE?
The amount of toxins (from wheat glutens) that individuals with celiac disease may consume without damaging the mucosa of the small intestine is unknown. (***Journal of the American Dietetic Association* 2001;101(12):1456-9)**

Sprouted grain *grasses* are very different foods than the grains themselves. Sensitivity that occurs from grains are not usually present when ingesting the sprouted grasses. So those who have reactions to wheat grains or barley grains, are unlikely to respond unfavorably to the grasses of these grains.

Modern wheat has been modified to such an extent that tens of millions of people in North America alone are allergic to it! The closer an agricultural product is to its naturally evolved beginnings, the less likely it is to cause an allergic response. So it is not surprising to find that many people who are allergic to products made from modern wheat grains are much less sensitive to foods made with more ancient types of grains.

This is yet another demonstration showing us that nature knows better than science, or better than human interference. High yield, resistance to pests and disease, suitability for mechanized harvesting and milling, even color for pasta manufacturing, are among the selection criteria. These attributes do not contribute to nutritional content, a factor that is rarely considered.

Pest resistance may have a particularly strong relation to allergic response. A pest-resistant plant is not simply a better and stronger plant. The resistance comes from higher levels of the plant's own natural pesticides. In some cases, our allergic response is a reaction to these natural poisons. It makes sense that ancient, unmodified species are less likely to trigger allergies.

Nature is abundant with animal species that thrive on newly sprouted grasses. But no animals have evolved to thrive on the part of the plant that modern humans choose to eat.

ALZHEIMER'S DISEASE

"They are waiting for tomorrow, but they are dreaming of yesterday – but that yesterday occurred a long time ago." I will never forget these words, told to me by an inhabitant of a nursing home as we passed a group of women with Alzheimer's disease in various stages of decline – all sitting quietly, seemingly lost in thought. My guide went on to say, "I am grateful that my problems are physical. My own husband was a brilliant lawyer. I cannot put into words what it was like to watch the slow deterioration of his incredible mental capacity."

We've learned a lot since the disease was given a name. But there are still so many unanswered questions. Why, for example, is the risk increased if you grow up in a large family? (*Neurology* **2000;54:415-420**) Why does the disease decline in the early 90s for men and later for women? (*Neurology* **2002;58:209-218.**) What is the connection between high cholesterol and high blood pressure in midlife and Alzheimer's in later life? (*British Medical Journal* **2001;322:1447-1451.**) We know one thing for certain: Alzheimer's disease is not an inevitable consequence of aging. *Healthy brain aging is possible.*

IN THIS SECTION:
- DIETARY TACTICS
- EARLY WARNING SIGNS
- ERT CONNECTION
- NATURAL REMEDIES & SUPPLEMENTS
- REDUCING RISKS

ALZHEIMER'S: DIETARY TACTICS

63. FAT, CALORIES & ALZHEIMER'S DISEASE

Think twice before reaching for chocolates, croissants, or ice cream! High fat and caloric intake are risk factors for Alzheimer's disease, while a diet of fruits and vegetables (five servings daily), fish, and a daily vitamin B supplement are protective against this disease for almost three-quarters of the population. High-fat intake (an amount greater than 40 percent of calories) when you're in your 40s and 50s is a major factor in this disease. And it's not only fat content, but also total calories that count.

About 1,000 older people with no signs of dementia were studied. A frightening number with the highest calorie and fat intake developed Alzheimer's within four years. The findings support the theory that caloric restriction can have an impact on age-related cognitive decline and dementia. The supplementary vitamin B helps to lower homocysteine levels in the blood, another factor correlated with Alzheimer's disease [as discussed in Hint #73],

Sources: *Archives of Neurology* **2002;59:1258-1263; 8th International Conference on Alzheimer's Disease & Related Disorders, Stockholm, Sweden, Jul 2002.**

WANT TO KNOW MORE?

[Your diet can be greatly improved by the simple addition of nutraceuticals and other dietary supplements, especially if you find it difficult to manage those five or more portions of veggies daily. See my book, *Everything I Know About Nutrition I Learned from Barley*, for a good introduction to this subject.]

ALZHEIMER'S: EARLY WARNING SIGNS

64. CLUES TO EARLY ALZHEIMER'S

Test yourself and your loved ones for these clues to early signs of Alzheimer's disease: difficulty managing finances and/or balancing a checkbook, frequently repeating stories and statements, getting lost while driving, forgetting the names of relatives, and using poor judgment. These clues overlap in the areas of learning and retaining new information (repetition), handling complex tasks (calculation), reasoning ability (judgment), and spatial ability and orientation (driving). Lack of recall is the symptom most consistent with the findings of a screening test for Alzheimer's.

Source: *Archives of Family Medicine* **2000;9:1066-1070.**

65. ALZHEIMER'S DISEASE & SENSE OF SMELL

If you have a hard time identifying smells but don't recognize this problem, you may be at risk for developing Alzheimer's disease. People with mild memory problems were asked to scratch open dozens of little capsules containing distinct scents, including menthol, peanut, and soap, and to identify these odors. A large number of those who thought they did well on the test but actually didn't, developed Alzheimer's disease in about two years. None of the people who scored well developed the illness.

Other studies also show that those at risk for developing Alzheimer's may perform more poorly on smell measures compared to those who are not at risk.

[It just may be that the very nutrients that protect our sense of smell, such as zinc, iron and niacin, may also protect brain cells.]

Source: *American Journal of Psychiatry* **2000;** *Neurobiological Aging* **2002;23(3):397-404.**

WANT TO KNOW MORE?

Those with Alzheimer's disease have elevated levels of copper. Checking for copper levels may be helpful in diagnosing the disease. (*Neurology* **2002;59:1153-1161**)

66. DEPRESSION AN EARLY SIGN OF ALZHEIMER'S

If Grandma or Grandpa show symptoms of depression, he or she may be at risk for Alzheimer's. These symptoms may foreshadow the disease by three years. Alzheimer patients are more likely to report a general lack of interest, concentration and memory problems, a loss of energy, and thoughts of death by as long as three years before a doctor's diagnosis identifies the disease.

Two symptoms – general lack of interest and thoughts of death – are especially pronounced. Looking for depression symptoms may be one way to identify those who will develop Alzheimer's within a few years.

Source: *Neurology* **1999;53:1998-2002.**

67. MEMORY RECALL TEST

Here's a quick memory test that may be useful in spotting a potential memory impairment. Ask the subject to study the list of words below for up to one minute. After a minute, take a 20-minute break. Then ask the subject to write down as many words from the list as possible. Recalling fewer than five words could indicate a problem with delayed recall. Words to use: dirt, gallery, lemon, vest, ambassador, snake, lump, mantle, elbow, kettle. About 40 percent of people 65 or older have age-associated memory impairment in the US. But only about one percent will progress to dementia each year. About 10 percent aged 65 years or older have mild cognitive impairment and nearly 15 percent of them develop Alzheimer's disease each year.

Source: *British Medical Journal* **2002;324:1502-1505.**

ALZHEIMER'S: ERT CONNECTION

68. ERT NO HELP AGAINST ALZHEIMER'S

The use of estrogen replacement therapy (ERT) by postmenopausal women does NOT reduce the risk of developing Alzheimer's disease. Over 112,000 postmenopausal women who used ERT were compared with women who had not used ERT. Nearly the same percentage of women in each group was afflicted with Alzheimer's disease.

Source: *Archives of Neurology* **2001;58:435-440.**

69. ERT ALSO WORSENS THE PROBLEM

Avoid ERT for anyone who already has Alzheimer's disease because it may worsen the memory dysfunction. Treatment with ERT impairs performance in test animals. The greatest impairment was observed in those animals who were treated the longest.

Source: Behavioral Neuroscience 2002;116:902-911.

WANT TO KNOW MORE?
[The deeper we study, the fewer advantages we see for ERT, and the more disadvantages – too many of them serious. On the other hand, we continue to hear excellent reviews about the use of natural progesterone cream (low dose) combined with small, safe amounts of tried-and-true Chinese herbs.

[See the *Menopause & HRT* section for more information on hormone replacement, as well as suggestions for healthier, natural alternatives.]

ALZHEIMER'S: NATURAL REMEDIES & SUPPLEMENTS
70. VITAMINS A, C & E AGAINST ALZHEIMER'S

Increasing your intake of antioxidants such as vitamins A, C, and E may protect against the onset of Alzheimer's disease. Concentrations of vitamins A and E found in those with Alzheimer's disease are lower than those found in non-afflicted people. Lower concentrations of these vitamins in normally nourished patients with Alzheimer's suggests that these antioxidant vitamins are consumed as a result of excessive production of free radicals. Vitamin C, also a powerful antioxidant, provides neuroprotection.

[Good sources of vitamin A are green, yellow, and orange vegetables and fruits, egg yolks, animal livers, and fish liver oils. Vitamin C is mainly found in (fresh and unprocessed) citrus fruits, kiwi, sprouts, broccoli, and cabbage. Important sources of vitamin E are grains (especially beneficial in sprouted wheat berries), nuts, and egg yolk. Tocotrienols are the best form of vitamin E, containing not only the alpha form, but other important factions, too.

See Hint #11 for more information on tocotrienols.]

Sources: *Age Ageing* **2001;30(3):23;** *Journal of the American Medical Association* **2002;287:3223-3237,3261-3263; Annual Meeting of the Gerontological Society of America, Washington, Nov 2000.**

71. DIDN'T MOM TELL YOU FISH WAS BRAIN FOOD?

Among older people who eat fish at least once a week, there is a significantly lower risk of developing dementia and Alzheimer's disease. The more fish you eat, the less chance of dementia. This beneficial effect of fish may be explained by the omega-3 polyunsaturated fatty acids contained in fish oils. These fatty acids have a protective effect against cardiovascular disease and thus they could contribute to reducing the vascular phenomena implied in vascular dementia but also in Alzheimer's disease. They could also have a specific effect on brain development and neuroprotection.

Source: *British Medical Journal* 2002;325:932-933.

72. SYSTOLIC PRESSURE AND CHOLESTEROL

Two treatable risk factors, high cholesterol and elevated systolic blood pressure, may be more important than other factors in the development of Alzheimer's disease. Solutions to these problems appear in the *High Cholesterol* and *Blood Pressure* sections.

Source: *Annals of Internal Medicine* 2002;137(3):149-55.

WANT TO KNOW MORE?
Since research shows that oxidative stress may contribute to Alzheimer's disease, it makes sense that the risk might be reduced by intake of antioxidants. The brains of patients with the disease contain lesions that are typically associated with exposure to free radicals. [The chief danger of free radicals comes from the damage they do when they react with cellular components such as DNA or the cell membrane. Antioxidants (also known as free-radical scavengers) function by absorbing a free radical. Free radicals come from rancid fats (salad dressings), foods heated at high temperatures, foods stored for long periods of time, etc.]

73. UP YOUR Bs FOR ALZHEIMER'S PROTECTION

Increasing B vitamins, which in turn decreases homocysteine, can help protect against an increased risk of developing Alzheimer's disease. [It can also help to improve your cognitive abilities as you age, as mentioned in Hint #10.] Low B vitamin concentrations (especially folate and B12) and high homocysteine concentrations are associated with cognitive decline or dementia (even if you are not considered deficient in these nutrients). Early diagnosis of these factors can help to prevent the onset of Alzheimer's disease.

Studies present compelling evidence of these relationships. In one, those with high homocysteine levels show a more rapid progression of Alzheimer's. In a second study, high homocysteine levels are associated with lower scores for cognitive thinking. A third three-year study demonstrates that low levels of both folate and B12 are related to *twice* the risk of developing Alzheimer's.

And yet another study that measured homocysteine concentrations up to 11 years before the onset of dementia shows that those with the highest levels are also at twice the risk compared with those at the lowest end of the scale.

If only ten percent of those with this problem could be stopped from developing Alzheimer's, several hundred thousand persons worldwide would benefit every year.

Sources: *Neurology* **2001;56:1188-1194;** *American Journal of Clinical Nutrition* **2002;75(5):785-786.**

WANT TO KNOW MORE?
Nondemented people 75 or older who are not currently taking vitamin B12 and/or folate supplements develop dementia within three years. Neither low levels of vitamin B12 nor folate alone significantly affect this risk. A clear association is detected only when *both* vitamins are taken into account.

The risk of dementia is found even in those who start off with good cognitive function, a very "unexpected" finding.

So monitoring B12 and folate levels in older people is important, even for those who are quite healthy in terms of cognition.

For good dietary sources of both folate and vitamin B12, see Hint #10 in the *Aging* section.

74. MORE PRAISE FOR VITAMIN E

The role of vitamin E as a protector against Alzheimer's disease is looking more and more concrete, so start increasing your dietary sources of this vitamin. The more vitamin E from food consumed, the lower your risk of developing Alzheimer's disease. Those in the top fifth of vitamin E intake have a 70 percent lower risk of developing Alzheimer's compared with those in the lowest fifth.

Subjects who use vitamin E are also less likely to receive low scores on cognitive tests, compared with those who do not use vitamin E. Vitamin E from food or supplements is associated with less cognitive decline with age.

Vitamin E supplements may even slow the progression of late-stage Alzheimer's disease.

Sources: Annual Meeting of the Gerontological Society of America, Washington, DC 2000; *Journal of the American Medical Association* **2002;287:3223-3237,3261-3263.;** *Archives of Neurology* **2002;59(7)L1125-32.**

75. TOCOTRIENOLS AGAINST ALZHEIMER'S

Add tocotrienol-rich foods to your diet or supplement regime to protect yourself from age-related diseases such as Alzheimer's disease. [Tocotrienols are natural compounds found in various foods and oils such as palm oil (one of the best sources), rice bran oil, wheat germ, barley, saw palmetto, and certain types of nuts and grains.] [The term vitamin E is now considered to be a generic name describing the bioactivity of both tocopherol (the vitamin E you are more familiar with) and tocotrienol derivatives.]

Tocotrienols have been shown to be a better form of vitamin E for the protection of neuronal cells.

Source: *Journal of Biological Chemistry*, Apr 2000.

WANT TO KNOW MORE?
Vitamin E, an antioxidant, may counteract the damage done to brain cells by free radicals, which are byproducts of normal body processes that damage tissue and have been linked to Alzheimer's disease.

Palm oil tocotrienols may also be effective in preventing Parkinson's disease and certain types of cancers, including breast cancer.

76. CURRY POWDER POWER

A spice found in curry powder possesses properties that may be protective against Alzheimer's disease. Curcumin (found in the curry spice turmeric) reduces the accumulation of substances associated with Alzheimer's Disease when fed to test animals.

There is also evidence of possible memory preservation, as the animals given curcumin perform much better in memory-dependent maze tests compared with those on normal diets.

Diets rich in curcumin may help explain why rates of Alzheimer's disease are much lower among seniors in India compared with their Western peers.

The compound has a long history of use as a dietary and herbal medicine. It is also a powerful antioxidant and anti-inflammatory agent, and curcumin appears to reduce Alzheimer's-related inflammation in neurologic tissue.

Chemicals from rosemary (rosmarinic acid) and ginger (vanillin and zingerone, also high in Indian diets) have similar structures.

Source: Annual Meeting of the Society for Neuroscience, San Diego, CA, Nov 2001.

77. GINKGO BILOBA FOR BRAIN PROTECTION

The herb ginkgo biloba protects against memory loss and Alzheimer's disease, and supplements of ginkgo *significantly* increase the activity of 10 genes involved in normal brain function. After ginkgo biloba supplementation, one gene in the brain's hippocampus and nine in the cortex increase in activity by more than three times. (The hippocampus is the center of learning and memory, whereas the cerebral cortex controls memory, speech, logical and emotional response, and voluntary movement.) All of the activated genes are involved in promoting normal brain activities, as well as protecting brain cells from damage.

Ginkgo biloba is an herb with powerful antioxidant effects, and its use in the treatment of many brain disorders has a clear molecular and genetic basis.

Source: *Proceedings of the National Academy of Science* **2001;98:6577-6580.**

ALZHEIMER'S: REDUCING RISK

78. KEEP BUSY AND FORGET ABOUT ALZHEIMER'S

Participating in leisure activities in midlife may substantially reduce your risk of developing Alzheimer's disease, especially if the activities involve intellectual stimulation. And if the activities are varied, your risk drops even further. Older men and women who participate in leisure activities are less likely to develop dementia, and these results have no relation to their racial, educational, or occupational group. In addition, there is an even further reduction (eight percent) for each additional activity they take part in.

People who are relatively inactive (either intellectually or physically) have about a 250 percent increased risk of developing Alzheimer's. Maintaining intellectual and social engagement through participation in everyday activities seems to buffer healthy individuals against cognitive decline in later life.

Sources: *Neurology* **2001;57;2236-2242;** *Proceeding of the National Academy of Science* **2001;98:3440-3445.**

WANT TO KNOW MORE?
Cholesterol lowering statins (the drugs commonly used to lower cholesterol) may increase the likelihood of developing Alzheimer's, so it is advisable for those taking statins to take coenzyme Q10 supplements. CoQ10 is reduced in statin consumers, and is a contributing factor to the development of this disease. (*British Medical Journal* **2002;325:851**)

79. LIFESTYLE, AGING & ALZHEIMER'S

To avoid Alzheimer's disease, make every effort to keep blood pressure, blood sugar, your weight, and cholesterol under control. These levels can and do influence this disease.

Controlling these lifestyle factors has a large role in preventing or delaying the onset of Alzheimer's. The research on exercise alone (which helps maintain blood pressure, cholesterol and blood sugar levels, as well as body weight) are striking.

Source: 8th International Conference on Alzheimer's Disease & Related Disorders, Stockholm, Sweden, Jul 2002.

WANT TO KNOW MORE?

Those with age-related macular degeneration are more than twice as likely as others to develop Alzheimer's disease. (***American Journal of Epidemiology* 1999;150:963-968**)

People who never marry are two to three times more likely to develop Alzheimer's disease, even compared with people whose spouses have died. (***Neurology* 1999:53:1953-1958**)

Those with very mild or mild Alzheimer's disease appear to drive as safely as their cognitively intact counterparts. (***Journal of the American Geriatric Society* 2000;48:18-22,100-102**)

Specific tell-tale brain activation patterns in Alzheimer's patients may be observed decades before the onset of the disease. (***New England Journal of Medicine* 2000;343:450-456;502-503**)

Smoking is another risk for memory loss as we age. One study found that smokers had double the risk of getting Alzheimer's disease compared with those who never smoked. However, when people quit smoking, at whatever age, they are able to reduce their risk.

Diabetes is a significant risk factor for cognitive decline in older women. (***Archives of Internal Medicine* 2000;160:141-143,174-180**) [See "Cognitive Decline" in the *Aging* section.]

The predicted number of individuals in the US who will have Alzheimner's disease in the year 2050 ranges from 11 to 16 million. There are an estimated 4.6 million Americans with the disease now. (**US Census Figures, presented at the 8th International Conference on Alzheimer's Disease and Related Disorders, Stockholm, Sweden, Jul 2002**)

ANEMIA

Iron deficiency is the most common nutritional deficiency worldwide, but anemia is not always the result of iron deficiency. Causes may range from dietary insufficiency to some unknown bleeding, or from chronic disease processes to destruction [or even lack of production] of red blood cells. (*Nurse Practitioner* **2002;27(3):38-40,42-5,49**) And sometimes, abnormal values for iron status may be caused by inflammatory conditions rather than by poor iron status.

If it is iron deficiency, the problem is greatest among toddlers aged one to three years and adolescent and adult females aged 12 to 49 years. (*Morbidity and Mortality Weekly Report* **2002;51:897-899**)

A significant number of women are iron-deficient, a seemingly neglected factor in women's health. Maternal iron-deficiency anemia might cause low birth weight and preterm delivery. (*Journal of the American Medical Association* **2002;288(17)**)

WANT TO KNOW MORE?
Runner's anemia is caused by the destruction of red blood cells and the release of hemoglobin from the pounding of feet on pavement. (*Journal of the American Medical Association* **2001 Aug 8;286(6):714**)

80. IRON ABSORPTION FRIENDS & FOES

Iron absorption decreases with dietary phosphate and increases with ascorbic acid [vitamin C], so decrease the former and increase the latter. Given the amount of phosphate in our diet, it's no wonder so many are so tired! Phosphate is served up in significant amounts in soft drinks, meats, cheeses, whole grains, and other high-protein foods.

However, ascorbic acid – the most commonly used vitamin supplement in our culture – has a pronounced enhancing effect on the absorption of dietary iron.

Source: *American Journal of Clinical Nutrition* **2001;73(1):93-98.**

81. RISK FACTORS FOR ANEMIA

Women with a menstrual period duration of more than eight days, or with a history of clots or flooding, have three to six times the increased odds of having iron-deficiency anemia, but vegetables and vitamin C can compensate. Low consumption of meat, vegetables, or vitamin C can increase your risk of having iron-deficiency anemia. Iron-deficiency anemia is defined as having low iron and specific low hemoglobin levels. In those taking nonsteroidal anti-inflammatory drugs and antacids, the odds of being iron=deficient are six to nine times higher. Watch your ingestion of nonsteroidal anti-inflammatory drugs or antacids, and if you are having menstrual difficulties as described, it's time to do something about it. If you require antacids, think about switching to probiotics instead.

[Nonsteroidal antiinflammatory drugs include aspirin, ibuprofen, and naproxen, among other analgesic substances.]

Source: *Saudi Medical Journal* 2001;22(6):490-496.

82. RED BEETS CAN REVEAL IRON DEFICIENCY

If you are among the 14 percent of the population whose urine is red after consumption of red beets (referred to as *beeturia*), there is a chance you have iron-deficiency anemia or malabsorption problems. The pigment responsible for the red color is betalaine, which is normally protected by reducing agents and decolorized by hydrochloric acid, ferric ions, and colonic bacteria.

Foods rich in oxylate, such as oysters, rhubarb, and spinach, may also promote "beeturia."

Source: *Pharmacogenetics* 1993;3(6):302-11.

83. UNIQUE SUPPLEMENT HELPS REGULATE IRON

Lactoferrin, a unique protein present in most human secretions (including human milk), is available in supplemental form to help regulate iron metabolism in the gut. Lactoferrin, in true adaptogenic fashion, has been postulated to both increase *and* to decrease intestinal iron absorption. Iron supplementation may increase free radicals, but this does not happen with the addition of lactoferrin.

[An adaptogen, unlike a drug, helps to normalize metabolic functions. A drug usually continues its action, regardless of the metabolism, whereas an adaptogen stops its action at the point of "mission accomplished."]

Remarkably, the lactoferrin protein transports iron to areas needed but also makes the iron unavailable to harmful infectious bacteria. So it is able to sequester and release iron under controlled conditions, helping to avoid harmful formations of oxidative reactions.

The newest techniques in cellular and molecular biology have allowed us to isolate lactoferrin from colostrum, and the results have been astounding.

Sources: *Advances in Experimental Medicine & Biology* 2001;501:233-9; *Journal of Infectious Diseases* 2003;23(1):178-85; *Pediatric Research* 2002;52(6):064-72; *Advances in Experimental Medicine & Biology* 1998;443:161-5; *Biochemical Society Transactions* 1997;25(2):315S.

ARTHRITIS

According to the Arthritis National Research Foundation, arthritis is progressive, erodes the physical endurance and pain tolerance of its sufferers, claims a new victim every 33 seconds, affects about 285,000 children in the US alone – often beginning very early in their young lives, and following them throughout adulthood.

And it's no fun. Arthritis, America's number one crippling disease, can cause grief in virtually every part of your body. Until recently, our traditional medical community has not been able to understand arthritis enough to make it go away. But new research is finally offering something better than drugs, which do little more than relieve pain, if that.

Arthritis and musculo-skeletal disorders are a more frequent cause of disability than either heart disease or cancer. They are responsible for 315 million physician visits per year in the US, and they are the second most common reason for visits to surgeons, the third most common to see a family doctor and the fourth most common reason for appointments to see a consultant. New musculo-skeletal complaints are the most time-consuming for physicians to evaluate and manage. (*Journal of Nutrition* **2002;132:341-346**)

By 2020, an estimated 18.2 percent of the population will suffer from arthritis, up 15 percent since 1995. Some states (West Virginia in particular) already experience higher percentages. Updated statistics tell us that nearly 70 million, or one in three US adults suffer from arthritis or chronic joint problems, causing disability in as many as eight million. (*Morbidity and Mortality Weekly Report*, **Oct 25, 2002**)

The prevalence of arthritis and joint problems increases with age, and is higher in women than men. People who are physically inactive or obese or overweight also have a higher incidence.

More than half of arthritis patients are under 65. Like so many other degenerative diseases of our time, the affliction is taking hold at earlier and earlier ages. The disease is most common among smokers and those who are separated, divorced, or unemployed.

Almost half the people who are not physically active suffer from arthritis or joint symptoms. (**Centers for Disease Control and Prevention, Nov 2002 Report**)

Osteoarthritis is the more common form. This disease is not necessarily what its name suggests. *Osteo* refers to bone, and you probably know that *itis* refers to inflammation. But this is something of a misnomer, because osteoarthritis does not always involve inflammation, while many other joint problems do.

Rheumatoid arthritis is an autoimmune disease in which the immune system attacks some of the same joint tissues that are involved in osteoarthritis. White blood cells mistakenly devour healthy cartilage in the joints. This is a chronic, inflammatory disorder causing stiffness and pain in joints and muscles, usually those of hands and feet, particularly knuckle and toe joints. Joints gradually become inflamed and swollen, leading to destruction of tissue and, in severe cases, deformity. Rheumatoid arthritis often occurs in young people, with predominance in women. Although genetic propensities may exist, these can be intercepted with lifestyle changes.

84. ICE IS NICE AGAINST ARTHRITIS

If you are suffering from arthritis pain, a simple application of ice on arthritic joints may bring relief. Patients with acute arthritis pain (typical of those suffering with gout) who use topical ice therapy along with inflammation-reducing steroids have *significantly* greater reduction in pain than those using steroids alone.

Joint circumference and synovial fluid volume (two other indicators of an arthritic joint) are also effectively reduced after one week of this combined therapy.

Source: *The Journal of Rheumatology* 2002;29:331-334.

85. ANTLERS AGAINST ARTHRITIS

If you are suffering from any form of arthritis, begin supplementing with velvet antler, a substance that has exceptional benefits for anyone with this condition. [Harvested from the antlers of deer and elk (without harming the animal), velvet antler is loaded with growth and immune factors, cartilage, glucosamine sulfate, chondroitin sulfate, and collagen. Several studies show that taking velvet antler can reduce or eliminate arthritis, and it has been used for millennia for arthritis relief.] Chondroitin sulfate and collagen type II [both found in velvet antler] have been scientifically substantiated to support healthy joint structure and function, in compliance with FDA regulations. Velvet antler is available at most health stores.

Sources: *Arzneim-Forsch Drug Research* 1990;40(1):319-323; First International Symposium on Antler Science and Product Technology, Banff, Canada, Apr 2000.

WANT TO KNOW MORE?
[To learn more about how velvet antler can help arthritis (and how it is better than isolated chondroitin and glucosamine sulfate), see my book, *The Remarkable Healing Power of Velvet Antler.*]

86. GREEN TEA FOR ARTHRITIS RELIEF

If you are suffering from any form of arthritis, drinking green tea may help. Compounds found in green tea have been shown to reduce inflammation in inflammatory arthritis and are protective to joint tissues. In studies with test animals, no toxic effects are seen with the use of these substances.

It is most likely the catechins (beneficial substances found in green tea) assist the arthritic patient by reducing inflammation and slowing cartilage breakdown.

Source: *Journal of Nutrition* 2002;132:341-346.

WANT TO KNOW MORE?

Next to water, tea is the most popular beverage in the world, and the preventive effects of green tea are currently the focus of considerable attention. As antioxidants, the polyphenols contained in green tea are potentially useful in preventing chronic diseases in humans. (*Life Sciences* **2003;72(9):1073-1083**)

Since catechins inhibit LDL oxidation (the bad kind of cholesterol), green tea is believed to be involved in reducing cardiovascular disease. (*Atherosclerosis* **2003;166(1):23-30**) It also possesses powerful anti-cancer properties. See the *Cancer* section for more information.

87.   ARTHRITIS RELIEF *CAN* BE FOUND

If you have arthritis, don't accept the fact that you must live with it (as do 99 percent of arthritis sufferers), but make an effort to learn about all the different things you can do to combat it – starting with the suggestions cited here. Adults suffering from arthritis are often depressed and report a substantially worse health-related quality of life than do people without the affliction, but many available interventions are sorely underused.

In a large group of over 32,000 Americans surveyed, as high as 29 percent reported having arthritis. But according to the Arthritis Foundation, helpful interventions reach less than *one percent* of arthritis sufferers.

Source: *Center for Disease Control, Morbidity & Mortality Report* **2000;49:366-369.**

88.   BEWARE ACETAMINOPHEN PAIN KILLERS

The use of acetaminophen to relieve arthritic pain, particularly in high doses, may be associated with gastrointestinal events. (Datril, Tylenol, Panadol, Tempra, and Anacin III are trademarks of brands of acetaminophen tablets.) Acetaminophen is often used to avoid the gastrointestinal toxicity associated with nonsteroidal anti-inflammatory drugs (NSAIDs, which are referred to as nonsteroidal because they are not steroids, which treat inflammation by suppressing the immune system).

However, high doses of acetaminophen also present problems. They are correlated with increased disturbed digestion or indigestion and, possibly, gastrointestinal bleeding.

Source: *Arthritis & Rheumatism* **2002;46:3046-3054.**

WANT TO KNOW MORE?

[The possible side effects of Ibuprofin (Motrin, Advil, Nuprin) include upset stomach, dizziness, drowsiness, headache, or ringing in the ears.]

ARTHRITIS: OSTEOARTHRITIS

Osteoarthritis is a degenerative joint disease, characterized by loss of the articular cartilage (which means narrowing of the joint space), hypertrophy (enlargement or overgrowth) of bone at the margins, and changes in the synovial membrane. Pain and stiffness accompany it, particularly after prolonged activity. It is caused by inflammation, breakdown, and eventual loss of cartilage of the joints.

IN THIS SECTION:
- ALTERNATIVE THERAPIES
- CAUSES & PRECURSORS
- EXERCISE THERAPY
- NATURAL REMEDIES & SUPPLEMENTS
- REDUCING RISK

OSTEOARTHRITIS: ALTERNATIVE THERAPIES

89. LEECHES FOR OSTEOARTHRITIS PAIN

Applying leeches to an osteoarthritic joint, an old-fashioned remedy, can actually provide significant pain relief that lasts almost a month. Considered quackery in recent years, this medieval-sounding practice proves to have real benefit and is regaining credibility. In one experimental study, four leeches placed around an arthritic knee joint resulted in pain relief that lasted at least 28 days! The one-time treatment took only 80 minutes, with no serious adverse effects.

There may be proteins in leech saliva that reduce swelling and inflammation, and something about the slow ooze of blood may also be involved.

Unlike other blood suckers, leeches don't seem to be vectors for diseases, so this treatment is probably harmless.

Source: *Annals of Rheumatic Disease* **2001;60:986.**

WANT TO KNOW MORE?
Very few of your bones actually touch each other. At least they shouldn't. A layer of an amazingly strong, slippery, and resilient material between your bones should absorb all the pressure and shock, yet remain almost totally frictionless as your joint moves. This material is *articular cartilage*. It is articular because it allows your joint to articulate or bend (creating a natural separation of joints), and it is 65 to 80 percent water.

Synovial fluid is transparent, resembling raw egg white. Without this lubricating and insulating fluid, movement would be difficult and painful. The fluid is contained by the synovial membrane, the tissue responsible for producing the nutrients that are transported to the joint tissue itself.

OSTEOARTHRITIS: CAUSES & PRECURSORS

90. MEN, EXERCISE & OSTEOARTHRITIS

If you are a man under the age of 50 who engages in high levels of physical activity (such as running 20 or more miles a week), you should know that you are at increased risk of developing symptomatic osteoarthritis. It is interesting to note that similar findings are not observed in women or in older men. In younger women, body-mass index and caffeine consumption, rather than high physical activity, are associated with the risk of osteoarthritis.

The incidence of osteoarthritis among those 50 years of age or older is actually higher among women, but under 50 it is nearly the same for both sexes. This does not mean, however, that you should not be exercising. Participation in *moderate*-intensity physical activity, at levels recommended by recent public health guidelines, is not likely to increase the risk of hip or knee osteoarthritis.

Source: *Journal of Clinical Epidemiology* 2000;53:315-322.

WANT TO KNOW MORE?
In persons over the age of 50, considerably more women are afflicted, but under the age of 50, the percentages are much closer between men and women.

91. UNFASHIONABLY PAINFUL

Ladies: Choose your footwear carefully! Certain kinds of shoes can lead to serious health conditions such as osteoarthritis. Beware high-heeled shoes. The altered forces at the knee caused by walking in high heels may lead to degenerative changes in the knee joint.

Osteoarthritis of the knee is twice as common in women as in men, and usually occurs in both knees. And now we know why – high-heeled shoes significantly alter the normal function of the ankle. Compensations occur at the knee and the hip to maintain stability and progression during walking, but most of the compensations occur at the knee. Wide-heeled shoes, too, may lead to similar problems, as women who wear wide-heeled shoes also have a higher risk of developing knee osteoarthritis, compared with women who wear narrow-heeled shoes. Increasing the width of a shoe's heel does nothing to lessen the problems caused by high heels. Neither type of heel is best for your knee health, but the narrow heel is the lesser of two evils. The wide heel increases the work of the quadriceps muscles, increases the strain through the patella tendon, and increases the pressure across the knee joint. These changes may put the knee at increased risk of degenerative joint changes.

Source: *Lancet* 2001;357:1097-1098.

OSTEOARTHRITIS: EXERCISE THERAPY

92. LESS BENEFITS TO EXERCISE OVER TIME

If you are exercising to improve osteoarthritis in your knees or hips, you should know that the early benefits of such exercise may decline and eventually disappear over time. After 24 weeks of moderate exercise, patients with osteoarthritis in the knee or hip experience small to moderate pain relief. However, by week 36, these benefits seem to disappear.

[This demonstrates the need for cure, in addition to symptom reduction. Consider velvet antler supplements as discussed in Hint #85.]

Source: *Annals of Rheumatic Diseases* **2001;60:1123-1130.**

OSTEOARTHRITIS: NATURAL REMEDIES & SUPPLEMENTS

93. HYALURONIC ACID FOR PAINFUL KNEES

If you have pain in your knees due to osteoarthritis, you should know about hyaluronic acid, which can greatly improve this condition. Hyaluronic acid is a natural substance that can reduce pain and improve joint function in people suffering from knee osteoarthritis. It may also be used successfully in those who fail to respond to or cannot tolerate conventional medical therapy.

Knee osteoarthritis can be a functionally and emotionally limiting condition. Six months after treatment with hyaluronic acid, participants demonstrate significant physical (and emotional) improvements, such as less pain while walking. These improvements occur regardless of age or body weight.

[Velvet antler (see Hint #85) is a good source of hyaluronic acid, which contains glucosamine and forms the core of a complex substance found in the cartilage matrix. Hyaluronic acid is essential for the lubricating and shock-absorbing properties of synovial fluid in the joints, and is also anti-inflammatory and analgesic.]

Sources: *Archives of Physical Medical Rehabilitation* **2000;81:479-483;** *Archives of Internal Medicine* **2002;162:292-298.**

94. VITAMIN C SLOWS DOWN OSTEOARTHRITIS

If you have osteoarthritis in your knee, supplement with vitamin C to decrease the progression of this condition considerably. High vitamin C intake is associated with a *threefold* reduction in the progression of knee osteoarthritis. Progression of both knee and hip osteoarthritis is also found to be faster in people with lower vitamin D concentrations.

However, it is not known if vitamin D supplementation is helpful. It is known, however, that high vitamin C intake reduces this progression.

Source: *British Medical Journal* 2000;321:882-885.

95. SAMe OLD SAMe OLD FOR SEVERAL SYMPTOMS

The benefit of SAMe in treating osteoarthritis was discovered when patients used SAMe for depression, and reported significant improvement in their osteoarthritis symptoms. More than 22,000 participants in 10 different studies confirm these results. SAMe has effects similar to those of the nonsteroidal anti-inflammatory drugs, but without the side effects. It appears to increase the chondrocyte activity.

[Velvet antler also increases chondrocyte activity. The word *chondro* as a prefix means *relating to cartilage*. Chondrocytes are the developed "living" cartilage cells. These cells are responsible for manufacturing collagen, and also for assembling and repairing the cartilage matrix. Part of the function performed by the chondrocytes involves destroying old cartilage to make room for new. Chondrocytes need to be active in order to keep the cartilage recycling and renewing.]

SAMe also increases concentrations of synovial fluid by three-to-fourfold. Synovial fluid is the fluid that lubricates your joints, and it enters and exits cartilage almost like water going in and out of a sponge that's continuously being compressed and released, which is why it's so important for joint health. Arthritics have lower synovial fluid.]

Sources: *Journal of Hepatology* 1999;30:1155-9,1081; *Drugs* 1990;40(supple):1-2.

96. GLUCOSAMINE FOR OSTEOARTHRITIS PAIN

If you have knee osteoarthritis, or osteoarthritis of the temporomandibular joint (TMJ), glucosamine sulfate can help improve joint function and reduce pain. Long-term use of glucosamine sulfate appears to prevent changes in joint structure in those with knee osteoarthritis. Patients receiving glucosamine have no significant joint-space loss even after three years. It also appears to be much more effective than ibuprofen in patients suffering from TMJ pain.

Glucosamine sulfate offers better control of functional pain and greater reductions in the effect of pain on daily activities, when compared with those taking only ibuprofen.

[Isolated glucosamine has been noted to have some side effects. Velvet antler is the safest and most holistic source of glucosamine sulfate, and it also contains additional beneficial constituents. It is far superior to taking isolated glucosamine supplements. See my book, *The Remarkable Healing Power of Velvet Antler*, for more information.]

Sources: *Lancet* **2001;357:251-256,247;** *Journal of Rheumatology* **2001;28:1347-1355.**

97. GINGER EXTRACT FOR KNEE PAIN RELIEF

Those suffering from knee osteoarthritis, take note: Treatment with a highly purified ginger extract may safely reduce symptoms. A group of patients (all with moderate-to-severe osteoarthritis knee pain) were given ginger extract, administered orally twice a day, or a placebo for six weeks. A significantly greater percentage of patients in the ginger group experienced pain reduction while standing and walking compared with those who received the placebo. [Ginger has a long history as a natural medicine. It is a powerful antioxidant and antimicrobial agent that is known to have anti-inflammatory properties.]

Source: *Arthritis and Rheumatism* **2001;44:2461-2462,2531-2538.**

98. GREEN-LIPPED MUSSEL FOR JOINT PAIN

New Zealand green-lipped mussel contains anti-inflammatory components that may enhance joint health. Shellfish supplements have been used for a long time as a traditional remedy for arthritis. Although the mechanism is not understood, the green-lipped mussel contains nutrients that benefit joint health. Unless special care is taken in processing, however, the efficacy is destroyed, so check your source carefully.

Source: *Journal of Nutrition* **2002;132:1634S-1636S.**

99. HELP FROM GREEN TEA CATECHINS

Consumption of green tea may be prophylactic for arthritis and may benefit the arthritic by reducing inflammation and slowing cartilage breakdown. Compounds found in green tea, called catechins, help to accomplish these dual roles.

Green tea differs from black tea in that there is no fermentation process involved, and therefore none of the associated changes in chemical composition take place.

Source: *Journal of Nutrition* **2002;132:341-346.**

OSTEOARTHRITIS: REDUCING RISK

100. JOINT INJURY? TAKE STEPS NOW!

If you have had knee or hip injuries and are still young, start healing therapy NOW to protect yourself from osteoarthritis later on. Having knee or hip injuries as an adolescent or young adult – or even in middle age – substantially increases your risk of developing osteoarthritis in the same joint later in life. But you can greatly benefit from learning about and beginning anti-arthritis treatments and therapies.

My recommendation for healing and prevention is the use of the supplement velvet antler (see Hint #85 for more information). The FDA agrees that two of the constituents in velvet antler – chondroitin and type II collagen – can support healthy joint structure and function.

Sources: *Annals of Internal Medicine* **2000;133:321-328; B. Kamen,** *The Remarkable Healing Power of Velvet Antler***; research conducted at Johns Hopkins University School of Medicine, Baltimore, MD.**

ARTHRITIS: RHEUMATOID ARTHRITIS

Rheumatoid arthritis is a chronic inflammatory disease in which there is destruction of joints. It is considered by some to be an autoimmune disorder (explained below) in which immune complexes are formed in joints and excite an inflammatory response. This in turn leads to the destruction of the synovial lining. But it can cause inflammation of tissues in other areas of the body as well (such as the lungs, heart, and eyes, and even nerves).

A chronic and progressive course is common with joint deformities.

Unlike osteoarthritis, which progresses steadily over time, rheumatoid arthritis is a condition that waxes and wanes. One may suffer either a single attack or several episodes, possibly leading to increasing disability. It is referred to as an autoimmune problem because the defense mechanisms of your immune system attack your joint tissues as if they were the enemy, a warlike reaction to normal body components, normally triggered by bacterial or viral infection. (*Arthritis and Rheumatism* **1998;41(2):191-194**)

IN THIS SECTION:
- ALTERNATIVE THERAPIES
- CAUSES & PRECURSORS
- DIETARY TACTICS
- NATURAL REMEDIES & SUPPLEMENTS

RHEUMATOID ARTHRITIS: ALTERNATIVE THERAPIES

101. ACUPUNCTURE FOR RHEUMATOID ARTHRITIS

If you are suffering from rheumatoid arthritis, you may want to consider acupuncture, which can result in a significant reduction of pain and the need for painkillers. New evidence suggests that acupuncture cuts the need for analgesia after just four sessions. In 73 percent of patients studied, pain is reduced by a third after acupuncture treatments, and by at least 50 percent in more than half of those afflicted. Analgesic use also declines significantly, from an average of 17 tablets per week to just six.

Source: *The Early Rheumatoid Arthritis Study*, Albans City Hospital, UK; Exeter University, UK; reported in *Reuter's Medical Health*, Jun 2001.

WANT TO KNOW MORE?
Nearly eight out of ten people with rheumatoid arthritis turn to complementary and alternative medicine to help relieve their symptoms. The most popular type of alternative treatments are vitamin supplements (73 percent of sufferers), acupuncture (45 percent), the wearing of a copper bracelet (42 percent), osteopathy (40 percent), aromatherapy (26 percent), and cod liver oil treatment (26 percent).

RHEUMATOID ARTHRITIS: CAUSES & PRECURSORS

102. DON'T MAKE MINE A DECAF

Avoid drinking decaffeinated coffee, which may increase your risk of developing rheumatoid arthritis. Drinking more than three cups of decaf coffee per day appears to increase the risk of developing rheumatoid arthritis, while the consumption of caffeinated coffee seems to have no effect on this particular disease. The link with decaffeinated coffee may be related to the direct application of industrial solvents to coffee beans, the method commonly used to extract caffeine.

In contrast, tea drinking may reduce the risk, perhaps due to its anti-inflammatory and antioxidant properties. [If you are avoiding caffeine in the first place, why not get into the more healthful habit of drinking herbal teas? Look for Rooibos ("redbush") tea, a lesser-known tea now gaining popularity for its many health-promoting properties such as relief from insomnia, depression, stomach cramps, constipation, allergy symptoms, and skin irritation. Rooibos tea is also chock-full of antioxidants and has anti-aging properties as well.]

Source: *Arthritis & Rheumatism* 2002;46:83-91.

103. GUM DISEASE? START SUPPLEMENTING

If you suffer from gum disease, it's time to consider anti-inflammatory supplementation, as you may also be at risk for rheumatoid arthritis. There is a *significant* association between rheumatoid arthritis and gum disease, which may result from an underlying dysfunction in inflammatory response. (However, the relationship is not causal; gum disease does not *cause* the rheumatoid arthritis. Again, it's the underlying dysfunction of the inflammatory response that's the culprit.)

Those with rheumatoid arthritis have more missing teeth and deeper gum pocketing compared with those who don't have this condition. Swollen joints are also associated with periodontal bone loss. [Velvet antler is among my favorite anti-inflammatory supplements, especially for joint problems. See Hint #85 for more information]

Source: *Journal of Periodontology*, 2001;72:779-787.

WANT TO KNOW MORE?
Possible causes of an increased cardiovascular disease risk among rheumatoid arthritis patients include side effects of medication, decreased mobility, adverse lipid profile (fat in the blood), increased homocysteine level, increased levels of thrombotic factors (clotting factors), and other inflammatory mechanisms. (*Arthritis Rheumatism* **2002;46:1714-1719**)

[Periodontal disease is also a risk factor for heart disease.]

104. RHEUMATOID ARTHRITIS & HOMOCYSTEINE

As high homocysteine levels are almost a given in those with rheumatoid arthritis, supplementing with folate, vitamins B6, and vitamin B12 is critical. Homocysteine is an amino acid produced naturally in your body, but high levels in the blood are associated with an increased risk of many health problems. Supplementing with folate (folic acid), B6, and B12 can help to reduce these levels.

The high homocysteine levels may be due to enzymatic defects in homocysteine metabolism due to chronic illness, disturbances of the gastrointestinal system, or impaired kidney function.

Research indicates that the immune system is involved in the development of atherosclerosis in rheumatoid arthritis patients.

[See the *Immune System Disorders* section for suggestions for enhancing immunity.]

Source: *Journal of Rheumatology* 2002;29:1619-1622; 875-82.

RHEUMATOID ARTHRITIS: DIETARY TACTICS

105. GO VEGAN FOR ARTHRITIS RELIEF

If you are suffering from rheumatoid arthritis, consider switching to an all-vegetable diet, which can significantly reduce your symptoms. A vegan diet, along with large amounts of living lactobacilli and chlorophyll-rich drinks consumed daily, decreases symptoms of rheumatoid arthritis, while a return to an omnivorous diet will aggravate symptoms. [Vegan means a strictly vegetarian diet: which also means no milk, butter, or eggs – nothing that comes from an animal.]

Some people may experience nausea or diarrhea at the start of such a diet [usually a sign of detoxification, which may happen to those who need such a diet the most]. The average person, however, experiences an immediate improvement in activity.

[From clinical experience, we know that this type of diet is helpful for all kinds of arthritis.] Such a diet also increases fiber intake, and eliminates the need for interventions such as gold, drugs, and steroids.

In Table Talk, this means a variety of vegetables, a high quality acidophilus, and a green mix. [My newest green find: packets of organic powdered young barley leaf, prepared from the whole leaf, rather than the juice-extracted variety, with both pre- and probiotics added to the mix.]

Source: *British Journal of Rheumatology*, 1998;37(3):274-281.

RHEUMATOID ARTHRITIS: NATURAL REMEDIES & SUPPLEMENTS

106 VITAMIN E AGAINST RHEUMATOID ARTHRITIS

Start supplementing with vitamin E to help reduce the symptoms of rheumatoid arthritis. Vitamin E, a known antioxidant, reduces inflammation and prevents joint destruction in those suffering from rheumatoid arthritis. (Inflammation is elevated in many disease conditions.)

In test animals with this disease, vitamin E seems to uncouple joint inflammation and joint destruction, with beneficial results.

In humans, those taking either vitamin E alone (400 IU of vitamin E three times daily) or antioxidants along with drugs experience an 80 percent reduction in symptoms, compared with only a 25 percent reduction in those taking drugs alone. Furthermore, people taking the vitamins benefit in just a month, twice as fast as the drug-only group.

[Dietary sources of vitamin E include butter, egg yolks, and liver. Vitamin E in the tocotrienol form is better absorbed than tocopherol vitamin E. Tocotrienols are found in various foods and oils such as palm oil, rice bran oil, wheat germ, barley, saw palmetto, and certain types of nuts and grains.]

Sources: *Arzneimittel Forschung Research* **(German) 2001;51:293-298;** *Arthritis & Rheumatism* **2002;46(2):522-532.**

WANT TO KNOW MORE?

[An inexpensive way to get extremely effective and bioavailable vitamin E is to consume a handful of sprouted wheat berries on a daily basis. The germ of the wheat is replete with vitamin E, and consuming the sprouted grain enhances the nutrient content even more! Wheat grains are easy to sprout, and offer a profusion of many other nutrients, too. It may be the only food you eat that is growing up to the minute of consumption. All you need is a glass jar, wheat berry grains, and your kitchen sink. Health stores carry many books with simple sprouting instructions.]

107. ELK ANTLER FOR RHEUMATOID ARTHRITIS

A dose of four to six capsules of elk velvet antler daily is safe and may lead to improvement in rheumatoid arthritis symptoms. In a study done on a group of stage II rheumatoid arthritis patients [meaning a more advanced stage of the disease], those taking six elk velvet antler capsules daily showed the greatest improvement, *double* that of those taking a placebo.

Elk velvet antler can be taken safely with concurrent rheumatoid arthritis medications. [You may find you don't require the medication after the velvet antler treatment is well under way.]

Source: Study conducted at the Faculty of Nursing, University of Alberta, Edmonton, Canada, and reported at the First International Symposium on Antler Science & Product Technology, Banff, Canada, Apr 2000.

WANT TO KNOW MORE?

[Velvet antler contains hyaluronic acid, which contains glucosamine and forms the core of the complex substance found in cartilage matix. One study showed that rheumatoid arthritis patients treated with hyaluronate improved, compared to a control group. Other studies demonstrating success with hyalyuronic acid are cited in Hint #93. Traditional treatment for rheumatoid arthritis includes advice to rest. However, exercise induces changes in circulating immune function that would appear helpful in regulating the inflammation. And there is evidence that rheumatoid arthrits patients can tolerate a program of regular moderate exercise, enhancing physicial performance without exacerbating the disease process.

To understand more about exactly how velvet antler helps repair joint function and alleviate symptoms in rheumatoid arthritis, see my book, *The Remarkable Healing Power of Velvet Antler.*]

108. SOD SPELLS RHEUMATOID ARTHRITIS RELIEF

If you have rheumatoid arthritis, you should know that a substance known as *superoxide dismutase* (SOD), found in most green plants, can help. Superoxide dismutase is a naturally occurring enzyme that reduces the chronic inflammation associated with rheumatoid arthritis. In test animals, SOD begins to ameliorate symptoms after just about a month. Inflammation, tissue and bone damage, and joint erosion are all reduced significantly.

[SOD can be found in barley and wheatgrass, broccoli, Brussels sprouts, cabbage, and most *uncooked* green vegetables (cooking destroys enzymes). It is also available in supplemental form, but whether or not it's useful this way is still a controversial topic.]

Source: *Arthritis & Rheumatism* **2001;44.**

109. CAT'S CLAW CONNECTION

A Peruvian plant called *Uncaria tomentosa*, or cat's claw, seems to be an effective treatment for acute rheumatoid arthritis. This Peruvian plant appears to be an effective treatment for acute rheumatoid arthritis and knee arthritis. Found in the Amazonian jungle, cat's claw has been widely used to treat inflammatory disorders. When given to rheumatoid arthritis patients, cat's claw safely reduces the number of swollen and tender joints, as well as morning stiffness (an effect not seen in those given a placebo).

Cat's claw is known to reduce the activity of several components of the immune system – including the proliferation of highly activated lymphocytes, which cause the autoimmune reaction that results in rheumatoid arthritis. The herb also has excellent antioxidant capability. In those with knee arthritis, cat's claw also significantly reduces pain associated with activity, with benefits seen as soon as the first week of therapy.

Sources: *Journal of Rheumatology* **2002;29:678-681;** *Phytomedicine* **2002;9(4):325-337;** *Inflammatory Research* **2001;50(9):442-448.**

110. COLLAGEN TYPE II: SWELL FOR SWELLING

Collagen Type II has been used with success against rheumatoid arthritis because it appears to stimulate immune cells to combat the problem. Sixty rheumatoid arthritics were divided into collagen and placebo groups. The group given collagen type II for three months reported significant reductions in joint swelling and pain, and a few patients even claimed complete remission. [Velvet antler contains collagen type II.]

Sources: *Arthritis & Rheumatism* **1998;41(2):191-194;** *Science* **1993;261:1727-1730.**

ASTHMA

Asthma continues to rise in industrialized countries worldwide. In England, patients experiencing asthma rose from about five percent to almost nine percent in a six-year period. Researchers conclude that it's the way we live as much as anything!

When we look at the list of risk factors associated with asthma, we have to wonder how anyone can escape being afflicted. These include: air pollution (***Thorax** 2002;57:687-693*); chronic migraine attacks (***British Journal of General Practice** 2002;52:723-727*); dog and cat allergies (***Journal of Allergy & Clinical Immunology** 2002;110:395-403*); acetaminophen taken by your mom during pregnancy (***Thorax** 2002;57:958-963*); exposure to tobacco smoke, gas stoves, and wood smoke (***Thorax** 2002;57:973-978*); systemic inflammation (***Annals of Allergy & Asthma Immunology** 2002;89:381-385*); eye drops used to treat glaucoma (***British Medical Journal** 2002;325:1396-1397*); travel and alcohol (***Archives of International Medicine** 2002;162:2421-2426*). And this is just the *short* list.

Information on childhood asthma is cited in the *Childhood Asthma* section before *Childhood Illnesses & Health Problems*.

IN THIS SECTION:
- CAUSES & PRECURSORS
- DIETARY TACTICS
- NATURAL REMEDIES & SUPPLEMENTS
- REDUCING RISK

ASTHMA: CAUSES & PRECURSORS

111. WINE MAY PROMPT ASTHMA ATTACKS

If you are asthmatic, avoid drinking wine – it can provoke an asthma attack. Alcoholic drinks, particularly wine, may be important triggers for asthmatic responses. About one-third of asthmatics questioned report that alcohol has been associated with their asthma attacks on at least two occasions.

Wines, both white and red, are most commonly cited as a cause, and reactions are seen in less than an hour. There are also significant associations between wine-induced asthma and asthma triggered by sulfite-containing foods or nonsteroidal anti-inflammatory drugs (NSAIDs) such as aspirin and ibuprofen. [Sulfites are commonly used to prevent or reduce spoilage or discoloration. They are frequently used on syrups and condiments, as well as in preserving fruits and vegetables, in wine making, and as a spray on restaurant salad bars.]

Source: *Journal of Allergy & Clinical Immunology* 2000;105:462-467.

112. MINERAL DEFICIENCIES IN ASTHMATICS

If you are asthmatic, make sure you are supplementing daily with essential minerals, especially magnesium. A significant percentage of asthmatics show low levels of this electrolyte. At least 85 percent of asthmatics have at least one mineral deficiency, and some have disturbances of two or three minerals.

(Please note: If your physician suggests bronchodilator therapy, steps should be taken to correct mineral disturbances *first* to avoid adverse results.)

Source: *Chest* **2001;120:431-436.**

113. ASTHMA CATCHES WOMEN WHO DON'T MOVE

If you have an inherited tendency to asthma, protect yourself by making sure to exercise regularly. Demonstrating once again that we CAN intercept heredity, it has been shown that asthma is likely to surface in women with an inherited tendency to the disease if they are sedentary, but not if they are physically active.

With the phenomenon of sedentary lifestyle increasing in our society nowadays, it is no surprise that asthma has also been increasing. Those with asthma (as well as their family members) are encouraged to exercise regularly, in accordance with their capabilities and physical limitations.

Source: *Chest* **2001;120:1434-1435,1474-1479.**

114. NSAIDs CAN TRIGGER ASTHMA ATTACKS

If you are asthmatic, avoid taking nonsteroidal anti-inflammatory drugs such as aspirin or Ibuprofen. A high percentage of those with asthma have asthma attacks following the ingestion of aspirin or other nonsteroidal anti-inflammatory drugs (NSAIDs) such as ibuprofen. The prevalence of aspirin intolerance is as high as 11 percent among asthmatics and 2.5 percent in non-asthmatics.

It's also been shown that asthmatics process perceptual information with less efficiency. Parents of obese children should be aware that these children are at high risk for asthma, one of the most common chronic childhood diseases. [See the *Childhood Asthma* section for more information.]

Sources: *Thorax* **2002;57:569-574;** *American Journal of Respiratory Critical Care Medicine* **2002;166(1):47-52;** *Archives of Pediatrics & Adolescent Medicine* **2002;156:269-275.**

115. CESAREAN BIRTH CAN LEAD TO ASTHMA

Adults with asthma are more likely to have been delivered by cesarean section compared with adults without asthma. Cesarean section is strongly associated with current physician-diagnosed asthma.

However, no strong relationships are observed between cesarean section and atopy (allergic reactions with family tendencies), hay fever, or atopic eczema. The reasons for the association remain unknown.

Source: *Journal of Allergy & Clinical Immunology 2001;107:732-733.*

ASTHMA: DIETARY TACTICS

116. AN APPLE A DAY...KEEPS *ASTHMA AWAY*

Protect yourself from asthma by eating apples, as well as by making sure to get enough selenium, an essential trace mineral. Asthma is less common and less severe in adults who consume more dietary antioxidants. Consumption of apples and selenium, both providing powerful antioxidants, is inversely associated with asthma in adults [that is, high apple and selenium intake = low asthma incidence]. Asthmatics have lower levels of serum selenium.

The association between apples and a reduced risk of asthma may indicate the protective effect of flavonoids [potent antioxidants found in apples, as well as in many plants] on respiratory health.

Interestingly, a particular catechin (a flavonol) found in green tea is also found in apples.

[Selenium can be found in brewer's yeast, broccoli, liver, butter, most fish, whole grains, and barley, among other sources. The amount of selenium found in food varies with levels in the soil.]

Sources: *American Journal of Respiratory & Critical Care Medicine 2001;164:1823-1828; Free Radical Biology & Medicine 2002;33(12):1693-702; Journal of Trace Elements in Medicine & Biology 2002;16(2):123-7*

.

WANT TO KNOW MORE?
[Selenium also has protective properties against several types of cancers. See Hint #158 for more information.]

ASTHMA: NATURAL REMEDIES & SUPPLEMENTS

117. PERILLA SEED OIL FOR ASTHMA

If you are asthmatic, consumption of perilla seed oil may help to reduce symptoms. Dietary supplementation with perilla seed oil, a supplement high in alpha-linolenic acid, may be beneficial for those with asthma. [Perilla is a member of the mint family.] Patients given perilla seed oil show *significant* improvement in as little as two to four weeks, and in addition to improved lung function they also have reduced cholesterol levels.

This is exciting news because so few single natural remedies have a beneficial effect for asthmatics.

Source: *International Archives of Allergy & Immunology* **2000;122:137-142**

WANT TO KNOW MORE?
[Alpha-linolenic acid is also found in flaxseed oil. We actually require higher amounts of alpha-linolenic acid than other fatty acids. That's why I recommend that everyone use a small coffee grinder to mince a tablespoon of flaxseed daily. The ground flaxseed has a light, nutty taste and is great sprinkled over cereal or salad. See Hint #180 and Hint #658 for more information.]

118. FISH OIL CAN HELP ASTHMA AS WELL

A derivative of docosahexaenoic acid (DHA), a compound found in fish oil, appears effective in reducing asthma. The incidence of asthma is extremely low in Greenland Inuits, who have a high dietary intake of marine oil, suggesting that these oils may have a protective effect against asthma. Test animals given DHA are shown to have a significant reduction in harmful cell numbers, while those given soybean oil do not. DHA treatment also reduces bronchial hyper-responsiveness.

Asthma patients experience a significant improvement in their breathing ability and better resistance to asthma attacks while on high fish-oil diets.

On the other hand, linoleic acid, found in vegetable oils such as safflower, sunflower and corn oils, exacerbate asthma symptoms.

[While fish oils are the most common source, DHA can also be found in egg yolks.]

Source: *International Archives of Allergy & Immunology* **2000;123:327-332;** *American Journal of Clinical Nutrition* **1997;1011-17.**

119. CoQ10 DEFICIENCY & ASTHMATICS

Supplementing with a natural substance known as coenzyme Q10 (CoQ10) may be beneficial against asthma. Concentrations of coenzyme Q10 are significantly lower in those with allergic asthma. Levels of alpha-tocopherol [vitamin E] are also significantly decreased in asthmatics. [Coenzyme Q10 and vitamin E actually perform similar actions in the body.] There are no differences observed, however, in levels of beta-carotene between asthmatics and non-asthmatics.

[Some dietary sources of CoQ10 are spinach, peanuts, beef, and oily fish such as mackerel and salmon.]

Source: *Allergy* 2002;57:811-814.

ASTHMA: REDUCING RISK

120. STOP COOKING WITH GAS

If you are an asthmatic, get rid of your gas stove, which releases nitrogen dioxide and may substantially aggravate asthma symptoms. Individuals who use a gas stove seven or more times per week are at *twice* the risk of seeking emergency room treatment for asthma exacerbations compared with less frequent users or nonusers of gas stoves.

Daily use of gas stoves is associated with a twofold increased risk of emergency room visits.

Source: *Thorax* 2002;57:973-978.

WANT TO KNOW MORE?
More asthma is seen among women with irregular menstruation. There are many causes of irregular menses, and some appear to be unrelated to asthma but others are known to be strongly related. A few women may have irregular periods as a consequence of the stress of severe asthma. Studies also show less asthma in postmenopausal women. **(12th Annual Congress of the European Respiratory Society, Stockholm, Sweden, Sep 2002)**

Although asthma is usually provoked by airbone allergens, responses can occur from inhalation of food allergens. **(***Allergy* **2002;57:713-717)**

121. YOU'LL HAVE CLEANER RUGS & RELIEF!

Asthma sufferers: Be sure to vacuum your rugs at least once a week to keep dust-mite allergen levels low in your home. Regular weekly rug vacuuming is more effective than monthly vacuuming in reducing allergen levels from house dust mites, which are associated with asthma and other allergic conditions. Weekly vacuuming results in a *significant* decrease in mite allergens.

Endotoxin concentrations, however, are not affected by this practice, possibly because vacuuming *stimulates* bacterial growth by releasing organisms from the base of the rug. [An endotoxin refers to a poisonous substance found in bacteria.]

Source: *Annals of Allergy, Asthma & Immunology* **2000;84:249-254.**

122. HEAT & STEAM AGAINST ASTHMA

If you or someone in your family is asthmatic, a onetime steam and heat cleaning of your home can be very helpful. A single steam and heat treatment of home furnishings reduces the dust-mite allergen load to below the risk level for sensitization – an advantage for asthmatics.

Treating carpets, upholstery, mattresses, and blankets with steam and heat causes reductions in bronchial hyper-reactivity. The reductions are very significant, and these improvements are sustained for many months (as long as 12 months in homes with bedroom ventilation units).

Source: *Journal of Allergy and Clinical Immunology* **2001;107:55-60.**

WANT TO KNOW MORE?
[For more helpful tips on reducing dust-mite allergens in your home, see the *Allergies* section.]

Exercise-induced bronchospasm in those with asthma is more intense in the evening than in the morning. (*Journal of Allergy & Clinical Immunology* **2002;110:236-240**)

Exposure to ozone increases the inflammatory responses of asthmatics. (*American Journal of Critical Care Medicine* **2002;166:1073-1077**)

People employed in the entertainment industry have a fivefold increased risk of occupational asthma. Researchers speculate that the high risk could be influenced by exposure to chemicals used in art, stage set production, makeup and photography. (*Occupational Environmental Medicine* **2002;59;505-511**)

123. ASTHMATICS: DON'T TAKE MELATONIN

If you are asthmatic, avoid taking supplemental melatonin, as it may exacerbate symptoms of asthma. Circulating melatonin (a pineal hormone) is elevated at night in all vertebrates. Air travelers who cross several time zones commonly use supplemental melatonin to prevent jet lag, which results from the body's internal rhythms being out of sync with the day-night cycle at the destination. But studies show an adverse effect of supplemental melatonin in asthma patients. There is also a possible interaction with warfarin (coumadin).

Because melatonin can act as either an antioxidant or a pro-oxidant on your liver (that is, beneficial or harmful), depending on the amount consumed, it is important not to overdose.

Sources: *American Journal of Respiratory Critical Care Medicine* **2002;166:1055-1061; Updated RefSource: Cochrane Database System, Review 2001;** *Life Science* **2000;68(4):387-399.**

124. ASTHMA INHALERS & ADRENAL PROBLEMS

If you are asthmatic and use an inhaler, be careful not to exceed the recommended dosage. Those who inhale corticosteroids for asthma may be at increased risk for compromised adrenal function, and children are especially susceptible. [Corticosteroids are any of the steroid hormones produced by the adrenal cortex or their synthetic equivalents.]

Some people experience severe symptoms even with prescribed amounts of corticosteroids, but it is especially essential not to exceed the suggested drug amount. Adrenal crisis associated with high-dose inhaled steroids is more common than previously thought. Among the symptoms of high-dose inhaled corticosteroids:

- acute hypoglycemia [low blood sugar]
- lethargy
- nausea

Adrenal crisis occurs when the body's production of cortisol is curtailed because of administration of an outside source of cortisol. And thus, your body's own adrenal reserve can become insufficient to respond to a respiratory infection.

[Any time we take any hormone from an outside source, our body begins to stop its own production of that same hormone.]

Sources: *Archives of Disease in Childhood* **2002;87:457-461;** *British Medical Journal* **2002;325:1261.**

WANT TO KNOW MORE?
Since steroid hormones are synthesized from cholesterol, it has also been suggested that taking statins – used to lower cholesterol – may predispose you to adrenal crisis.

ATHLETE'S FOOT

Athlete's foot is a contagious fungal skin infection that usually affects the feet, especially the skin between the toes. It is characterized by itching, blisters, cracking, and scaling. It's a benign pathology, but more common than previously recognized, especially in children.

Feet can become infected by bacteria, which could spread to other parts of the body. Fungal infections are usually very difficult to cure, so we are delighted to offer two safe and natural potential remedies. (*Archives of Pediatric Adolescent Medicine* **2002;156(11):1149-52;** *Drug therapy Bulletin* **2002;40(7):53-4)**

125. LACTOFERRIN FOR ATHLETE'S FOOT

If you are suffering from athlete's foot, try supplementing with lactoferrin (a protein component of colostrum, the first milk produced for newborns by mammals). A placebo-controlled double-blind study demonstrated that oral intake of lactoferrin works to treat athlete's foot. Doses of either 600 mg or 2,000 mg of lactoferrin, or a placebo, were orally administered daily for 8 weeks to adults who were judged to have mild or moderate *tinea pedis* (athlete's foot).

The potential usefulness of lactoferrin as a treatment for tinea pedis was seen for the first time in this study. There were no adverse events and no one withdrew from the study because of any discomfort.

Source: *Mycoses* **2000;43(5):197-202**

WANT TO KNOW MORE?
[I have been writing about lactoferrin for some time now, and it is an extraordinary supplement. But this is exciting news because there are so few natural products that work to eliminate any fungus. Lactoferrin is safe.]

126. TEA TREE OIL TO THE RESCUE

Tea tree oil proves to be effective for treating athlete's foot. A randomized, controlled, double-blinded study showed that tea tree oil works for athlete's foot! Patients applied the solution twice daily to the affected areas for four weeks.

There was a marked clinical response seen in 68 percent of patients using a 50 percent solution of tea tree oil, and even an excellent response in those using only a 25 percent solution.

Source: *Australas Journal of Dermatology* **2002;43(3):175-8.**

ATHLETIC INJURIES

Strenuous exercise produces an overload of harmful free radicals that can damage healthy cells. Antioxidants neutralize the free radicals and limit their destructive impact. so the best advice for the athlete, whether professional or weekend only, is to be sure you are getting enough supplemental antioxidants (including vitamins C and E in particular).

Most injuries are caused by overuse. Their gradual onset, coupled with the intense competition for professional positions, often results in injuries being ignored, and not treated until late in their course. (*Occupational Medicine* **2001;16(4):609-18, iv**)

Some sports injuries are assumed to be inevitable. For example, foot injuries are frequent at higher levels of sport climbing. For optimal performance, climbers wear shoes that are too tight and have an unnatural shape. Custom shoes conforming to the form of your foot are available. (*Applied Ergonomics* **2001;32(4):379-87**)

127. NUTRIENTS FOR TENNIS ELBOW RELIEF

A combination of essential fatty acids and antioxidants appears to be an effective alternative treatment for repetitive-motion injuries such as "tennis elbow" and "golf elbow." The results of research confirm that inflammatory injuries can be treated *without* the use of NSAIDs (nonsteroidal anti-inflammatory drugs). In addition, athletes are able to continue to train while receiving treatment.

The treatment is a combination of omega-3 (fish oil), omega-6 (borage oil), vitamins A, B6, C and E, plus selenium and zinc. Most patients respond positively to the treatment in a matter of two to three weeks, depending on the severity of the injury. The bad cases require the use of intensive ultrasound and certain massage techniques in addition to the antioxidants and essential fatty acids, but in the milder cases the use of nutrients alone is adequate.

Source: *Reuter's Medical Health Report*, Apr 2000.

128. NO STRETCHING BEFORE EXERCISING

Contrary to conventional wisdom, it has now been validated that there is *no* advantage to stretching before or after exercising. The long-held beliefs about the benefit of this common practice have now been questioned, and several studies show that stretching before or after exercising produces non-significant reductions in muscle soreness, injury risk, and even sporting performance.

A few studies even suggest that stretching is harmful. These findings are supported by a large randomized controlled trial. The results are contrary both to what many athletes and coaches believe and what is common practice.

Researchers conclude that the findings are not too surprising if we consider the complex mechanical properties of biological soft tissues.

Source: *British Medical Journal* 2002;325:468.

WANT TO KNOW MORE?
Other commonly held views are also coming into question, such as applying ice or compression bandages to sore muscles. (Early movement gives the best result.) There is, however, evidence to show that taping or bracing can reduce the incidence of recurrent ankle sprains. But the protective effect of taping seems to be limited to people with previous injury.

Furthermore, there is evidence that balance training can improve sensorimotor control in athletes with previous injuries.

129. FROZEN PEAS MAKE PERFECT ICE PACKS

A simple bag of frozen peas, used as an ice pack, is ideal to ease the swelling or pain of injuries caused by muscle sprains, strains, or from any other cause because it can mold to the shape required. One warning, however: A bag of frozen peas will remain colder for a longer period of time than a normal ice pack, and if left on too long could potentially cause frostbite. Frostbite in the gym is not as rare as one might think!

The experts suggest that cold packs should be wrapped in a towel, and should never be applied to the skin for more than 20 minutes at a time. Those with nerve problems or diabetes should be more careful, since they may not be able to feel the temperature accurately.

Source: *British Journal of Sports Medicine* 2000.

130. CAPSAICIN FOR PAIN RELIEF

Capsaisin can be helpful in relieving the pain of various injuries. Topical capsaicin has been known as an effective pain management adjunct for many problems. Recent studies and case reports confirm that it is also helpful for pain incurred from general athletic injuries. It can decrease the use of analgesics that have side effects.

Other problems for which capsaicin offers pain relief include rheumatoid arthritis, osteoarthritis, neuralgias, diabeteic neuropathy. inflammation of the airways, and urinary tract infections. Capsaicin is also considered an antimicrobial factor.

Source: *Clinical Journal of Pain* 1998;14(2):97-106; *Bioscience, Biotechnology, & Biochemistry* 2002;66(3):532-6..

AUTISM

There is a troubling increase in autism worldwide. It is about ten times as common in the US today as it was in the 1980s. Teachers, pediatricians, and social workers describe soaring numbers. The US education department reported a 544 percent increase in autistic students from 1992 to 2000, and now includes this condition as a category for special education services. Individuals with autism have unusual social, communicative, and behavioral development and may have abnormalities in cognitive functioning, learning, attention, and sensory processing.. (*Journal of the American Medical Association* **2003;289:49-55;** *British Medical Journal* **2003;326:71**) Food, vaccination and pathogens have all been suggested to play a role. Maternal viral infection may also increase autism in the offspring, sometimes not even showing until adulthood. (Mom's viral infection during pregnancy is assumed to have an effect on the maternal immune response of the fetus.) (*Journal of Neuroscience* **2003;23(1):297-302**) It is not unusual for children who develop autism after a normal period of growth to have a history of food allergy, antibiotic use, ear infection, and vaccine exposure.

131. IMPROVING AUTISTIC SYMPTOMS WITH DIET

Elimination of dairy, gluten and other food components from the diet can dramatically improve the symptoms of children and adults with autism. More than 50 percent of autistic children show *significant* improvements when dairy products and gluten are eliminated from their diet. Poorly-degraded food proteins may leak from the gut into the blood, and peptides with opioid activity adversely affect brain function. [Many parents with autistic children are already aware of this. All parents are encouraged to eliminate the traditional snack of milk and cookies].

During the first phase of a three-month intervention trial, milk and dairy products, food colorings, grains, caffeine, and other food components were eliminated from the diet. Sometimes these foods actually mask other food sensitivities. Additional problem foods can be soy products, peanuts, buckwheat, and grapes.

This study was extremely tight and very dependable, totally controlling the diets at a resident facility. Improvement was seen in cognition, sociality, and alertness.

Source: 12th International Conference on Autism, Durham University, UK, Apr 2001.

132. NUTRIENTS THAT HELP

Nutrient supplements that may be beneficial for autistics and are well tolerated in children include dimethylglycine, vitamin B6, magnesium, vitamins A, B3, C, folic acid, the minerals calcium and zinc, cod liver oil, and digestive enzymes. Current pharmaceuticals fail to help the primary symptoms and can have adverse effects.

Source: *Alternative Medical Review* **2002;7(6):472-99.**

BACK PAIN

Back pain is a major economic burden. Increasing numbers of people are looking for alternatives, including acupuncture to replace or to accompany traditional medical treatment. (*British Journal of Nursing* **2002;11(21):1395-1403**) Many people with chronic back pain suffer from depression. In fact, psychological distress more than doubles the later risk of back pain. (*Archives of General Psychiatry* **2002;60(1):39-47**)

Because of the fear of inciting pain, levels of physical activity in chronic back pain patients are low. This has an impact on bone mass, and only exacerbates the problem after awhile. Chronic low back pain patients have an increased incidence of osteopenia and osteoporosis. (*Clinical Rehabilitation* **2002;16(8):867-70**)

Lower back pain in children is a common problem. Contrary to belief, heavy school bags are not always associated with this pain. Psychosocial factors, rather than mechanical factors, are more significant in our younger population. (*Archives of Diseases of Childhood* **2003;88(1):12-7**) If you are under doctor's care for lower back pain, you might ask for B12 injections. Intramuscular vitamin B12 may safely lower the pain. (*European Review of Medical Pharmacology Science* **2000;4(3):53-8**) And the same capsicum that helps relieve the pain of athletic injuries can help here, too. (See Hint #130.)

133. WILLOW BARK FOR ACHING BACKS

If you are suffering from back pain, try taking extract of willow bark, a traditional herbal medicine. Willow bark was compared with a placebo in a trial in patients with chronic back pain. The startling results showed significant improvement. Thirty-nine percent of patients given a high dose of willow bark extract reported pain completely relieved, compared with only six percent of those given the placebo. Side effects were few and researchers concluded that willow bark extract may be a useful alternative for patients who cannot tolerate NSAIDs (nonsteroidal anti-inflammatory drugs).

Source: *American Journal of Medicine* **2000;109:9-14.**

WANT TO KNOW MORE?
Buying a pharmaceutical analgesic off the shelf is considerably easier and more convenient – and far less expensive – than seeing a doctor and going through the process of getting a prescribed drug.

Unfortunately, the average American does not realize that a drug purchased over the counter (OTC) may be associated with the same adverse effects as the same drug purchased by prescription. In the case of OTC NSAIDs, adverse reactions may include kidney damage, hypertension, and gastrointestinal (GI) symptoms ranging from mild dyspepsia to serious or even fatal GI bleeding. GI disease associated with NSAIDs has been reported as the most common serious adverse drug effect in the US. NSAIDs can exacerbate underlying disease or cause new lesions.

NSAIDs include aspirin, Tylenol, ibuprofen (Advil, Motrin IB, Nuprin), indomethacin, diclofenac, ketoprofen, piroxicam, naproxen (Aleve), sulindac, choline subsalicylate, diflunisal, fenoprofen, meclofenamate, salsalate, tolmetin, and magnesium salicylate.

134. AIR MATTRESS FOR BACK PAIN RELIEF

If you suffer from chronic lower back pain, sleeping on an adjustable air mattress rather than on a conventional innerspring mattress may provide some relief. Aside from the common cold, lower-back pain is the single biggest cause of lost work time among adults in the US, affecting nearly 40 million Americans. The fact that sufferers can adjust the firmness of an air mattress to their liking seems to make a difference when it comes to sleeping comfort and relief.

According to the American Academy of Orthopedic Surgeons, four out of five persons experience back pain in their lifetime, but risk can be reduced by exercising regularly, maintaining proper posture, using proper lifting techniques, avoiding smoking, and maintaining proper body weight.

Source: Kenny Institute Chronic Pain Rehabilitation Program, Minneapolis, MN, reported by CBS "HealthWatch" Sep 2000.

BRITTLE NAILS

Although about 20 percent of the population has brittle nails (with women overtaking men), few reports exist about their occurrence. The problem is age-related, and could be used for disease prognosis. Wet working conditions increase nail brittleness, but do not cause it. Frequent alternating periods of hydration and drying also increase the incidence. (*Dermatology* **1992;185(2):120-2**)

135. CAULIFLOWER FOR STRONGER NAILS

If you suffer from frail or brittle nails, biotin (one of the B vitamins) can thicken your fingernails to help prevent them from splitting and cracking. [Cauliflower is a rich source of biotin, as are legumes such as lentils. You are better off getting your B nutrients from food, rather than in any isolated form (which can set your need for other B vitamins askew).

I sprout a tablespoon of lentils daily and add them to salads. Just a day or two of sprouting in a jar does the trick. Biotin is also produced by healthy intestinal bacteria, so regular consumption of good probiotics can be helpful, too.]

Source: *Cutis* 1993;51(4):303-305.

BRONCHITIS

Bronchitis is among the most common respiratory tract infections. It is also among the top seven common conditions that benefit from alternative therapies. (The others are: stress/anxiety, headaches/migraine, back pain, insomnia, cardiovascular problems, and musculo-skeletal problems.)

Good thing we have alternatives, because antibiotics, as indicated in our hint below, offer little, if any, relief for bronchitis. (*Complementary Therapeutic Medicine* 2001;9(3):178-85) Plans to combat antibiotic resistance were recently proposed by the World Health Organization, but the experts predict that the problem is here to stay. (*Medical Journal of Australia* 2002;177(6):325-9)

Bronchitis is usually viral-initiated, so, unlike bacteria, *a virus cannot be killed with antibiotics.* A virus can't reproduce without entering a host cell as a parasite. Viruses alter the DNA of a cell in order to produce more viruses, subverting the cell's normal function. Not very good for anyone's overall health!

Because making treatment decisions often includes diagnostic uncertainty, meeting insurance expectations, and concern in case of litigation, the physician tends to err on the side of prescribing antibiotics even if the chance of bacterial infection is low. Nor does antibiotic use for viral respiratory infection minimize or prevent the development of secondary bacterial infections. (*Journal of the American Medical Association* 1998;279:944; *Clinical Infectious Disease* 1998;27(S):S5)

Scattered throughout the hints are many suggestions for keeping your immune system at optimum performance so that your body has the armamentarium to fight ailments such as respiratory infection.

136. BRONCHITIS NOT HELPED BY ANTIBIOTICS

Most adults with acute bronchitis who consult their general practitioner will receive antibiotics, but for many, antibiotics will do *nothing* to change the natural course of this disease. Doctors should be sharing with their patients the current uncertainty about the benefits of antibiotics, and the extensive risks under many conditions. Overuse of antibiotics encourages antibiotic resistance and is often a waste of money. Antibiotic therapy must be limited to syndromes in which bacterial infection is the predominant cause and should attempt maximal reduction in bacterial load. It's important to emphasize the difference between bacterial and nonbacterial infections.

Sources: *British Medical Journal* 2002;324:91; *Archives of Internal Medicine*, 2002;162:41-47; *Journal of Antimicrobial Chemotherapy* 2002;49(1):31-40.

WANT TO KNOW MORE?
[The use of antibiotics can decimate your body's stores of health-promoting bacteria normally living in your digestive tract. Replacement with probiotics containing friendly bacteria such as *Lactobacillus acidophilus* is therefore essential once the antibiotics are finished.]

BURNS

Few injuries are more traumatic to the victim than a burn. Scientists are still sorting out the biochemical and cellular pathways that result in the production of scar tissue. We do know that there is a disruption of normal healing in the presence of a burn, and a very significant impact on oxidative stress. (*Journal of Surgical Research* **1998;75(1):74-80**)

There appears to be a wide variation in the basic approach to the first-aid and pre-hospital care of burn patients. (*Burns* **2002;28(2):135-42**)

137. HELPFUL TIPS FOR BURNS

Do NOT apply butter. A greasy substance traps the heat and can retard the natural healing process.

Just in case – it's a good idea to know about emergency treatments for burns:

- Place the inside of banana peel or avocado peel on the wound. These oils and special nutrients found close to the skins of bananas and avocados have amazing healing properties. Raw potatoes, too, can be helpful.

- Vitamin C in large amounts (10,000 mgs) supports the immune system to ward off infection for anyone with second- or third-degree burns. It also helps the body to cope with toxic effects of damaged tissues.

- If the wound is not open, breaking open a vitamin E capsule onto the burn improves healing and reduces scarring.

- Silica can also promote skin healing. [I keep a bottle of liquid silica in my kitchen.]

- Aloe vera gel can soothe intense pain from the heat of burns, so that's in my kitchen, too. It's a good idea to have the actual aloe vera plant on hand, as well. (The gel in the leaves is effective when the plant is three years old or older.)

- Tea tree oil can be used when the wound is partially healed and dry.

- A poultice of green tea has antiseptic properties and can help to prevent skin-cell damage.

Sources: Wisdom of the ages and *Encyclopedia of Natural Healing* (Burnaby, BC, Canada: Alive Books, 1998), 541-544.

138. ANTIOXIDANTS HASTEN BURN REPAIR

Treatment with alpha tocopherol immediately after thermal skin injury prevents vitamin E reduction and membrane damage. There is strong evidence that alpha-tocopherol and glutathione deficiencies contribute in part to the changes in red blood cells caused by a burn. The deficiencies of these two substances potentiate the susceptibility of red blood cells to oxidative membrane injury.

There is a marked, long-lasting oxidant/antioxidant imbalance in burned patients, in accordance with the severity of the injury, which is also reflected as systemic oxidant stress. The oxidative stress may contribute to secondary tissue damage and impaired immune function.

In very serious cases, antioxidants given post-burn can help to restore antioxidant defenses and prevent death, indicating that oxidants are likely the cause of mortality.

Source: *Acta Physiologica et Pharmacologica Bulgarica* **1988;23(2):55-9,** *Burn Care Rehabilitation* **1997;18(3):187-92;** *Free Radical Research* **2000;33(2):139-46.**

139. DIETARY L-ARGININE SPEEDS HEALING

Oral dietary L-arginine supplementation can shorten the time for burn-damaged epithelial tissue to heal and help the collagen repair process to take place. [This makes sense because L-arginine is an amino acid that controls a wide range of growth, healing, and immune functions. It can also stimulate the production of growth hormone.]

Source: *Chinese Medical Journal* **1999;112(9):828-31.**

140. COOL WATER, NOT ICE, FOR BURNS

Although applying an ice cube immediately after a burn may do more harm than good, running the burned area under cool water can be helpful. Many studies show the benefits of treating burns by the immediate application of cool water. Early cooling prevents a significant percentage of superficial burns from progressing to deep burns. It also reduces the risk of other consequences.

Running serious burns under cool water should be considered at least as important as subsequent medical and surgical treatment.

Source: *Burns* **2002;28(2):173-6.**

CANCER (GENERAL)

Although some experts believe that dietary modifications may prevent up to 32 percent of all cancer deaths, the range varies from as low as 10 percent to as high as 70 percent. What are the food recommendations for people to eat to avoid cancer? Must we make drastic lifestyle changes? Unfortunately, the study of nutrition and cancer is less developed than that of nutrition and cardiovascular disease. But there are answers, and we do know that the role of nutrition may vary with the type of cancer involved. (*American Journal of Clinical Nutrition* 2002;76(4): 701)

While the scientists are making up their minds, let's never forget that what you put in your mouth every day of your life affects the length and quality of your entire life.

IN THIS SECTION:
- CAUSES & PRECURSORS
- DIETARY TACTICS
- NATURAL REMEDIES & SUPPLEMENTS
- REDUCING RISK

CANCER: CAUSES & PRECURSORS

141. NO GRAVY, THANKS...

Go easy on the gravy during meals, as it contains dangerous levels of cancer-causing substances.

Gravy made from meat drippings contains substantial amounts of carcinogenic chemicals. Cooking muscle meats (beef, pork, fowl, and fish) at high temperatures creates chemicals that are not present in uncooked meats. In fact, at least *17* different chemicals resulting from the cooking of muscle meats may pose human cancer risk.

Those who eat beef four or more times a week have more than twice the risk of developing stomach cancer, partly because these methods use high temperatures. An increased risk of colorectal, pancreatic, and breast cancer is associated with frequent intakes of well-done, fried, broiled, or barbecued meats.

Oven roasting and baking are done at lower temperatures, and stewing, boiling, steaming, or poaching creates negligible amounts of these chemicals. Regardless of cooking method, foods cooked a long time ("well-done" instead of "medium") will also form slightly more of the chemicals.

Milk, eggs, tofu, and organ meats such as liver have very little or none of these carcinogenic chemicals, either naturally or when cooked.

Sources: *Advances in Experimental Medical Biology* **1995;369:211-220**; *Japanese Journal of Cancer Research* **1990;81:10-14**; *Journal of Agricultural Food Chemistry* **1983;31:18-21**; *Food Chemical Toxicology* **1994;32(6):505-515**; *Cancer Research* **1995;55(20):4516-4519**; *Cancer* **1994;74:1070**.

142. MELATONIN, LIFESPAN & TUMORS

A warning about melatonin: It may promote the growth of tumors. From early on until their natural deaths, test animals were given melatonin with their drinking water (20 mg/l) for five consecutive days every month. Melatonin increased the body weight of the older animals; it did not influence physical strength or the presence of fatigue; it decreased locomotor activity and body temperature. The good news is that it inhibited free radical processes in the blood, brain, and liver; it slowed down age-related hormone changes; and it actually increased lifespan. The bad news is that the melatonin also increased spontaneous tumor incidence!

Source: *Journal of Gerontology & Biological Science Medicine* **2001;56(7):B311-323.**

WANT TO KNOW MORE?
[The use of melatonin may also exacerbate asthma symptoms. See Hint #123 in the *Asthma* section for more information.]

143. RISK FROM MOTHBALLS & DEODORIZERS

Naphthalene, the chemical that gives mothballs and public restroom deodorizers their distinctive aroma, causes cancer in test animals – and humans run the same risk. Test animals that breathed naphthalene fumes developed cancer at a rate high enough to worry scientists at the National Toxicology Program. The test animals were exposed by inhalation, just as most people are, in doses comparable to some human consumer and workplace exposures.

Chemicals that cause tumors or other diseases in test animals are often eventually found to cause similar if not identical problems in humans. German workers exposed to naphthalene developed larynx, gastric, nasal, and colon cancers.

Source: US Govt. Researchers, National Institute of Environmental Health Sciences,

WANT TO KNOW MORE?
Chemicals that have been restricted include carbon tetrachloride (once used in home cleaning fluids), benzene (an ingredient in gasoline) and phenolphthalein (once an active ingredient in most over-the-counter laxatives).

The National Toxicology Program Report for January 2003 "Report on Carcinogens" (US Govt. Researchers, National Institute of Environmental Health Sciences) includes sun lamps and tanning beds, wood dust created in cutting and shaping wood, and nickel compounds among the 228 items in their list of carcinogenic substances.

144. HIGH IRON STORES & CANCER RISK

Beware excessive iron intake, which can lead to elevated iron stores, putting you at risk for cancer. High iron intake from more than 21 servings of fruit juice a week, or more than four servings of red meat a week, or more than 30 milligrams of supplemental iron daily, can elevate your body's iron stores. And even *moderately* elevated iron stores may increase your risk of cancer (as well as diabetes and heart disease).

Fruit and fruit juices are rich dietary sources of organic acids such as vitamin C, citric, malic, and tartaric acids, and the combined effects of vitamin C and these other organic acids may enhance iron bioavailability [meaning the degree to which iron can be used by the body].

Although red meat increases the risk, poultry and seafood do not.

Source: *American Journal of Clinical Nutrition* 2002;76(6):1375-1384.

WANT TO KNOW MORE?
Your body has a considerable capacity to store iron. Among older people especially, intakes of highly bioavailable iron promote high iron stores, whereas foods containing phytate (whole grains) decrease these stores. (Phytate and calcium, as found in flour used in sweet baked products, inhibit iron absorption.)

145. CREATINE COULD LEAD TO CANCER

If you use or know an athlete using creatine (popular for increasing muscle bulk), be warned: It is considered a potential carcinogenic risk. Creatine is sold over the counter in many countries, and is used by many leading athletes. It is not banned by the International Olympic Committee, and is often described as a "legal steroid."

But evidence now associates creatine use with digestive, muscular, and cardiovascular problems, and it is banned in France.

Source: The French Agency of Medical Security for Food, a regulatory agency.

146. AIR OUT YOUR DRY-CLEANED CLOTHES

Because clothes that are dry-cleaned may emit carcinogenic fumes from the substances used in the cleaning process, remove the plastic bags immediately, and let garments air in front of an open window for a few hours before placing in closets.
There is growing evidence that solvents used in the dry-cleaning industry are carcinogenic. Dry-cleaning workers have an excess mortality from several types of cancer.

Perchloroethylene (PCE), used in dry cleaning, is a known animal carcinogen and probable human carcinogen. A petroleum-based dry-cleaning solvent can also increase risk. Obviously, those who work in dry-cleaning establishments are at greater risk, but why not be cautious and air out your dry-cleaned clothes before storing or wearing!

Source: *American Journal of Industrial Medicine* 2001;39:121-132.

147. FEAR OF FRYING

Steer clear of carbohydrate-rich fried foods such as potato chips and french fries to protect yourself from a dangerous carcinogen. Researchers at Stockholm University (in cooperation with the government food safety agency) have discovered that this substance (called *acrylamide*, a well-known carcinogen) is formed in very high concentrations when carbohydrate-rich foods such as rice, biscuits and bread, potatoes, and cold cereals (eaten daily by millions of people around the world) are fried or baked, but not boiled. Acrylamide is known to cause damage to the human nervous system, and the International Agency for Research on Cancer says it has been found to induce gene mutations and cause stomach tumors in animals. There is also an indication that acrylamide is mutagenic to sperm at fairly reasonable exposure levels, affecting fertility. The amount increases in heated food.

An ordinary bag of potato chips may contain up to 500 times more acrylamide than the maximum concentration allowed in drinking water by the World Health Organization! French fries sold at some fast food restaurants contain 100 times the allowable concentration.

These alarming findings have caught the attention of both the FDA and the WHO, and both agencies are now warning people worldwide to minimize their intake of these foods. Some food safety advocacy groups have even started planning lawsuits against fast-food companies, arguing that the companies should be placing cancer-warning labels on their products.

Studies have also been done at the Institute for Biomedical and Pharmaceutical Research in Nuremberg, Germany, concluding that pregnant and nursing mothers should sharply limit or even cease consumption of french fries and potato chips. Blood-brain barriers in fetuses and newborn infants are not fully developed, and are particularly susceptible to this toxin.

Sources: *Reuter's Medical Report* Jan 2003, May 2002; *Journal of the American Medical Association* 2002;288(17):2105-2106; *Nature* 2002;419:448-450.

WANT TO KNOW MORE?
Acrylamide can be created when foods are heated above 120° C (245° F), whether oven-cooked or fried, because of a reaction between amino acids (such as the asparagine found in potatoes and cereals) and natural sugars in the foods. Acrylamide levels can vary within a particular food due to heating levels, time spent cooking, and other factors such as water and starch content. Acrylamides are also used to produce plastics and dyes, as well as to purify drinking water, so there are non-food sources of this substance as well.

CANCER: DIETARY TACTICS

148. CRUCIFEROUS BEST AGAINST CANCER

Increasing your intake of cruciferous vegetables may *greatly* reduce your risk of developing many kinds of cancers. Cruciferous vegetables [such as cabbage, cauliflower, Brussels sprouts, broccoli, kale, turnip greens, and spinach] may be more effective than total fruit and vegetable consumption in reducing cancer risk at several organ sites, and three or more servings of cruciferous vegetables a week slashes prostate cancer risk almost in half! Evidence supports the view that substances in these vegetables are highly effective in reducing susceptibility to carcinogens. In addition to detoxifying, cruciferous vegetables exercise long-lasting antioxidant protection.

Sources: *Journal of Nutrition* 2001;131:3027S-3033S; *Journal of the National Cancer Institute* 2000;92:61-68.

149. AN APPLE A DAY...KEEPS *CANCER* AWAY

Turns out Grandma was right. An apple a day really *does* keep the doctor away. Phenolic acids and flavonoids, natural antioxidants found in fresh apples, seem to combine to inhibit the proliferation of tumor cells. Researchers extracted material from fresh Red Delicious apples to treat a colon-cancer cell line. They found that tumor proliferation was inhibited 57 percent with an extract containing apple skin and 40 percent by extract not containing skin. [Didn't I always tell you to eat the skin?]

About one serving (100 grams) of fresh apple provides antioxidant activity equal to that of 1,500 mg of vitamin C. But because the amount of vitamin C in an apple is only about 5.7 mg, almost all the antioxidant activity must come from a synergistic effect between the *many* phytochemicals found in the fruit. (Apples contain almost 100 known phytochemicals.)

Source: *Nature* 2000;405:902-904.

150. ANTIOXIDANTS ARE *ANTI*-CANCER

It's simple: The higher your antioxidant intake, the lower your risk of developing cancer (even in smokers and those infected with *H. pylori*). In people exposed to abnormal toxic loads, such as smokers and H pylori-infected individuals (the bacterium implicated in ulcers), the increased need for antioxidants is especially important. Antioxidants can significantly reduce the risk of cancer for both of these conditions [and many others].

Different plant foods have different antioxidant potential. [Some of the best sources of antioxidants are leafy greens, cruciferous veggies such as broccoli and cabbage, garlic, and the vitamins A, E, and C.]

Source: *Gastroenterology* **2002:123:985-991.**

WANT TO KNOW MORE?
People who never smoke and who have the highest antioxidant intake have the lowest cancer risk.

151. DON'T SKIP BREAKFAST!

Be sure to have a light breakfast in the mornings, which can help reduce your risk of developing cancer. Consumption of a light breakfast – defined as anything other than a traditional fry-up – seems to have a protective effect on cancer development, while consumption of a cooked breakfast does not (and NO breakfast is the worst offender!). Women who eat a traditional cooked breakfast are *twice as likely* as light-breakfast eaters to develop cancer, but women who skip breakfast altogether have the highest risk.

Also, women who eat a traditional cooked breakfast or consume large quantities of hot tea appear to have an increased risk of developing esophageal cancer specifically. (The quantity and temperature of tea consumed are directly related to this risk.)

Consumption of salads, in addition to light breakfasts, is also linked to reduced cancer risk.

Source: *British Journal of Cancer* **2001;85(11):1667-70.**

WANT TO KNOW MORE?
If you are uncertain about anti-cancer kitchen strategy, there are places you can go where you can learn the very best dietary measures. Spas and detoxification facilities abound, but I have a favorite. It is affordable (by comparison), and has a long history of incredible teaching and healing results.

It is the *Optimum Health Institute* (OHI) of Lemon Grove, a suburb of San Diego in California. Aside from the fact that OHI attracts exciting people from all over the world, just being there offers an opportunity to see *first hand* how nature uses its magic to turn sickness around when given the right nutrients with which to work.

There is no stove top or oven in the OHI kitchen. The diet is comprised of sprouts and very specific juiced vegetables and fruits, and includes sun-dried natural goodies, some of which are churned into special, delicious spreads. In addition tobeing fed this raw-foods, anti-disease diet (which, by the way, also includes pro- and prebiotics), classes by highly trained professionals are available all day long.

Most everyone leaves OHI looking radiant – having left pot bellies, pale complexions, fatigue, and toxic cellular molecules behind. To follow this quintessential anti-cancer diet at home is no easy task, but a week or two at OHI gives you the best head start..

CANCER: NATURAL REMEDIES & SUPPLEMENTS

152. E PROTECTS AGAINST RADIATION DAMAGE

If you are undergoing radiation therapy for cancer, vitamin E can help to protect you. Although radiation therapy generates large numbers of free radicals to destroy cancer cells, the antioxidant vitamin E protects normal cells from destruction, while not affecting the destruction of the cancer cells.

[Some dietary sources of vitamin E are butter, egg yolks, and liver.

Tocotrienols, a superior form of vitamin E, are natural compounds found in various foods and oils such as palm oil, rice bran oil, wheat germ, barley, saw palmetto, and certain types of nuts and grains.] Natural vitamin E may also help to interrupt or stop the growth of cervical, ovarian, breast, and lung cancer cells.

Source: *Nutrition & Cancer* **1999;35:189-194.**

153. CURCUMIN AGAINST CANCER

A spice found in curry powder may possess properties that are protective against cancer. Curcumin, the yellow pigment in the common curry spice turmeric, has been shown to have anti-carcinogenic properties and to suppress tumor growth in test animals. When combined with carotenoids, it's an even more powerful cancer preventive.

Curcumin acts as a free-radical scavenger, which means that this phytochemical helps prevent oxidative damage-related diseases. Curcumin can block colon tumor and skin tumor promotion, and also has anti-inflammatory properties.

When curcumin is added to the diet, it achieves drug levels in the colon and liver sufficient to explain its pharmacological activities. The good news is that this mode of administration may be preferable for the prevention of colon cancer.

Sources: *Clinical Cancer Research* **2001;7(5):1452-1458;** *Proceedings of the National Science Council of the Republic of China* **2001;25(2):59-66.**

WANT TO KNOW MORE?
[Curcumin may also possess properties that are protective against Alzheimer's disease. See Hint #76 for more information.]

154. GINSENG IS ANTI-CARCINOGENIC

Supplementing with ginseng can help reduce your risk of developing a wide variety of cancers. Ginseng has anti-carcinogenic effects on human cancers, with decreasing risk as the frequency and duration of ginseng intake increases. Cancers of the lip, oral cavity, pharynx, esophagus, stomach, colorectum, liver, pancreas, larynx, lung, and ovary are all significantly reduced with ginseng.

As for the type of ginseng, cancer risk decreases *significantly* among those taking fresh ginseng extract, either alone or together with other ginseng preparations. [My favorite ginseng is Siberian ginseng, which, in addition to exhibiting anti-cancer properties, can also lower cholesterol, moderate insulin levels, reduce pain, and increase energy].

Source: *Journal of Korean Medical Science* 2001;Suppl:S19-S27.

155. GLUTAMINE, THE TUMOR KILLER

Dietary supplementation of the amino acid glutamine can improve immune function and reduce the growth of tumors. The precise way in which oral supplemental glutamine suppresses tumor growth remains unclear, but it may be related to a faster immune response or a better natural cytotoxic [cell-killing] activity directed at the tumors. Although glutamine concentrations in plasma are not increased with supplementation, the nutrients necessary for glutamine production are.

[Glutamine is classified as a nonessential amino acid, which means you don't have to eat it – your body already makes it. However, research indicates that glutamine becomes essential when the demand for it exceeds the amount available. Raw spinach and parsley are good dietary sources.]

Source: *The Journal of Nutrition* 1997;127(1):158-166.

156. (GREEN) TEATIME INCREASES LIFETIME

Drinking green tea regularly may significantly reduce your risk of developing many kinds of cancers. Green tea is now accepted as a cancer preventive. Studies show that plant extracts found in green tea (specifically, catechins and polyphenols) have powerful anti-cancer properties. These substances can halt the progression of and even destroy cancer cells. They can also inhibit harmful pro-oxidation and other processes that undermine your health.

There is an apparent delay of cancer onset/death associated with increased consumption of green tea, specifically in ages before 79. In addition to prevention of cancer, green tea has an anti-metastic activity, helping to prevent cancer from spreading.

[Do be aware that green tea does contain a small amount of caffeine, unlike most herbal teas.]

Source: *Journal of Molecular Medicine* **2000;78(6):333-336;** *Aging Research Review* **2003;2(1):1-10;** *Laboratory Investigations* **2002;82(12):1685-93.**

WANT TO KNOW MORE?
[Green tea has also been shown to reduce inflammation in inflammatory arthritis. See **Hint #86** for more information.]

157. MUSHROOMS AS MEDICINE

Mushrooms used in traditional Asian medicines can reduce the side effects of chemotherapy and radiotherapy, and significantly improve the quality of life for patients with advanced cancers. Certain mushroom extracts can prolong survival of cancer patients, and mushroom-derived substances have shown anti-tumor activities. Lentinan, an extract from shiitake mushrooms, seems to activate the immune system, maintaining its anti-tumor property even with oral administration. A compound from maitake mushrooms has been shown to kill cancer cells. The lentinan maintains its anti-tumor property with oral administration.

Sources: London, *Cancer Research UK, Reuter's Medical Report* **Aug 2002;** *Journal of Alternative & Complementary Medicine* **2002;8(5):581-9.**

WANT TO KNOW MORE?
[For more information on the power of mushroom extracts, see my latest book, *Everything I Know About Nutrition I Learned from Barley*, in which I cite the studies showing how mushroom extracts can both prevent cancer and help to alleviate the side effects of the disease.]

There are 140,000 mushrooms on Earth, yet only about 10 percent are known, with 14,000 named species. Mushrooms comprise a vast and yet largely untapped source of powerful new nutraceutical products. They represent an unlimited source of polysaccharides with antitumor and immunostimulating properties. (*Applied Microbiology & Biotechnology* **2002;60(3):258-74.**

158. SELENIUM AGAINST CANCER

Selenium, an essential trace mineral, has protective properties against several types of cancers. In test animals, selenium can prevent breast and colon cancers, and the use of this mineral may help prevent prostate and lung cancer in humans.

The cancer-preventive effects of selenium seem to result from its ability to activate a certain protein that suppresses tumors. Human lung cancer cells treated with the major component of dietary selenium appear to activate this protein. By enhancing this activity, cells are better equipped to repair DNA damage and prevent cancer from progressing.

Other antioxidants may also activate additional tumor suppressors, so there could be an additive anti-cancer effect by consuming several different types of minerals.

[The amount of selenium in our food varies with levels in the soil. Brewer's yeast, liver, butter, and most fish contain adequate amounts. Whole grains and barley are also good sources.]

Source: *Proceedings of the National Academy of Science* **Sep 2002; early edition.**

159. CHILI PEPPERS REDUCE TUMORS

Capsaicin, the pungent constituent of hot chili peppers, helps to kill tumor cells.
Hot peppers are a good source of dietary antioxidants, including widespread compounds such as flavonoids, phenolic acids, carotenoids, vitamin A, ascorbic acid, and tocopherols, as well as specific constituents such as the pungent *capsaicinoids* (capsaicin), which protect linoleic acid against free-radical damage.

Capsaicin also selectively induces death in malignant cancer cells without affecting normal cells.

Sources: *International Journal of Cancer* **2003;103(4):475-482;** *Journal of the National Cancer Institute* **2002;94:1263-1265,1281-1292;** *Journal of Agriculture & Food Chemistry* **2002;50(25): 7396-7401.**

WANT TO KNOW MORE?
[Topical application of capsaicin is also helpful in relieving itchy skin (pruritis). See Hint #360 in the *Dermatological Problems* section for more information.]

160. OMEGA-3s FOR CANCER PATIENTS

Supplementing with omega-3 fatty acids may be very beneficial for those with cancer.
The consumption of omega-3 fatty acids helps to slow the growth of cancer in test animals, increase the efficacy of chemotherapy, as well as reduce the side effects of chemotherapy – and even the cancer itself.

The multiple benefits of omega-3 fatty acids include a decrease in both the proliferation of cancer cells and tumor promotion. After appropriate cancer therapy, consumption of omega-3 fatty acids might slow or stop the growth of metastatic cancer cells, increase longevity of cancer patients, and improve their quality of life.

[Omega-3 fatty acids can be found in fatty fish and fish oil, as well as in flaxseed and walnuts.]

Source: *Journal of Nutrition* **2002;132:3508S-3512S.**

161. AGED GARLIC EXTRACT FIGHTS CANCER

Significant increases in natural killer cell and killer cell activities are observed in test animals given aged garlic extract. Aged garlic has a variety of pharmacologic effects, including the inhibition of tumor cell growth and the enhancement of detoxification.

Suppression of tumor-cell growth may be one of the most important mechanisms in the prevention of cancer. Maintenance of balanced immune stimulation can significantly reduce the risk of cancer.

Long-term extraction of garlic (up to 20 months) ages the extract, creating unusual antioxidant properties. The aged garlic exerts its effect by enhancing the antioxidant enzymes – the ones that are so crucial in helping us get rid of the harmful free radicals.

Heating may inactivate a substance in garlic that is responsible for its anti-cancer properties.

Sources: *Journal of Nutrition* **2001;131:1041S-1045S,1054-1057,1075S-1079S.**

162. AGED GARLIC REDUCES CHEMO DAMAGE

Aged garlic supplementation has been shown to protect the small intestine of test animals from the anti-tumor drug-induced damage. Many anti-tumor drugs induce intestinal damage. This is a serious side effect of cancer chemotherapy. A study examined whether or not aged garlic extract protects against damage from these anti-tumor drugs. Interestingly, the absorption of the toxic chemotherapy drug administered to test animals was depressed in those animals fed a diet containing the aged garlic. The aged garlic is also effective against the side effects of UV radiation.

Source: *Journal of Nutrition* **2001;131:1071S-1074S.**

WANT TO KNOW MORE?
Just as specific foods and supplemental nutrients are beneficial for all forms of cancer, there are foods and supplemental nutrients that are helpful for all forms of degenerative diseases. But there are also very specific nutrients that may be helpful for a particular disease state.

In addition, there are specific foods and environmental factors that will have adverse effects on various degenerative diseases. For example, excessive iron intake, as indicated above, which can lead to elevated iron stores in your body, places you at risk for cancer, diabetes, and heart disease. (*American Journal of Clinical Nutrition* **2002;76(6):1375-1384**) See Hint #144 for more information.

CANCER: REDUCING RISK

163. SUNLIGHT ACTUALLY *PREVENTS* CANCER

Contrary to what you may believe, staying OUT of the sun may increase your risk of developing cancer. Insufficient exposure to sunlight may be an important risk factor for cancer in Western Europe and North America, mainly because of insufficient levels of vitamin D in people who avoid the sun.

Years ago, the sun was especially effective in restoring a degenerated hip, before surgery was an effective option. The sun facilitates the construction of vitamin D in your skin, and your body can stockpile a supply of this nutrient over the summer to help you through a cold, dark winter.

Deaths from various cancers of the reproductive and digestive systems are about twice as high in New England as in the Southwest, despite a diet that varies little between these two regions. The same geographical trend affects black Americans, whose overall cancer rate is significantly higher. Darker skinned people require more sunlight to synthesize vitamin D.

There are 13 malignancies that show this inverse correlation (*high* sunlight = *low* cancer risk), mostly reproductive and digestive cancers. The strongest inverse correlation is with breast, colon, and ovarian cancer. Other cancers apparently affected by sunlight include tumors of the bladder, uterus, esophagus, rectum, and stomach.

Source: *Cancer* **2002;94:1867-1875.**

WANT TO KNOW MORE?
[Vitamin D is also essential for proper bone mineralization, and its deficiency is recognized as a risk factor for hip fracture. See the *Osteoporosis & Other Skeletal Problems* section for more information on this topic.

Adequate intake of vitamin D is unlikely to be achieved through dietary means. (*Medical Journal of Australia* **2002;177(3):149-52**) Vitamin D deficiency is a major unrecognized health problem. Ongoing deficiency may have dire effects on cancers of the colon, prostate, breast, and ovary. There needs to be a better appreciation of the importance of vitamin D for overall health and well-being, and for cancer prevention. (*Journal of Cell Biochemistry* **2003;88:296-307**)

Antioxidants are effective in minimizing ultraviolet damage to the skin. Consumption of such antioxidants (especially lycopene, beta-carotene, vitamin E, and vitamin C) help the skin to withstand ultraviolet rays. (*Free Radical Biology & Medicine* **2002;32:1293-1303**)

CANCER, BLADDER

IN THIS SECTION:
- CAUSES & PRECURSORS
- REDUCING RISK

BLADDER CANCER: CAUSES & PRECURSORS

164. DON'T DYE FOR YOUR HAIR

If you use permanent hair dye to color your hair, you may be putting yourself at risk of developing bladder cancer. Evidence supports a causal link between the use of hair dye and the risk of developing bladder cancer. This risk is affected by the frequency of use, duration of use, cumulative total times of use, as well as the speed in which the carcinogen involved is eliminated from the body. The shade of the dye also plays a role: dark brown and black dyes are worse than blonde. Although most shades are comprised of essentially the same chemicals, there are more of these chemicals in darker dyes.

Typically, the US Food and Drug Administration requires safety testing of all coloring agents used in cosmetics and food. However, hair dyes have historically been exempt from this requirement. [Natural, nonpermanent dyes are available in every hair color in health stores, and are much safer.]

Sources: *Reuter's Report*, Keck School of Medicine, University of Southern California, Jan 2001 (to be published in February issue of *International Journal of Cancer*); 93rd Annual Meeting of the American Association for Cancer Research, Apr 2002.

WANT TO KNOW MORE?

Women who use permanent hair dye at least once a month are twice as likely to develop bladder cancer than women who don't. And women who have regularly used hair dye for at least 15 years are *three times* as likely to develop it compared with nonusers. Hairstylists and barbers are 50 percent more likely to have bladder cancer than those who do not have this occupational exposure. Those who are exposed to hair dye for at least 10 years are *five times* more likely to develop this disease. [To encourage elimination of carcinogens from the body, fiber supplementation, dehydrated sprouted grass drinks, and the algae chlorella can all be very beneficial.]

165. SMOKING: A CONFIRMED RISK

Women who smoke significantly increase their risk for urinary bladder cancer. Compared with women who never smoke, the risk of developing bladder cancer among smokers is evident. Each 20-pack years increase in smoking is associated with an increased risk. The good news is that for women who stop smoking for more than 15 years, the risk is similar to that of nonsmokers.

Diabetes is also associated with bladder cancer risk. as are reduced physical activity and obesity. These results were concluded from data collected from 37,459 women over a period of years.

Source: *Cancer* 2002;95:2316-2323.

BLADDER CANCER: REDUCING RISK

166. VITAMIN E AGAINST BLADDER CANCER

People who take vitamin E regularly are less likely than those in the general population to suffer from bladder cancer. Researchers tracked nearly one million US adults over a period of 16 years, interviewing them about their diets. Those who had been taking vitamin E supplements for at least 10 years are less likely to die from bladder cancer, compared with adults who report shorter durations of use.

Just how vitamin E offers this protection is not known yet. We do know that vitamin E is a powerful antioxidant. One of its major functions is to neutralize the free radicals that damage DNA.

Vitamin E may also be helpful by preventing the formation of carcinogenic nitrosamines. Only effective immune systems offer this kind of protection. Nitrosamines are compounds formed from nitrites and nitrates found in foods. The transformation into carcinogenic nitrosamines takes place in your digestive tract.

Salt-cured meats like ham and bacon, smoked meats, hot dogs, and luncheon meats all contain these compounds.

Source: *American Journal of Epidemiology* 2002;156:1002-1010.

167. AGED GARLIC AGAINST BLADDER CANCER

Aged garlic extract is reported to inhibit the development of tumors in the bladder. Bladder cancer is one of the few human malignancies that responds so well to immunotherapy. But aged garlic extract is even more effective! There is no observed toxicity with aged garlic treatment for bladder cancer.

Source: *Journal of Nutrition* 2001;131:1067S=1070S.

CANCER, BREAST

IN THIS SECTION:
- BONE-DENSITY LINK
- CAUSES & PRECURSORS
- CHOOSING A DOCTOR
- DIETARY TACTICS
- HORMONE REPLACEMENT THERAPY CONNECTION
- MAMMOGRAMS
- NATURAL REMEDIES & SUPPLEMENTS
- REDUCING RISKS
- AFTER THE FACT

BREAST CANCER: BONE-DENSITY LINK

168. LOWER BONE DENSITY = LOW CANCER RISK

There appears to be a significant connection between bone-mineral density in women and the development of breast cancer, so think twice about taking drugs to increase your bone-mineral density. Women with *lower* amounts of bone mineral density appear to have a major health advantage because they are at the lowest risk for breast cancer, while *higher* bone density is associated with an increased risk. In fact, one study shows that senior women with high bone density are *twice* as likely to develop this disease.

Bone-mineral density can be an accurate marker of the body's response to estrogen, and it's no news that estrogens are linked to breast cancer. Women with higher bone density are thought to be physiologically more sensitive to the hormone's effects than women with lower bone density.

Another theory is that the higher incidents of breast cancer have to do with an accumulation of estrogen exposure, either from the environment or from hormone replacement therapy. [Another reason to think twice about HRT.]

Bone-mineral density remains one of the most powerful predictors of breast cancer.

Sources: *Journal of the National Cancer Institute* **2001;93:930-936;** *British Medical Journal* **Jun 2001;322:1566;** *Journal of Clinical Epidemiology* **2001;54:417-422.**

WANT TO KNOW MORE?
[The important lesson here is that it is not necessarily bone density that is as significant as the cause for its increase.

A weak bridge structure paved over with heavy concrete is not going to make the bridge stronger. Neither will bone density that is the result of drug reactions and/or abnormal metabolism. For more information on the link between bone-mineral density and breast cancer, see my book, *Hormone Replacement Therapy: Yes or No? How to Make an Informed Decision.*]

BREAST CANCER: CAUSES & PRECURSORS

169. BEEF ADDITIVE & BREAST CANCER RISK

Here's another good argument for eliminating beef from your diet: It most likely contains additives that may lead to breast cancer. Residual amounts of a growth promoter (Zeranol) used in beef cattle may have an estrogenic effect on the growth of normal and cancerous breast cells in humans. Serum, muscle extract, and adipose extract of cattle exposed to Zeranol *significantly* elevates DNA synthesis in both normal and cancerous cells. This compound acts like estrogen at the molecular level.

[This is one more compelling motive to stop eating beef, which is definitely not in your best health interest.]

Source: Department of Defense Breast Cancer Research Program meeting, reported in *Reuter's Medical News*, Atlanta, GA, Jun 2000.

WANT TO KNOW MORE?
The FDA-approved levels of Zeranol are 150 ppb (parts per billion) for meat, 300 ppb for liver, 450 ppb for kidney and 600 ppb for fat tissue.

170. THE DANGERS OF WELL-DONE MEAT

When eating red meat, avoid meat that is "very well done" – it contains a carcinogen that may lead to breast cancer. Mutagens formed in meats cooked at high temperatures have been demonstrated as mammary carcinogens in animals, and they increase the risk of breast cancer in humans. Women who consistently consume "very well done" hamburger, beefsteak, or bacon have a *significantly* higher risk of breast cancer than women who consume these meats cooked rare or medium well. And this risk is further elevated with increased intake of over-cooked meat.

So if you must eat red meat, pay attention to how it is cooked. The consumption of well-done meats (and exposures to the mutagens formed during high-temperature cooking) may play an important role in the development of breast cancer.

Source: *Journal of the National Cancer Institute* 1998;90(22):1724-1729.

WANT TO KNOW MORE?
Red meat cooked at high temperatures has also been associated with the increased risk of many other kinds of cancers, such as colorectal cancer and pancreatic cancer. See Hint #199 for more information on this topic.]

171. POWER LINES, MELATONIN & BREAST CANCER

If you live close to power lines AND you are also taking medications that affect melatonin levels, be warned: You may be at increased risk of developing breast cancer. The effect of magnetic field exposure is greater for women who use medications known to affect melatonin levels (such as beta-blockers, calcium-channel blockers, and psychotropic medications), thereby increasing the risk of breast cancer.

This issue has been highly controversial. Now, two research teams conclude that high magnetic fields in the vicinity of high power electric lines can have a deleterious effect in women taking the drugs cited above.

The level of melatonin was found to be similar in those who live near and those who live far away from power lines, except for women on the specific medications noted.

The decrease is higher during summer months, and the negative effects increase with age and with high body mass.

Source: *American Journal of Epidemiology* 2001;154:591-609.

172. NIGHT LIGHT, MELATONIN & BREAST CANCER

Avoiding night shifts and keeping your bedroom very dark at night may help to protect you from breast cancer. It has been found that women exposed to light at night are more likely to develop breast cancer than are women who are not exposed. Women who do not sleep at night (when melatonin levels are typically highest) also have an elevated risk. (Interrupted sleep accompanied by turning on a light does not increase this risk, but sleeping in a brighter bedroom does.)

An elevated breast cancer risk is also seen in women who work "graveyard" shifts, and the risk is directly related to the number of years and the numbers of hours per week worked. Women who have been on the job at least three night shifts per month, in addition to their usual day and evening shifts, have a moderately increased risk of breast cancer.

Light at night may be associated with an increased risk of this disease because electromagnetic fields released by light suppress the normal nocturnal production of melatonin, which could increase the release of estrogen by the ovaries. This factor would explain why industrialized societies have *five times* the risk of breast cancer.

Sources: *Journal of the National Cancer Institute* 2001;93:1513-1515,1557-1568; "Era of Hope," Department of Defense Breast Cancer Research Program meeting, Orlando, FL, Sep 2002.

WANT TO KNOW MORE?
Studies show slight increases of breast cancer risk for flight attendants and rotational shift nurses, but half the risk for blind women.

173. GO ORGANIC TO AVOID HIDDEN PCBs

High levels of PCBs, chemicals that linger in the food chain (particularly in fatty foods), have been linked to breast cancer, which is why it is advisable to buy organic foods whenever possible. Similar in structure to dioxin, these contaminants mimic hormones or alter hormone metabolism, thereby increasing the risk of breast cancer. Although banned in the US and Canada two decades ago, these chemicals are still present in our food chain.

Levels of specific PCBs (polychlorinated byphenols) are linked to a 60 to 80 percent greater risk of breast cancer. Women exposed to combinations of these toxins are *twice* as likely to have breast cancer.

[As explained in my well-researched book, *She's Gotta Have It!,* products containing PCBs include old fluorescent lighting fixtures and electrical appliances with PCB capacitors. They persist in our environment and enter fat stores of plants and animals, easily migrating into our food chain. PCBs keep piling up and are retained in our tissues, where they promote tumors and affect the nervous system.]

Sources: *American Journal of Epidemiology* **2002;155:629-635; B. Kamen,** *She's Gotta Have It!*

174. YOUNG SMOKERS HEADED FOR BREAST CANCER

If you know an adolescent girl who smokes, make sure she knows this alarming fact: Smoking while young may lead to breast cancer in adulthood. Women who start smoking in early adolescence appear to have a *significantly* increased risk of developing breast cancer compared with women who start smoking later in life.

Among premenopausal women, the risk for developing breast cancer is greatly increased in those who started smoking early (as well as in those who smoked 20 or more cigarettes a day and who have smoked for 20 years or more).

Breast cancer in very young women is a disease that may differ in its causes and progression compared with breast cancer that is diagnosed later on.

Source: *Lancet* **2002;360:1033-1034,1044-1049.**

WANT TO KNOW MORE?
[For many helpful tips on protecting yourself from the damage caused by smoking, as well as some great quitting strategies, see the *Smoking & Nicotine Addiction* section.]

175. DON'T DRINK TO BREAST CANCER!

Keep your consumption of alcohol to a minimum, as even one drink a day increases your chances of developing breast cancer. The results of 53 studies worldwide show that daily consumption of alcoholic beverages (equivalent to 10 grams a day) raises your chances of developing breast cancer. This analysis includes data on 150,000 women, and shows a clear link between alcohol and risk of this disease. The link may involve changes in estrogen levels.

[I wrote about this association more than 10 years ago in my book, *Hormone Replacement Therapy: Yes or No? How to Make an Informed Decision*. Every drink you take causes thiamine and folate loss, impaired B6 activation, and increased magnesium excretion. And if you are on hormone therapy, one or two glasses of wine causes a *threefold* increase in estrogen circulating in your blood, and the levels begin to rise within 10 minutes after drinking. This increased estrogen heightens the risk of breast cancer.]

Sources: *British Journal of Cancer* 2002;87:1234-1245; B. Kamen, *Hormone Replacement Therapy: Yes or No? How to Make an Informed Decision* (2002 ed).

WANT TO KNOW MORE?
Drugs used to treat psychotic illnesses and other conditions may also increase a woman's chance of getting breast cancer. Anti-psychotics can raise blood levels of prolactin, which has been shown to promote tumor growth in test animals. (*Archives of General Psychiatry* 2002;59:1147-1154)

Women who get breast cancer are more likely to have begun menstruating before age 11. (*Pediatrics* 2002;119:43)

In March 2002, the International Breast Cancer Intervention Study recommended that women should no longer be prescribed tamoxifen for the prevention of breast cancer. (Another statement included in my book on hormone therapy, written 10 years ago.)

Pressure on breasts does not cause breast cancer or make women more susceptible to it. Breast lumps grow very slowly and can take years to become noticeable. A knock to the breast could not be the cause.

BREAST CANCER: CHOOSING A DOCTOR
176. BREAST CANCER? FIND A FEMALE DOCTOR

If you have been diagnosed with early-stage breast cancer, it's advisable to see a female physician, as she is more likely than her male peers to recommend lumpectomy rather than mastectomy. Surgery is frequently performed when there is no indication for such radical treatment. It is shown that physicians recommend mastectomy to 45 percent of women who have no apparent clinical indication for this surgery. (This is especially true for older women patients.)

The most common reason cited by patients for choosing a mastectomy is fear of recurrence. To increase the use of lumpectomy, fear of recurrence needs to be addressed with improved education and counseling.

Source: *Archives of Surgery* **2001;136:185-191.**

BREAST CANCER: DIETARY TACTICS
177. GO VEGGIE TO REDUCE BREAST CANCER RISK

You can reduce your risk of developing breast cancer by adopting a vegetarian diet. Lifelong vegetarianism may provide a small reduction in the risk of breast cancer, but this is associated with an increased consumption of vegetables rather than the absence of meat in the diet.

When compared with lifelong meat-eaters, lifelong vegetarians have a lower risk of developing breast cancer, while women in the top 75 percent of meat consumption have higher odds of developing the disease.

There is also a "strong inverse trend" with increased vegetable and pulse (peas and beans) consumption, meaning the more of these foods consumed, the lower the risk.

While there is the possibility that abstaining from meat may also play a role, there is evidence that a lifelong diet rich in vegetables may be protective against this cancer.

Source: *International Journal of Cancer* **2002;99:238-244.**

178. THE POWER OF WHITE BUTTON MUSHROOMS

Protect yourself against breast cancer by consuming organic white button mushrooms, which contain a substance that is preventive against this disease. The white button mushroom (*Agaricus bisporus*) reduces an estrogen-converting enzyme (aromatase) that plays a large role in breast cancer development. Estrogen is a major factor in its development, but the production of estrogen by this enzyme can be inhibited with certain natural phytochemicals, including flavones and isoflavones.

These mushrooms suppress the activity of aromatase in a dose-dependent manner (meaning the more consumed, the greater the inhibition.) This action helps to reduce the proliferation of breast cancer cells.

[Caution: Commercial mushrooms are often heavily treated with pesticides because of the way they are grown. Be sure the mushrooms you consume are *organic*.]

Sources: *Journal of Nutrition* **2001;131(12):3288-3293;** *Recent Progress in Hormone Research* **2002;57:317-338;** *Toxicology Application in Pharmacology* **2002;179(1):1-12;** *Journal of Endocrinology* **2002;172(1):31-43.**

WANT TO KNOW MORE?
Pesticides can *stimulate* this negative aromatase activity, as can retinoic acids [acids derived from vitamin A, often used in the treatment of acne].

179. WHOLE SOY BETTER THAN SOY ISOFLAVONES

If you are a premenopausal woman, you can lower breast cancer risk by eating foods that contain soybean products (but not by consuming isolated soy isoflavones). Isoflavones are shown to be ineffective in deterring mammary tumor growth in test animals. In fact, research shows that isoflavone dietary supplements may actually be harmful and *promote* breast tumor growth. [This is in keeping with my belief that whole foods and whole-food supplements are far superior to their extracted and isolated constituents.]

These findings suggest that isoflavones themselves are not the soy component involved in suppressing mammary tumor growth. The anti-tumor activity of a soy mixture may result instead from the production of enzymes that eliminate free oxygen radicals.

Source: 91st Meeting of the American Association of Cancer Research, University of Illinois, Chicago, Apr 2000.

WANT TO KNOW MORE?
[Isoflavones are unique to soybeans, and have structures very similar to the body's natural estrogens.]

180. LNA-RICH FOODS AGAINST BREAST CANCER

Increase your consumption of foods rich in linolenic acid, such as flaxseed and fish, to lower your risk of breast cancer. Women with high levels of alpha-linolenic acid (LNA) in their adipose (fatty) breast tissue have a 60 percent lower risk of developing breast cancer than do women with low levels of this nutrient.

Linolenic acid is the most important essential fatty acid in humans. (Essential means you must eat it; your body doesn't make it.) This omega-3 fatty acid is the precursor of the protective oils now known to be in fish and flaxseed, and also in black currant seed, canola, and soybean oils.
Please note: High amounts of isolated linolenic acid can be inflammatory, especially if vitamins A and E are depleted. But when taken in food form, high amounts are NOT inflammatory.

[Because all seed oils get rancid quickly, it's a good idea to buy whole flaxseed at the health food store and grind a tablespoon to sprinkle over your salads. (A small, inexpensive coffee grinder works well.) And when you eat fish, don't forget to eat the skin – that's where those fatty acids hang out.]

Source: *European Journal of Cancer* **2000;36:335-340.**

WANT TO KNOW MORE?
Alpha-linolenic acid is the only fatty acid associated with reduced breast cancer risk.

181. DIET CHANGES & BREAST CANCER SURVIVAL

If you have been diagnosed with breast cancer, making simple changes to your diet might increase your chances of survival. Replacing red meat with poultry, dairy, and fish and increasing vegetable intake may increase survival odds of breast cancer patients, especially if the diet is high in protein.

Women with the highest intake of protein show a 35 percent lower risk for mortality. These findings are strongest in women without metastases [secondary growths of malignant tumors], although some benefit is also observed in women with metastatic cancer.

Source: *Clinician Reviews* **1999;9(11):45-56.**

BREAST CANCER: HRT CONNECTION

182. HORMONE REPLACEMENT & BREAST CANCER

If you are a woman undergoing estrogen replacement therapy (ERT), you are putting yourself at *serious* risk of developing breast cancer. Postmenopausal use of estrogen therapy, particularly when it includes progestin (the synthetic progesterone), significantly increases the risk that a woman will develop breast cancer by the age of 70.

In women who use unopposed postmenopausal estrogen from ages 50 to 60, the cumulative risk increases by 23 percent, compared with women who never use hormones. And the risk increases by *67 percent* in those who use estrogen plus progestin. And alcohol worsens the situation:

Alcohol use increases the cumulative risk by seven percent in women 18 and over who report one drink per day, compared with nondrinkers.

Source: *American Journal of Epidemiology* **2000;152:950-964.**

WANT TO KNOW MORE?
[There are safer and more natural alternatives to HRT/ERT out there. See the *Menopause & Hormone Replacement Therapy* section for many helpful hints.]

BREAST CANCER: MAMMOGRAMS
183.   NO SURVIVAL BENEFIT TO MAMMOGRAMS

If you are a woman over the age of 40, you should be aware that annual mammograms to detect breast cancer do little to reduce the risk of death from this disease. Recent US recommendations call for mammograms every one to two years for women, beginning at age 40. But for women in this age group, adding mammography to careful physical examinations does not reduce the mortality rate from breast cancer when compared with self-examination or physician examination alone.

Since the mid-1980s, more than 39,000 women have been assigned either to annual physical examination or to examination plus mammography. Although breast cancer detection does occur some two years earlier with mammography, tumors detected by mammography are more likely to be small and are less likely to be lymph node-positive.

Michael Baum, MD, from London's University College points out that many of these "cancer" lesions would not progress to an invasive type if left undiscovered, and that screening 1,000 women over a period of 10 years may be helpful for only one woman. The screening, however, leads to more aggressive treatment, with the number of mastectomies and tumorectomies increased by about 30 percent. An extensive review of half a million women failed to find a decrease in breast cancer mortality, or reductions in death from any other causes.

Sources: *Journal of the National Cancer Institute* 2000;92:1490-1499; *Lancet* 2001;358:1284-1285,1340-1342; *Annals of Internal Medicine* 2002;137(5):305-312,344-346,361-362,363-364.

WANT TO KNOW MORE?
Mammograms actually cause harm due to increased rates of mastectomy and lumpectomy. The US has the highest mastectomy rate in the world.

The ability to accurately interpret screening mammograms varies widely among radiologists. Younger, recently trained radiologists are more likely to make mistakes.

Agreement between radiologists interpreting the same set of mammograms is known to be low. Independent double reading has been implemented in 22 countries, but not in the US. (*Journal of the National Cancer Institute* 2002;94:1346-1347;1373-1380)

184. PHYSICIAN EXAM BETTER THAN MAMMOGRAM

Women, take note: Physicians and surgeons are much more effective in identifying breast lumps compared with detection by mammography, and ultrasound is the best noninvasive way of determining whether lumps are benign or malignant. General practitioners successfully identified lumps in 78 percent of cases, while breast surgeons were found to be slightly better with an 82 percent success rate. Mammography, in contrast, only proved sensitive in 63 percent of patients. However, in clinical examinations general practitioners were only able to determine if lumps were benign or malignant in two out of five cases. Breast surgeons had a 78 percent success rate. Ultrasound is very effective for this determination, and less invasive than mammography.

Source: 7th Nottingham International Breast Cancer Conference, London, England, Sep 2001.

WANT TO KNOW MORE?
A large, well-conducted randomized controlled trial from Shanghai shows conclusively that teaching women how to examine their breasts does not lead to a reduction in mortality due to breast cancer. However, women should become familiar with changes in their breasts at different times of the month and with age, looking and feeling for any variations from normal. (*Journal of the National Cancer Institute, Cancer Spectrum* **2002;94:1445-1457**)

185. HRT CAN LEAD TO MAMMOGRAM ERRORS

If you are a menopausal woman considering HRT, you should be aware that such therapy can produce false-positive mammogram results. An increase in breast density is common among women receiving continuous HRT, an unwanted side effect. This hampers mammographic diagnosis.

Source: *American Journal of Obstetrics & Gynecology* **2002;186(4):717-22;** *Surgery* **1997:122(4): 669-73.**

186. NO MAMMOGRAMS FOR OLDER WOMEN

If you are a woman over the age of 69, you should know that continuing routine mammography has little value. Continuing biennial mammography after age 69 may extend life by just three days. Continuing testing after 79 spares only an additional 1.4 deaths per 10,000 women screened and extends life expectancy by a mere 0.3 day. The miniscule gain and potential false-positive result should be important factors to consider when older women are deciding about screening.

Source: *Journal of the American Medical Association* **1999;282.**

WANT TO KNOW MORE?

[See my book, *Hormone Replacement Therapy: Yes or No? How to Make an Informed Decision*, for a good introduction to this topic. Also see the *Menopause & Hormone Replacement Therapy* section for many helpful hints on natural alternatives to HRT.]

Concern has been growing over the safety and effectiveness of the government-approved mammography screening centers in the US. Every year, more than 40 percent of our nation's 9,500 mammography clinics have been cited for violating one or more federal rules governing their operation. Many experts say that our federal government's standards are too low, resulting in poor quality mammograms. Our federal rules require that doctors read at least 960 mammograms every two years, while many experts think that 5,000, the number required in the United Kingdom and Canada, is necessary for proficiency. (***British Medical Journal 2002;3947-3955***)

The risk of a woman contracting breast cancer at some point during her life is now one in eight, against one in 22 just 50 years ago.

BREAST CANCER: NATURAL REMEDIES & SUPPLEMENTS

187. VITAMIN D AGAINST BREAST CANCER

Supplementation with vitamin D may reduce your risk of developing breast cancer. Vitamin D protects against breast cancer and, in some forms, may even be used to shrink existing tumors. According to the Cancer Research Campaign, a great deal of research into vitamin D and its effects on cancer has already been done, and some potential new treatments are based on this vitamin. [Unfortunately, very few foods contain vitamin D. Those that do include egg yolks, liver, fatty fish, and fish liver oils.]

Source: *British Journal of Cancer* **2001;85:171-175.**

WANT TO KNOW MORE?

[Sunlight also helps to produce vitamin D in the body. See Hint #163 for information on how some daily sunlight can actually help to *reduce* the risk of some cancers.]

188. PALM TOCOTRIENOLS FIGHT BREAST CANCER

Consumption of palm tocotrienols [a form of vitamin E found in palm oil] has been shown to prevent and reduce the risk of breast cancer. The more cancerous the mammary cells, the more susceptible these cells are to annihilation by the palm tocotrienol complex. Tocopherols [the more commonly used form of vitamin E] do not have this effect.

It's the delta faction, found in significant quantities only in palm tocotrienols, that has this beneficial cancer-fighting effect. These palm tocotrienols not only curtail the proliferation of cancer cells, they have even been shown to destroy them.

Source: *Journal of the Proceedings for Experimental Biology & Medicine* 2000;224.

BREAST CANCER: REDUCING RISK

If you live in San Francisco or Nassau County, New York, pay special attention to the next section. Northern California in particular has seen breast cancer diagnoses skyrocket. At long last, the experts are beginning to look at environmental chemicals as one of the most likely causes of this sudden increase in risk. The increase has paralleled the proliferation of synthetic chemicals since World War II. Only seven percent of the estimated 85,000 synthetic chemicals registered for use in the US has been subjected to toxicological screening. **(Dr. Ana Soto, Tufts Medical School, reported in *Reuter's Medical Health*, Oct 2002)**

189. 7 HOURS A WEEK AGAINST BREAST CANCER

Exercising seven hours or more per week may diminish your risk of developing breast cancer by nearly 20 percent, compared with those who exercise less than one hour a week. Walking appears to be just as effective as more strenuous activities such as jogging, bicycling, and swimming.

These figures are the result of the Nurses' Health Study, which followed more than 121,000 women over a period of 16 years, and which was one of the largest studies to address the relationship between breast cancer and physical activity.

Source: *Clinician Reviews* 2000;10(1):35-48.

190. POSTMENOPAUSAL WOMEN: KEEP BUSY!

Postmenopausal women take note: Keeping busy, even if it's just around the house, can reduce your risk of developing breast cancer. Household and occupational activities (rather than recreational, such as sports or exercise classes) provide the most protection against breast cancer in postmenopausal women. Women of this age with the highest levels of activity are 30 percent less likely to be diagnosed with breast cancer than are those women with the lowest activity levels.

The benefit of such physical activity is greatest for those active postmenopausal women who also don't smoke or drink alcohol, or who have never given birth.

Source: *American Journal of Epidemiology* 2001;154:336-347.

WANT TO KNOW MORE?

Pregnancy can confer a lifelong twofold reduction in breast cancer risk. No, it's not because your child keeps you busy (the risk reducer suggested in the previous hint). It's because certain mammary cells develop during pregnancy that are theorized to have a role in risk reduction. This population of cells increases with multiple pregnancies, possibly augmenting the anti-cancer effect. **(42nd Annual American Society for Cell Biology, San Francisco, Dec 2002)**

191. FLAME-BROILED BREAST CANCER RISK

Barbecue lovers beware: Women who consume flame-broiled food more than twice a month have an increased risk of developing breast cancer compared with those who do not. These findings are based on a study done at Johns Hopkins Hospital, which also found that this risk is increased in women with a particular type of genetic predisposition, present in 45 percent of the population.

While flame-broiling food is a common cooking method, it is also a modifiable risk factor – just start avoiding it.

[And if you have had your share of barbecued meat, start protecting yourself with antioxidant-rich supplements such as young barley leaf powder. See Hint #1,047 for more details.]

Source: *Reuter's Medical News* **Apr 2000.**

192. DAILY SUNLIGHT PREVENTS BREAST CANCER

Daily exposure to sunlight, which elevates the body's supply of vitamin D, may be protective against the development of breast cancer. The sun's ultraviolet rays spur the production of vitamin D.

[Foods containing vitamin D are dairy products, eggs, and fish liver oils.] Breast cancer rates are higher in the Northeast than in the Southwest, a pattern suggesting the role of sun exposure and vitamin D.

[For decades I have been encouraging women to get out in the sun for about 20 minutes a day. These findings are not new, but unfortunately, the negative press about sunlight continues to influence us.]

There is also an association between breast cancer and diets heavy in animal fats. Diets marked by a higher fraction of animal products, such as meat, are associated with a higher risk of this disease. Diets rich in vegetables, fruits, grains and fish, on the other hand, are correlated with a decreased risk.

Source: *Cancer* **2002;94:272-281.**

193. REDUCED TISSUE = REDUCED CANCER RISK

Women who undergo breast reduction surgery can reduce their risk of developing breast cancer later on. Regardless of a woman's age at surgery, the more tissue removed during breast reduction, the less likely she is to be at risk for breast cancer later on. Among over-endowed women who have at least 800 grams of tissue removed, the risk of breast cancer is lower than among those who have less than 400 grams of tissue removed from either breast. The theory is that breast cancer risk declines with the reduction in the number of potential glandular structures that could become future sites of cancer development. These findings should reassure women concerned that such procedures could increase breast cancer risk or potentially obscure early detection.

Source: *Cancer* 2001;91:478-483.

194. BREAST IS BEST, FOR *MOM*, TOO!

Pooled data from 47 epidemiological studies found that the risk of breast cancer decreases by 4.3 percent for every 12 months in which women engage in breastfeeding. So the longer you breastfeed, the more you are protected against breast cancer. The short duration of breastfeeding typical of women in the US and other developed countries makes a major contribution to the high incidence of breast cancer in these countries. It works both ways: If you were breastfed, you have a reduction in risk, albeit a weak one.

Source: *Lancet* 2002:360:187-195, *British Journal of Cancer* 2001;85(11):1685-94.

195. BREAST CANCER, DAUGHTERS & STRESS

If you are a daughter of a woman with breast cancer, learning hope to cope with stress can help protect YOU from the disease. Coping techniques to reduce stress levels may help daughters of breast cancer sufferers decrease their own risk of breast cancer onset, as stress itself can increase the risk of cancer (as indicated by measurements of immune function and stress hormones).

Daughters of breast cancer patients may be under persistent increased emotional distress, causing adverse reactions. Emotional stress affects several immune functions and the secretion of stress hormones. Consequently, natural killer-resistant cells become impaired, increasing the risk of disease. So learning a few stress-coping exercises can be extremely helpful. [It should be noted that genetic predisposition to breast cancer is not as significant as lifestyle and other factors.]

Sources: *International Journal of Cancer* 2002;100:347-354; *Statistics in Medicine* 1997;16(1-3):133-151; *Breast Journal* 2001;7(1):34-39; *Journal of the National Cancer Institute* 2002;94(16):1238-1246.

BREAST CANCER: AFTER THE FACT

196. EXERCISE FOR BREAST CANCER SUFFERERS

If you are diagnosed with breast cancer, physical exercise can greatly improve your overall quality of life. Women with breast cancer who exercise demonstrate increased fitness, vigor, more positive thinking, decreased distress, enhanced well-being, and improved functioning.

Those treated for cancer often experience higher levels of emotional distress than the general population, but physical activity can increase life quality in many ways. (Moderate physical activity over the course of a lifetime can reduce a young woman's risk of developing breast cancer by 33 percent, and the risk of breast cancer after menopause by 26 percent.)

Sources: *Psychooncology* 2002;11(5):447-456; Department of Defense Breast Cancer Research Program, Orlando, FL, Sep 2002.

197. PROGESTERONE PROTECTION

Applying progesterone transdermally (directly to the skin) may help to curtail the proliferation of breast cancer cells. Accumulating evidence shows that progestins (synthetic hormones) produce unwanted and hazardous increases in the number of cells in breast tissue.

The use of small quantities of *progesterone* (the natural form) seems to be of great benefit when applied directly to the breast. This direct application increases breast cell progesterone levels, which in turn significantly *decreases* breast-cell proliferation. Transdermal progesterone seems to be well absorbed by the skin.

Sources: *Fertility & Sterility* 1995;63:785-791; *Breast Cancer Research & Treatment* 2001;65(2):163-169; *British Medical Journal* 1985;290:1617-1621.

WANT TO KNOW MORE?
[Not only does use of natural progesterone prevent breast cancer, it also plays a critical role in female sexuality. Women who have lost interest in sex often also have water retention, fibrocystic breasts, depression, wrinkled and dry skin, and irregular, heavy periods. Is it any coincidence that these are the symptoms of progesterone deficiency? (***Journal of Steroid Biochemistry & Molecular Biology*** 2000;74:30)

Progesterone can help reduce, prevent, or reverse the endometrial cancer caused by estrogens. Progesterone receptors are essential for effective sexual behavior. (***Proceedings of the National Academy of Sciences*** USA 2001;98(3):793-5)

Both exogenous (that is, from an outside source) estrogen and testosterone cause cell death in the thymus, but progesterone not only inhibits this reaction, it also influences T cell development and thereby immune responses. (*International Journal of Immunopharmacology* **2000;22(11):955-65**)

Progesterone participates in practically every physiological process (in both women *and* men). Biochemically, it provides the material out of which other steroid hormones, including *cortisone*, *testosterone*, *estrogen*, and even the salt-regulating hormone *aldosterone*) can be made as needed.

By helping to balance hormone ratios, progesterone may compensate for xenoestrogens (those outside environmental chemicals), helping to prevent the risks associated with estrogen overload. Because it is a master hormone, it gets shunted into other hormone pathways when the body's need for progesterone is fulfilled. That's one reason why progesterone therapy increases libido. (Excerpted from my book on female sexuality, *She's Gotta Have It!*) See the section on *Female Sexual Problems* for more information.

198. SURVIVING BREAST CANCER DIAGNOSIS

Breast cancer sufferers, take note: Diets high in vegetables and fruit (and related micronutrients), plus physical activity, are associated with a significant increased likelihood of survival after diagnosis. Obesity is an important negative factor in the disease prognosis. Evidence strongly supports an inverse relationship between relative body weight and survival in women who have been diagnosed with breast cancer (that is, the more excess weight, the lower the survival odds).

A marginal inverse result is associated with the intake of high-fiber foods such as vegetables and fruit. [The relationship may be higher if better high-fiber foods are consumed. Those of you who have read my book, *New Facts About Fiber*, know that most commonly consumed fruits and veggies are not high-fiber foods!]

Total fat intake is *significantly* inversely associated with survival or treatment failure – so watch your fat intake.

As stated earlier, physical exercise has a positive effect on the quality of life after a breast cancer diagnosis, including physical and functional well-being as well as psychological and emotional well-being.

Source: International Research Conference on Food, Nutrition & Cancer, given by the American Institute for Cancer Research and the World Cancer Research Fund International in Washington, DC, July 2002.

WANT TO KNOW MORE?
Breast cancer currently accounts for 31 percent of cancer cases and 15 percent of cancer deaths among women in this country. But the good news is that lifestyle can modify the results – *even after diagnosis*!

CANCER, COLON

IN THIS SECTION:
- CAUSES & PRECURSORS
- DIETARY TACTICS
- FIBER LINK
- NATURAL REMEDIES & SUPPLEMENTS

COLON CANCER: CAUSES & PRECURSORS

199. RED MEAT & COLORECTAL CANCER RISK

Reduce your consumption of red meat and increase your consumption of vegetables to help reduce your risk of developing colorectal cancer. The world's largest study of the role of diet in the development of cancer confirms a link between the consumption of red meat (mainly beef, but not poultry and fish) and colorectal cancer.

Other studies show that red meat consumption is significantly associated with an elevated risk of intestinal tumors.

In one large group of patients studied, the risk of cancer was increased by 40 percent in those with the highest levels of red meat consumption, while the risk was *reduced* by 40 percent in those with the highest levels of vegetable consumption.

These studies confirm what researchers have known for ten years [and what those involved in nutrition have known for many decades]: A diet high in fruits and vegetables can help prevent cancer.

Sources: International Agency for Research on Cancer, WHO, Sep 2000; *Journal of Nutrition* **2001;131:170S-175S.**

WANT TO KNOW MORE?
One important point: Although the association with cancer risk (beneficial for fruit and veggies; negative for meat) can be considered to be reasonably well established, no definitive explanation yet exists for the biological mechanisms involved, even though a large number of experimental studies have been carried out and many different possibilities have been tested. We can only guess at the causes.

Food frequency and nutrient intake patterns vary considerably between black and white South Africans. The lower prevalence of colon cancer in black South Africans compared with white South Africans appears to be the *absence* of "aggressive" factors in the diet (Westernized foods), rather than the *existence* of protective factors. (*American Journal of Gastroenterology* **1999;94:1373-1380**)

200. FRANKLY, HOT DOGS CAUSE COLON CANCER

Avoid both beef and pork hot dogs, as there is evidence that eating them can lead to colorectal cancer. Compounds found in the colon caused by the consumption of processed meat (such as hot dogs) are associated with colorectal cancer, and the problem is dose-related.

Fiber, in the form of vegetables or bran, does not reduce the level of these substances formed, although fiber can reduce transit time and increase fecal weight.

[Transit time refers to the time it takes for your food to go from ingestion to elimination. For information on how to measure your transit time, see Hint #1,082. The equivalent amount of white meat, however, has no effect on this harmful metabolic process.]

Source: *Journal of Nutrition* **2002;132:3522S-3529S.**

WANT TO KNOW MORE?
Red and processed meats are also a risk factor for childhood cancer and type 2 diabetes. The culprit substances found in beef and pork hot dogs are directly mutagenic [meaning they cause mutation]. See Hint #212 for the link between hot dogs and leukemia.

COLON CANCER: DIETARY TACTICS
201. A CLOVE A DAY KEEPS COLON CANCER AWAY

Eating a lot of garlic seems to be protective against colorectal cancer. Data combined from 22 different studies suggests that a high consumption of raw or cooked garlic decreases the risk of colorectal cancer by 30 percent. (The amount that needs to be consumed to achieve this effect is about six cloves a week.)

Of the many beneficial actions of garlic, inhibition of the growth of cancer is perhaps the most remarkable.

Source: *American Journal of Clinical Nutrition* **2000;72(4):1047-1052;** *Journal of Nutrition* **2001;131:1054S-1070S.**

WANT TO KNOW MORE?
[Garlic also may be protective against stomach cancer as well. See Hint #258 for more details.]

202. LUTEIN: AN ANTI-CANCER CAROTENOID

The more spinach, broccoli, lettuce, tomatoes, oranges, carrots, celery, and greens you consume, the less chance you have of developing colon cancer. The common denominator in all these foods is the carotenoid *lutein*. Taking lutein in supplemental form, however, is not as effective. Look at the list of foods again, and think about how many of them you actually consumed today. (You need more than one or two of them to get an effective level of lutein.)

Lutein appears to be more potent than other carotenoids in preventing colon cancer (although zeaxanthin also shows a protective effect). High intakes of the other carotenoids (alpha-carotene, beta-carotene, lycopene, and beta-cryptoxanthin) do not seem to greatly affect colon cancer risk. Lutein is more protective than other carotenoids at the membrane level, which may influence permeability of tissue to oxygen and other molecules (and which may account for its greater cancer-preventive effects). The protective effects of lutein and zeaxanthin also appear to be enhanced in younger people.

Source: *American Journal of Clinical Nutrition* **2000;71:575-582.**

WANT TO KNOW MORE?
[Lutein has other benefits, too. It acts as an antioxidant, protecting cells against the damaging effects of free radicals. There is also a lower risk of cataracts and macular degeneration seen in those with higher intakes of this nutrient. See the *Eye & Vision Problems* section for more information.]

203. PINTO BEANS INHIBIT COLON CANCER

Eating pinto beans may help to reduce your risk of developing colon cancer. Scientific studies validate that the low incidence of colon cancer in many Latin American countries is due to the high consumption of dry beans such as pinto beans.

Test animals fed a bean diet and exposed to cancer-causing toxins have significantly less colon cancer than do animals fed a casein diet and exposed to the same toxins, indicating that pinto beans contain anti-carcinogenic compounds capable of inhibiting induced colon cancer. But it still remains unclear whether dietary fiber, phytochemicals, or other components within dry beans are primarily responsible for their anti-carcinogenic properties.)

Source: *Journal of Nutrition* **1997;127(12):2328-2333.**

204. EAT LESS FOR BETTER BOWEL HEALTH

Smaller portions and healthier food choices may be the key in keeping your gut and your colon cancer-free. Obviously, this one is not easy, even though the researchers refer to "the simple act of cutting back!" The fact is that cancer-prone test animals fed either a restricted-calorie diet or a diet rich in olive oil, fruits and vegetables is significantly less likely to develop pre-cancerous colon polyps.

Adding exercise to the regimen also helps curtail polyp growth, just as high-fat diets encourage such growth. The conclusion is that low-calorie, plant-based diets may alter levels of hormones that initiate cancer development.

Source: Annual Experimental Biology 2002 Conference, New Orleans, LA, Apr 2002.

COLON CANCER: FIBER LINK

205. HIGHER FIBER = LOWER CANCER RISK

A high consumption of dietary fiber (30 to 40 grams per day) lowers your risk of death from colorectal cancer, and its protective influence even appears to outweigh the deleterious effects of a high-fat diet. Dietary fiber intake in the US is less than one-third of the level required for adequate protection against colorectal cancer. The American Gastroenterological Association has awakened to the fact that we need 30 to 40 grams of fiber a day to reduce the risk of colorectal cancer.

Higher intake of plant foods (including fruits, vegetables, potatoes, and grains) is only marginally related to a reduced risk of colorectal cancer. That's because it is virtually impossible to get that much fiber from these foods. An apple contains only two grams of fiber, a serving of white rice little more than 1/2 a gram, and a total of five heads of lettuce would give you only six grams.

The solution for most of us (in addition to watching our food intake) is the right kind of fiber supplement – one that contains a mix of fibers. [Good fiber supplements are available in health food stores.]

Vitamin B6 and alpha-tocopherol [a form of vitamin E] consumption are also inversely related to colorectal cancer mortality [that is, more of these two nutrients = reduced mortality risk], but higher fiber intake is the key. Cereal fiber can act very rapidly to slow down colon cancer, even after initial signs have been diagnosed.

Sources: *International Journal of Cancer* 1999;81:174-179; *Gastroenterology* 2000;118:1233-1257; B. Kamen, *New Facts About Fiber*.

WANT TO KNOW MORE?
New Yorkers and Copenhagen Danes have a much higher colon cancer risk than rural Finns, even though all three groups have similar fat intakes – but the Finns consume about 80 percent more fiber, due to the consumption of a coarse rye bread popular in Finland. Their incidence of colon cancer is reported to be less than one-third that of the United States, despite fat intake in Finland ranking among the highest in the world.

COLON CANCER: NATURAL REMEDIES & SUPPLEMENTS

206. FOLATE AGAINST COLORECTAL CANCER

An adequate intake of the B vitamin folate (also known as folic acid) may lower the risk of developing colorectal cancer. Women with the highest intakes of folate are 40 percent less likely to develop colorectal cancer than are those who consume the lowest amounts. Folate and folic acid may protect against certain cancers by helping with DNA synthesis and repair. Other studies show the same applies to men.

The US recommendation for daily folate intake is 400 micrograms.

Long-term folic acid supplementation may also reduce the risk of colorectal cancer in those who get recurrent polyps of the colon.

[This nutrient derives its name from the Latin word for foliage because it is found in leafy green veggies such as spinach, kale, and beet greens. But folic acid is very sensitive and is easily destroyed by light, heat, cooking, and storage. The best source is from fresh, unprocessed food.]

Source: *International Journal of Cancer* **2002;97:864-867;** *Gut* **2002;51:195-199;** *Cancer* **2002;95:1421-1433.**

WANT TO KNOW MORE?
[Folate is also crucial for pregnant women as it prevents birth defects. See the *Pregnancy & Childbirth* section for more information.]

207. TURMERIC FOR BOWEL CANCER PREVENTION

Turmeric, a spice used in curry powder, may be helpful in the prevention and treatment of bowel cancer. Turmeric is a member of the ginger family, and is believed to have medicinal properties because it inhibits production of a pro-inflammatory enzyme.

This enzyme is abnormally high in certain inflammatory diseases and cancers. Turmeric may possess both *chemotherapeutic* and *chemopreventive* effects, meaning that it may play a role in both the prevention of colon cancer as well as its treatment.

One note: You would have to eat a huge amount of curry to get the same effect as you would get from the isolated turmeric product.

Source: *University of Leicester School of Medicine & Biological Sciences*, **England, reported in** *Reuter's* **2001.**

WANT TO KNOW MORE?
[Turmeric has been used in cooking for thousands of years, and may also be helpful in reducing the risk of Alzheimer's disease. See Hint #76 for more information.]

208. VITAMIN D REDUCES COLON CANCER RISK

If you consume a diet high in fat, vitamin D may help to reduce your risk of developing colon cancer. High-fat diets result in the production of certain substances that interfere with the detoxification process, and this, in turn, can initiate cancerous conditions. Supplementing with vitamin D can be protective.

[However, this does not mean that we should continue consuming high-fat diets, thinking that vitamin D will protect us. Remember that the best way for you to lower your cancer risk is by modifying your diet.

Some good dietary sources of vitamin D are dairy products, eggs, and fish liver oils. Exposure to sunlight also allows the body to produce vitamin D.]

One note of warning: The protective powers of vitamin D do come at a cost – high intake of this vitamin can lead to abnormally high concentrations of calcium in your bloodstream.

Source: *Science* 2002;296:1313-1316.

209. B6 STOPS GROWTH OF COLON CANCER CELLS

Taken in large quantity, vitamin B6 may prevent colon cancer cells from reproducing, thereby preventing the growth of tumors. A significant increase of vitamin B6 can suppress colon tumors by reducing cell proliferation. It won't cause the tumor cells to die, but it will prevent their continued growth.

[Our stores of vitamin B6 are easily depleted by stress, as well as by the use of oral contraceptives. The processing, cooking, and storage of foods also reduces this nutrient. Be certain to take a supplement or food containing the full range of B vitamins whenever you take one of the isolated factions. When I take vitamin B6, I am sure to take soluble rice bran and chlorella to cover all bases.]

Source: *Journal of Nutrition* 2001;131:2204-2207.

WANT TO KNOW MORE?
Colon cancer is the second most frequently diagnosed cancer among both men and women in the United States and the second most common cause of cancer death. Between 133,000 and 160,000 new cases of colorectal cancers are diagnosed each year.

210. PROBIOTICS AGAINST COLON CANCER

Consuming probiotics ("friendly" bacteria) can help to inhibit the development of precancerous lesions and tumors that can lead to colon cancer. Your diet is one factor you can control to reduce the risk of colon cancer. The ingestion of probiotics (particularly *Lactobacillus bulgaricus* and *Streptococcus thermophilus*) leads to the excretion of urine with low concentrations of components that are toxic in human colon cells, helping to protect against this disease. If taken with *prebiotics* (such as fructooligosaccharides or inulin), a reduced load of toxic agents in the gut plus an increased production of agents that deactivate toxic components can result. One such protective agent (butyrate) is associated with lowering cancer risk.

Much attention has been focused recently on decreasing colon cancer risk through increasing intake of dietary fiber, and we can now add probiotics to the list.

Sources: *Journal of Nutrition* 2000;130:410S-414S; Institute for Nutritional Physiology, Karlsruhe, Germany.

WANT TO KNOW MORE?
A probiotic is defined as a "a viable microbial dietary supplement which beneficially affects the host through its effects on the intestinal tract." It was first discovered that test animals fed fermented milk had reduced colon tumors.

211. GARLIC AGAINST COLON CANCER

Epidemiologic studies link increased garlic consumption with a reduced incidence of colon cancer. The underlying mechanisms may involve both the initiation of the cancer and its promotion phases.

Colorectal cancer remains the second leading cause of cancer deaths in the US. Affluent lifestyle with its sedentary tendency is the strongest risk factor of colon cancer. Extensive sitting causes less diffusion of bacterial heat. A very slight rise in colon temperature over decades may promote tumor growth, according to these researchers.

Sources: *Cancer Research* 2001;61(2):725-31; *Nutrition & Cancer* 2000;38(2):255-64; *Journal of Korean Medical Science* 2001;16 Suppl:S81-6; *Medical Hypotheses* 2002;54(3):469-71.

WANT TO KNOW MORE?
Treating ulcerative colitis helps to reduce the risk of colon cancer. (**100th Annual Meeting of the American Gastroenterological Association, Orlando, FL, May 1999**) And obesity is linked to increased risk of colon cancer death, especially in men. (***American Journal of Epidemiology* 2000;152:847-854**)

CANCER, LEUKEMIA

212. HOT DOGS & LEUKEMIA DANGER IN KIDS

Keep your child's diet free of hot dogs, which are linked to an increased risk of developing leukemia. Hot dogs and other processed meats contain substances called nitrosamines, long known to be carcinogenic. There is a significant association between the consumption of 12 nitrate-laden hot dogs a month and an increased risk of leukemia in children.

Luncheon meats such as bologna also contain nitrates (the precursors of nitrosamines). There is also no evidence that consumption of fruit (an inhibitor of nitrosamine compounds) provides any protection. Fruit is not the protector that vegetables may be. [See hint #200 for the link between hot dogs and colorectal cancer.]

Source: *Cancer Causes & Control* **1994;5(2):195-202.**

CANCER, LUNG

IN THIS SECTION:
- CAUSES & PRECURSORS
- DIETARY TACTICS
- NATURAL REMEDIES & SUPPLEMENTS

LUNG CANCER: CAUSES & PRECURSORS

213. WHERE THERE'S SMOKE, THERE'S LUNG CANCER

Is knowing that your risk of lung cancer can be 20 to 30 times greater than a non-smoker enough to make you quit? Well, if that's not enough, you should also know that more than half of lung cancer patients also develop survival problems with at least three other disease states. These include: HIV/AIDS, tuberculosis, metastatic cancer, thyroid/glandular diseases, electrolyte imbalance, anemia, other blood diseases, dementia, neurologic disease, congestive heart failure, asthma, pulmonary fibrosis, liver disease, gastrointestinal bleeding, renal disease, connective tissue disease, osteoporosis, and peripheral vascular disease.

Ninety percent of lung cancer cases are tobacco-related. The only good news is that the risk of lung cancer decreases with time elapsed since smoking cessation.

Sources: *Lancet Oncology* **2003;4(1):45-55;** *International Journal of Cancer* **2003;103(6):792.**

214. RED MEAT & LUNG CANCER

Start cutting out red meat from your diet to reduce your risk of developing lung cancer. The consumption of red meat, especially fried or well-done red meat, is associated with an increased risk of developing this disease.

There is already a well-established association between red and well-done meat and both colon and breast cancer. Studies done at the National Cancer Institute in Bethesda, Maryland indicate that we can also add lung cancer to this list.

Source: *Cancer Causes & Control* 1998;9(6):621-630.

215. ESTROGEN & LUNG TUMOR GROWTH

If you are currently undergoing estrogen replacement therapy, you may not be at risk merely for breast cancer, but for *lung* cancer as well. While the role of estrogen in breast cancer has long been recognized, new research findings now suggest that this hormone may also contribute to the development of non-small-cell lung cancer.

Lung cancer cells contain a great number of estrogen receptors, strongly suggesting that estrogen enhances lung tumor growth. A key new finding is that rather than being concentrated in the breast, estrogen receptor levels are high in the ovaries, brain and lungs.

When exposed to estrogen, both lung cancer cells and normal cells increase their cell-division activity. And in test animals with weakened immune systems, lung tumor volume increases with chronic estrogen exposure but decreases with anti-estrogen treatment.

These findings suggest one possible reason why women are more susceptible than men to lung cancer.

Tamoxifen, no longer a favored drug for breast cancer, has anti-estrogen effects in breast tissue, but actually has estrogenic effects in other organs.

Source: University of Illinois, Chicago, IL, 91st Meeting of the American Association of Cancer Research, Apr 2000

WANT TO KNOW MORE?

Lung cancer is the most deadly cancer among women in the US, causing more deaths than breast and colon cancers combined. Symptoms do not appear until advanced stages. Even though more men smoke cigarettes, women's risk for lung cancer is three times higher than that of men with the same exposure. **(Weill Medical College, Cornell University study, 2002)**

216. RADON AND RISK

You may want to check the radon level of your house and workplace because it may lead to a twofold or greater increase in the risk of lung cancer. We all know that a reduction in smoking serves everyone's best interest in lung cancer prevention, but considering the results of recent research, let's look at radon levels, too.

Even levels of radon exposure substantially below official guidelines are associated with increased risk of lung cancer. Radon detectors were placed in the homes of 163 patients with lung cancer, and an even larger control group.

There is no question about the association. A synergistic effect between radon and smoking is also noted. Smokers with a high radon exposure have a 46 times greater risk of developing lung cancer compared with nonsmokers exposed to lower radon concentrations.

Source: *American Journal of Epidemiology* **2002;156:549-555.**

LUNG CANCER: DIETARY TACTICS
217. LYCOPENE FOR YOUR LUNGS

Increase your consumption of lycopene-rich foods to protect yourself from lung cancer. Diets high in bioavailable lycopene [meaning in a form that can be used by your body] appear to lower the risk of lung cancer in both smokers and nonsmokers. [Lycopene is a carotenoid, a class of compounds related to vitamin A. It is the red pigment that gives tomatoes their color, and can also be found in fruits such as pink grapefruit and watermelon.]

The inverse association between lycopene and the risk of lung cancer [high lycopene consumption = low lung cancer risk] is stronger than for most other phytochemicals, but other phytochemicals may also be important in reducing carcinogenesis. This is the primary rationale for having fruit and vegetables at the base of the food pyramid – to increase the number of phytochemicals consumed in the interest of disease prevention.

Source: *American Journal of Clinical Nutrition* **2000;72:901,990-997.**

WANT TO KNOW MORE?
[Lycopene is also beneficial for those suffering from both atherosclerosis and colitis. See Hint #491 and Hint #520 for more information.]

218. NOT A SMOKER? YOU'RE STILL AT RISK

Even if you are not a smoker, you may still be at risk for developing lung cancer – but the good news is that eating vegetables can help to protect you. Although we associate lung cancer with smokers, lung cancer risk in nonsmoking women increases with passive exposure to secondhand smoke (from coworkers or from a spouse), as well as those with a prior diagnosis of pneumonia or tuberculosis. Women who work for more than 10 years in jobs with known or suspected lung carcinogens also have an increased risk for this disease. [Of course the same applies to men. It was just women who were studied here.]

It is interesting to note that neither a family history of lung cancer nor residential radon levels is associated with an increased risk.

And more good news is that a diet rich in fresh vegetables appears to protect against lung cancer. [Make sure you are getting several servings a day, and if you can't, be sure to add a supplemental green drink, such as young barley grass powder, to fill in the blanks.]

Source: *International Journal of Cancer* 2002;100:706-713.

219. ORDER SUSHI FOR PROTECTION

Eating fresh fish, particularly sushi, may protect you against lung cancer. People who eat the most fresh fish are *half* as likely to develop lung cancer as are those who eat the least. Fish rich in omega-3 PUFA [polyunsaturated fatty acid] modifies the risk of this disease.

Even though Japan and the UK have an equal rate of smoking, lung cancer rates in Japan, where fresh fish is a dietary staple, are only two-thirds as high.

However, dried and salted fish are not associated with any protective effect. In fact, the consumption of Cantonese-style salted fish has been found to be associated with the risk of nasopharyngeal cancer.

Obviously, quitting smoking is the most important thing you can do to reduce your risk of developing lung cancer. But for those who find themselves unable to quit, adding lots of fresh fish to the diet is a useful way to moderate risk.

Sources: *British Journal of Cancer* 2001;84:00-00; *Journal of Nutrition* 2001;131:170S-175S.

WANT TO KNOW MORE?
Soybean curd [tofu] consumption is also associated with a lower risk of lung cancer in women.

LUNG CANCER: NATURAL REMEDIES & SUPPLEMENTS

220. SMOKERS: TAKE YOUR VITAMIN E

Supplement with vitamin E to reduce your risk of developing lung cancer. If you are a male smoker, you should know that high serum levels of alpha-tocopherol (vitamin E) are associated with a decreased incidence of lung cancer. [Commercial vitamin E supplements are usually in the form of alpha-tocopherol.]

Source: *Journal of the National Cancer Institute* **1999;91:1738.**

221. OTHER ANTIOXIDANTS FOR SMOKERS

Significant reductions in the risk of lung cancer occurs with the consumption of the dietary antioxidants that include carotenoids, vitamin E, glutathione, and flavonoids. These dietary antioxidants are associated with a marked protective effect in lung carcinogenesis. This conclusion was reached after studying 540 hospitalized patients and an equal number of controls. Diet can positively raise or lower the risk of lung cancer.

For vitamin A intake, a protective effect was observed only for its fruit and vegetable component (carotenoids) among current smokers.

When vitamin E, vitamin C, and carotenoid intakes were examined in combination, a strong protective effect was observed. While smoking *avoidance* is the most important behavior to reduce lung cancer risk, the daily consumption of a variety of fruits and vegetables that provides a combination of these nutrients and other potential protective factors may offer the best dietary protection against lung cancer.

Source: *American Journal of Epidemiology* **1997;146(3):231-43;** *Annals of Thoracic Surgery* **2001;71(3):929-35,** *International Journal of Cancer* **2002;100:706-713.**

WANT TO KNOW MORE?
Currently, only 15 percent of lung cancers are detected in the earliest stage. Men's hormones break down carcinogens in tobacco faster and more efficiently than women's. In addition, women retain the cancer-producing substances in tobacco and transform them into more toxic substances that produce precancerous changes in cells. Even nonsmoking women have a *threefold* greater risk of developing lung cancer than do their male counterparts.

CANCER, ORAL

222. DON'T GET DOWN IN THE MOUTH!

To reduce oral cancer, curtail your consumption of alcohol and cigarettes, both of which place you at increased risk for oral cancer. Mouth cancer is one of the most common cancers worldwide, and your diet plays a role: meat and meat products, plus alcohol and smoking are the culprits. However, consumption of cereals, antioxidants in fruit and vegetables, added lipids (from quality oils), and wholesome dairy products can help to reduce the occurrence.

The prevalence of oral cancer increases with age and is more common in men. The general condition of the mouth (as indicated by gum bleeding, tartar deposits, and mucosal irritation) is worse among oral cancer cases. No differences are detected in sexual practices (including oral sex).

Over the last two decades, little progress appears to have been made in reducing the incidence and number of deaths associated with oral cancer. An oral cancer screening done by a dentist is not invasive and provides a good opportunity for early detection [another important reason not to neglect your dental checkups!]

Sources: *Cancer* 2002;94:2981-2988; *Cancer & Epidemiology Biomarkers of Prevention* 2002;11(2): 155-8; *Clinical Oral Investigations* 2001;5(4):207-213; *Journal of Nutrition* 2002;132(4):762-767; *British Journal of Cancer* 2000;83(9):1238-1242; *Dental Update* 2000;27(8):404-8.

WANT TO KNOW MORE?
The role of nutrition in mouth cancer is not well understood, and there has been little improvement in survival rates in 30 years.

Because most oral malignancies are asymptomatic, they may mimic benign conditions. (***Nurse Practitioner*** **1997;22(6):109-10;113-5passim)**

Alcohol consumption is a more implicated factor in oral cancer than tobacco, especially in those who have the highest cancer incidence in the floor of the mouth and tongue. This demonstrates that alcohol and tobacco affect very specific sites in the mouth in the initiation of oral cancer. (***West African Journal of Medicine*** **2002;21(2):142-5)**

Family members of patients with oral cancer are also at high risk and therefore should be aware of those factors that reduce risk.

Retinoids, the natural and synthetic derivatives of vitamin A may block the cancer cell cycle or actually cause these cells to die off. Positive effects have been observed in early stages of oral cancer. (***Oral Oncology*** **2002;38(6):532-42)**

CANCER, OVARIAN

IN THIS SECTION:
- CAUSES & PRECURSORS
- DIETARY TACTICS
- NATURAL REMEDIES & SUPPLEMENTS
- HORMONE REPLACEMENT THERAPY CONNECTION

OVARIAN CANCER: CAUSES & PRECURSORS

223. MEAT, STARCH, SUGAR & OVARIAN CANCER

Avoid eating red meat, starchy foods, and sugar, all of which place you at higher risk of developing ovarian cancer. The frequent consumption of red meat and starchy foods is associated with an increased risk of ovarian cancer, while the consumption of vegetables and fish appears to protect against this disease.

There is also a significant increased risk associated with the frequent consumption of bread and sugar. An inverse relationship is seen between ovarian cancer and consumption of fish, peas and beans, raw vegetables, and cooked vegetables [that is, high consumption of these foods = low incidence of ovarian cancer.]

Source: *International Journal of Cancer* **2001;93:911-915.**

224. LACTOSE MALABSORPTION INCREASES RISK

If you are lactose intolerant, restrict your diet to lactose-free foods, because lactose malabsorption may increase the risk of ovarian cancer in women by more than 2.5 times. Populations with high rates of lactose intolerance also appear to have higher than average rates of ovarian cancer. In one study, nearly one-third of ovarian cancer patients were characterized as "lactose malabsorbers." This indicates that lactose ingestion and lactase persistence may play a role in the development of ovarian cancer.

(Foods high in lactose are milk and cheese products.)

Source: *American Journal of Epidemiology* **1999;150:183-186**.

WANT TO KNOW MORE?
Removal of benign ovarian cysts is not necessarily associated with reduced risk of ovarian cancer. In other words, ovarian cancer does not arise from benign cysts. Most benign cysts in middle-aged women would probably do no harm if they were left in place. (***Lancet* 2000;355:1028-1029,1060-63**)

OVARIAN CANCER: DIETARY TACTICS

225. CARROTS FOR OVARIAN CANCER PREVENTION

Make sure you are eating enough fruits and vegetables high in both carotene and lycopene weekly – they may protect you from ovarian cancer. Consuming five carrots a week, plus a few tomatoes and other foods high in carotene (sweet potatoes, apricots, cantaloupe) and lycopene (pink grapefruit, watermelon) may help reduce your risk of developing ovarian cancer.

Because of the high mortality from ovarian cancer, women should consider increasing carotenoids in their diet. Several studies show that high carotene intake significantly reduces this risk. High lycopene is also associated with a reduced risk of this disease.

[One tip: Always try to buy organic produce when possible. It has been shown that organic foods contain higher amounts of nutrients. Organic crops contain significantly more vitamin C, iron, magnesium, and phosphorus and less nitrates than conventional crops, plus better quality protein. And although it's best to get the nutrients from fresh food, palm oil tocotrienols contain a significant amount of carotene, too.]

Source: *International Journal of Cancer* 2001;94:128-134; *Journal of Alternative & Complementary Medicine* 2001;7(2):163-173..

OVARIAN CANCER: NATURAL REMEDIES & SUPPLEMENTS

226. LEARNING FROM OTHER CULTURES

The high carbohydrate Mexican diet is associated with a risk of ovarian cancer, but there is protection when retinal and vitamin D intakes are high, and the Chinese diet shows a decline in risk with an increased consumption of vegetables and fruits, but vice versa with high intakes of animal fat and salted vegetables. A case-controlled study in Mexico City did demonstrate the beneficial association with retinal and vitamin D; and a negative outcome with high carbs, but it did not show any tie-in with ovarian cancer and tortilla intake.

The study in Zhejiang, China showed an increased risk in ovarian cancer for those women preferring fat, fried, cured, and smoked food. Vegetables were found to be more protective than fruits.

Sources: *Oncology* 2002;63(2):151-157; *British Journal of Cancer* 2002;86(5):712-717.

227. TIME FOR TEA – AGAIN!

Ovarian cancer risk declines with increasing frequency and duration of overall tea consumption. Women who drink tea daily have a decreased risk of ovarian cancer compared with women who are non-tea drinkers. The response relationships are quite dramatic, especially with the consumption of green tea. [See Hint #86 for more information on green tea.]

Source: *Cancer Epidemiology Biomarkers & Prevention* 2002;11(8):713-718.

228. C AND E AGAINST OVARIAN CANCER

Combining the vitamins C and E is associated with a reduced risk of ovarian cancer. Getting these antioxidants from your diet is unrelated to risk. But more than 343 mgs of *supplemental* C and more than 75 mgs of supplemental vitamin E daily is associated with reduced risk. The levels of C and E offering the protective effects are well above the current US Recommended Daily Allowances.

Source: *Nutrition & Cancer* 2001;40(2):92-09.

OVARIAN CANCER: HRT CONNECTION

229. HRT & THE HIGH RISK OF OVARIAN CANCER

If you are a woman who is considering or currently undergoing estrogen replacement therapy (ERT), you should be aware that you are putting yourself at high risk of developing ovarian cancer. Postmenopausal women who use estrogen replacement therapy for 10 years or more have *double* the risk of death from ovarian cancer compared with women who have never used HRT. The number of years that a woman uses HRT also increases this risk.

Source: *Journal of the American Medical Association* 2001;285:1460-1465.

WANT TO KNOW MORE?
[See my book, ***Hormone Replacement Therapy: Yes or No? How to Make an Informed Decision*** for a good introduction to this subject. Also see the *Menopause & Hormone Replacement Therapy* section of this book for many informative hints.]

CANCER, PANCREATIC

230. EXERCISE LOWERS PANCREATIC CANCER RISK

Regular exercise may do more than make you look good – it may also reduce your risk of developing pancreatic cancer, one of the most serious forms of cancer. In men, physical activity appears to have a protective effect against the development of pancreatic cancer.

In women, there is also a relationship seen between increasing strenuous activity and a lower risk of this disease. However, there is *twice* the increased risk of pancreatic cancer among men with high body mass.

Similarly, weight loss is also protective. Weight loss of at least 2.9 percent in men or 12.5 percent in women (from maximum lifetime weight) *significantly* reduces the risk of pancreatic cancer compared with those reporting no weight loss or a smaller change.

Source: *International Journal of Cancer* 2001;94:140-147.

WANT TO KNOW MORE?
[Consumption of red meat has been linked to pancreatic cancer, along with various other kinds of cancers including stomach cancer and breast cancer. See Hint 253 in the *Stomach, Gastric & Esophageal Cancer* section for more details. As usual, consumption of fruits and vegetables decreases risk. (*Hematology/Oncology Clinics of North America* 2002;16(1):1-16)

231. BUTT OUT TO DECREASE RISK

Quitting smoking offers one of the best strategies against pancreatic cancer. Smoking doubles your risk of developing this disease. Since pancreatic cancer is a leading cause of cancer-related mortality, reconsider smoking habits. The mortality rates from pancreatic cancer have increased in 37 countries around the world.

Only five to ten percent of cases can be linked to inherited susceptibility. Heavy alcohol consumption is another risk factor.

Diabetes is also a risk factor. And because obesity and physical inactivity have their impact on insulin resistance, these become risk factors, too. As stated above, however, physical activity may reduce the risk for those who are overweight.

Sources: *Oncology* 2002;16(12):1615-22;1631-2; *Hematology/Oncology Clinics of North America* 2002;16(1):1-16; *Epidemiology* 2003;14(1):45-54.

232. HOW TO AVOID PANCREATIC CANCER? GO FISH!

Fatty acids derived from fish oil can alter the proinflammatory progression of acute-phase pancreatic disease. A group of pancreatic cancer patients received a supplement consisting of two grams of eicosapentanoic acid (EPA) and one gram of docosahexanoic acid (DHA), daily, for four weeks. Researchers concluded that the enriched fish-oil supplement lessens the progression of negative responses to weight loss with advanced pancreatic cancer.

Source: *Journal of Nutrition* **1999;129:1120-1125.**

CANCER, PROSTATE & TESTICULAR

IN THIS SECTION:
- CAUSES & PRECURSORS
- DIETARY TACTICS
- NATURAL REMEDIES & SUPPLEMENTS
- REDUCING RISK
- SCREENING FOR

PROSTATE CANCER: CAUSES & PRECURSORS

233. DAIRY FOODS & PROSTATE CANCER RISK

Men with diets high in dairy foods, be warned: You may be at increased risk of developing prostate cancer. A high calcium intake, mainly from dairy products, may increase prostate cancer risk by lowering concentrations of the hormonal form of vitamin D (1,25-dihydroxyvitamin D), thought to protect against prostate cancer. Men who consume more than 600 mg of calcium a day from skim milk have lower plasma D3 concentrations than do those men consuming less than 150 mgs.

These are the results of the 11-year Physicians' Health Study. They support the hypothesis that dairy products and calcium are associated with a greater risk of prostate cancer.

Sources: *Physicians' Health Study*, Harvard University and Brigham Women's Hospital, Apr 2000; *American Journal of Clinical Nutrition* Oct 2001;74(4):549-554.

WANT TO KNOW MORE?
[This research is not new. I wrote about too much calcium depleting D3 years ago in my booklet, *Startling New Facts About Osteoporosis*.]

234. MILK & TESTICULAR CANCER RISK

Watch your consumption of milk, as high levels are thought to be linked to increased risk of testicular cancer. Men with testicular cancer are found to have consumed significantly more milk during adolescence than population controls. The incidence of testicular cancer – as well as undescended testes – increases for each quarter pint of milk consumed. [This is believed to be caused by the estrogens that wind up in our milk.]

Adding synthetic vitamin D3 to milk further decreases its health value. Risk of illness from vitamin D fortification rises with increased milk consumption because it helps to activate an enzyme that can wreak havoc on heart health.

The upper limit for vitamin D added to milk and the current monitoring of the process are unsatisfactory, and research validates that there are errors in fortified-milk products all across the US milk industry.

Sources: *New England Journal of Medicine* **1992;326:1173-1177;** *American Journal of Health* **1995;85:656-659;** *British Journal of Cancer* **1996.**

235. HIGH-FAT DIETS & PROSTATE CANCER

If your diet is too high in fat, be warned: You could be at a *significantly* increased risk of developing prostate cancer. When fat in the diet exceeds 30 percent of total caloric intake, prostate cancer risk increases *tenfold*. A high-fat diet may set off a reaction that somehow motivates the disease to grow.

[While this study did not look at what kind of fat was being consumed, chances are that when dietary fat is *that* high, a good percentage of it comes from products that are hydrogenated, causing the production of free radicals, which can lead to cancer.

Hidden fats can be a major culprit. Hidden fats include those added during preparation and cooking, and are generally found in cakes, biscuits, chips, processed meats, fried foods, mayonnaise, etc. Hidden fats may also be present in the membranes of the plant and animal tissues we consume.

Hidden fats and oils are usually inedible in their original forms, so processing is necessary to make them more palatable. Processing starts with the use of solvents for extracting the fats and oils from their raw material beginnings (the farm animal or plant crop). Heating, dehulling, pressing, bleaching, alkali refining, and deodorizing follow. Hidden fats and oils are so widely used today that they are produced on an industrial scale. So perhaps this hint should really read: *Beware processed foods: they may promote prostate cancer.*]

Source: Fred Hutchinson Cancer Research Center, Seattle, WA, Oct 2000; *Obesity Reviews* **2002; 3(4):303-8;** *Cancer Epidemiology Biomarkers & Prevention* **2002;11(8):719-25.**

236. FATHER'S AGE INFLUENCES *SON'S* RISK

Sons of older fathers, be warned: You may be at increased risk of developing prostate cancer, so all the more reason to improve your dietary and lifestyle habits NOW to protect yourself. Older paternal age at birth is associated with an increased risk and earlier occurrence of prostate cancer in male offspring. The incidence rate of prostate cancer increases as the father's age at birth increases.

This relation seems to be stronger in early-onset cases rather than late-onset cancer. Those with early-onset of prostate cancer (before the age of 65) had fathers who were 4.5 years older when they were born compared with the fathers of those men without prostate cancer.

Maternal age at birth does not seem to be related either to the incidence of prostate cancer or its onset.

Source: *American Journal of Epidemiology* **1999;150:1208-1212**.

237. VITAMIN D & PROSTATE CANCER

If you are a man under the age of 51 with a deficiency in vitamin D, be warned: You could be at increased risk of developing prostate cancer, so consider vitamin D supplementation. A deficiency of vitamin D may increase risk for both the initiation and progression of prostate cancer in men up to about 51 years of age (the age before andropause, the male menopause, sets in).

Androgens are male hormones. During andropause, these male hormones begin to decline. And once they do, this vitamin D deficiency is not particularly associated with prostate cancer risk. The risk is instead highest in younger men (40-51 years old) who have a vitamin D deficiency. This suggests that vitamin D has a protective role against prostate cancer only before andropause.

In addition, the lowest concentrations of vitamin D in younger men are associated with more aggressive prostate cancer.

High vitamin D levels delay the appearance of clinically verified prostate cancer by 1.8 years.

Source: *Journal of Steroid Biochemistry & Molecular Biology* **2001;76(1-5):125-134.**

WANT TO KNOW MORE?
[Some good dietary sources of vitamin D are dairy products, eggs, and fish liver oils. Exposure to sunlight alsoallows the body to produce vitamin D. Full spectrum lighting does not.]

PROSTATE CANCER: DIETARY TACTICS

238. VEGGIES AGAINST PROSTATE CANCER

Increasing your consumption of fresh vegetables – especially *cruciferous* vegetables – can help reduce your risk of prostate cancer. Men who eat 28 or more servings of vegetables a week have a significant advantage for prostate health over those who consume fewer than 14 servings a week. Vegetable intake, particularly of cruciferous vegetables such as cauliflower and broccoli, *substantially* lowers the risk of prostate cancer.

Even after accounting for total vegetable intake, those who eat three or more servings of cruciferous vegetables have an even greater advantage over those who eat less than one serving per week. Cruciferous vegetables are high in *isothiocyanates*, substances that activate enzymes present in all cells. Their purpose is to detoxify carcinogens. [And remember, we're talking *vegetables* here, not fruit. Prostate cancer risk is not particularly reduced by the consumption of fruit.]

Source: *Journal of the National Cancer Institute* **2000;92:61-68.**

239. NO MEAT, NO DAIRY = REDUCED RISK

A diet free of meat or dairy products may reduce the risk of developing prostate cancer.   Meat-eaters are defined as men who eat meat most days of the week. Prostate cancer rates are generally lower in countries were consumption of meat and dairy products is low. Prostate cancer is the second most common cancer in British men. Each year, the disease kills about 9,500 men, and about 21,000 new cases are diagnosed. The incidence of prostate cancer has been even greater here in the US, where it is still steadily increasing year by year.

Source: Report of the Imperial Cancer Research Fund, Oxford, England, as reported in *Reuter's Medical News,* **Jun 2000.**

WANT TO KNOW MORE?
Charcoal-cooked red meat and fish have been demonstrated to contain heterocyclic amines that are carcinogenic in test animals. Some of these amines have been shown to induce cancers in mammary glands and in the prostate.

240. TOMATO SAUCE & PROSTATE CANCER

You may be able to reduce your risk of developing prostate cancer by eating tomatoes and tomato products such as tomato sauce. We know that the risk of prostate cancer is lower in men with a higher consumption of tomatoes, and now we know that those *already suffering* with prostate cancer are also helped by tomato consumption.

Men with prostate cancer given a short-term tomato sauce-based diet have reduced levels of prostate-specific antigen (PSA), significantly lower prostatic tissue DNA damage, and significant increases in lycopene concentrations – both in their blood and prostate gland. Oxidative DNA damage in prostate tissue is also reduced. [Lycopene is a carotenoid, a class of compounds related to vitamin A. It is also the pigment that gives tomatoes their red color.]

Source: *Journal of the National Cancer Institute* **2001;93:1872-1879.**

241. BETA-CAROTENE & PROSTATE CANCER

High intakes of carotenoids may reduce your risk of prostate cancer. [Carotenoids are compounds related to vitamin A, of which beta-carotene is the most well known. Others include alpha-carotene, lycopene, and lutein.] Carotenoids are found in spinach, broccoli, kale, asparagus, parsley, lettuce, carrots, sweet potatoes, winter squash, yams, pumpkin, red cabbage, apricots, peaches, mango, cantaloupe, papaya, cherries, and watermelon. However, those who are diabetic or have low thyroid function have a lowered ability to convert beta-carotene to vitamin A.

Source: *Journal of Nutrition* **2000;130:728-732.**

WANT TO KNOW MORE?
High intake of all types of carotenoids, not just lycopene, may reduce prostate cancer risk. In addition to lycopenes and carotenoids, micronutrients such as selenium, zinc, isoflavones, carotenoids, and vitamins E and D have been listed. (*Toxicology* **2002;181-182:89-94**)

242. BORON REDUCES PROSTATE CANCER RISK

You can reduce your risk of prostate cancer by increasing your consumption of boron, a trace element found in fruits, nuts, and alfalfa. The more boron-rich foods and beverages consumed, the greater the risk reduction. Three and a half servings of boron-rich fruits and one serving of nuts a day are recommended.

[Good sources of boron include organic grapes, grape juice, avocados, kelp, and alfalfa. It's interesting to note that elements found in large quantities in humans are found in large quantities in plants and animals, just as those required in traces by us are found in traces in plants and animals. A trace element is defined as one occurring in amounts less than 0.01 percent of the human body. It's difficult to imagine such a small percentage of *anything*, yet this definition attests to a certain uniformity in nature.]

Source: *Experimental Biology* **meeting, Orlando, FL, 2001.**

WANT TO KNOW MORE?
[As explained in my booklet, *Startling New Facts About Osteoporosis*, one of boron's roles is the balance of hormones, which may be why it's helpful for the prostate. Fluoride in drinking water also negatively alters the efficiency of boron.]

243. FISH REDUCES PROSTATE CANCER RISK

Eating certain kinds of fish can help you to reduce your prostate cancer risk. Men who consume moderate-to-high amounts of fatty fish, such as salmon, herring and mackerel (which contain high levels of omega-3 fatty acids) appear to have a significantly reduced risk of developing prostate cancer. Men who eat a lot of fish are also more likely to be physically active, to be non-smokers, and to consume fruits and vegetables.

High fish consumption is inversely associated with eating red or processed meat (that is, high fish intake = low red or processed meat intake, and vice versa). Men who do not eat fish are at a two- to threefold increased risk of developing prostate cancer compared with men who eat moderate-to-high amounts.

Source: *Lancet* 2001;357:1764-1766.

WANT TO KNOW MORE?
[Although tuna is the most consumed fish in the US, it is suspected to contain dangerously high levels of mercury due to environmental pollution, and the FDA urges women who are pregnant to limit their intake to protect developing fetuses. See Hint #840 for more details.]

PROSTATE CANCER: NATURAL REMEDIES & SUPPLEMENTS
244. VITAMIN E AGAINST PROSTATE CANCER

Taking supplemental vitamin E may help reduce the incidence of prostate cancer. Vitamin E interferes with the ability of prostate cancer cells to progress, and also decreases the receptor cells that contribute to the problem. And the good news is that treatment with vitamin E produces no side effects, whereas commonly used drugs can impair the role of testosterone.

Among men, prostate cancer is the second leading cause of death from cancer and the most commonly diagnosed form of this disease.

Sources: *Proceedings of the National Academy of Sciences* 2002;99:7408-7413; *Annals of New York Academy of Sciences* 2001;952:145-52; *The Prostate* 2000;44:287-295.

245. SELENIUM & PROSTATE CANCER

Supplementing with selenium, an essential mineral, may be helpful in reducing prostate cancer risk. Low levels of selenium are associated with a four- to fivefold increase in the risk of prostate cancer.

It is interesting to note that blood selenium levels decrease with age, and there is a direct connection between selenium and prostate cancer. But older men with higher levels of selenium are at lower risk.

[Western states in the US generally have more selenium in their soil than eastern states. Brewer's yeast, butter, liver, most fish, lamb, whole grains, nuts, and many vegetables contain selenium. The herb Astragalus accumulates selenium from the soil.]

Source: *Journal of Urology* **2001;166:2034-2038.**

246. ISOFLAVONES & PROSTATE CANCER

Supplementing with isoflavones, derived from soybeans or red clover, may reduce the risk of prostate cancer. The types of isoflavones differ slightly between the two. Red clover contains the precursors of genistein and daidzein, similar isoflavones extracted from soybeans.

[The closer to a natural source, the better, so my vote is for the red clover isoflavones. You can take this a step further and buy red clover seeds at the health food store, and sprout them – an inexpensive, beneficial sprout to add to your salads. Some stores sell red clover seeds already sprouted.

Isoflavones are a subfamily of plant antioxidants. These can easily be incorporated into breakfast cereal. Tempeh (fermented soybeans) is another food that contains isoflavones which are easily absorbed. So here's another natural food source, again – my recommendation over anything extracted and isolated.]

It's interesting to note that these same isoflavones also help to reduce the risk of breast cancer.

Source: *Journal of Nutrition* **2002;132:2199-2202.**

WANT TO KNOW MORE?
Because of their safety and the fact that they are not perceived as "medicine," food-derived products are highly interesting for development as chemopreventive agents that are finding widespread, long-term use. Many food-derived agents are extracts, containing multiple compounds or classes of compounds. [But beware the ones that become too isolated.] (***Journal of Nutrition* 2000;130(2S Suppl):467S-471S**)

The crop year and the location affect isoflavone content of soybeans, which can account for differences in results.(***Journal of Agriculture & Food Chemistry* 1994;42:1674-1677**)

PROSTATE CANCER: REDUCING RISK

247. SUNLIGHT AS PROSTATE CANCER PROTECTION

Exposure to ultraviolet radiation (such as sunlight) appears to be *protective* against prostate cancer. There is a link seen between latitude and prostate cancer mortality, indicating a possible protective effect of the sun's ultraviolet radiation against the development of this disease.

A history of childhood sunburn, regular foreign holidays, and sunbathing exposure are all found to be protective against prostate cancer, and many – rather than few – childhood sunburn events seem to increase this effect.

Men with low ultraviolet radiation exposure also seem to develop prostate cancer at a younger age than do those men with higher exposure.

Source: *Lancet* 2001;358:641-642.

WANT TO KNOW MORE?
[Avoiding the sun totally is NOT in your best health interest, and insufficient exposure may be a risk factor for cancer in Western Europe and North America, mainly because of insufficient levels of vitamin D. For more information on the connection between cancer and sunlight, see Hint #163.]

PROSTATE CANCER: SCREENING FOR

248. PROSTATE CANCER SCREENING: WORTHWHILE?

If you are a man and concerned about prostate cancer, you should be aware that annual screenings to detect this disease do little to reduce the death rate. The reasons for supporting the test include the belief that early diagnosis reduces mortality and that quality of life is improved with testing.

But epidemiologists assert that widespread PSA (prostate-specific antigen) screening leads to many false-positives and unnecessary treatment while doing little to lower the rate of death from the disease.

In the US, the incidence rate of prostate cancer increased sharply in the early 1990s after widespread adoption of PSA testing. In Great Britain, where PSA testing is relatively uncommon, the incidence rate increased only slightly, and is now less than half the US rate.

As a common saying goes: "Men tend to die *with* prostate cancer, not from it." In other words, most men have some degree of prostate cancer, but the extent of the disease is not usually significant enough to cause death. [And while surgery may or may not save lives, it can cause incontinence and impotence.]

Sources: *Journal of the American Medical Association* 2002;287(8):PAGES; *British Medical Journal* 2002;325:725-726,737-743.

WANT TO KNOW MORE?

One study compared more than 200,000 men, aged 65 to 79, living in either Seattle or Connecticut. The subjects in Seattle were 5.39 times more likely to undergo PSA testing and 2.20 times more likely to undergo prostate biopsy. In addition, radical prostatectomy and radiotherapy were used more often in Seattle than in Connecticut. But despite more intensive screening and treatment in the Seattle group, the prostate cancer mortality rates of the two groups remained comparable.

Men with prostate cancer who decide not to have surgery and instead opt only for treatment of the symptoms of their disease do as well as men who have surgery, at least in the first six or seven years after diagnosis. Watchful waiting appears to be as good as surgery for prostate cancer. (*British Medical Journal* 2002;325:613.

249. FREQUENCY OF PSA SCREENING QUESTIONED

Another note about PSA tests: Intervals as long as four years may be adequate between screenings for prostate cancer, rather than the recommended annual testing. Although the American Cancer Society has recommended annual prostate-specific antigen (PSA) screening since 1993, *no* studies have established this as the optimum interval. PSA values predict the amount of tumor in biopsy specimens during the first round of screening but not during the second round.

A substantial decrease is seen in both the amount and the grade of screen-detected prostate cancers four years after an initial screen. Relatively few advanced tumors are found after a four-year interval, which is not long enough for most large tumors to develop.

In December of 2002, the US Preventive Services Task Force concluded that there is insufficient scientific evidence to promote routine prostate cancer screening for all men and inconclusive evidence that early detection improves health outcomes. The task force's recommendation was based on a review of studies regarding the effect of screening, including both the prostate-specific antigen test and digital rectal exams, to prevent death in men 40 or older.

Statistics indicate that 15 percent of American men eventually will be diagnosed with prostate cancer, 75 percent after age 65.

Sources: *Journal of National Cancer Institute* 2001;93:1153-1158; *Annals of Internal Medicine,* 2002;137:917-929.

CANCER, SKIN

IN THIS SECTION:
- CAUSES & PRECURSORS
- NATURAL REMEDIES & SUPPLEMENTS

SKIN CANCER: CAUSES & PRECURSORS

250. SUNSCREEN GIVES FALSE SECURITY

Sunbathers take note: Using sunscreen to stay out in the sun longer may actually *increase* your risk of developing skin cancer. Unfortunately, the use of sunscreen is not associated with a reduced risk of melanoma.

Several studies suggest an association between sunscreen use and an increased risk of skin cancer. People who use sunscreen also tend to stay in the sun longer than those who don't use sunscreen, and those who spend more time sunbathing have a greater incidence of malignant melanoma.

[However, *some* sunlight daily is good for you and may actually help to prevent cancer. There is a happy medium! See Hint #163 for more information on this subject.]

Source: *International Journal of Cancer* **2000;87:145-150.**

WANT TO KNOW MORE?
Alcohol consumption is possibly associated with the risk of melanoma. (*American Journal of Epidemiology* **1990;131:597-611**)

SKIN CANCER: NATURAL REMEDIES & SUPPLEMENTS

251. GREEN TEA CAN PROTECT YOUR SKIN

When going out into the sun, apply green tea and spearmint to your face to protect yourself from skin damage. Substances found in both green tea and spearmint work to shield your skin from ultraviolet light reactions, so applying green tea (especially with added spearmint) to your face before going out in the sun can be protective.

Spearmint is also an effective agent against oxidative stress, toxicity, and other damaging effects.

Green tea is known to have cancer preventive effects, and we now know that actually applying green tea to your skin can inhibit damaging sun exposure, or what is known as *photocarcinogenesis*. This topical application of green tea and spearmint is recommended as a novel chemopreventive tactic to reduce UV-induced skin cancer risk.

Sources: *Clinical Cancer Research* **2000;6(10):3864-9;** *Food Chemistry Toxicology* **Oct 2000;38(10):939-948.**

WANT TO KNOW MORE?
[*Drinking* green tea can also protect you from many forms of cancer. See Hint #156 for more details.]

252. BETA-CAROTENE & VITAMIN E PROTECTION

If you spend long periods of time in the sun, supplement with both beta-carotene and vitamin E to protect yourself against skin damage. Beta-carotene has been shown to modify sunburn damage, and vitamin E may increase the benefit.

With the number of diagnosed melanomas doubling in the US since 1973, protection of the skin against ultraviolet radiation damage has become a priority health issue.

Beta-carotene has been widely used as an oral sun protectant. Clinical evidence shows that sunburn intensity is *significantly* reduced in those who take vitamin supplements over a 12-week period while being exposed to UV radiation.

[Some good dietary sources of beta-carotene are spinach, broccoli, Brussels sprouts, carrots, pumpkin, peaches, papaya, cherries, and many other foods, including most orange or yellow fruits and vegetables. Some sources of vitamin E are butter, egg yolks, liver, palm oil, rice bran oil, wheat germ, barley greens, saw palmetto, and certain types of nuts and grains.]

Source: *American Journal of Clinical Nutrition* **2000;71:795-798.**

WANT TO KNOW MORE?
A complete palm oil tocotrienol is the best source of supplemental carotenoids and vitami E (instead of just the beta-carotene).

A 100 percent five-year survival rate was reported in patients with stages I and II melanoma. (These are advanced stages.) These patients were committed to the Gerson diet therapy, which includes a lactovegetarian diet. It also emphasizes low sodium, low fat and (temporarily) low protein, but high potassium, fluid, and nutrients – with hourly raw vegetable and fruit juices. Of 17 with stage IIIA (regionally metastasized) melanoma, 82 percent were alive at five years, considerably higher than those reported elsewhere. **(Gerson Research Organization, San Diego, CA, reported in** *Alternative Therapy & Health Medicine* **1995;1(4):29-37)**

CANCER,
STOMACH, GASTRIC & ESOPHAGEAL

IN THIS SECTION:
- CAUSES & PRECURSORS
- DIETARY TACTICS
- NATURAL REMEDIES & SUPPLEMENTS

STOMACH CANCER:
CAUSES & PRECURSORS

253. RED MEAT & DIGESTIVE SYSTEMS CANCERS

Beware red meat: it has been linked to colorectal, stomach and pancreatic cancers.
Studies show that patients with high red meat intake are found to be the ones at risk for these cancers.

Such research confirms previous studies from the US Department of Agriculture and the UK Committee on the Medical Aspects of Food and Nutrition Policy (among others), all of which indicate that the consumption of red meat plays a large role in the development of human cancer.

Source: *International Journal of Cancer* **2000;86:425-428.**

WANT TO KNOW MORE?
[Cooking red meat at high temperatures is especially dangerous, as it can produce potentially carcinogenic chemicals not present in uncooked meat. See Hint #170 to learn more.]

254. HEARTBURN LINKED TO ESOPHAGEAL CANCER

If you suffer from chronic heartburn, be warned: This condition can greatly increase your risk of developing esophageal cancer, so think about improving your digestion.
Patients with longstanding, severe heartburn have a 43.5 times higher risk of developing adenocarcinoma of the esophagus. Those who experience heartburn, regurgitation, or *both* at least once weekly have eight times the risk, and those with symptoms of reflux at night have nearly 11 times the risk. [All of this underscores the importance of improving your digestion if you are subject to this problem. Some possible solutions: Natural digestive aids such as liquid probiotics, or drinking an herbal tea containing fennel, anise, and caraway – herbs known to help digestion. See Hint #570 in the *Heartburn* section for more details on this tea.]

Source: *New England Journal of Medicine* 1999;340:825-831.

255. SMOKING LINKED TO *STOMACH* CANCER TOO

It's not just your lungs you need to worry about — cigarette smoking and use of other tobacco products significantly increases your risk of *stomach* cancer. Men who are former cigarette smokers (or current or former users of more than one type of tobacco) are also at increased risk for stomach cancer mortality.

Women who are current or former cigarette smokers are also at significantly increased risk.

Men who smoke cigarettes or cigars, and who have a history of chronic indigestion or gastroduodenal ulcers, have substantially higher rates of death from stomach cancer compared to men without such a history.

These conditions are strongly associated with chronic and recurrent *H. pylori* infection [the bacteria that have been implicated in the development of duodenal and gastric ulcers]. So *H. pylori* and tobacco smoke may act together to increase the risk of stomach cancer.

Note: Stomach cancer death rates are also higher among current smokers who are aspirin-users.

Source: *International Journal of Cancer* **2002;101:380-389.**

WANT TO KNOW MORE?
[See the *Smoking & Nicotine Addiction* section for helpful tips on protecting yourself from smoking-related damage, as well as some useful quitting strategies.]

STOMACH CANCER: DIETARY TACTICS

256. ONIONS AGAINST STOMACH CANCER

Consumption of allium vegetables such as onions may considerably reduce your risk of developing stomach cancer. A large-scale Netherlands Cohort Study on diet and cancer, which started in 1986 with 120,000 subjects, shows that the rate of stomach carcinoma in those consuming at least half an onion per day is only *half* that of those eating no onions.

Source: *Gastroenterology* **1996;110(1):12-20.**

WANT TO KNOW MORE?
[Other allium vegetables include chives, leeks, shallots, and, of course, garlic, which also has associations with reduced risk for many cancers, including colorectal cancer. See Hint #201 for more information.]

257. STRAWBERRIES AGAINST ESOPHAGEAL CANCER

Eating strawberries may reduce your risk of developing esophageal cancer. Test animals fed a diet comprised of freeze-dried strawberries have significantly less incidence of esophageal cancer. Those with a diet comprised of five percent strawberries have a 25 percent reduced incidence of this disease, while those fed a diet that is 10 percent strawberries have as high as a 50 percent reduced incidence.

The freeze-dried strawberries inhibit the development of substances used to induce esophageal tumors, and one or more components in the berries seems to prevent DNA damage from taking place.

Source: *Carcinogenesis* **2001;22(3):441-446.**

258. 6 CLOVES A WEEK AGAINST STOMACH CANCER

A high intake of raw or cooked garlic may reduce your risk of developing stomach cancer. Data combined from 22 different studies suggests that a high consumption of raw or cooked garlic decreases the risk of stomach cancer by as much as 50 percent. (The amount that needs to be consumed to achieve this effect is about six cloves a week.) And the good news is that eating more has no side effects.

Source: *American Journal of Clinical Nutrition* **2000;72(4):1047-1052.**

WANT TO KNOW MORE?
[Garlic also may be protective against colorectal cancer as well. See Hint #201 for more details.]

STOMACH CANCER: NATURAL REMEDIES & SUPPLEMENTS

259. VITAMIN C AGAINST GASTRIC CANCER

The use of a vitamin C supplement at least once a week for six months or longer lowers your risk of developing cancer of the esophagus and the stomach. In those with precancerous gastric lesions, antioxidant supplementation with ascorbic acid (vitamin C) appears to be effective in curing gastric cancer. This is an important lead to a potential way to reduce the toll of stomach cancer, still the second most common malignancy on a global scale. (Beta-carotene also proved to be effective, but combining both nutrients does not increase the success of this therapy.)

Vitamin C deficiency is a significant factor contributing to the progression of precancerous lesions to gastric cancer. Additional factors are *H. pylori* infection (the bacteria that have been implicated in the development of duodenal and gastric ulcers) and cigarette smoking.

Saturated fat, as well as substances found primarily in animal products – cholesterol, animal protein, and vitamin B12 – all raise the risk of both gastric and esophageal cancers. (And intake of salt and nitrites are each linked with risk of one form of gastric cancer.) But intake of fiber, beta-carotene, folate, vitamin C, and vitamin B6 are all associated with a lower risk of these cancers.

Sources: *Journal of the National Cancer Institute* **2000;92:1607-1612,1868-1869,1881-1888;** *Cancer Epidemiological Biomarkers & Prevention* **Oct 2001.**

An area of China with the world's highest rates of gastric cancer was studied for more than four years. Patients with progression to cancer had ascorbic acid serum levels 40 percent lower than those without progression, and patients with the highest amounts had only 20 percent the risk of those with the lowest concentrations.

260. FIBER & UPPER DIGESTIVE TRACT CANCERS

Higher intake of dietary fiber may help to protect you against oral, pharyngeal, and esophageal cancer. The reduced risk is similar for vegetable fiber, fruit fiber, and grain fiber. [Unfortunately, the American diet is sorely lacking in fiber. In addition to efforts to include high fiber vegetables and grains (most fruits are actually rather low in fiber), a good fiber supplement has become a necessity for optimal health. Look for one in your local health food store, and make sure it includes an assortment of fibers rather than just one fiber source.]

Source: *International Journal of Cancer* **2001;91:283-287.**

WANT TO KNOW MORE?

Dietary Fiber in Popular Foods

Food	Portion	Grams of Dietary Fiber
apple	1 small	2.8
avocado	1/2 average	2.8
banana	1 medium	2
beans (kidney)	1 cup	11
chestnuts (raw)	1 cup	14.5
chickpeas	1/2 cup	6
cucumber	10 thin slices	0.7
figs (fresh)	1	2
green beans	1/2 cup	2.1
lamb chop	1	0
oatmeal	1/2 cup	7.7
pear	1 medium	6
sauerkraut	1/2 cup	1.5

[The doctors tell us we need at least 35 grams of fiber a day, and the alternative physicians agree that even better results are accomplished with 50 to 65 grams.. You can see the need for supplementation. To learn more about fiber, see my book, *New Facts About Fiber.*]

CARPAL TUNNEL SYNDROME

Carpal tunnel syndrome is a constellation of symptoms associated with compression of a particular nerve at the wrist. (*Clinical Neurophysiology* **2002;113(9):1373-81**) Its pathophysiology is not fully understood, but the researchers do offer a few very beneficial hints.

IN THIS SECTION:
- ALTERNATIVE THERAPIES
- NATURAL REMEDIES & SUPPLEMENTS

CARPAL TUNNEL SYNDROME: ALTERNATIVE THERAPIES

261. YOGA FOR CARPAL TUNNEL SYNDROME

If you are a carpal tunnel syndrome sufferer and have not found relief, consider taking up yoga – it has been showing promising results. Very simple yoga exercises can be used to achieve the improved flexibility, strength, and endurance that can help relieve symptoms of carpal tunnel syndrome such as weakness, pain, or loss of sensation in the hands. The exercises should be done at the start and at the end of each day.

Yoga is an ancient form of exercise that can reduce stress and relieve muscular tension and pain. Stress is certainly one of the factors leading to musculo-skeletal disorders, including carpal tunnel syndrome. You may find that back pain, shoulder or neck tension, eye strain, or headaches may also be relieved with the practice of yoga. [Many gyms and health clubs now offer yoga classes as part of their regular exercise class programs.]

Sources: *Work* **2002;19(1);3-7;** *Lancet* **1999;353:691.**

262. AEROBICS FOR CARPAL TUNNEL SYNDROME

If you have carpal tunnel syndrome, starting an aerobic exercise program may be as good for your *hands* as it is for your heart. A 10-month aerobic exercise program significantly improves nerve function and reduces hand symptoms such as pain, tightness, and hand clumsiness in those suffering from carpal tunnel syndrome. Increased physical fitness and reduced body fat lead to improved blood circulation and oxygen delivery to tissues, which may improve nerve function.

Many people with carpal tunnel syndrome are overweight and physically inactive, suggesting a possible link between this problem and physical fitness. Other specific symptoms of carpal tunnel syndrome include numbness, tingling, and nocturnal awakening.

Source: *Journal of Occupational & Environmental Medicine* **2001;43:10:840.**

CARPAL TUNNEL SYNDROME: NATURAL REMEDIES & SUPPLEMENTS

263. VITAMIN B6 FOR CARPAL TUNNEL SYNDROME

Protect yourself from carpal tunnel syndrome by increasing your consumption of vitamin B6, as a low level of this vitamin may increase the risk of developing this condition. If you are already suffering from carpal tunnel syndrome, new research shows that taking vitamin B6 can help.

Because many different factors can affect vitamin B6 levels – including age, sex, weight, and certain diseases and medications – previous research was unable to detect the link between this vitamin and carpal tunnel syndrome.

Another factor contributing to the confusion is that many people who develop the problem start taking vitamins as treatment. But new research done with subjects who do not take vitamins confirms that low vitamin B6 levels increase the risk of symptoms.

[Although vitamin B6 (also known as pyridoxine) can be found in almost all foods, heating significantly decreases its bioavailability. So when foods are cooked, the B6 cannot be utilized optimally by your body. Heating also affects the *quality* of the vitamin, Dehydration and concentration result both in diminished quality and quantity of vitamin B6. Some of the best sources are brewer's yeast, carrots, chicken, eggs, fish, meat, spinach, and walnuts.]

Sources: *Journal of Occupational & Environmental Medicine Oct 1997; Dec 1997.*

WANT TO KNOW MORE?
Excessive computer keyboard force may contribute to the severity of hand and wrist symptoms in those suffering from carpal tunnel syndrome. People with symptoms tend to hit the keys harder than those not suffering from this condition.

The computer keyboard is not the only culprit. The problem is associated with many disease conditions and other work-related stressors. These include heavy equipment mechanics and sheet metal workers (who have the highest rates, by the way).

Construction workers may begin developing carpal tunnel syndrome before or during their apprenticeship. Few beginning construction workers seek medical attention for hand symptoms characteristic of carpal tunnel. But in terms of lost work time and restricted workdays, surgery, and rehabilitation, carpal tunnel syndrome is one of the most costly occupational musculo-skeletal disorders. (*American Journal of Industrial Medicine* **2002;42(2):107-16**)

CHILDHOOD ASTHMA

Asthma is the most common chronic disease in children. In the past 25 years, the prevalence of asthma has increased in children under the age of four by 160 percent and in children aged five to 14 by 74 percent. (*Archives of Pediatrics & Adolescent Medicine* 2002;156:269-275) This disease is significantly more common among children born to asthmatic mothers than among children born to non-asthmatic mothers. Breastfeeding for less than four months creates another risk factor. (*Journal of Allergy & Clinical Immunology* 2002;110:65-67) Current literature supports the use of self-management plans in childhood asthma. (*Nursing Standards* 2002;17(10):38-42)

IN THIS SECTION:
- ALTERNATIVE THERAPIES
- CAUSES & PRECURSORS
- DIETARY TACTICS
- NATURAL REMEDIES & SUPPLEMENTS
- REDUCING RISK
- TESTING FOR

CHILDHOOD ASTHMA: ALTERNATIVE THERAPIES
264. HYPNOSIS THERAPY FOR ASTHMATIC KIDS

Hypnosis may be helpful in the treatment of asthma symptoms, particularly in children. Studies have shown *significant* effects with the use of hypnosis. Relaxation-oriented self-hypnosis therapy seems to have positive effects in children. It results in reductions in symptom severity, as well as in emergency room visits.

Source: *Journal of Asthma* 2000;37:1-15.

CHILDHOOD ASTHMA: CAUSES & PRECURSORS
265. CHILDHOOD ASTHMA RISKS & ASSOCIATIONS

- Being part of a large family does *not* reduce the risk of developing asthma (although it does reduce the risk of developing hay fever and eczema).

- The more infections a child has had, the greater the likelihood of developing asthma. (Although having had measles offers a modest measure of *protection*.)

- Children with a history of allergy to pets are 24 times more likely to have asthma.

- Exposure to tobacco smoke, the use of a gas stove or oven for heat, or improperly used cooking devices in the home also increase the risk of asthma significantly.

- An increase in allergic disease and asthma has been recorded in many countries that have become more prosperous, and changes in the diet of pregnant women in these countries may result in the birth of children predisposed to allergy and asthma.

- Children with the lowest intakes of vitamin C are at a twofold increased risk of adult-onset wheezy illness, and a sevenfold increased risk of bronchial hyper-reactivity. Kids with the lowest intakes of vitamin E are at a fivefold increased risk of adult-onset wheezy illness.

- Kids with the lowest intakes of saturated fats have a tenfold *reduced* risk of developing bronchial hyper-reactivity.

- The elimination of household allergens and pollutants could potentially reduce asthma by 39 percent in young children.

Sources: *Pediatric Allergy & Immunology* 2000;11 (Suppl13):37-40; *Pediatrics* 2001;107:505-511; *Chest* 2002;122:304-396,409-414.

266. PLASTIC WALL COVERINGS & ASTHMA

Plastic wall coverings in homes may have adverse effects on lower respiratory tracts and place young children at risk for asthma. Plastic wall coverings are present in the homes of a significant number of children with symptoms of persistent wheezing, coughing, and phlegm. However, given the large number of chemicals present in plastics and other building materials, it is difficult to measure all of the relevant compounds in indoor air, so it is difficult to identify specific culprits in the plastic.

Source: *American Journal of Public Health* 2000;90:797-799.

CHILDHOOD ASTHMA: DIETARY TACTICS

267. KIWI FRUIT REDUCES WHEEZING IN KIDS

If you have a child suffering from wheezing or other asthma symptoms, fresh fruit rich in vitamin C, especially kiwi fruit, may help. The beneficial effect of fresh fruit on lung function has been observed in several studies. The consumption of fruit rich in vitamin C (such as kiwi fruit) shows a positive effect on wheezing and other respiratory symptoms, such as nocturnal cough or chronic cough. In most cases the protective effect is evident even among children who eat as little as one to two servings of fruit weekly. (The effect is somewhat stronger in those with a history of asthma.) Intake of fruit five to seven times a week is a highly significant protective factor against wheeze.

Although other dietary components cannot be excluded, the consumption of fruit rich in vitamin C, even at a low level of intake, may reduce wheezing symptoms in children, especially among already susceptible individuals.

But please note: while the temperature and storage time of kiwi fruit increases, vitamin C and chlorophyll content decrease.

Source: *Thorax* **2000;55:283-288;** *Archives of LatinoAmerican Nutrition* **1999;49(4):351-357.**

WANT TO KNOW MORE?
In asthmatic children who eat vitamin C-rich fruit once a week, the one-year occurrence of wheeze is 29.3 percent compared with 47.1 percent in similar children who eat fruit less than once a week.

268. NO MILK, SEAFOOD, OR PEANUTS FOR BABY

Protect your infant from asthma by keeping his/her diet free from cow's milk, seafood, and peanuts. The elimination of these three foods during the first year of a baby's life can cut the risk of developing asthma *dramatically*. Other suggested tips to reduce asthma risk:
~ breastfeed for at least four months
~ fit box springs and mattresses with vapor-impermeable covers
~ treat upholstery and carpets to control dust mites
~ remove furry pets from the home
~ do not smoke inside the home or anywhere in the presence of an infant.

Source: *Archives of Pediatric & Adolescent Medicine* **2000;154:657-663.**

269. SUGAR, FAT & CHILDHOOD ASTHMA

Another reason to watch your child's diet: A diet high in sugar and fat may be a contributing factor in the development of asthma in children with common allergies.
Children with airway hyper-responsiveness eat 23 percent more refined sugar and 25 percent more high-fat foods than do those without these symptoms. (This is an important finding because the prevalence of asthma has increased more than 66 percent since 1980.)

Obesity or excess weight also obstructs lung function in children with airway hyper-responsiveness. However, it has also been suggested that the children studied are eating differently because the healthier children are outside playing, while the children with the airway condition are sitting home and therefore more likely to snack.

Source: International Conference of the American Lung Association/American Thoracic Society, New Orleans, LA, 1996.

CHILDHOOD ASTHMA:
NATURAL REMEDIES & SUPPLEMENTS
270. PROBIOTICS AGAINST ASTHMA & ALLERGY

Probiotics given to both pregnant moms and infants can help protect children from a variety of allergic diseases. Given prenatally to mothers, as well as to children in infancy, probiotics can help to prevent many allergic diseases, including asthma, eczema, and rhinitis.

[Probiotics are food supplements that *promote* the growth and proliferation of healthful bacteria in your body, such as the *Lactobacillus acidophilus* found in viable, cultured yogurt.]

Pregnant women given probiotics during their pregnancy are half as likely to bear children with allergic eczema than are those women given a placebo, even though they may have a first-degree relative or partner with allergic eczema, allergic rhinitis, or asthma.

Sources: *Lancet* **2001;357(9262):1057-1059.**

WANT TO KNOW MORE?
Gut microflora may be an unexplored source of natural immunomodulators [substances affecting immune system function] for prevention of allergic diseases such as asthma, eczema, and allergic rhinitis. The increase in atopic [allergic] disease is attributed to a reduced microbial exposure in early life. Reversing allergic disease frequency would be an important breakthrough for health care and modern society.

CHILDHOOD ASTHMA:
REDUCING RISK
271. VENTILATE YOUR BABY'S BEDROOM

If you have an infant in the house, protect him/her from asthma by making sure the bedroom is properly ventilated. Poor indoor air quality may play an important role in the development of childhood asthma, with the air quality of the immediate sleeping environment of particular importance.

Infants exposed to home gas heating or environmental tobacco smoke have an increased risk of developing asthma. Infants whose parents do not smoke in the same room as them appear to be at lower risk. Ventilation of the infant's bedroom can have a significant effect.

Source: *Epidemiology 2000***;11:128-135.**

272. EXTENDED BREASTFEEDING PREVENTS ASTHMA

If you are breastfeeding, make sure to continue for at least four to six months (preferably nine) to protect your baby from developing asthma. Studies show that breastfeeding children for more than nine months protects against asthma and wheeze. Children breastfed for less than nine months are at higher risk of developing this increasingly common childhood ailment.

Children fed exclusively on breast milk (rather than other milk) for at least the first four months of life have a *significant* reduction in risk at the age of six. Asthma, wheezing, and wheeze-related sleep disturbances increase in those children introduced to other milk before the age of four months.

In addition, the potential for having at least one allergy is high. Increasing the breastfeeding rate can help to reverse the current trend of an increasing incidence of childhood asthma. Too many women in this country stop breast-feeding within a few weeks. [More health benefits of breastfeeding are discussed in detail in the *Pregnancy & Childbirth* section.]

Source: *Archives of Pediatric & Adolescent Medicine 2001;155:1261-1265.*

273. CAT ALLERGENS GO TO SCHOOL TOO

If you have an asthmatic child with a cat allergy, you should be aware that he/she may be exposed to high amounts of allergens even if your family does not own a pet. Asthmatic children who are allergic to cats may not have pets themselves, but indirect exposure to pet allergens clinging to classmates' clothing could increase their asthmatic symptoms. Children between the ages of six and 12 (with no furred pets of their own) in classes with many cat-owning students run a ninefold higher risk of increased asthma symptoms. But in classes with few cat owners, no such effects are seen. A cat owners' clothing is a major source of cat allergens. [If you are concerned seriously enough about your child's respiratory health, you may want to discuss this issue with your child's teacher or school principal.]

Source: *American Journal of Respiratory & Critical Care Medicine 2001;163:694-698.*

274. DON'T BUNK DOWN WITH CHILDHOOD ASTHMA

If your child sleeps in a lower bunk bed, and has any suggestion of respiratory problems or asthma, move that child to a single-unit bed. There is a tendency towards higher allergen levels in those who sleep in the bottom section of bunk beds. The prevalence of asthma is *significantly* higher in those who occupy the bottom bunks.

Source: *Annals of Allergy & Asthma Immunology 1999;82(6):531-3.*

275. FEATHER BEDDING BEST FOR ASTHMA

If you have a child with asthma or dust mite allergies, switch to feather pillows and bedding for his/her bed. The use of feather bed quilts is associated with reduced house dust mite levels and dust-mite sensitization. Feather bedding is also associated with less severe asthma and respiratory symptoms, as well as reduced wheezing episodes among children.

Mite-sensitive kids sleeping under non-feather bedding are *significantly* more likely to have severe symptoms, compared with non-sensitive kids sleeping under the same non-feather bedding.

There is also an inverse relationship between feather quilt use and both inhaled steroid medication use and hospital visits [that is, those kids with feather bedding are less likely to use medications or need to visit the emergency room for an asthmatic episode.]

The reason for the lower mite allergen levels in feather bedding is because of the more tightly woven casings used to contain the feathers.

Source: *Journal of Clinical Epidemiology* **2002;55:556-562.**

WANT TO KNOW MORE?
[See the *Allergies* section for more helpful information on protecting yourself and your family from house dust mites and their allergens, specifically Hints **#40, #41, and #42.**]

276. BUCKWHEAT PILLOWS LEAD TO ASTHMA

Here's another hint about kids and proper bedding: avoid buckwheat pillows! Small amounts of buckwheat flour found in buckwheat-husk pillows [a recently popular Japanese-style pillow] may induce buckwheat sensitization and nocturnal asthma in children sleeping on them.

Several children using these pillows for six months developed nighttime wheeze and cough, and the pillows were found to be the culprits. And although not sensitive to buckwheat prior to the pillow exposure, the children later showed positive skin reactions to buckwheat sensitivity skin tests. However, once the pillows were removed, night wheezing and awakening disappeared after the first day, and coughing gradually disappeared.

Asian folklore suggests that children and adults use such pillows as a traditional means to improve health and intelligence. But as buckwheat is a known food and occupational allergen, it may also be a hidden domestic allergen.

Source: *Allergy* **2001;56:703-704,763-766.**

277. PETS MAY *PROTECT* KIDS FROM ASTHMA

Pets may be more than just fun to have around; they may actually protect infants from childhood asthma and allergies. Swedish researchers have discovered that children exposed to dogs and cats during the first year of life have a lower frequency of allergic rhinitis (inflammation of nasal mucus membranes) at age seven to nine, and of asthma at age 12 to 13. In addition, children with early exposure to cats show fewer cat-positive skin tests when they are 12 to 13 years old.

Source: *Pediatric Allergy & Immunology* 2002;13(5):334-41.

CHILDHOOD ASTHMA: TESTING FOR

278. ONLINE TEST FOR DIAGNOSING ASTHMA

If you are not sure whether or not your child has asthma, go online to http:// allergy.mcg.edu, where a 21-question self-test can help you to determine the facts. This test was developed in response to the increasing prevalence of undiagnosed and untreated childhood asthma. This Kids' Asthma Check can be instrumental in controlling the disease and preventing long-term lung damage. The test is available in two versions, one of which is for children ages eight to 14 to answer themselves. The other is designed to be completed by parents of younger children.

Further details of the nationwide asthma-screening program are also available at the site.

WANT TO KNOW MORE?
Asthma frequently worsens during travel. Alternative therapies should be intensified if you are planning any trips with asthmatic children. (***Archives of Internal Medicine*** 2002;162:2421-2426) Respiratory problems are estimated to make up about 11 percent of in-flight emergencies. (***British Medical Journal*** 2002;325:1186-1187)

Heavy fetal exposure to acetaminophen (over-the-counter mild pain or fever treatments, such as tylenol) late in pregnancy may influence the inception of persistent wheezing in early childhood. This suggests that childhood asthma begins in utero. (***Thorax*** 2002;57:958-963)

The single best predictor for asthma is sensitivity to mite allergens. Such sensitivity is also seen in more than half of children with atopic eczema. (***Archives of Pediatric Adolescent Medicine*** 2002;156:1021-1027)

The risk for asthma is increased if Mom smoked during pregnancy. (***American Journal of Epidemiology*** 2002;156:954-961)

CHILDHOOD ILLNESSES & HEALTH PROBLEMS

It's no secret that we are raising a generation of overweight children and adolescents. It's also no surprise that this places our next generation of adults at risk for cardiovascular disease, among other serious problems. We're not going to change the obesity statistics overnight, but there are a few strategies that can help to keep our children in the best of health. We know, for example, that reducing obese children's sedentary activities has the same effect as increasing exercise. (*Archives of Pediatric & Adolescent Medicine* **2000;154:220-226**) Let's look at other good-health game plans.

IN THIS SECTION:
- BEHAVIORAL PROBLEMS
- CHILD SAFETY
- CHILDHOOD CANCER
- CHILDHOOD OBESITY & EXERCISE
- CONSTIPATION
- DRUG & MEDICATION CAVEATS
- EAR INFECTIONS
- INFANTS & TODDLERS
- NUTRITION

279. CHILDHOOD DISEASES, ADULT DISEASES

Illnesses and diseases in childhood increase the risk of diseases in adulthood, so if your child has a history of childhood illnesses, NOW is the time to maximize his or her health through lifestyle changes. Childhood infectious diseases such as scarlet fever, pneumonia, measles, and tuberculosis are strongly associated with the development of chronic obstructive lung disease in adulthood.

And those who have childhood noninfectious conditions – such as anemia, scoliosis, or heart murmurs – are found to have a higher incidence of cancer, arthritis, or rheumatism as adults.

Source: *Reuter's Health News* **Aug 2000.**

CHILDREN: BEHAVIORAL PROBLEMS
280. EYE PROBLEM MISDIAGNOSED AS ADHD?

If your child has attention deficit hyperactivity disorder (ADHD), have your eye doctor check for convergence insufficiency (an inability to keep both eyes focused on a close target), a problem now associated with this syndrome. It is not known whether children are being misdiagnosed with ADHD when they really have convergence insufficiency or vice versa. Nor is it known if medications used for ADHD cause convergence insufficiency. In any case, checking this potential association is a good idea.

Convergence insufficiency makes it more difficult to concentrate on reading, which is also one of the ways doctors diagnose ADHD. Convergence insufficiency may not be well known outside the field of eye care specialists.

Source: Meeting of the American Academy of Pediatric Ophthalmology & Strabismus, San Diego, CA, Apr 2000.

281. GET THE LEAD OUT!

If you child suffers from developmental or behavioral problems, have him/her tested for exposure to lead. Children with developmental and behavioral problems appear to have high blood concentrations of lead, so kids with such difficulties should be tested for lead toxicity. The good news is that lead is a *treatable* toxin, and inexpensive and simple control measures can be effective in reducing children's blood lead concentrations.

To avoid the problem, here are a few precautions:

~ Children should not have access to ceramics, as the use of glazed ceramic dishes can be a risk for lead toxicity.
~ Food should not be stored in glazed ceramics.
~ Don't allow children to play in areas that are exposed to automobile exhaust.
~ Invest in a good water filter to filter out lead from faucets.

Studies with animals show that the developing nervous system is more susceptible to lead exposure, and humans are more sensitive to lead than many test animals.

Sources: *Archives of Diseases of Childhood* 2001;85:286-288; *Occupational Medicine* 2001; 16(4):563-575; *Toxicology* 2001;165(2-3):121-131.

282. BETTER NUTRITION = BETTER BEHAVIOR

Young adults who consume adequate amounts of essential nutrients are less likely to engage in antisocial behavior, including violence. Dating as far back as 1942, there is evidence linking nutritional deficits to antisocial behavior. Young adult prisoners who received supplements of vitamins, minerals, and essential fatty acids committed fewer offenses than those who received a placebo. No reduction was seen in a placebo group at all. So the dietary requirements for good health may also be supportive of social behavior.

[Although prisoners were used in this study, it is obvious that meeting nutrient requirements can help many of us in terms of our behavioral reactions.]

Source: *British Journal of Psychology* 2002;181:22-28.

CHILDREN: SAFETY

283. KEEP NEWBORNS LYING DOWN

Keep newborn infants out of car seats, swings, or other upright seating devices for the first month or two of life, as such a position can affect their ability to breathe properly. Babies need to be watched when they are in a position that is not natural for them. Only 15 minutes in an upright position can cause an infant's oxygen saturation levels to decline *significantly*. Babies breathe better when they are lying down.

If an infant is slouched down, they do not have any way of pulling themselves out of that position. This is particularly important if the baby has a cold, is having problems spitting up, or is sitting in a seat for a long period of time.

Preterm infants are at additional health risks when sitting in an upright position before they are ready, and this time period should be extended for these babies until they have attained good head and neck control.

Source: *Pediatrics* **2001;108:647-652.**

284. PUT BABIES TO SLEEP ON THEIR BACKS

Protect babies from Sudden Infant Death Syndrome (SIDS) by always putting them to sleep on their *backs*, rather than their stomachs or sides. Research has found that babies normally put to sleep on their backs who are then put to sleep on their stomachs have a higher rate of death from SIDS. In addition, keep the baby's room sufficiently warm but keep pillows, stuffed animals, and other soft objects OUT of the crib.

SIDS is believed to affect babies who already have existing, underlying health problems — such as a difficulty regulating breathing, body temperature, or blood pressure. When such infants are placed face down in a crib, they can breathe the carbon dioxide-rich air that collects under their nose, possibly resulting in death.

Source: *Journal of the American Medical Association* **2002;288(21).**

WANT TO KNOW MORE?
There are approximately 3,000 SIDS deaths annually in the US, most occurring between the ages of two to four months. Other factors that contribute to risk of death from SIDS include low birth weight, insufficient prenatal care, a mother who smokes, drinks alcohol, or uses drugs while pregnant, smoking in the baby's presence, and a mother who is younger than 20 years of age.

285. KEEP BABIES OUT OF ADULT BEDS

Make sure never to place an infant alone in an adult bed, which can put them at risk of accidental death from falls or suffocation. Between 1999 and 2001, more than 100 infants under the age of two died while sleeping in a bed made for adults. Many parents believe that pushing a bed against a wall or surrounding a napping baby with pillows makes it a safe place for infants to sleep, but this places them at risk of suffocation.

Babies have been found suspended between the mattress and the wall, and have also died by falling from a bed and suffocating on piles of clothing or plastic bags.

Needless to say, when the parents are in the bed with the baby, that's another story.

If using a crib, parents should be sure to use only the mattress that came with the crib and be certain the set-up has a tight-fitting sheet.

Source: US Consumer Product Safety Commission, reported in *Reuter's Medical Health* Sep 2002.

286. SOCCER RISKS FOR KIDS

If you have a child who plays soccer, you should be aware that this activity could lead to a variety of cognition problems. Studies suggest long-term brain deficits among soccer players. These athletes score *significantly* lower on tests that measure visual and verbal memory, visual analysis and planning, and mental flexibility.

Soccer has been growing in popularity in the US, but it is not 100 percent safe. "Heading" a soccer ball does not usually cause enough trauma to injure a player's head, but such trauma may result from player collisions.

According to the American Youth Soccer Organization, children under 10 should never head the ball.

Source: *Reuter's Medical Report*, Physician's Online, May 2002.

287. CHECK WEIGHT OF YOUR CHILD'S BACKPACK

Check the weight and construction of your child's school backpack to see if it is too heavy, which could potentially lead to back problems. Back pain complaints from children rise with increasing use of heavy backpacks. A backpack that weighs more than 20 percent of your child's body weight could potentially cause injury, and should be replaced with one equipped with a frame and hip straps to keep the heavy weight off the spine and shoulders.

Because some schools have eliminated lockers for security reasons, backpacks are more and more common. Wide padded shoulder straps, a padded back and a hip strap, or even a backpack on wheels, make good sense for children who must carry heavy loads.

Source: American Academy of Orthopedic Surgeons, reported in *Reuter's Medical News* Oct 1999.

288. CELL PHONES PUT KIDS AT RISK

Think twice before giving mobile phones to kids – there is evidence that the radiation such phones emit has subtle biological effects, including memory loss and even Alzheimer's, and children may be at higher risk. An independent expert group in Great Britain comprised of medical and engineering teams recommends "a precautionary approach" to cell phone use. They claim that mobile phone use could be linked to memory loss and even Alzheimer's disease.

Children may be more vulnerable because of their developing nervous system, the greater absorption of energy in the tissue of the head, and a longer lifetime of exposure.

The group advises that widespread use of mobile phones by children for non-essential calls be discouraged.

The researchers also advise that signs be placed around hospitals warning people to switch off phones while on the grounds so as not to affect hospital equipment.

And they also advise consumers not to rely on mobile phone shields as protection against radiation until scientific research is conducted into their efficacy.

Source: Report of the Independent Expert Group on Mobile Phones (IEGMP). The full text of the report is available at www.iegmp.org.uk.

CHILDREN: CANCER

289. HEAD & NECK CANCERS ON THE RISE

Make sure your kids are consuming an adequate amount of antioxidants in the form of fresh vegetable or nutritional supplements, to protect them from the alarming increase in head and neck cancers seen in American children. Childhood cancer has been on the rise over the past couple of decades in the US and elsewhere, but cancers of the head and neck appear to be outpacing other cancers among American children.

Well-established environmental factors implicated in pediatric head and neck cancers include:
- ~ exposure to ionizing radiation
- ~ excessive sunlight
- ~ certain chemotherapy drugs.
- ~ environmental pollution, infection
- ~ parental exposure to toxins are also suspected.

Premature birth and low birth weight have also been associated with a higher-than-average risk of childhood cancer.

Lymphoma is the most common type of head and neck cancer, affecting 27 percent of children in the national database. The next most common cancers include neural tumors, thyroid malignancies and soft tissue sarcomas.

Source: *Archives of Otolaryntology of the Head & Neck Surgery* **2002;128:655-659.**

WANT TO KNOW MORE?
[See Hint #212 for information on children and leukemia.]

CHILDREN:
CHILDHOOD OBESITY & EXERCISE
290. GIRLS, OBESITY & HIGH CHOLESTEROL

We know that obesity causes high cholesterol, but at least for girls, high cholesterol may be a marker of obesity to come. It appears that a high level of cholesterol in girls ages five and six acts as a marker of altered metabolism, and the body mass index of high-cholesterol girls increases at a greater rate than in girls with normal cholesterol. By age 11 to 12, 45.2 percent of high-cholesterol girls are overweight or obese, compared with 21.6 percent of normal-cholesterol girls.

This effect is *not* observed in boys.

Associations between weight and risk factors for cardiovascular disease (such as blood pressure, insulin, and blood lipids) are more pronounced with age, and in some cases are stronger in high-cholesterol children and girls. Increased relative weight, even at an early age, can increase these risk factors.

Source: *American Journal of Clinical Nutrition* **2002;76:730-735.**

WANT TO KNOW MORE?
[See the *High Cholesterol* section for many helpful tips on combating this condition.]

291. EXERCISE & ASTHMATIC/OBESE KIDS

Participation in an exercise program can be very beneficial – both physically *and* psychologically – for asthmatic or overweight kids. Children who have asthma or who are obese (or both) are more fit and report a better sense of well-being after just two months in a structured exercise program. After eight weeks of biweekly 40-minute workouts, children ages 10 to 15 show statistically significant gains in flexibility, strength, and aerobic fitness.

Activities include careful warm-ups and cool-downs to help prevent asthma episodes, as well as martial arts, weight lifting, and step aerobics.

After workouts, the children sit in a circle for a 20-minute "rap session," which includes discussion of coping with asthma and obesity.

Source: *Reuter's Health Report* **Mar 2000.**

WANT TO KNOW MORE?
[If you child is asthmatic, see the *Childhood Asthma* section for lots of helpful information on this condition.]

292. SPORTY GIRLS = FITTER WOMEN

Girls who participate in organized sports during childhood and adolescence are more likely to be physically active as adults — and therefore, less likely to be obese. Promoting the involvement of girls in athletics may be an avenue to prevent obesity, which is essential given the difficulty of obesity treatment today.

Since not all girls are interested, or have the skills necessary to participate in traditional competitive sports, programs that target these girls in particular would be beneficial.

[Although boys are more likely to be involved in sports, some kind of physical activity should also be encouraged for more inactive boys. And let's not forget that we all learn better by example — so, at the very least, get out and take a walk with your kids on a daily basis. Make it mandatory.]

Source: *Preventive Medicine* **2002;34:82-89.**

293. INCREASING BONE DENSITY IN KIDS

Physical activity can help to increase bone density in children as young as four years of age. Preschoolers who are the most active have five percent greater hipbone density compared to the least active. And increased television viewing is associated with lower bone-mineral content and bone-mineral density, particularly in girls.

Parents are encouraged to do everything possible to help their children optimize bone development, so that they will be better able to preserve their skeletons later in life. Peak bone mass is a major determinant of osteoporosis in later years, and peak bone mass is largely determined by age 20. Activities such as jumping, running, and tumbling should be encouraged.

Source: *Pediatrics* **2001;107:1387-1393.**

WANT TO KNOW MORE?
[For more information on improving bone density, especially as it pertains to adults, see the *Osteoporosis & Other Skeletal Problems* section.]

CHILDREN: CONSTIPATION

294. ACUPUNCTURE FOR CONSTIPATED KIDS

If you have a child who is suffering from chronic constipation, acupuncture might be able to help. The frequency of bowel movements in children with long-lasting constipation improves after only 10 acupuncture sessions, performed once a week. However, for some reason, the frequency of bowel movements in boys increases more gradually compared with girls receiving the same treatment.

[Despite the use of ultra-fine needles, unlike injections, acupuncture is completely painless and few children are bothered by the experience.]

Source: *Digestive Diseases & Science* Jun 2001;46(6):1270-1275.

295. FIBER FOR CONSTIPATED KIDS

Protect your kids from childhood constipation by making sure they are getting adequate amounts of daily fiber. Children with daily fiber intakes below minimum recommended levels are at risk for chronic constipation. To calculate this minimum amount, start with five grams of fiber and add another gram for each year of the child's age (so a seven year old, for example, would require at least 12 grams of fiber daily). Constipated children also tend to have a lower caloric and nutrient intake, lower body weight, and a higher prevalence of reported anorexia.

Sources: *Journal of Pediatric Gastroenterology Nutrition* Aug 1999;29(2):132-135; *Journal of Pediatric Gastroenterology & Nutrition* Feb 1999;28(2):169-174.

WANT TO KNOW MORE?
[Foods we believe to be high in fiber, including many fruits and vegetables, actually offer very little fiber. See my book, *New Facts About Fiber*, for a good introduction to this subject.]

CHILDREN: DRUG & MEDICATION CAVEATS

296. HOW TO SWALLOW A PILL

Here are a few hints for the recalcitrant pill, tablet, or supplement swallower (child *or* adult):

~ Coat tablets with butter, and they will slide down more easily.
~ Place tablets in applesauce or some mashed banana.
~ Grind the tablets and mix them into food or liquid.
~ And credit for the best trick of all goes to my mom, who practiced this for years at the dinner table before finally convincing any of her family members (including me!) to try it: Put some salad or other food in your mouth and while chewing, slip the pill in on one side. The pill will magically disappear down the hatch! Once you and your children master this technique, you will never need liquids or other tricks for swallowing tablets again.

Children should be taught that the food available to us no longer has all the nutrients needed for optimal health, and taking supplements is an attempt to replace what should have been there to begin with.

And here's a helpful trick for getting eye drops into the eyes of children: Drop the eye drop into a *closed* eye – when the child blinks a few times, most of the drop will reach the eye.

297. FEVER IS A SYMPTOM, NOT AN ILLNESS

If your child has a fever, do not overdo efforts to reduce it – such as overdosing him/her with anti-fever drugs. The idea that fever is a disease rather than a symptom or sign of illness leads to many children being overdosed with anti-fever medication, as well as being given other unnecessary and harmful treatments. "Fever phobia" is a problem we can't seem to shake. Ninety percent of parents report concern about fever. In fact, many even fear death if fever is not normalized. Fourteen percent of parents were found to give Tylenol every three hours or less, and 44 percent to give Motrin every five hours or less – both of which are NOT recommended doses for these medications.

Other problematic behaviors include waking children to give them drugs, checking temperature every hour or even more frequently, and administering sponge baths with cool water or alcohol. Fever actually plays a positive role in the get-well process.

Source: *Pediatrics* 2001;107:1241-1246.

298. DON'T ALTERNATE ANTI-FEVER DRUGS!

If your child has a fever, be careful not to alternate between anti-fever drugs. Acetaminophen and ibuprofen are commonly given by pediatricians in an alternating manner to treat fever in children, but this practice may actually cause harm.

Fifty percent of pediatricians advise parents to alternate acetaminophen and ibuprofen for children with fever. However, there is *no* scientific data indicating that this is a beneficial thing to do – but there *is* data indicating that this is potentially harmful.

Source: *Pediatrics* **2000;105:1009-1012.**

WANT TO KNOW MORE?
[As discussed in Hint #297, fever is *not* something to be afraid of (something that most people involved in alternative medicine already know). Fever is a signal that something is wrong and is often an indication that the immune system is working. That doesn't mean it should be neglected, but parents should learn about safe ways to bring fever down only if it is dangerously high.]

299. ANALGESICS & COLA = HEADACHES

The most common reasons for headaches in children and adolescents: the misuse or prolonged use of analgesics, and the consumption of cola. When analgesics have ceased being effective for a child's headache, medical experts say that the child must no longer be given the drug. Children who consume more than 1.5 liters of cola a day may suffer from caffeine-induced daily headaches. Withdrawal headache can be avoided if children stop drinking cola gradually.

Source: 2000 World Headache Conference, London, England.

WANT TO KNOW MORE?
[For many more helpful tips on headaches, including some natural and alternative remedies, see the *Headaches & Migraines* section.]

CHILDREN: EAR INFECTIONS

300. EAR INFECTIONS & ANTIBIOTICS

Think twice about giving your child an antibiotic for an ear infection: the percentage of middle ears that contain no harmful bacteria is as high as 70 percent. Five percent of people polled think that antibiotics will also be helpful for other conditions such as colds, flu, herpes, measles, and tonsillitis, but these are all *viral*, not bacterial.

Source: *Archives of Otolaryngology* **1988.**

301. PACIFIERS CAN CAUSE EAR INFECTIONS

Limit pacifier use to the moment when an infant falls asleep to decrease his/her risk of developing acute *otitis media* [infection and inflammation of the middle ear space and eardrum]. Otitis media is a frequent cause of fever and discomfort in young children, and can even lead to diminished hearing. Children who do not use a pacifier continuously have 33 percent fewer episodes than children who do.

To prevent otitis media, researcher recommend that ideally children use a pacifier freely until the age of six months, only when falling asleep or on special occasions between the ages of six and 10 months, and then decrease or stop use after 10 months. *Limiting* pacifier use, rather than complete stoppage, appears to be enough to prevent disease.

Source: *Pediatrics* **2000;106:483-488.**

CHILDREN: INFANTS & TODDLERS

302. THE DANGERS OF DISPOSABLE DIAPERS

Use cloth diapers instead of disposable ones: they may be linked to both respiratory illnesses such as asthma and to problems with male fertility. Chemical emissions from disposable diapers cause pulmonary irritation and other symptoms in test animals. Analysis of these emissions revealed several chemicals with documented respiratory toxicity. So disposable diapers should be considered as one of the factors that might cause or exacerbate asthmatic conditions, in both children and parents. In fact, asthmatic mothers are advised not to handle them at all.

The increased use of disposable, plastic-lined diapers may also be directly related to a decline in male fertility in recent decades. Scrotal temperature is significantly higher when infant boys wear disposable diapers, indicating that the natural testicular cooling mechanism is greatly affected by the insulating properties of modern plastic-lined diapers. (Increased testicular temperature in infancy can have an impact on later sperm production.) Be especially wary about disposable diapers when a child has fever.

Sources: *Archives of Environmental Health* **1999;54:353-358;** *Archives of Diseases of Childhood* **2000;83:281-282,364-368.**

303. PROTECT YOUR BABY FROM RICKETS

Protect infants from the alarming increase in rickets by giving them supplemental vitamin D, as well as avoiding the use of sunscreen. The prevalence of rickets in infants and toddlers appears to be on the rise, due in part to an increase in the use of sunscreen, a warning that adults should pay attention to as well. [Rickets is a deficiency disease that affects developing bones.]

Cases of rickets have occurred in children who were exclusively breastfed for at least seven to 19 months and who did not receive vitamin D supplementation. (Human milk, unfortunately, has very little vitamin D.) One reason for the apparent increase in rickets may be the trend toward protecting babies from sunlight [which, without supplementation, may be their only major source of vitamin D].

To offset the increasing rickets trend, the American Academy of Pediatrics (AAP) will probably recommend that all breastfed infants receive vitamin D supplements.

Source: American Academy of Pediatrics meeting, Chicago, Oct 2000.

WANT TO KNOW MORE?
[I have long been against the use of sunscreen, and an advocate of a half hour of sunlight daily, which can also be preventive against many other diseases, including cancer, multiple sclerosis, and osteoporosis. See Hints #163, #730, and #800 for more details.]

304. WALK AWAY FROM BABY WALKERS

Parents: Keep your babies out of baby walkers, as they can significantly delay your infant's locomotor development. Infants who use baby walkers have delayed normal development of locomotor milestones [those important first steps!], as well as an increased risk of injury. Parents and grandparents of young children should be aware of the associations between the amount of baby-walker use and the extent of developmental delay – including raising the head, rolling over, sitting with support, sitting alone, crawling, standing with support, walking with support, standing alone, and walking alone.

Because baby walkers enable infants to "walk" long before they are able, they are often viewed in terms of early enrichment. But walkers actually *prevent* the baby from seeing their own moving limbs, which normally plays a critical role in the development of their motor systems. Each 24-hour use of a baby walk is associated with a 3.3-day delay in walking alone, and a 3.7-day delay in standing alone.

And infants between six and 15 months who use walkers also score lower on mental development as well as motor development, so it appears that the risks of baby walkers far outweigh the benefits.

Source: *British Medical Journal* 2002;324:1494.

305. LACTOBACILLUS PROTECTS BABY'S SKIN

Children from families with a history of atopic disease [allergic skin rashes] may be protected by the early administration of probiotics. Atopic dermatitis is a long-lasting disease that affects the skin. Atopic refers to a group of diseases that run in families and often occur together – including asthma, allergies such as hay fever, and atopic dermatitis. (In atopic dermatitis, the skin becomes extremely itchy and inflamed, causing redness, swelling, cracking, weeping, crusting, and scaling.)

Eczema is the main sign of atopic disease in the first years of life. Scientists estimate that 65 percent of patients develop symptoms in their first year, and 90 percent develop symptoms before the age of five. People who live in urban areas and in climates with low humidity seem to be at an increased risk for developing atopic dermatitis.

But we now have the validation that probiotics such as *Lactobacillus acidophilus* can protect very young children whose parents have the disease. [Liquid *acidophilus* is found in the refrigerated section of most health food stores.]

Source: *Lancet* **2001;357:1057-1059,1076-1079.**

WANT TO KNOW MORE?
[Probiotics are helpful against a host of maladies. I have been recommending the use of large amounts of *Lactobacillus acidophilus* for years to teenagers suffering with acne, and have endless reports of great success. See Hint #352 in the *Dermatological Conditions* section for more information.]

306. INFANTS, TODDLERS & DENTAL HEALTH

Healthy teeth begin to be formed long before they emerge, so it's a good idea to wet some gauze or a little towel and wipe your baby's mouth, palette and gum pads to reduce plaque and to start building dental habits. Your child's first visit to the dentist should be within six months of the first tooth. When your baby's molars come in, it's time to start thinking about a toothbrush.

Toothpaste can be used after age two [although a moistened toothbrush can serve the same purpose without introducing the possible toxins or additives used in toothpaste]. Healthy teeth mean trips that are more pleasant for your child – *and* the dentist. Thumb- and pacifier-sucking habits will generally only become a problem if they go on for a very long period of time, and most children stop these habits on their own. One last helpful note: Try to avoid expressing your own anxieties about going to the dentist in front of your children, as it can cause them to form negative attitudes early on.

Source: American Academy of Pediatric Dentistry, Chicago, IL.

WANT TO KNOW MORE?
The higher the oral bacteria count in you, the higher the percentage of your oral bacteria affecting your child. [See the *Dental Disorders* section for helpful tips on adult dental health, including a simple and natural way to reduce cavities.]

307. VITAMIN D FOR BABY GIRLS

If there is an infant girl in your family, encourage vitamin D supplementation because it will increase her bone density later in life. Girls who receive vitamin D supplements during their infancy have increased bone-mineral content and bone-mineral density later in childhood [and therefore a decreased risk of osteoporosis and other skeletal health problems later in life].

Source: *The Journal of Clinical Endocrinology & Metabolism.*

308. VITAMIN D FOR YOUNG GIRLS TOO

Help ensure that young girls attain their peak bone mass by making sure to give them supplemental vitamin D. Pubertal girls who are vitamin D deficient seem to be at risk for not reaching maximum peak bone mass, particularly in lumbar [lower] region of the spine. Either dietary enrichment or supplementation with vitamin D should therefore be considered for pre-pubertal girls, to ensure an adequate vitamin D status.

[Unfortunately, very few foods contain vitamin D. Some good dietary sources are dairy products, eggs, and fish liver oils. Exposure to sunlight also allows the body to produce vitamin D.]

Source: *American Journal of Clinical Nutrition* Dec 2002;76(6):1446-1453.

WANT TO KNOW MORE?
[As mentioned in Hint #307, supplemental vitamin D is also recommended for baby girls as well, to help increase bone density later in life. In addition, vitamin D may also help to protect *all* children from the alarming increase in rickets in this country, as explained in Hint #303.]

309. MUSIC HEARD IN WOMB IS REMEMBERED

Children recognize and prefer music they are exposed to while in the womb, for at least one year after birth. All babies seem to show a significant preference for the pieces of music they were exposed to in utero over very similar tunes that they had not previously heard.

It has been demonstrated that the fetus is able to hear fully as early as 20 weeks after conception, and babies can remember and prefer music they heard before they were born even 12 months after birth. This preference is based on long-term memory.

These results indicate that environmental factors experienced by the fetus may have a long-term influence on its development, and that the prenatal period is more important than previously thought.

Source: School of Psychology at the University of Leicester, England, reported in *Reuter's Medical* Jul 2001.

WANT TO KNOW MORE?
When some babies recognized a tune, they turned to their mothers, indicating that the music played some sort of role in developing an emotional bond.

CHILDREN: NUTRITION

310. KIDS & NUTRIENT DEFICIENCIES

Make sure to monitor your child's diet, and consider adding nutritional supplements if you suspect they are missing out on key nutrients. Zinc deficiency is most likely to occur in children who get most of their nutrition from milk and cheese.

[A deficiency in zinc can result in many health problems, including acne, frequent colds and flu, greater susceptibility to infection, hair loss, and growth impairment.]

Vitamin A deficiencies most often show up in adolescents who live on meat, potatoes, and fast foods, and who shun vegetables and eggs.

[A vitamin A deficiency can also result in acne, frequent colds, and growth impairment, as well as night blindness.]

Source: J. Beasley, J. Swift, *The Kellogg Report*, The Bard College Center, 1989;144.

311. FRUIT JUICES SHOULD BE LIMITED

A warning to parents: Avoid giving your kids too much fruit juice, as it can cause nutritional and gastrointestinal problems. In its most extensive policy statement to date on fruit juice consumption, the American Academy of Pediatrics recommends that fruit juice consumption be limited to four to six ounces a day for children between the ages of one and six, and eight to 12 ounces for children between the ages of seven and 18. [Adults should not be consuming fruit juices in quantity, either.]

Fruit juice should not be given to infants before six months of age and, after six months, infants should not be given juice from bottles or cups that allow them to consume juice easily throughout the day.

In addition, infants should not receive fruit juice at bedtime. Fruit juice does not contain any significant amounts of protein, fat, minerals or vitamins other than vitamin C – but it does contain a large amount of carbohydrate, which can result in diarrhea, abdominal pain, bloating and flatulence. Most juices do not contain fiber, so they offer no real nutritional advantage over whole fruits.

Source: *Pediatrics* **2001.**

WANT TO KNOW MORE?
Fruit juice consumption can also cause tooth decay if children are allowed to hold a bottle, cup, or box of juice in their mouth throughout the day or at bedtime. [See Hint #338 in the *Dental Disorders* section for more information about this.]

COLDS & FLU

Minor illnesses, such as colds and influenza, are frequent, widespread, and a major cause of absenteeism from work and school. Colds and flu have selective effects on performance; even sub-clinical infections can produce performance impairments; performance may be impaired during the incubation period of the illness; and performance impairments may still be observed after the clinical symptoms are gone.

When it comes to colds and the flu, there's a high level of self-care. Only about one percent of the population see a physician when they have a cold. So prescription use is low; over-the-counter drugs high! (*Canadian Family Physician* **1999;45:2644-6, 2649-52**) Approximately 50 percent of episodes of the common cold are caused by rhinoviruses. Bacterial infections are rare, supporting the concept that the common cold is almost exclusively a viral disease.

312. COLD OR FLU? HERE'S A CLUE

Coming down with something? Here's how to tell whether you have a cold or whether you have the flu. In general, a cold starts gradually. At worst you will have a slight temperature for 24 hours. Your appetite is normal, and your headaches are minimal. Prominent symptoms are sneezing, a runny nose, and a sore throat. There are about 400 different viruses that cause the common cold, and the average person catches three to four colds a year.

The flu, in contrast, starts rapidly. Your temperature increases quickly and lasts for up to five days. Your headaches can be severe, and your joints and muscle also ache. You lose your appetite and feel nauseous, often vomiting. Whereas people with a cold feel tired, those with the flu feel *exhausted*.

Source: *The Times Online,* **Times Newspaper, Ltd., Jan 2002, reported by the** *British Medical Journal* **Jan 2002.**

313. DON'T SHAKE HANDS WITH A VIRUS

Be careful about shaking hands with lots of people, a common way to catch a cold. The cold virus is more easily transmitted through contact with the nose and eyes than through the mouth, so it's not as important to focus on not sharing drinks or utensils, or not kissing someone with a cold.

Colds are caused by contact with a *virus*, so you can't catch one by not wearing enough clothes in cold weather or by going outside with wet hair. And because colds are viral, and not bacterial, antibiotics are useless against them.

Source: **Annual Meeting of the Infectious Diseases Society of America, San Francisco, CA, Oct 2001.**

314. ASPIRIN & ACETAMINOPHEN NO HELP

If you come down with a cold, do not take aspirin or acetaminophen for it. Several studies show that these medications may *increase*, rather than decrease, symptoms of a cold. The use of aspirin and acetaminophen is associated with the suppression of neutralizing immune responses, and aspirin is associated with an increase of nasal symptoms such as nasal obstruction in the presence of a rhinovirus (a cold).

Children infected with chickenpox who received a placebo rather than acetaminophen recovered faster than did children who were given the true medication.

Source: *Southern Medical Journal* **2001;94(1):26-32.**

315. PROBIOTICS AGAINST COLDS

Including probiotics with your multivitamin and minerals supplements can be an even better way to avoid the common cold. The beneficial effects of multivitamins and minerals on the immune system are enhanced when probiotics are added. [Probiotics are food supplements that *promote* the growth and proliferation of healthful bacteria in your body, such as the *Lactobacillus acidophilus* found in viable, cultured yogurt.] People taking vitamin and mineral supplements as well as probiotics had significantly fewer colds compared with those who took only the vitamin and mineral supplements alone.

Source: *The Times Online*, **Times Newspaper, Ltd., Jan 2002, reported by the** *British Medical Journal* **Jan 2002.**

316. ECHINACEA & THE COMMON COLD

At the first signs of a cold, start taking echinacea, a common herbal supplement that is indeed helpful in reducing the length of the common cold. People who take echinacea are sick for fewer days, compared with those taking placebos. In addition, almost two-thirds of those taking echinacea feel that their cold was "shorter than usual."

Source: *Arzneimittel-Forschung/Drug Research* **2001;51:563-568.**

317. KNOCK IT OUT WITH MYCELIZED VITAMIN A

High-level doses of mycelized vitamin A at the first sign of a cold or flu can help to knock out the infection right from the start. Vitamin A is a potent all-around immune stimulant that helps to maintain the integrity of the cells lining the lungs. Several alternative physicians recommend 200,000 to 300,000 IU daily *for two to three days only* to stop the infection before it can take hold. [Since large doses of vitamin A may be toxic, it is imperative to use the high doses only for a few days. If you are under a doctor's care, you may be told to use higher doses for longer to knock out the infection.]

High-level vitamin A enhances T-helper cells and other immune functions. Smaller doses can be effective for bacterial and parasitic infections, but larger doses in this particular form of vitamin A are essential for this nutrient to work in the presence of a cold or flu virus.

Source: *Journal of Nutrition* **2000;130(5):1132-9.**

318. CRANBERRY JUICE TO AVOID THE FLU

If you are concerned about a flu bug that seems to be going around, drinking cranberry juice may help reduce your risk of coming down with it. A substance found in cranberry juice (proanthocyanidins) appears to have an inhibitory effect on several varieties of influenza, and may also reduce the risk of respiratory infections in children.

One caveat: We know that eating fruits and vegetables is healthful, but excessive consumption of fruit juices can contribute to obesity, the development of cavities, diarrhea and other gastrointestinal problems, such as excessive gas, bloating and abdominal pain.

Source: **Annual Meeting of the Infectious Diseases Society of America, Chicago, IL, Oct 2002.**

WANT TO KNOW MORE?
[Cranberry juice is also a great natural remedy for urinary tract infections. See Hint #994 for more information.]

CONSTIPATION

Constipation is a common condition affecting millions of people throughout the world. Americans alone spend more than $300 million a year on constipation remedies. As you will see, the solution is so simple and so inexpensive! As for causes, intake of fiber below the minimum recommendation is a risk factor. (*Journal of Pediatric Gastroenterology* **1999;29(2):132-5**) Dementia and being bed- or chair-bound also greatly increase the risk of chronic constipation. Excessive laxative use is another cause. (*Nursing Times* **1997;93(4):35-6**)

Despite common medical advice to consume extra fluid for constipation, extra fluid intake in normal healthy people does *not* produce a significant increase in stool output. (*Journal of Clincial Gastro-enterology* **1999 Jan;28(1):29-32**)

[For a helpful tip on alleviating constipation in seniors, see Hint #14. For tips on constipation in children, see Hints #294 and #295.]

IN THIS SECTION:
* DIETARY TACTICS
* NATURAL REMEDIES & SUPPLEMENTS

CONSTIPATION: DIETARY TACTICS

319. ADDING FIBER IS THE KEY

If you are constipated, make sure you are getting enough dietary fiber, as drinking lots of water and other fluids will have no effect without it. Constipation is a common health phenomenon, associated with our modern habits of diet and lifestyle. It is one of the most chronic digestive disorders, *but* it can be overcome overnight. Many studies show that lack of fiber and insufficient water intake are the causes of constipation. However, in the absence of fiber, fluid is simply absorbed from the bowel and excreted in urine. High-fiber foods provide moisture-retaining bulk so that waste matter in your colon won't become dry and tightly packed.

Some food that encourage constipation: over-processed foods, cheese, meat, boiled milk, hot drinks, foods containing tannin (tea, cocoa, red wine), cloves, hard-boiled eggs. Foods that absorb moisture readily: celery, radishes, carrots, and lettuce.

Foods that are slightly laxative: raw figs, raw spinach, strawberries, sesame seeds, watermelon, garlic (prescribed for constipation by Hippocrates 2,500 years ago), dandelion leaf tea, flaxseed, brewer's yeast, rice polishings, and the herb cascara sagrada.

Source: B. Kamen, *New Facts About Fiber.*

320. BUCKWHEAT FOR CONSTIPATION

If you are constipated, eating buckwheat may help to alleviate the problem. Buckwheat proteins have a unique amino acid composition with special biological actions that improve constipation by acting as a dietary fiber. These same proteins can also help to lower cholesterol and blood pressure, and even help to control obesity. Buckwheat has also been shown to improve diabetes.

One caveat: If not cooked thoroughly, buckwheat can cause digestive problems.

Source: *Critical Review of Food & Scientific Nutrition 2001;41(6):451-464.*

CONSTIPATION: NATURAL REMEDIES & SUPPLEMENTS

321. PREBIOTICS & PROBIOTICS TO THE RESCUE

If you are suffering from chronic constipation, try adding prebiotics and probiotics to your diet to improve your overall gastrointestinal health. There is a high level of evidence that some pre- and probiotics can alleviate constipation, as well as colon cancer, intestinal infection, inflammatory bowel disease, lactose intolerance, antibiotic-associated intestinal disorders, and gastroenteritis.

[Probiotics are food supplements that *promote* the growth and proliferation of healthful bacteria in your body, such as the *Lactobacillus acidophilus* found in viable, cultured yogurt.

Prebiotics are non-digestible food ingredients that can stimulate the growth or activities of probiotic-like bacteria, which colonize the colon and can improve health.

Oligosaccharides, one type of prebiotic, are found naturally in foods such as wheat, onions, bananas, honey, garlic, leeks, and artichokes.]

The potential nutritional advantages of probiotics and prebiotics consist of preventive – and sometimes curative – effects against certain diseases. The evidence supporting such advantages is rapidly increasing.

Source: *British Journal of Nutrition May 2002;87(Suppl2):S153-157.*

WANT TO KNOW MORE?
[Pre- and probiotics are explained in detail in my book, *Everything I Know About Nutrition I Learned from Barley*.]

322. TRY INULIN AGAINST CONSTIPATION

Supplementing with inulin, another kind of prebiotic, is an excellent and safe way to combat constipation. [A nondigestible fiber, inulin is a prebiotic that helps promote the growth of "good" bacteria in the colon. Historically, humans have eaten significantly large amounts of inulin. The highest food concentrations occur in dahlia tubers, burdock roots, chicory roots and greens – foods that are not traditionally eaten in large amounts nowadays. Sixteenth century Europeans consumed about 35 grams of inulin daily, while 19th century Central and South Americans consumed up to 100 grams daily. In contrast, the average American today consumes only about three grams, unless he or she takes inulin in supplemental form, or is on an unusually prudent diet.]

Inulin has a better laxative effect than lactose, and it can safely and successfully reduce functional constipation.

Source: *American Journal of Clinical Nutrition* **1997; 65(5):1397-1402.**

323. PADMA FROM TIBET: SAFE & EFFECTIVE

Padma Lax, a complex Tibetan herbal formula for constipation, is found to be both safe and effective. Patients with constipation-predominant irritable bowel syndrome were recruited from the gastroenterology department of a clinic. More than half were given Padma Lax, a well known Tibetan herb, and the rest were given a placebo in this double-blind, randomized study.

Significant improvement was seen after three months in the Padma Lax group compared to the placebo group in terms of constipation, severity of abdominal pain and its effect on daily activities, incomplete evacuation, abdominal distension, and flatulence. Many more Padma Lax patients rated the Padma treatment superior to previous therapies they had been given for irritable bowel.

There were no significant side effects, and most patients preferred this method to their current multi-drug approach.

Source: *Digestion* **2002;65(3):161-71.**

WANT TO KNOW MORE?
Herbal medicines are now used by up to 50 percent of the Western population for the treatment or prevention of digestive disorders. (*Alimentary Pharmacology & Therapy* **2001;15(9):1239-52**)

Constipation with no identifiable causative factor is very common. Most constipation problems respond to fiber therapy, and this is one area where people can self-manage the problem. (*Ostomy Wound Management* **2002;48(12):30-41**)

CONTRACEPTION CAVEATS

A well-known medical journal described contraceptive drugs as creating pathology (abnormality that characterizes a disease) by turning normal fertility into an "abnormal sterile state," and warned that "contraceptives are toxins which paralyze the reproductive system and render it inoperative." Risk associations with the use of oral contraceptive drugs include antibiotic interactions, breast cancer, cardiovascular problems, high cholesterol, liver disease, and skeletal problems.

324. ANTIBIOTICS & THE PILL: A WARNING

If you are on oral contraceptives, you should know that taking antibiotics at the same time increases your risk of pregnancy. More often than not, physicians who prescribe antibiotics to women taking oral contraceptives neglect to inform them of the risk of pregnancy while taking this drug combination. But antibiotic use can *significantly* diminish the effectiveness of oral contraceptive medication.

Source: *Journal of Accidental & Emergency Medicine* **1999;16:265-270.**

WANT TO KNOW MORE?
[Did you know that the use of antibiotics can decimate your body's stores of health-promoting bacteria normally living in your digestive tract? Replacement with probiotics containing friendly bacteria such as *Lactobacillus acidophilus* is therefore essential once the antibiotics are finished.

325. CONTRACEPTIVES & BREAST CANCER RISK

Warning: Using oral contraceptives for ten years or more increases breast cancer risk later in life. Women over 55 with a 10-year or longer history of oral contraceptive use have *double* the risk of developing breast cancer. The elevated risk is associated with women with the highest level of oral contraceptive use.

Since breast cancer development is related to many factors, it is possible that the use of hormone replacement therapy adds to the risk.

Source: *International Journal of Cancer* **2000;87:591-594.**

WANT TO KNOW MORE?
[See the *Breast Cancer* section for many informative and helpful hints about this disease.]

326. DEPO-PROVERA CAN LEAD TO HEART DISEASE

If you are currently taking the contraceptive drug Depo-Provera, be warned: This drug may increase your risk of developing heart disease when taken for more than a year. Many have found this long-acting contraceptive drug useful, as it does not have to be taken daily, but Depo-Provera (depot medroxyprogesterone acetate) can put your health at serious risk. The drug impairs responsiveness to increased blood flow as a result of cell abnormality, which can then lead to heart disease.

Before beginning oral contraceptives, a blood pressure check is essential. There is a strong association between oral contraceptives and stroke or heart disease in women with hypertension, diabetes, obesity, and a history of smoking.

Sources: *British Medical Journal* **Sep 2002;325:513;** *Medscape Women's Health eJournal* **Aug 2002.**

WANT TO KNOW MORE?
Twenty-three percent of reproductive-age women in the US use oral contraceptives as their method of contraception. Adverse effects associated with oral contraceptive use – such as stroke and myocardial infarction (heart attack) – were reported soon after their introduction to the market in the early 1960s. New formulas have been developed over the years, creating new health problems.

327. CONTRACEPTIVES & RISK OF STROKE

If you are currently taking oral contraceptives, be advised that the risk of suffering an ischemic stroke is increased with these drugs, even with low-dose formulations. Ischemic refers to a decrease in blood supply caused by constriction or obstruction of blood vessels. While the risk for ischemic stroke is reduced with lower-dose estrogen, the risk for contraceptives of any dose is still "significantly elevated." The relative risk of stroke is the same for women with hypertension, those who are smokers, or those who suffer from migraines.

Source: *Journal of the American Medical Association* **2000;284:72-78.**

328. CONTRACEPTIVES & HIGH CHOLESTEROL

Teen girls and adult women, beware: The use of oral contraceptives raises blood cholesterol levels, which can have *serious* consequences on your cardiovascular health, including an increased risk of heart disease, strokes and heart attacks. In teenage users of oral contraceptives, total cholesterol levels are found to be significantly higher than in teenage nonusers.

And adult women who use oral contraceptives have significantly greater increases in total cholesterol, LDL cholesterol (the negative kind), and triglycerides.

Studies also show an increased risk of thrombosis (blood clotting leading to stroke), even as a result of some of the newer formulas.

Sources: *Contraception* 2000;62:113-116; *Obstetrics & Gynecology* 2002;100:235-239; *Stroke* 2002; 33(5):1202-1208; *Australian Family Physician* 1998;27(7):578.

329. ORAL CONTRACEPTIVES & LIVER DISEASE

If you are taking oral contraceptives, you should know that *once again* the association between this medication and the risk of developing serious liver disease has been confirmed. Women with this disease were studied, and 83 percent of them reported using oral contraceptives. And the risk increased when women used oral contraceptives for three years or more.

Source: *American Journal of Obstetrics & Gynecology* 2002;186:195-197.

WANT TO KNOW MORE?
[See the *Liver Disease* section for some helpful hints on how to protect your liver.]

330. ORAL CONTRACEPTIVES & BONE DENSITY

If you are a woman who is currently taking oral contraceptives and you are also concerned about skeletal health problems such as osteoporosis, you should know that premenopausal women who take these drugs have lower bone-mineral density than do women who don't take them. Bone-mineral density is 2.3 to 3.7 percent *lower* in oral contraceptive users than it is in women who have never used them. This lower density is not related to the duration of oral contraceptive use, nor is it related to the age of first use.

Source: *Canadian Medical Association Journal* 2001;165:1023-1029.

WANT TO KNOW MORE?
[Low bone-mineral density can lead to serious conditions such as osteoporosis. See the *Osteoporosis & Other Skeletal Problems* section for lots of helpful hints on protecting your skeletal health.]

331. LOSING OUT ON BONE MASS IMPROVEMENTS

If you are a younger woman who exercises regularly but uses oral contraceptives, you may not get the boost in bone strength seen in women who exercise but don't

use them. Regular resistance training and aerobic exercise strengthens bones in women aged 18 to 31 over a two-year period. However, oral contraceptives appear to prevent the build-up of bone in the spine seen in women who exercise.

So it seems that the use of oral contraceptives may negate the benefit of exercise in building bone.

If you exercise but continue to take oral contraceptives, you may be compromising your chances of attaining peak bone mass at key sites in your body [and this may have serious health consequences later on, such as osteoporosis.]

Source: *Medicine & Science in Sports & Exercise* **2001;33:873-880.**

332. CONTRACEPTIVES & MICROALBUMINURIA

Here's another negative to add to the growing list for oral contraceptives: Their use is associated with an increased risk of microalbuminuria (early stages of albumin in the urine), which in turn increases the risk of cardiovascular disease. In premenopausal women, oral contraceptive use is more prevalent in those with microalbuminuria than in those without. In fact, oral contraceptive use in premenopausal women increases the risk of microalbuminuria by as high as *90 percent*!

Source: *Archives of Internal Medicine* 2001;161:2000-2005.

WANT TO KNOW MORE?
[In postmenopausal women, an increased microalbuminuria risk is also associated with the use of hormone replacement therapy (HRT). See Hint #714 in the *Menopause & Hormone Replacement Therapy* section for more details.]

Choosing a method of contraception is an important decision. The diaphragm as a contraceptive device was invented in the nineteenth century. Margaret Sanger helped to popularize it, but it lost favor in the 1960s with the discovery of the Pill.

The diaphragm comes in different sizes, so you must be fitted for a proper one for you by a physician or physician assistant. it requires more care than simply taking the Pill, but it is withoug side effects.

Although it is suggested that the diaphram be used with spermicides, some practitioners believe that spermicides offer no additional contraceptiv eprotection. (*Cochrane Database System ReviewI* **2003;(1):CD002031**) The contraceptive sponge was developed as an altlernative to the diaphragm, but allergic-type reactions are more common with the sponge. (*Contraception* **2003;67(1):15-8**)

DEMENTIA

Dementia affects about five percent of our seniors over the age of 65 and has an unexplained predominance in women, and a low rate in some cultures. Different forms of dementia are now distinguished. Alzheimer's disease is only one form, but the different dementias are believed to have a common underlying neuropathology. (*Lancet* 2002;360(9347):1759-66)

Increased risk is associated with age. The rates of dementia nearly triple from the 75-to-79-year and 80-to-84-year age groups, but the relative increase is much less thereafter. Although gender is associated with dementia in general, it is not associated with Alzheimer's onset. Educational level (more than 15 years vs less than 12 years) is associated with a decreased risk of Alzheimer's disease. (*Archives of Neurolology* 2002;59(11):1737-46)

Although gait abnormalities are not associated with Alzheimer's disease, they are associated with other forms of dementia. (*New England Journal of Medicine* 2002;347:1761-1768)

IN THIS SECTION:
* ALTERNATIVE THERAPIES
* NATURAL REMEDIES & SUPPLEMENTS

DEMENTIA: ALTERNATIVE THERAPIES
333. AROMATHERAPY CAN HELP WITH DEMENTIA

For treating agitation among patients with dementia, aromatherapy with essential oils may be very effective. Sixty percent of patients receiving lemon balm or lavender oil aromatherapy (applied as a lotion or inhaled) have a 30 percent improvement compared with only five percent receiving a placebo. Quality of life also improves greatly among those receiving aromatherapy, with less time spent socially withdrawn and more time spent in constructive activity. Aromatherapy with essential balm oil appears to be safe, well tolerated and highly effective.

Sources: *Journal of Clinical Psychiatry* 2002;63:553-558; *British Medical Journal* 2002;325:1312-1313.

334. BRIGHT-LIGHT THERAPY FOR DEMENTIA

Bright light may help reduce the agitation and sleep disturbances experienced by older people with dementia. People with dementia are among the most vulnerable in our society. Drugs commonly used to treat them can be hazardous and are often poorly tolerated, frequently causing treatment to be terminated.

Bright-light therapy may be an effective alternative treatment because it helps patients to sleep longer and more soundly. This method is safe and effective and may have an important role in managing behavioral problems in this growing population of our society.

Source: *British Medical Journal* 2002;325:1312-1313.

DEMENTIA: NATURAL REMEDIES & SUPPLEMENTS
335. GINKGO BILOBA AGAINST DEMENTIA

The dietary supplement Ginkgo biloba can improve memory and function in people suffering from dementia, and may slow down cognitive degeneration. Ginkgo contains a number of organic biologically active components, including *ginkgolides*, which are unique to the Ginkgo tree, and may contribute to Ginkgo's beneficial qualities. The medicinal effects of Ginkgo are believed to be gained by causing blood vessels to dilate, improving blood flow to the brain, and through thinning the blood and making it less likely to clot.

Ginkgo biloba appears to be safe, and without any excessive side effects. It probably also has some antioxidant effects, protecting nerve cells against biological "rusting."

Source: Alzheimer Society of Britain, Oct 2002.

DENTAL DISORDERS

Silver amalgam in dentistry has been used for over a hundred years, and for just as long controversy has accompanied its use. Many health care professionals believe that dental amalgam restorations are a factor in a host of diseases and conditions because of mercury leakage concerns. The American Dental Association, however, still supports the use of amalgam. (*Journal of the American Dental Association* 2001;132(3):348-56)

The mercury vapor release from amalgam is dependent on many factors, including operator experience, operator techniques, and restoration design. (*Operative Dentistry* 2002;27(1):73-80)

But silver amalgam has become a less attractive dental restorative material for restoration of primary teeth. After many decades of controversy, use of silver amalgam for primary teeth is waning, not because of its mercury content but because dentistry has come up with more suitable materials. (*Quintessence International* 1998;29(11):697-703)

Until recently removable prostheses were the only form of treatment for those who had lost all or most of their natural teeth. (*Primary Dental Care* 2002;9(3):81-5)

336. GREEN TEA HELPS PREVENT CAVITIES

A cup of green tea after a meal can help to reduce the risk of dental cavities. Green tea is abundant in polyphenol catechins, phytochemicals found in plants that stabilize collagen and prevent capillary fragility. Polyphenols have powerful antioxidant properties, and are the major health-promoting active ingredient found in green tea.

More good news is that these catechins also inhibit cariogenic bacteria (the microbes that cause cavities) from adhering to your tooth surfaces. They do so in a dose-dependent manner, meaning the more tea you drink, the more protection you have. In addition, catechins prevent actions that could otherwise lead to periodontal disease.

Mouth rinsing with water containing green tea polyphenols also results in significant reduction in dental plaque formation. [Make sure you select a pure, high-quality green tea.]

Source: A.S. Nadu, "Phytoantimicrobial (PAM) agents as multifunctional food additives," *Phytochemicals as Bioactive Agents*, **W.R. Bidlack, ed., (Technomic Publications, 2000), p. 120.**

WANT TO KNOW MORE?
[Green tea has many remarkable qualities, including protective properties against diseases such as arthritis and cancer. See Hints #86, #156, and #227 for more information.]

337. SPECIAL GUM FOR HYPERSENSITIVE TEETH

If you suffer from painful, hypersensitive teeth, daily use of a chewing gum containing potassium chloride may bring relief. Dental hypersensitivity has been observed in an increasing number of younger patients over the past few decades. The reasons for this include poor tooth-brushing techniques, abrasions caused by bruxism [the unconscious gritting or grinding of the teeth], or orthodontic procedures.

But the daily use of a potassium chloride-containing chewing gum proves to be a useful, non-invasive method for reducing dental hypersensitivity over an extended period of time. Patients who use the gum (in conjunction with a sensitivity-reducing toothpaste) experience *significant* decreases in tooth hypersensitivity.

Source: *European Journal of Medical Research* **2001;6(11):483-487.**

338. FRUIT JUICES CAN ERODE TEETH

Protect your teeth by limiting your consumption of fruit juices and beverages made with citrus fruits, which can erode your teeth. Most juices or beverages made with grapefruit, lemon, or lime are more erosive on teeth than those prepared with fruits such as apple or peach. (Among non-juice beverages, sport drinks generally have the greatest demineralizing effect, while beer has the least.)

Susceptibility to erosion is virtually the same for all types of teeth and dental surfaces.

The erosive capacity of fruit juices and beverages is related to their pH balance — as the pH falls, their erosive capacity rises.

Source: *Acta Odontology LatinoAmerica* **1998;11(1):55-71.**

WANT TO KNOW MORE?
[Excessive consumption of fruit juices can also contribute to obesity, diarrhea and other gastrointestinal problems, such as excessive gas, bloating, and abdominal pain.]

339. ANTIBIOTICS NO HELP FOR DENTAL PAIN

If you are taking antibiotics for any dental pain, you should be aware that these medications will probably not help this problem. The most commonly prescribed drugs for dental pain are antibiotics, yet there is *no* evidence that antibiotics reduce dental pain, even in the case of an acute abscess with related signs of infection.

Source: Report given by Dr. Richard Walton at the 56th Annual Session of the American Association of Endodontists, Atlanta, GA, as reported in *Reuter's Health*.

340. ORTHODONTIC HELP & HINDRANCE

Wearers of braces, be warned: Fluorides can cause a reduction of tooth movement during orthodontic procedures, thereby delaying results. Orthodontic tooth movement and bone remodeling activity are dependent on factors such as nutrition, metabolic bone diseases, age, and use of drugs. Anything that increases bone mineral content (such as fluoride) decreases the rate of bone resorption, and so tooth movement slows down. [Important side note: The bone mineral increase caused by fluoride is not in your best health interest anyway.]

Nonsteroidal anti-inflammatory drugs [NSAIDs] can also reduce bone resorption, and therefore should also not be administered for long periods of time to those undergoing orthodontic tooth movement.

Thyroid hormones, however, may aid in a more rapid tooth movement during orthodontic therapy (although they have a less stable orthodontic result).

Source: *Quintessence International* **May 2001;32(5):365-371.**

DEPRESSION

Depression is a serious and extensive problem in this country, and it has become a very serious mental health issue. Unfortunately, mental health services focus on care, rather than cure. (*Nursing Standards 2002;16(26):33-6*) A large group of antidepressants commonly used can cause the loss of libido, among other health-endangering problems.

Although we generally think of depression as a strictly emotional state, nutrition can and does play a major role in maintaining our mental health.

Sleep disturbance has attracted considerable attention as an early indicator of depression.

IN THIS SECTION:
- ALTERNATIVE THERAPIES
- CAUSES & PRECURSORS
- DRUG WARNINGS & SIDE EFFECTS
- EXERCISE THERAPY
- NATURAL REMEDIES & SUPPLEMENTS

DEPRESSION: ALTERNATIVE THERAPIES

341. "LIGHTEN UP" AGAINST DEPRESSION

If you are suffering from *nonseasonal* depression, bright-light therapy (phototherapy) may be helpful. Phototherapy *significantly* improves clinical symptoms of depression, independent of the time of therapy. In those suffering from affective disorder, circadian rhythms of body temperatures are more sensitive to the corrective effects of bright light compared with normal subjects, but these effects are *not* related to any clinical improvement.

The bright-light exposure seems to have an antidepressant effect on patients with nonseasonal depression, but this effect is unlikely to be mediated via the same circadian system that regulates body temperature. (Dim-light therapy, by the way, has no effect.)

Source: *Biological Psychiatry* Jun 1995,37(12):866-873.

342. COMEDY THERAPY FOR DEPRESSION

Simply watching a funny video can have a *considerable* beneficial effect on depression, stress, tension, and other emotional states that can negatively affect your health. Watching a funny video can decrease tension by 60 percent, confusion by 75 percent, fatigue by 87 percent, and depression and anger by as much as 98 percent. Vigor can increase by 37 percent immediately following the viewing, and can actually increase by 12 percent *before* the viewing (just the positive anticipation of humor can begin the process). Vigor indicates more energy and better disease resistance, unlike negative mood categories, which are known to increase stress hormone levels and reduce the effectiveness of the immune system.

Source: Meeting of the Society for Neuroscience, San Diego, CA, Nov 2001.

DEPRESSION: CAUSES & PRECURSORS

343. LOW CHOLESTEROL & DEPRESSION LINKED

If you are a middle-aged man with naturally low cholesterol, you could be at risk for depression. Middle-aged men with naturally low serum cholesterol levels are *significantly* more likely to have symptoms of severe depression than men whose cholesterol levels are higher. (There is an essential difference between cholesterol levels that are naturally low and those that have been deliberately lowered.)

It is not clear how naturally low cholesterol levels might predispose individuals to depression, but changes in serotonin metabolism may occur as a result of tryptophan [an essential amino acid] depletion in the brain. This may result when fatty acid levels are low. There is also an association seen between chronically low cholesterol levels and death from violent causes, especially suicide.

Source: *Psychosomatic Medicine* 2000;62:205-211.

344. MARIJUANA & MENTAL HEALTH

The link between cannabis (marijuana) and psychosis is well established, and it is now confirmed that there is also a link between the use of marijuana and depression. In some countries, the use of cannabis among young people is now becoming more common than the use of tobacco. The ready availability of the drug, the increasing social disapproval of cigarette smoking, strict drunk-driving laws, and perceptions that cannabis is safe or less harmful than cigarettes or alcohol may explain these changes.

The use of marijuana during adolescence increases the risk of schizophrenia, the length of exposure predicting the severity of the psychosis. And the evidence in relation to depression is growing: Young people who use cannabis three times or more by the age of 18 are more likely to have a depressive disorder at the age of 26. Early use (by age 15) confers greater risk than later use (by age 18), and this link appears to be stronger for young women than for young men.

Source: *British Medical Journal* Nov 2002;325:1183-1184;1212-1213.

DEPRESSION:
DRUG WARNINGS & SIDE EFFECTS
345. PROZAC MAY LEAD TO BRAIN TUMORS

If you are taking Prozac, be warned: This drug may lead to brain tumors. Prozac, a medication commonly prescribed to treat depression, may stimulate the growth of brain tumors by blocking the body's natural ability to kill cancer cells. The drug actually prevents cancer cells from "committing suicide," thereby leading to a more vigorous growth of tumors. These results may initiate a global re-evaluation of the drug's long-term safety.

The drug, along with many other antidepressants, works by preventing serotonin from being quickly reabsorbed by nerve cells in the brain. Paxil and Celexa also have this same stimulating effect on tumor growth.

Source: *Blood* **2002;99(7);2545-2553.**

346. GINKGO BILOBA FOR A SEXUAL RECHARGE

If you are experiencing sexual dysfunction as a side effect of antidepressant medication, Ginkgo biloba may be able to help. Ginkgo biloba extract, derived from the leaf of the Chinese ginkgo tree, is noted for its cerebral enhancing effects. But it is also found to be 84 percent effective in treating antidepressant-induced sexual dysfunction, a common side effect of SSRI drugs. (SSRI is the acronym for "selective serotonin reuptake inhibitor," and refers to antidepressive drugs such as Prozac and Paxil that promote transmission of nerve impulses along pathways using the neurotransmitter serotonin.)

Women are more responsive to the sexually enhancing effects of Ginkgo biloba than men, with relative success rates of 91 percent versus 76 percent. Ginkgo biloba generally has a positive effect on all four phases of the sexual response cycle: desire, excitement (lubrication), orgasm, and resolution (afterglow).

Source: *Journal of Sex & Marital Therapy* **1998;24(2):139-143.**

WANT TO KNOW MORE?
The study of the sexual-enhancing effects of Ginkgo biloba originated from the observation that a geriatric patient taking ginkgo biloba for memory enhancement noted sexual improvements.

In the study, dosages of Ginkgo biloba extract ranged from 60 milligrams daily to 120 milligrams twice a day (average = 209 mg a day). Generally, more than 240 milligrams a day is necessary.

DEPRESSION: EXERCISE THERAPY

347. AEROBICS CAN LIFT DEPRESSION

If you are suffering from depression, take note: Aerobic exercise may be a simple and healthy solution. A basic program of regular aerobic exercise (only 30 minutes a day) can *substantially* improve depression in patients with moderate to severe major depression, even despite prior failures with drug therapy. Walking on a treadmill for just 30 minutes a day can lead to a significant drop in depression after just 10 days.

[This is something you CAN try at home, kids – if you don't have access to a gym, aerobic videos of every kind are available for you to exercise in the comfort of your own home.]

Isn't a half hour of exercise daily an alternative worth trying before resorting to drugs, with all their drastic side effects?

Source: *British Journal of Sports Medicine* **2001;35:114-117.**

DEPRESSION: NATURAL REMEDIES & SUPPLEMENTS

348. ST. JOHN'S WORT AGAINST DEPRESSION

If you are suffering from depression, the remarkable herb St. John's wort should be your first choice of treatment. St. John's wort proves to be as beneficial as the antidepressant drug imipramine in the treatment of mild-to-moderate depression, but it is far better tolerated. When St. John's wort was compared with a full therapeutic dose of imipramine, scores on a standard depression scale decreased from 22.4 to 12.00 among those taking the herb, and from 22.1 to 12.75 among those taking the drug.

In addition, the rate of adverse effects was greater in the imipramine group (63 percent) than in the St. John's wort group (just 39 percent).

Source: *British Medical Journal* **2000;321:536-539.**

WANT TO KNOW MORE?
Among the negative side effects of imipramine: It may induce or exacerbate an arrhythmia [irregular heartbeat]or lead to low blood pressure. It should be used with caution in hyperthyroid patients and in those on thyroid medication because of the possibility of cardiovascular toxicity. It may produce urinary retention and should be used with caution in patients with urinary problems, particularly in the presence of prostatic problems. Newborns

whose mothers have taken imipramine up until delivery have shown symptoms such as breathing difficulties, lethargy, colic, irritability, high or low blood pressure, tremor, or spasms.

[Given this long list of side effects, the recommendation of using St. John's wort over imipramine should be seriously considered.]

349. SAMe EFFECTIVE AGAINST DEPRESSION

The antioxidant supplement SAMe (S-adenosylmethionine) is as effective in treating depression as some conventional antidepressant drugs. SAMe is well tolerated and relatively free of adverse side effects, and it may even accelerate the effects of conventional antidepressants.

Although some people require higher doses, 200 to 1,600 milligrams of SAMe daily can be very effective, and most people improve within a few days to two weeks. SAMe appears to have a faster onset of action than conventional antidepressants, and it may also protect against the deleterious effects of Alzheimer's disease.

The production of SAMe in your body relies in part on adequate levels of the vitamins folate and B12, two vitamins that Americans are generally deficient in. Deficiencies of these vitamins have long since been linked to depression [see Hint #350].

Because homocysteine is a byproduct of SAMe metabolism, some have been concerned that SAMe supplementation can cause homocysteine elevations. But research shows that homocysteine is removed naturally in the bodies of healthy people.

[SAMe is also helpful against alcoholic liver damage. See Hint #38 for more details.]

Sources: World Congress of the Oxygen Club of California, Santa Barbara, CA, Mar 2001; *American Journal of Clinical Nutrition* **2002;76(5):1158S-1161S.**

WANT TO KNOW MORE?
Major depression remains difficult to treat, despite the wide array of antidepressants available. Between 19 and 34 percent of depressed people do not respond to acute antidepressant treatment. Depression affects almost twice as many women as men.

350. FOLIC ACID DEFICIENCY & DEPRESSION

Depression may be linked to a folic acid deficiency, and folic acid treatment may be helpful in reducing symptoms. Folic acid has particular effects on mood and cognitive and social function, and depression is common in those that have a deficiency of it. (There is a strong link between folic acid and homocysteine, aging, depression, dementia, Alzheimer's disease, and vascular disease.) But depressive mood can improve with only 15 milligrams of folic acid given daily for four months, and 50 milligrams of folic acid daily is as effective in improving depressive symptoms as 100 milligrams daily of the standard antidepressant trazodone. Although important for all ages, in older people folic acid deficiency contributes to aging brain processes and increases the risk of Alzheimer's disease and vascular dementia. Patients with impaired intellectual function are *strikingly* improved after six to 12 months of folic acid therapy.

Source: *British Medical Journal* **2002;324:1512-1515.**

WANT TO KNOW MORE?
Factors causing folate deficiency can include:
  ~ drugs
  ~ chronic illness
  ~ increased demand
  ~ malabsorption

[The best dietary sources of folic acid (also known as folate) are green leafy vegetables such as spinach, kale, and beet greens, as well as beets, chard, asparagus, broccoli, bean sprouts (lentil, mung, and soy), and brewer's yeast.]

351. FISHY TREATMENT FOR DEPRESSION

Daily treatment with *eicosapentoic acid* (EPA), an omega-3 fatty acid, may help to reduce symptoms of clinical depression. Low blood levels of EPA are found in depressed patients, but administration of this fatty acid (one gram a day) is found to be effective in treating those who remain depressed despite adequate standard therapy.

EPA appears to have beneficial effects against depression, anxiety, sleeplessness, lassitude, low libido, and suicidal tendencies.

In one case, administration of EPA (four grams daily) led to rapid improvement – including the cessation of suicidal tendencies and lessening of social phobia – within a month. This benefit was progressive, and after nine months, symptoms had disappeared entirely. (The patient's depressive symptoms had previously continued to worsen, despite adequate trials with a range of standard medications. But EPA turned things around.)

Additionally, a mixture of EPA and *docosahexaenoic acid* (DHA), previously reported to improve depression and the course of illness in bipolar disorder, may also be helpful in the treatment of unipolar depression.

[Fish such as mackerel, sardines, and salmon are all good sources of both these fatty acids.]

Source: *Archives of General Psychiatry* **2002;59(1):913-919.**

DERMATOLOGICAL CONDITIONS

The growing resistance of skin conditions to antibiotics should encourage the use of more natural solutions. Dermatitis symptoms usually signal a nutrient deficiency or food sensitivity. Treatment of any skin condition is always more effective when the intestinal tract is free of disease-producing toxins.

IN THIS SECTION:
- ACNE
- DERMATITIS
- ECZEMA

- ITCHY SKIN (PRURITIS)
- PSORIASIS

DERMATOLOGICAL CONDITIONS: ACNE

352. ACIDOPHILUS AGAINST ACNE

Here's a safe and effective treatment for acne (especially for teens): consume a half-pint of liquid *acidophilus* every day for two weeks, followed by one to two tablespoons after every meal from then on. Anyone on this regimen will probably enjoy far better health in all areas, not just limited to clearer skin. At the start of the program, acne may worsen, but will quickly clear with continued use. [Liquid *acidophilus* is a form of *Lactobacillus acidophilus*, health-promoting bacteria also found in viable, cultured yogurt. Liquid *acidophilus* can be found in the refrigerated sections of health food stores. It is also my favorite quick fix for upset stomachs as well.]]

Sources: *Archives of Dermatology* 2002;138(12):1584-1590; *Proceedings of the Nutrition Society* 2002;61(3):397-400; *American Journal of Clinical Nutrition* 2000;71(1):367S.

353. NO MORE ANTIBIOTICS FOR ACNE

Antibiotics should NOT be used to treat acne; they are ineffective and contribute to the development of resistant strains of bacteria. Physicians are now being asked to rethink the practice of prescribing antibiotics for acne, a treatment used for several decades. The lack of effectiveness of antibiotics in treating acne has now been confirmed, and resistant strains of bacteria are found in a significant number of acne patients treated with antibiotics (far less than the amount found in an untreated control group). The increased number of antibiotic-resistant strains being seen underscores the need for alternative regimens to treat acne.

Source: 11th European Congress of Clinical Microbiology & Infectious Diseases, Sweden, Apr 2001.

DERMATOLOGICAL CONDITIONS: DERMATITIS

354. DERMATITIS & CHEAP STAINLESS STEEL

Dermatitis sufferers, be advised: Inexpensive stainless steel pots may emit nickel into foods, which may exacerbate this condition. Nickel-sensitivity is not an uncommon problem, and nickel ingestion can cause increased dermatitis in patients who are already nickel-sensitive. There is a significant difference in nickel intake between glass and stainless steel saucepans. However, the emission from the stainless steel pots is not significant, provided the stainless steel pots are of good quality.

Source: *Contact Dermatitis* 1998;38(6):305-310.

355. NUTRIENTS AGAINST DERMATITIS

If you have dermatitis, you can benefit from supplements of vitamin C, omega-3 fatty acids, iodine, and calcium. Those with dermatitis symptoms are usually nutrient-deficient, and a lower food intake in general is found in those suffering from this condition. The following are among the foods included on the low-intake list: dairy products, fish, eggs, pork, oranges, fruits in general, apples and kiwis in particular, green or red peppers, and hazelnuts. Consuming more of these foods may therefore be beneficial.

Source: *European Journal of Dermatology* 2001;11(3):199-202.

DERMATOLOGICAL CONDITIONS: ECZEMA

356. VITAMIN "E" FOR "ECZEMA RELIEF"

Supplementing with vitamin E – 400 IU (268 milligrams) once a day for eight months – is a very effective treatment for atopic dermatitis (eczema). Eczema is a chronic itchy, inflammatory skin disease that is extremely difficult to treat. Effective therapeutic agents are limited in number, and may have long-term toxic side effects. It is a common disease that appears to be increasing in frequency over the last few decades.

[Some dietary sources of vitamin E are butter, egg yolks, and liver. Tocotrienols, a superior form of vitamin E that I recommend, are natural compounds found in various foods and oils such as palm oil, rice bran oil, wheat germ, barley, saw palmetto, and certain types of nuts and grains.]

Sources: Dermatologists at the University of Siena, Italy; *Skin Therapy Letters* **2002;7(2):1-5;** *Journal of Allergy & Clinical Immunology* **2001;108(6):929-937;** *British Journal of Dermatology* **2002;146(4):631-635.**

WANT TO KNOW MORE?
Eczema is a common precursor to the development of asthma.

357. CLEAR UP YOUR SKIN WITH FIBER

Seborrheic eczema (the kind that causes excessive discharge from the sebaceous glands) and other skin conditions may be relieved with the use of a good fiber supplement. Our Western diet is associated with an increased incidence of acne. Rapid clearing of acne can follow with the intake of one ounce daily of a high fiber cereal (or a good high-fiber supplement).

Treatment of any skin condition is always more effective when the intestinal tract is free of disease-producing fungi.

Vegetable fiber is recommended to reduce yeast colonies between your intestinal villi – the threadlike projections covering the surface of the mucous membranes lining your small intestine, which serve as the absorption sites of nutrients.

Fiber also helps to prevent yeast cells from invading your lymph tract and circulating blood.

Source: B. Kamen, *New Facts About Fiber.*

358. ECZEMA WORSENED BY DUST MITES

If you suffer from eczema, take steps to decrease dust-mite allergens in your home, as they can worsen eczema symptoms. Dust mites, which feed on the dead skin that sloughs off our bodies as well as food crumbs, are the single most important allergen in the exacerbation of eczema, affecting many more children (and adults) than food allergies.

These microscopic monsters lurk quietly under our beds, inside sofas, and in carpets. They live their whole lives in dark corner dust bunnies – hatching, growing, eating, defecating, mating, and laying eggs. It's their bathroom habits that make us itch and wheeze: many people develop severe allergies to dust mite droppings. Lie on a rug where they live and you might get itchy red bumps all over your skin. Breathe in dust and you may have more serious symptoms like difficulty breathing or even a severe asthma attack.

Good treatment includes the use of polyurethane-coated cotton encasings for bedding, a high-powered vacuum cleaner, and a spray containing benzyl alcohol and tannic acid to kill mites and denature allergens.

Sources: *Allergology & Immunopathology* May-Jun 2002;30(3):126-134; *Allergy* May 2001;56(5):451.

WANT TO KNOW MORE?
Dust mites are in the arachnid family, which also includes spiders, scorpions, and ticks. [For more information on lowering dust-mite allergens in your home, see the *Allergies* section.]

359. BETTER BEDDING FOR ECZEMA SUFFERERS

If you suffer from eczema, making simple changes to your bedding can be very helpful. Encasing mattresses and pillows in cotton reduces symptoms for those with allergic dermatitis, regardless of sensitivity to house dust mite or cat allergen. Bedding made of cotton that is coated on one side with polyurethane works even better than bedding with plain cotton covers. (Both types of covers have an allergen-reducing capacity.)

During the last six months of a 12-month study, autoimmune-initiated levels of trouble-making cells (IgE, T-helper cells, and antigen CD30) decreased *significantly* with this practice.

Washing blankets once a month as seems to help, as does vacuuming carpets and mattresses.

Source: *Allergy* 2001;56:152-158.

DERMATOLOGICAL CONDITIONS: ITCHY SKIN (PRURITIS)

360. CAPSAICIN FIGHTS ITCHY SKIN

If you have itchy skin, topical application of capsaicin can help, regardless of the cause. Patients were treated with topical capsaicin (four to six times daily, for periods of two weeks up to 10 months), and all patients had completely recovered after 12 days of treatment. (The topical capsaicin application was in doses ranging from 0.025 percent to 0.3 percent.) Some reported localized burning and itch during the first three to five days of treatment, but all of these symptoms disappeared within 20 to 60 minutes after application.

[Capsaicin is a natural compound obtained from hot chili peppers.] It is also effective for promoting the gradual healing of skin lesions. In general, longer-term application of capsaicin and higher concentrations are associated with a better response.

Itchy skin (pruritis) can be caused by drugs, food allergies, parasites, aging, dry skin, poison ivy, or even unknown sources.

Source: *Journal of the American Academy of Dermatology* 2001;44:471-478.

DERMATOLOGICAL CONDITIONS: PSORIASIS

361   DIETARY TIPS FOR PSORIASIS RELIEF

If you are suffering from psoriasis, eliminating fruits (especially citrus fruits), nuts, corn, and milk may help to relieve and even eliminate the condition. In addition, eliminating acidic foods such as coffee, tomatoes, soda, and pineapple can also help. One study shows a possible benefit of supplemental vitamins A and E, and some patients are helped by a gluten-free [wheat-free] diet.

Psoriasis is a common chronic and recurrent inflammatory skin disorder that has been associated with oxidative stress, abnormal plasma lipid metabolism, and with high frequency of cardiovascular events. The disease is rarely found in blacks, Indians, or Asians, and never in Eskimos. Psoriasis most commonly develops between the ages of 20 to 50, that is, during the most active period of life.

Sources: *Clinical Chim Acta* Jan 2001;303(1-2):33-39; *British Journal of Dermatology* Jan 2000;142(1):44-51; *Acta Med Croatica* 1998;52(4-5):199-202.

362.   ALOE VERA GEL FOR PSORIASIS

Psoriasis, normally difficult to treat, may be helped and possibly eliminated with a stabilized 200 percent aloe vera gel. Many scientific studies validate the effectiveness of aloe for psoriasis. The quality of the product used, however, is extremely important. Aloe treatment is well tolerated, with no reported adverse effects. One study shows a cure rate of 83.3 percent compared to 6.6 percent for a placebo.

Psoriasis appears as raised red patches and silvery scales on the skin. It most commonly occurs around the elbows and knees – at hard or stressed surfaces. But it may also appear around the scalp or, in fact, anywhere on the body. Although we don't fully understand psoriasis, we do know that it represents rapid cell division – skin that is growing too fast.

Sources: Deborah's Collection, Abeline, TX; *Tropical Medicine & International Health* 1996;1(4): 505-550.

DIABETES (GENERAL)

The number of Americans diagnosed with diabetes is projected to increase by 165 percent over the next 50 years – but getting more people to change their diet and exercise habits could help slow the trend. According to the US Centers for Disease Control and Prevention in Atlanta, 29 million Americans will be diagnosed with diabetes in 2050, compared with about 11 million today. This report may actually *underestimate* future rates of diabetes because as many as one third of those with diabetes are not diagnosed. (***Diabetes Care 2001;24:1936-1940***)

The most common alternative medicines taken by the diabetic patient are garlic (11.6 percent), echinacea (8.9 percent), herbal mixtures (8.5 percent), chromium (5.8 percent), and glucosamine sulfate (5.8 percent). Diabetic patients spend almost as much on OTC medications and alternative medications – approximately $300 per year – as they spend on their prescription medications. Control individuals believe that alternative therapies are as effective as their prescribed medications. (**59th Scientific Sessions of the American Diabetes Association, 1999**)

IN THIS SECTION:
- CAUSES & PRECURSORS
- DIETARY TACTICS
- INSULIN RESISTANCE

- NATURAL REMEDIES & SUPPLEMENTS
- REDUCING RISK

DIABETES: CAUSES & PRECURSORS

363. HIGH IRON STORES & DIABETES RISK

Beware excessive iron intake, which can lead to elevated iron stores in the body, putting you at risk for diabetes. High dietary iron intake can elevate your body's stores of iron, and even *moderately* elevated iron stores may increase your risk of diabetes (as well as cancer and heart disease).

Consuming more than 21 servings of fruit juice a week can lead to elevated iron stores. Fruit and fruit juices are rich dietary sources of organic acids such as vitamin C, citric, malic, and tartaric acids, and the combined effects of vitamin C and these other organic acids may help to enhance iron bioavailability [meaning the degree to which iron can be used by the body] – leading to increased iron stores.

More than four serving of red meat a week (but not poultry or seafood) may also contribute to this problem, as well as more than 30 mg of supplemental iron daily.

Source: *American Journal of Clinical Nutrition* 2002;76(6):1375-1384.

WANT TO KNOW MORE?
You have a great capacity to store iron. Among older people especially, intakes of highly bioavailable forms of iron promote high iron stores, whereas foods containing phytate (whole grains) decrease these stores. (Phytate and calcium, as found in flour used in sweet baked products, inhibit iron absorption.)

DIABETES: DIETARY TACTICS

364. SALAD VEGGIES = LOW DIABETES RISK

It's so simple, with bags of organic greens readily available in most good markets: Frequent salad vegetable consumption throughout the year is associated with a reduction in the risk of diabetes. This reduced risk is maintained after adjusting for age, gender, and family history. BUT the key here is vegetable consumption *year-round* – consumption during the summer months alone has a much weaker association.

Source: *Journal of Clinical Epidemiology* Apr 1999;52(4):329-335.

365. DIABETICS: EAT MORE FISH!

Diabetics, take note: High fish consumption can reduce the excretion of albumin, one of the more serious side effects of diabetes. The excretion of albumin is known as *albuminuria*. Diabetics with the highest intake of fish protein (about nine grams a day) have a *significantly* decreased risk of elevated urine albumin levels compared with those who consume an average of only 2.7 grams of fish protein per day. (The amount of protein consumed, as well as vitamin usage and intake of calories, fat, and carbohydrate were similar between the two groups of diabetics studied.) Fish protein may decrease renal [kidney] workload, which in turn reduces the risk of developing diabetic nephropathy.

Source: *Diabetes Care* 2001:24:805-810.

366. CEREAL FIBER LOWERS DIABETES RISK

Eating cereal fiber may lower your risk of developing diabetes – and the higher your intake, the higher the protection. Cereal fiber intake is found to be inversely associated with the risk of diabetes (that is, high intake = low risk, and vice versa).
Given the explosion in diabetes rates worldwide that is following closely on the heels of the obesity epidemic, we need to work harder in developing programs to prevent both of these health problems.

Source: *Diabetes Care* 2002;25:1715-1721.

DIABETES: INSULIN RESISTANCE

367. WHOLE GRAINS & INSULIN RESISTANCE

Consuming a diet rich in whole grains can help to improve insulin resistance, which can reduce your risk for diabetes. Insulin sensitivity is improved in overweight and obese adults when they consume a diet rich in whole-grain foods, thereby reducing their risk of diabetes. In one group studied, insulin levels were 10 percent lower and blood glucose levels were slightly reduced when the same individuals ate a whole grain-rich diet compared with when they ate a refined-grain diet.

The USDA recommends people consume six to eleven servings of carbohydrates daily, including servings from whole grain sources.

Source: *American Journal of Clinical Nutrition* 2002;75:848-855.

WANT TO KNOW MORE?
[Insulin sensitivity refers to the ability of the cell to receive insulin. Insulin resistance refers to the insensitivity of tissue to insulin. For more information on these concepts and their relation to diabetes and heart disease, see my book, *The Chromium Connection: A Lesson in Nutrition.*]

368. GLUCOSAMINE & INSULIN RESISTANCE

Stay away from supplemental glucosamine sulfate, as it may lead to insulin resistance. The use of isolated glucosamine sulfate supplements may contribute to insulin resistance in diabetics or in those at risk for diabetes.

Fasting blood insulin levels – but not fasting glucose levels – are *significantly* higher in subjects taking glucosamine than in those taking a placebo. In diabetics the effect may be even worse.

Source: Experimental Biology Conference, San Diego, CA, Apr 2000; *Experimental Biology* **2000.**

WANT TO KNOW MORE?
[This is another example of the disadvantages of isolated nutrients, and another reason to use velvet antler (which contains glucosamine in small quantities, but in a natural context). The velvet antler offers the same benefits sought with the use of glucosamine, and research continues to demonstrate the superiority of food-type supplements over their isolated components. See Hint #1,108 in the *Healthier Living* section for more information.]

369. ZINC AGAINST INSULIN RESISTANCE

If you are insulin resistant, supplementing with the mineral zinc may be helpful.
Zinc supplementation in overweight, insulin-resistant women improves insulin sensitivity, even in the absence of zinc deficiency. [Insulin resistance refers to a condition in which insulin is present in the body to escort glucose into your cells, but your cells refuse to admit the glucose.]

Only a short period of zinc supplementation appears to be necessary to improve insulin sensitivity.

Source: American Diabetic Association Annual Meeting, Abstracts 1644-P, 569-P. June 16-17, 2002.

WANT TO KNOW MORE?
[Insulin resistance is common in those who are overweight. To learn more about this subject, see my book, *The Chromium Connection: A Lesson in Nutrition*.]

DIABETES: NATURAL REMEDIES & SUPPLEMENTS

370. VITAMIN C MAY PREVENT DIABETES

Increasing your intake of ascorbic acid (vitamin C) may be helpful in reducing your risk of developing diabetes. There is an increasing prevalence of diabetes today, and an inverse association is seen between blood ascorbic acid levels and this disease (that is, those with lower vitamin C levels are more likely to be diabetic, while those with high levels are less likely). Therefore, increasing your plasma vitamin C through dietary measures is an important strategy for reducing your risk.

[Vitamin C is one of the least stable vitamins, and cooking can destroy much of it. Some good dietary sources of vitamin C are citrus fruits, strawberries, green peppers, broccoli, dark leafy greens, and tomatoes.]

One important note: What prevents can also help. Vitamin C supplementation can be beneficial to both type 1 and type 2 diabetics, helping to restore impaired vasodilation [widening of the blood vessels].

Sources: *Diabetes Care* 2000;23(6):726-732; *Circulation* 2001;103(12):1618-1623.

WANT TO KNOW MORE?
[Vitamin C may also be protective against several chronic diseases and health problems such as arterial disease (see Hint #515), cataracts (Hint #428), diseases of the gallbladder (Hint #480), gastric cancer (Hint #259), osteoarthritis (Hint #94), and more.]

371. VITAMIN E PROTECTION FOR DIABETICS

If you are diabetic, supplementing with vitamin E may help you to reduce your risk of developing cardiovascular disease. Twelve hundred IU of vitamin E daily for three months reduces the oxidation of bad cholesterol (LDL) in diabetics and improves white cell abnormalities. It also improves insulin sensitivity when consuming sugar.

Vitamin E is currently being touted as an anti-inflammatory for diabetics. Diabetics develop cardiovascular disease at an earlier age, and also have higher levels of free radicals. Inflammation, particularly of blood vessel walls, contributes to cardiovascular disease.

Supplements of vitamin E reduce free-radical levels, free- radical oxidation of cholesterol, and inflammation in diabetics. Vitamin E supplementation promises to be a safe and inexpensive means of controlling these functions, both in diabetics as well as others at risk for cardiovascular disease.

Source: *Circulation* **2000;102:191-196,** *Journal of Nutrition* **1997;127:103-107.**

372. FOLATE FOR DIABETES COMPLICATIONS

If you are diabetic, you should know that folate [folic acid] therapy could be helpful in preventing vascular complications. Endothelial dysfunction is seen early in the development of vascular disease in diabetes, as is a high level of homocysteine. [The endothelium is the covering of internal and external surfaces of the body, including the lining of vessels. Homocysteine is an amino acid produced naturally in your body, but high levels in the blood are associated with many health problems.]

Folate status is an important determinant of endothelial function both in youngsters with type I diabetes and in those with late-onset (type 2) diabetes. Folate consumption is associated with better endothelial function, and may therefore protect against the long-term vascular complications of the diabetes.

[Folate is a form of vitamin B, and gets its name from "foliage" as can be found in green leafy vegetables. The best sources of folate are spinach, kale, and beet greens, as well as beets, chard, asparagus, broccoli, bean sprouts (lentil, mung, and soy), and brewer's yeast.]

Source: *Diabetes* **2002;51:2282-2286.**

373. CHROMIUM POLYNICOTINATE & DIABETES

Supplementation with one form of chromium may be helpful for both non-insulin-dependent and insulin-dependent diabetics. *Chromium polynicotinate* in supplemental form may help non-insulin-dependent diabetics get off medication entirely, and may help insulin-dependent patients to reduce their insulin need by *significant* amounts. In the presence of optimal amounts of biologically active chromium (identified as the organic GTF-chromium complex), much lower amounts of insulin are required. (Niacin-bound chromium polynicotinate is absorbed significantly faster and better than chromium chloride or chromium picolinate.) According to the US Department of Agriculture, almost every American is deficient in chromium.

Glucose intolerance, related to insufficient dietary chromium, appears to be widespread. Adequate intake of chromium (50 to 200 micrograms daily) can help this problem. In fact, improvements in glucose metabolism (for hypoglycemics, hyperglycemics, and diabetics) and cardiovascular disease following chromium supplementation are well documented.

Source: B. Kamen, *The Chromium Connection: A Lesson in Nutrition.*

374. GINSENG HELPS LOWER BLOOD SUGAR

Ginseng may hold promise as an adjunct to conventional diabetes therapy and perhaps as a preventive treatment for this disease. Ginseng reduces the glycemia [blood sugar level] that usually occurs following a meal in most people, whether diabetic or not. In diabetics, this glycemia reduction is *significant*, whether taken before or during a "glucose challenge" [meaning the ingestion of foods that induce blood sugar levels to rise]. In non-diabetic subjects given ginseng during a glucose challenge, this effect does not differ significantly from a placebo. But when given beforehand, glycemia is significantly lowered 45 and 60 minutes after the glucose challenge.

Animal research also suggests that ginseng has a positive effect on carbohydrate metabolism and diabetes, and it has been shown to reduce the concentrations of sugar in the urine of diabetic animals.

Sources: *Archives of Internal Medicine* 2000;160:1009-1013; *American Journal of Clinical Nutrition* 2001;73:1101-1106; B. Kamen, *Siberian Ginseng: The Latest Research on the Fabled Tonic Herb.*

WANT TO KNOW MORE?
[Traditionally, ginseng was considered part of the daily diet and taken in relatively low doses over a long period of time. The purity and potency of ginseng products varies, and are not always representative of what is on the label, so you should try to get your ginseng from a company you trust. My preferred form is Siberian ginseng.]

375. GINSENG BERRY EXTRACT FOR DIABETES

If you are diabetic, supplementing with ginseng berry extract may help to normalize your blood glucose levels. Extract of ginseng berry [as opposed to ginseng root, the more commonly consumed form] has effects on the symptoms of diabetes by completely normalizing blood glucose levels. The researchers studying this extract were surprised at how different the berry is from the root, as well as how effective it is in correcting the metabolic abnormalities associated with diabetes.

Source: University of Chicago study, Chicago, IL, as reported in *The Daily Mail*, UK, May 2002.

WANT TO KNOW MORE?
[Ginseng berry may also help you to lose weight. See Hint #749 in the *Obesity* section for more details.]

376. RICE BRAN HELPFUL FOR DIABETICS

Diabetics, take note: Rice bran shows remarkable promise in the controlling of blood glucose levels. Specially developed rice bran products may have significant potential as nutritional support in the management and control of blood glucose in diabetes. Fasting glucose levels in both type 1 and type 2 diabetics are reduced by 33 percent after taking rice bran products for about eight weeks (20 grams daily, 10 before breakfast, and 10 after dinner).

Diabetic patients are in need of strong antioxidant defenses to modulate the consequences of hyperglycemia, and rice bran appears to meet those needs. Rice bran and rice bran products may not only help to stabilize diabetes, but may also have a role in preventing diabetic complications.

Sources: R. Cheruvanky, "Bioactives in Rice Bran and Rice Bran Oil," *Phytochemicals as Bioactive Agents*, W.R. Bidlack, ed. (New Jersey: Technomic Publications, 2000), p. 234.

377. ANTIOXIDANTS AGAINST DIABETES

Administering vitamins A, C, E, and barley leaf extract during treatment of some diabetic side effects may help to minimize associated complications. Oxidative stress plays an important role in the chronic complications of insulin-dependent diabetes, which can lead to an increase in free radicals [atoms that can cause cell damage]. Antioxidant vitamins such as A, C, and E administered during such treatment could be beneficial in minimizing oxidative stress and possibly both the acute and chronic complications of insulin-dependent diabetes mellitus.

Barley leaf extract may also help to scavenge these free radicals and inhibit negative cholesterol oxidation. In type 2 diabetics, this supplement may protect against vascular diseases as well.

Sources: *Journal of Diabetes Complications* 2002;16:294-300; *Nutrition* 2001;17(10):824-834; B. Kamen, *Everything I Know About Nutrition I Learned from Barley*.

WANT TO KNOW MORE?
[To learn more about young barley leaf extract and the remarkable qualities of this important nutritional supplement, see Hint #1,109 in the *Healthier Living* section.]

DIABETES: REDUCING RISK

378. DIABETES & RISK OF HIP FRACTURE

If you are a diabetic woman, be warned: You are at increased risk for hip fracture.
Women with diabetes have an increase risk of hip fracture, and they may benefit from strategies to prevent such clinical outcomes of osteoporosis. In addition, regular exercise, a healthy diet, and supplementing with both chromium and soluble rice bran are all concrete steps you can take to protect yourself.

[Keep these facts in mind: The USDA confirms that almost every American is deficient in chromium. Chromium deficiency has been correlated with diabetes. Less insulin is required to keep glucose controlled when adequate chromium is present. Exercise binds glucose without the need for insulin. An hour and a half after a single exposure to sugar, there are marked increases in chromium excretion.]

The use of insulin or oral diabetes medications is also associated with a significantly increased risk of hip fracture relative to those without diabetes.

Sources: *Diabetes Care* **2001;24:1192-1197;** **B. Kamen,** *The Chromium Connection: A Lesson in Nutrition.*

WANT TO KNOW MORE?
[See the *Osteoporosis & Other Skeletal Problems* section for useful information on hip fracture, as well as lots of informative tips on how to prevent.]

379. UNDIAGNOSED DIABETES IS COMMON

If you are older and are overweight or have hypertension, you could be diabetic without realizing it. Up to one third of older Americans with diabetes are undiagnosed, so the time to consider lifestyle change is NOW, regardless of how young you are — especially if you are overweight and/or have hypertension.

Undiagnosed diabetes cases are more likely among men and those who are overweight or have hypertension. Since there is a higher risk of undiagnosed diabetes found in those also at risk for heart disease, monitoring glucose [sugar] levels in these individuals is important.

The prevalence of diabetes in developed nations is expected to jump by 42 percent over the next 25 years.

Source: *Diabetes Care* **2001;24:2065-2070.**

WANT TO KNOW MORE?
[As discussed in Hint #376, supplements like soluble rice bran are scientifically demonstrated to keep blood sugar under control. It should be added to your regimen if you fit the pattern described above, or think you are at risk for any other reason.]

DIABETES TYPE 1

IN THIS SECTION:
- CAUSES & PRECURSORS
- NATURAL REMEDIES & SUPPLEMENTS
- REDUCING RISK

DIABETES 1: CAUSES & PRECURSORS

380. RAPID EARLY GROWTH & DIABETES 1

If you have a child experiencing rapid early growth, be warned: He/she may be at increase risk for type 1 diabetes. Rapid growth in early childhood – measured by height, weight, or body mass index – is a risk factor for childhood-onset diabetes. Among patients with type 1 diabetes, scores for height and weight are *significantly* higher one month after birth compared with controls. The maximum difference occurs between one and two years of age.

An important note to new moms: Breastfeeding is associated with a reduction in the risk for this type of diabetes.

Source: *Diabetes Care* 2002;25:1755-1760.

381. OLDER MOMS = DIABETES 1 RISK FOR KIDS

Older mothers, be warned: Your children are at an increased risk of developing childhood (type 1) diabetes. The risk of type 1 diabetes in childhood is *strongly* associated with increasing maternal age at delivery. The higher age of the mother can influence maturation of the child's immune system, possibly increasing a predisposition to type 1 diabetes later in life.

This risk increases progressively with the age of the mother: For mothers older than 40 the risk is *three time greater* than for mothers younger than 20. Diabetes 1 risk increases by 25 percent for each five-year increase in the mother's age.

As people in many parts of the world are tending to start their families later in life, this may be a partial explanation for the increase in childhood diabetes seen in many countries today. Experts claim that the trend of increasing maternal ages between 1970 and 1996 accounts for an 11.4 percent increase in the incidences of childhood diabetes.

But this can only partly explain an increase of this magnitude, and other as yet unknown factors must be involved.

Source: *British Medical Journal* **2000;321:420-424.**

WANT TO KNOW MORE?
Diabetes 1 risk for children is also linked, although less strongly, to higher paternal age and earlier birth order. Risk increases nine percent for each five-year increase in the father's age, and increasing birth order decreases the relative risk: after the firstborn, each subsequent child faces a 15 percent lower risk of diabetes.

DIABETES 1: NATURAL REMEDIES & SUPPLEMENTS

382. VITAMIN D REDUCES DIABETES 1 RISK

Giving your child supplemental vitamin D may reduce their risk of developing type 1 diabetes. Children who receive regular vitamin D supplementation are 88 percent less likely to develop type 1 diabetes compared to children who receive no supplementation. (In fact, even *irregular* supplementation is tied to a reduced risk of 84 percent.)

[Given that vitamin D acts as an immunosuppressant and type 1 diabetes is considered an autoimmune disease, these findings are not surprising. Ensuring that infants receive adequate vitamin D supplementation might help reverse the increasing incidence of type 1 diabetes.]

Source: *Lancet* **2001;358:1500-1503;** *Journal of Endocrinology* **2001;169(1):161-8.**

WANT TO KNOW MORE?
Children thought to have rickets during infancy are three times more likely to develop diabetes than other children. [Rickets is a deficiency disease that affects developing bones, and is also related to vitamin D deficiency. See Hint #303 in the *Childhood Illnesses & Health Problems* section for more information on this disease.]

383. IGF-1 FOR ADOLESCENT DIABETICS

Supplementation with the hormone *insulin-like growth factor 1* (IGF-1) is helpful for those with type 1 diabetes. The addition of IGF-1 improves control in adolescent diabetics *without* increasing weight (as is seen with intensive insulin therapy).

IGF-1 is found in significant quantities in velvet deer antler and colostrum supplements.

Source: Meeting of the Endocrine Society, San Diego, CA.

WANT TO KNOW MORE?
[See Hints #1,110 and #1,108 in the *Healthier Living* section for more information on colostrum and velvet antler.]

DIABETES 1: REDUCING RISK

384. RETINOPATHY IN TYPE 1 DIABETICS

Taking steps to reduce hypertension and high cholesterol may help protect those with type 1 diabetes from the progression of a diabetes-related eye disease. Diastolic blood pressure and, possibly, cholesterol levels may play important roles in the progression of retinopathy in patients with type 1 diabetes mellitus. [Retinopathy, a common side effect of diabetes, is an eye disease involving damage to the blood vessels of the retina.] As expected, hyperglycemia [high blood sugar] is significantly associated with retinopathy progression. But two newly recognized factors, *diastolic blood pressure* and *cholesterol*, also appeared to predict the progression of retinopathy.

Source: *American Journal of Medicine* 1999;107:45-51.

DIABETES TYPE 2

IN THIS SECTION:
- CAUSES & PRECURSORS
- DIETARY TACTICS
- NATURAL REMEDIES & SUPPLEMENTS
- REDUCING RISK

DIABETES 2: CAUSES & PRECURSORS

385. A SIDE ORDER OF INFLAMMATION?

Eating too much fast food is not just linked to heart disease and obesity – you are also putting yourself at risk for diabetes. If you eat a fast-food-type meal every three or four hours [as many Americans do], you spend most of your time in a pro-inflammatory state, which is now linked to the onset of type 2 diabetes (in addition to heart disease).

The act of eating induces an inflammatory state in everyone, but normally this inflammation occurs for three or four hours and then tapers off. But McDonald's-type meals every three or four hours can put you into a nearly continuous pro-inflammatory state, which can damage healthy tissue.

Anti-inflammatory treatment may help prevent the onset of diabetes and/or heart disease. [There are many natural substance with anti-inflammatory properties such as curcumin, ginger, and velvet antler, to name a few.]

Source: 62nd Annual Meeting of the American Diabetes Association, San Francisco, CA, Jun 2002; *Journal of the American Medical Association* **2001;286:327-334.**

WANT TO KNOW MORE?
The association between higher levels of inflammatory markers and the onset of type 2 diabetes was found after a decade-long study involving more than 10,000 people.

386. OVERWEIGHT YOUNG ADULTS AT RISK

If you are a young adult who is overweight, be warned: You are at risk of developing diabetes by middle age. Body mass indexes at 25, 35, and 45 years of age are all *strongly* associated with the risk of diabetes. In men, being overweight at the age of 25 strongly predicts diabetes risk at middle age (largely through its association with remaining overweight at middle age.)

Source: *Archives of Internal Medicine* **1999;159:957-963.**

WANT TO KNOW MORE?
[If you are overweight, the time to make lifestyle changes is now! See the *Obesity* section for helpful advice on this problem, and start lowering your risk today.]

387. GROWTH HORMONE & DIABETES RISK

The use of human growth hormone (with or without sex steroid supplementation) may lead to diabetes and glucose intolerance, as well as other serious health problems.
In healthy men and women, positive changes in body composition (specifically in lean body mass) are directly related to the use of human growth hormone. But despite some potential benefits, adverse effects are frequent, the most serious being diabetes and glucose intolerance. Other side effects can include peripheral edema in women, and carpal tunnel syndrome and arthralgia [joint pain] in men. Growth hormone supplementation has also long been associated with increased risk of malignant tumor development, especially leukemia.

Sources: *Journal of the American Medical Association* **2002;288:2282-2292;** *Archives of Physical Medical Rehabilitation* **2000;81(12):1594-1595;** *Endocrinology Journal* **2000;47(4):471-473;** *Clinical Journal of Sports Medicine* **2002;12(4):250-253.**

WANT TO KNOW MORE?
Although lean body mass increases with the use of human growth hormone, there is no evidence of increased muscle strength in those trained athletes who take it.

388. CIGARETTES INCREASE DIABETES RISK

Yet another important reason to quit: Smoking cigarettes can lead to diabetes.
Smoking is associated with a substantial increase in the incidence of adult-onset (type 2) diabetes. Smoking increases blood glucose levels after an oral glucose challenge [meaning the consumption of something that causes blood sugar levels to rise] and may impair insulin sensitivity [which can be a precursor to diabetes]. Compared with those who had never smoked, smokers of 20 or more cigarettes daily a 2.1 relative risk of diabetes, while smokers of less than 20 cigarettes daily have a 1.4 relative risk. (Former smokers have a 1.2 relative risk.)

Source: *American Journal of Medicine* **2000;109:538-542.**

WANT TO KNOW MORE?
[See the *Smoking & Nicotine Addiction* section for helpful quitting strategies and tips on protecting your health from the effects of cigarette smoking.]

389. LESS SLEEP = HIGHER DIABETES RISK

A chronic lack of sleep may cause far more serious problems than a tendency to nod off the next day, including increased risk of diabetes. Sleep deprivation, which is becoming commonplace in industrialized countries, may play a role in the current epidemic of type 2 diabetes. The National (US) Sleep Foundation has documented a steady decline in the number of hours Americans sleep each night. In 1975, the average American slept 7.5 hours, down from nine hours in 1910. Today, adults sleep about seven hours a night.

How does this affect blood sugar? Healthy adults who average 316 minutes of sleep a night (about 5.2 hours) over eight consecutive nights secreted 50 percent more insulin than those who averaged 477 minutes of sleep a night (about eight hours). As a result, the "short sleepers" were 40 percent less sensitive to insulin. So chronic sleep deprivation — 6.5 hours or less of sleep a night — has the same effect on insulin resistance as aging.

Source: **Annual Meeting of the American Diabetes Association, Philadelphia, PA, Jun 2001.**

390. SNORING & THE RISK OF DIABETES

Another sleep-related hint: If you are a snorer, you should be aware that you could be at risk of developing diabetes. Because people who regularly snore have an increased risk of developing type 2 diabetes, lifestyle modifications that reduce the risks of snoring *and* diabetes (such as physical activity, smoking cessation, and weight loss) are all strongly recommended.

Source: *American Journal of Epidemiology* **2002;155:387-393.**

391. ERECTILE DYSFUNCTION & DIABETES

If you are a man suffering from erectile dysfunction, be warned: You may have undiagnosed diabetes. Erectile dysfunction is a marker symptom for diabetes, so all men with this problem should have their fasting blood glucose tested.

The prevalence of undiagnosed diabetes in men with erectile dysfunction is much higher than previously believed. While many studies have investigated the prevalence of erectile dysfunction in diabetic men, few have assessed the incidence of undiagnosed diabetes in men with erectile dysfunction.

Important note: Dipstick testing for diabetes is not accurate, and in fact can miss 80 percent of men with the disease. Instead, fasting blood glucose levels should be tested in the presence of erectile dysfunction.

Source: *BJU International* **2001;88:68-71.**

DIABETES 2: DIETARY TACTICS
392. A VEGAN DIET HELPS DIABETES

If you are a type 2 diabetic, a vegan diet will help you to improve metabolic control and will even help you to lose weight. A low-fat, vegetarian diet can help improve glycemic control in those with type 2 diabetes, and reduce the need for oral hypoglycemic medication even in the absence of exercise or controlled energy consumption. [Vegan refers to a strict, vegetable-only diet — so no milk, butter, cheese, or eggs. Nothing that comes from an animal source.]

In addition, those who adhere to the vegan diet lose more weight than those consuming a conventional low-fat diet for 12 weeks.

Source: *Preventive Medicine* **1999;29:87-91.**

WANT TO KNOW MORE?
In one study, fasting serum glucose dropped an average of 28 percent in patients on the low-fat vegan diet, compared to only 12 percent in those given a conventional low-fat diet. Average weight loss was 7.2 kg in the vegan group and 3.8 kg in the low-fat group.

393. WHOLE GRAINS REDUCE DIABETES RISK

Eating three or more servings of whole grain foods per day could substantially reduce your risk of developing type 2 diabetes, and fiber supplements can minimize diabetes side effects. **Cereal fiber found in whole grains and other foods helps to slow digestion, thus slowing the release of glucose into the blood. This, in turn, helps to reduce the insulin response that occurs after eating.**

Current dietary guidelines recommend six to 11 servings of grains per day, and suggest several of those servings come from the whole grains group. But most Americans consume far less whole grains than recommended.

Fiber can also lower cholesterol and triglyceride values and promote weight loss. High-fiber diets can lead to discontinuance of insulin therapy in about 60 percent of non-insulin-dependent diabetics, and significantly reduce doses in the other 40 percent. Long-term use of fiber supplements may prevent or delay the vascular complications usually associated with diabetes.

Water-soluble fibers (as found in oat bran, apples, beans, and psyllium seed husks) are much more effective in lowering glycemia than insoluble fibers (as found in processed or non-whole grain cereals and certain vegetables).

Sources: *American Journal of Clinical Nutrition* 2002;76:390-398; B. Kamen, *New Facts About Fiber*.

394. DIABETICS: CUT OUT ANIMAL PROTEIN!

If you have type 2 diabetes, limiting your intake of animal protein and sugar may greatly improve your health. Type 2 diabetics who limit their intake of animal protein (*all* animal protein, including fish and poultry) and sugar may *significantly* improve their health — and may even prevent the disease from taking hold.

Remarkable improvements are seen in patients following a special six-month diet: Reduction of animal protein (from two to three times daily to once every other day, replacing it with vegetable protein) and the elimination of sugar results in some being able to reduce insulin by 50 percent, or even discontinue it altogether. Important improvements are also seen in many other areas, including a 32 percent decrease in cholesterol and a 60 percent decrease in triglycerides. (Calories in this study remained the same to prevent weight loss.)

Animal protein contains essential amino acids, which stimulate pancreatic insulin secretion. This increased insulin then increases adrenaline levels, which is thought to induce insulin resistance.

Source: 83rd annual meeting of the Endocrine Society, University of South Florida, Tampa, FL, Jun 2001.

395. NUTS AGAINST TYPE 2 DIABETES

Eating nuts can help to prevent the development of type 2 diabetes. Major constituents of nuts – unsaturated fatty acids, magnesium, and fiber – have been inversely associated with the risk of type 2 diabetes. Women who eat nuts less than once a week are at greater risk than those who eat nuts four times weekly. Women who eat nuts more than five times weekly are at the least risk.

The protective effects of nuts seem to be independent of the amount of fruit or vegetables consumed.

Source: Annual Meeting of the American Diabetic Association, abstracts 1644-P, 569-P, Jun 2002.

WANT TO KNOW MORE?
[Eating nuts can also help protect you against heart disease and cardiovascular disease. See Hints #542-544 for more information.]

DIABETES 2: NATURAL REMEDIES & SUPPLEMENTS

396. TAKE YOUR VITAMINS!

Adults who use vitamin supplements may be at reduced risk of developing diabetes. In an analysis of over 9,500 US adults between the ages of 25 and 74 who participated in the study, 1,010 (nearly 10 percent) developed diabetes during 20 years of follow-up. Roughly 21 percent of those who developed diabetes reported using vitamins in the month prior to entry compared with 33.5 percent of participants who did not develop diabetes.

In addition, people who reported taking vitamins regularly had larger reductions in risk than people who reported taking vitamins irregularly, suggesting a dose-response relationship.

Source: *American Journal of Epidemiology* 2001;153:892-897.

397. ANTIOXIDANTS AGAINST TYPE 2 DIABETES

Increasing your intake of antioxidants such as vitamin E, beta-carotene, alpha-carotene, and lutein may help protect you against type 2 diabetes. Higher blood levels of oxidation products [such as free radicals] and lower levels of antioxidants are found in people long before they develop obvious adult-onset (type 2) diabetes. When levels of glucose, insulin, lipid oxidation products, and antioxidants are studied in healthy, non-diabetic subjects, a strong association is seen between oxidation products, high glucose levels, and higher blood pressure – a common complication of diabetes.

Higher glucose levels are also associated with lower levels of vitamin E, as well as carotenoids such as beta-carotene, alpha-carotene, and lutein. [Vitamin E can be found in butter, egg yolks, liver, palm oil, rice bran oil, wheat germ, and barley. Carotenoids can be found in spinach, broccoli, asparagus, lettuce, carrots, sweet potatoes, peaches, cantaloupe, and cherries, among many other sources. (However, those who are diabetic or have low thyroid function have a lowered ability to convert beta-carotene to vitamin A.)]

Source: *American Journal of Clinical Nutrition* 2000;72:776-779; *Journal of Nutrition* 2000;130:728-732; *Free Radical Biology Medicine* 1999;27:449-455.

WANT TO KNOW MORE?
[Free radicals refer to atoms or groups of atoms that can cause damage to healthy cells, and can result from many things, including a diet high in fat or fried foods. Antioxidants act as free-radical scavengers, protecting the body from these harmful particles.]

398. CHROMIUM LOWERS GLUCOSE LEVELS

If you have type 2 diabetes, supplementing with chromium can help decreases your glucose and fat levels. Subjects given 200 micrograms of chromium twice a day for three weeks (in addition to receiving standard diabetes treatment) have significant decreases in their fasting blood glucose and triglyceride levels.

Chromium appears to work by increasing the sensitivity of the patients' insulin receptors, so they are able to use the insulin more effectively.

Source: Gerontological Society of America, cited in *Reuter's Medical Report* Nov 2000.

WANT TO KNOW MORE?
[*Chromium polynicotinate* may help non-insulin-dependent diabetics get off medication entirely, and insulin-dependent patients to reduce their insulin needs by significant amounts. See Hint #373 for more details. And for a good introduction to the subject of chromium, see my book, *The Chromium Connection: A Lesson in Nutrition.*]

399. SOLUBLE RICE BRAN FOR DIABETES

A good daily fiber supplement, such as soluble rice bran, can be protective against diabetes. Increasing dietary fiber can be a major factor in helping to curtail the onset of diabetes type 2, and using fiber supplementation [such as soluble rice bran] is the easiest way to accomplish this goal. Fiber supplementation has few side effects, and can help to reverse factors associated with diabetes. It is an easy lifestyle intervention that promotes health in general (reducing blood pressure and lipids), empowers people, makes us less reliant on medicine, and helps to improve quality of life.

Although we should all strive to make several lifestyle changes – regular exercise, consumption of organic whole foods, and so on – increasing intake of dietary fiber is one of the easiest ways to help prevent diabetes from taking hold because of the availability of excellent high-fiber supplements.

Source: *British Medical Journal* 2001;323:63-64.

400. AMINO ACID ARGININE FOR DIABETES

If you are diabetic, supplementing with the amino acid arginine may be helpful. Long-term treatment with L-arginine improves insulin sensitivity in patients with type 2 diabetes. [The "L" simply denotes the chemical structure of the molecule.] L-arginine, which increases nitric oxide (NO) levels, is known to stimulate insulin secretion.

Patients treated with L-arginine (three grams given three times a day), have reductions in systolic blood pressure and significantly increased forearm blood flow. Compared with placebo-treated patients, those receiving L-arginine have a 34 percent increase in glucose disposal and significant improvement in liver insulin sensitivity.

Source: *Diabetes Care* 2001;24:875-880.

WANT TO KNOW MORE?
[A vaginal cream containing L-arginine can help to increase sexual enhancement in women with libido problems, one demonstration of how supplemental arginine can benefit health systemically. See my book on female sexuality, *She's Gotta Have It!*, for more details.]

401. GUAVA LOWERS GLUCOSE LEVELS

A traditional Chinese medicine comprised of guava fruit and leaves ground into a powder appears to lower blood glucose levels in patients with type 2 diabetes, without any side effects. Improvement is seen after two months of therapy in which two to three grams of guava extract is taken three times a day.

Source: *Reuter's Medical Report*, 1999.

402. COENZYME Q10 AGAINST DIABETES

Supplementing with a natural substance known as coenzyme Q10 (CoQ10) may be beneficial against type 2 diabetes. Treatment with 100 milligrams of CoQ10 twice daily may help adults with type 2 diabetes to stabilize blood glucose levels and lower their blood pressure. (There is a threefold increase in plasma CoQ10 concentration as a result of the 200-milligram daily supplementation.)

We have known that CoQ10 therapy can reduce blood pressure in those with hypertension, and now we know that CoQ10 supplementation may also control long-term blood sugar in type 2 diabetes.

[Some dietary sources of CoQ10 are spinach, peanuts, beef, and fish such as mackerel and salmon.]

Source: *European Journal of Clinical Nutrition* **2002;56:1137-1142.**

WANT TO KNOW MORE?
[CoQ10 may be also be beneficial for a variety of other health problems, including asthma (see Hint #119), hypertension (Hint #626), and migraines (Hint #508).]

403. FISH OIL PROTECTS AGAINST DIABETES

If you are overweight and in danger of developing diabetes, supplementing with a fatty acid found in fish oil may be protective. Docosahexaenoic acid (DHA) is an omega-3 fatty acid found in fish and fish oil. Daily consumption of 0.6 grams of fish oil – or two servings per week of cold-water fish such as halibut, herring, mackerel or salmon – appears to improve insulin function in overweight individuals who are vulnerable to type 2 diabetes.

Three months of daily supplementation with DHA produces a "clinically significant" improvement in insulin sensitivity in overweight people. The omega-3 found in whale blubber are believed to contribute to the lack of diabetes in Greenland Eskimos, despite their obesity.

An important note: DHA has a slight blood-thinning effect, so those on heart medication should check with their physician before increasing doses of fish oil.

Source: Annual Conference of Experimental Biology, New Orleans, LA, Apr 2002.

404. ALPHA-LIPOIC ACID AGAINST DIABETES

The antioxidant alpha-lipoic acid (ALA) can help to prevent insulin resistance and may reduce your risk of diabetes. Alpha-lipoic acid prevents insulin resistance and oxidative stress when given to test animals, and could reduce the development of diabetic complications.

The hypoglycemic effects of alpha-lipoic acid seem to be associated with its antioxidative properties.

[Dietary sources of alpha-lipoic acid are slim, but it can be found in broccoli, spinach, and organ meats.]

Source: *Hypertension: Journal of the American Heart Association* **2002;39:303-307.**

WANT TO KNOW MORE?
[Alpha-lipoic acid also prevents rises in systolic blood pressure and can be used to treat hypertension. See Hint #625 in the *Hypertension* section for more details.]

DIABETES 2: REDUCING RISK

405. LOWERING RISK FOR HIGH-RISK FOLKS

If you are worried about diabetes, you should know that the most common type of this disease may be prevented simply by changes in eating and exercise habits – even for those at high risk. In people at high risk for type 2 diabetes, lifestyle modification reduces the incidence of the disease by 58 percent. (Those at risk for type 2 diabetes are those who are overweight, those with diabetes in the family, those with hypertension, and women with prior gestational diabetes.) Losing only 10 pounds, eating a healthful diet, and exercising moderately is all it takes, even despite serious glucose-tolerance problems. Equal benefits are seen in both men and women when these changes are seriously implemented.

Using lifestyle changes to prevent type 2 diabetes was a concept originally recommended by Dr. Elliott Joslin in the *Journal of the American Medical Association* way back in 1921, but to date there have only been a handful of related studies.

Source: American Diabetes Association's 60th Annual Scientific Sessions, San Antonio, TX, as reported in MedscapeWire, Jun 2000.

WANT TO KNOW MORE?
Although an increasing number of children and teenagers around the world are developing type 2 diabetes due to obesity and sedentary lifestyles, the disease (formerly called non-insulin-dependent or adult-onset diabetes) usually arises because of insulin resistance, in which the body fails to use insulin properly, combined with some level of insulin deficiency. It was formerly more typical in those older than 45 and overweight.

406. EXERCISE AWAY YOUR DIABETES RISK

A combination of a low-fat diet and a half hour of exercise daily (walking or other moderately intensive exercise) is an effective way of reducing your risk of diabetes. Exercise alone can play an important therapeutic role in patients with type 2 diabetes by contributing to glucose control and beneficial carbohydrate metabolism, as well as reducing insulin sensitivity. Patients vulnerable to the disease can cut their risk of developing it in half with this diet and exercise program.

Regular exercise correlates "positively and significantly" with glycemic (blood sugar) control. However, most adults with the disease do not exercise regularly.

The association of exercise with diabetic control is independent of age, body mass index, race, smoking, alcohol intake, diet, and diabetic medications.

Sources: *British Medical Journal* **2001;323:359;** *Southern Medical Journal* **2002;95:72-77.**

WANT TO KNOW MORE?
Studies done on people with impaired glucose tolerance show that those at risk of type 2 diabetes can prevent the disease more effectively with diet and exercise than with metformin, a drug frequently prescribed to diabetics. (A full report of this study is available on the National Institutes of Health website at www.nih.gov).

407. WEIGHT TRAINING HELPFUL FOR DIABETICS

If you are diabetic, training with weights may be protective against a variety of diabetes-related complications. High-intensity progressive resistance training reduces hyperglycemia [high blood sugar], and in diabetics could also reduce the long-term risk of such diabetes complications as retinopathy, neuropathy, and kidney problems.

Resistance training with free weights and weight machines, three 45-minute sessions weekly, offers surprising results comparable to those typically seen with diabetes drugs. Lean body mass increases, while weight and waist circumference decrease.

Resistance training should be included as part of a well-rounded exercise program for all people with type 2 diabetes.

Source: *Diabetes Care* **2002;25:1729-1736.**

408. DIETING REDUCES YOUR DIABETES RISK

Overweight men and women who intentionally lose weight can *significantly* reduce their risk of developing diabetes. Overweight people who try to lose weight and succeed are less likely to develop diabetes than overweight people who do not try to lose weight. And the more weight a person loses, the less likely they are to develop this disease.

On average, for every 20 pounds lost, men decrease their rate of diabetes by 11 percent, and women by 17 percent.

Source: *American Journal of Public Health* **2002;92:1245-1248.**

409. DIABETES: AVOIDING SIDE EFFECTS

Blood pressure, but not glucose levels, appears to influence the risk of some complications in type 2 diabetics, including macular degeneration. Vascular complications were analyzed in the medical records of almost 3,000 patients with newly diagnosed type 2 diabetes. Blood pressure, but not glucose level, was *directly* related to the risk of stroke and cardiovascular disease. High cholesterol levels were found to increase the risk of coronary artery disease and retinopathy.

Simple dietary advice for keeping blood pressure under control includes garlic (which can also aid in blood thinning), hawthorn berries, potassium tonics (to help balance the high sodium content of prepared and restaurant foods), fish such as salmon, cod, and mackerel, maitake and reishi mushrooms, and of course, regular exercise.

Sources: *Journal of Diabetes Complications* **2002;16:271-276;** *Alternative Medicine: Definitive Guide*, **2nd ed., 2002),773-781.**

410. OLDER DIABETIC WOMEN & MEMORY PROBLEMS

If you are an older woman with diabetes, you could be at increased risk of developing memory problems. Senior women with type 2 diabetes may be at greater risk of developing memory problems compared to other elderly women, but diabetes treatment may help prevent a decline in cognitive function.

Female type 2 diabetics score lower than non-diabetic women on tests for mental acuity, and increased duration of diabetes increases the risk of poor test scores. Having diabetes is equivalent to aging *four years* in terms of scores on one of the four tests given.

Source: *Diabetes Care* **2001;24:1060-1065.**

WANT TO KNOW MORE?
[Gingko biloba is a remarkable herb that protects against memory loss and diseases such as Alzheimer's. See Hint #77 for more details.]

411. HEART DISEASE LINK AWARENESS TOO LOW

Diabetics, take note: Few with diabetes understand they are at very high risk for heart disease and stroke. Many people with diabetes need to increase their awareness of heart disease as a problem they may ultimately face, since nearly *two thirds* of type 2 diabetics experience some form of cardiovascular disease. In addition, many also lack a broader understanding of just how insulin resistance contributes to heart disease.

Awareness of the link was lowest among seniors and among Hispanics, two groups at higher risk for this disease. Sixty percent of diabetics surveyed said they did not feel that they were at high risk for high blood pressure or elevated cholesterol. But as many of *60 percent* of diabetics have hypertension, and *almost all* have one or more cholesterol abnormality!

When people are diagnosed with diabetes there is great emphasis on controlling blood sugar and the metabolic issues, but we haven't done as thorough a job emphasizing heart disease and its contributions to morbidity and mortality in this group.

A recent survey of diabetic subjects found the following:

- Only 53 percent of the subjects ate recommended amounts of fruits and vegetables, and only 33 percent exercised on a regular basis.

- 28 percent had high cholesterol levels.

- 83 percent did not know the correct definition of "insulin resistance."

- 43 percent using glitazone class drugs did not know if the medication treated insulin resistance and 33 percent had never heard of the term.

- 33 percent were overweight, with nearly half being obese or morbidly obese.

Source: American Heart Association Survey, released May 2001.

412. EXERCISE FOR HYPERTENSIVE DIABETICS

If you have hypertension as well as type 2 diabetes, consider exercise before going on drugs to control your sugar and blood pressure levels. These two problems, if co-existing, can result in abnormalities that are damaging to your heart health. Most of the advice you get usually focuses on drugs or remedies to control your sugar and reduce your blood pressure. But exercise can be directly effective for resolving these problems. It can reduce your total fat and your abdominal fat, and such changes in body composition actually result in improvements in insulin sensitivity, blood pressure, and heart function.

So exercise can go beyond the recognized benefits of glycemic [sugar] control and blood pressure reduction, accomplishing the goal of the drugs without the side effect of drugs.

Source: *Journal of the American Medical Association* **2002;288:1622-1631.**

WANT TO KNOW MORE?
[See the extensive *Hypertension* section for helpful advice on treating high blood pressure through diet, exercise, and nutritional supplementation.]

DIARRHEA

Reports of diarrhea outbreaks have increased in the last decade. Transient diarrhea can occur for many different reasons, and there are quick-fix solutions. *Chronic* diarrhea demands more serious attention. The first cause of chronic diarrhea is usually ulcerative colitis; the next, celiac disease; followed by colitis. (*Saudi Medical Journal* **2002;23(6):675-9**)

IN THIS SECTION:
- CAUSES
- DIETARY TACTICS

- NATURAL REMEDIES & SUPPLEMENTS

DIARRHEA: CAUSES

413. SWIMMING POOL WATER & DIARRHEA RISK

To avoid a common source of diarrhea, don't swallow swimming pool water and avoid standing under a swimming pool sprinkler. Cryptosporidium infection from swallowing swimming pool water may be an under-recognized source of diarrhea infections. Activities that increase the risk for pool water getting in the mouth (such as standing under a pool sprinkler) increase the risk for illness by about 8.4-fold.

Young children should be taken on regular bathroom breaks, and those with diarrhea are advised to refrain from swimming for at least a two-week period after cessation of the problem. Chlorine does not kill everything!

Although bacteria are susceptible to chlorine, parasites are more resistant.

Source: Centers for Disease Control & Prevention (CDC) *Morbidity and Mortality Weekly Report* **2001;50:406-412.**

414. SAUCES ON THE SIDE, PLEASE...

In addition to unpurified water and fresh fruit and vegetables, travelers to Mexico should stay away from condiment sauces (such as guacamole, pico de gallo, and green and red salsas), all of which could be heavily contaminated with diarrhea-causing bacteria. Two-thirds of the sauces studied in restaurants in Guadalajara, Mexico, were found to be contaminated with thousands of bacteria per gram, including *E. coli*, a primary cause of diarrhea. [As a point of reference, a gram is about a fifth of a teaspoon, so you can see that it doesn't take much to cause problems.]

Sauces served in Houston, Texas, were also found to be contaminated, even though sauces are usually refrigerated before served. The number of bacteria found in Texas, however, was far less than found in Mexico, and not as devastating, but those who are especially sensitive could still be affected.

[In general, when ordering food in *any* country, it's a good rule to ask that your sauces be served on the side. Since bacterial infection is often dose-related, by asking that sauces be served on the side, YOU control the amount you are consuming. In addition to bacteria, you may also be getting a nice portion of rancid oils.]

Source: *Annals of Internal Medicine* **2002;136(12):884-887.**

WANT TO KNOW MORE?
[As explored in my newest book, *Everything I Know About Nutrition I Learned from Barley*, probiotics and prebiotics can modify the metabolic activity of bacteria. So be sure you get them on a daily basis, whether you are traveling or not.]

DIARRHEA: DIETARY TACTICS
415. EAT NORMALLY TO RECOVER FROM DIARRHEA

Children with diarrhea who are given food will recover sooner and with a better body weight than those who are fasted. The preferred nutritional treatment for diarrhea should be a diet as close to the normal as possible. The maintenance of fluid and electrolyte balance in a child is vital, and fluid intake should be increased as soon as diarrhea begins.

Oral feedings should be resumed as soon as they are tolerated to help maintain bowel function.

When a child's nutritional status has been jeopardized by poor intake or excessive nutrient losses due to diarrhea, nutritional therapy becomes even more important for recovery.

The following are helpful for diarrhea: red raspberry, yarrow, oak bark, bayberry bark, garden sage, nettle, strawberry leaves, ginger, and plantain (not the banana, but the herb).

Baked potatoes and apple peel are also binding foods.

Source: B. Kamen, *Kids Are What They Eat: What Every Parent Needs to Know About Nutrition* (available at www.publishingonline.com).

DIARRHEA: NATURAL REMEDIES & SUPPLEMENTS

416. ZINC FOR INFANT DIARRHEA

Twenty milligrams of supplemental zinc can be helpful for young children with persistent diarrhea. The US recommended dietary allowance for zinc is one mg/day for infants up to one year of age and 10 mg/day for children until adolescence. Doubling, or even tripling, this recommended amount of zinc reduces the duration of acute and persistent diarrhea. This applies to any child who experiences severe diarrhea, although the children who benefit most have a zinc deficiency beforehand. (American children in general often consume less than the recommended amounts of zinc.)

This effective and inexpensive supplement helps reduce the common and unnecessary antibiotics and other drugs usually prescribed for diarrhea.

Sources: *Journal of Pediatrics* **1999;135:208-217;** *American Journal of Clinical Nutrition* **2000;72.** *Pediatrics* **2002;109(5):898-903**

417. LACTOBACILLUS FOR DIARRHEA RELIEF

Lactobacillus supplements (the "friendly" bacteria commonly found in real yogurt) can help to shorten bouts of diarrhea in children. Childhood diarrhea is a worldwide problem, but nine different studies demonstrate the effectiveness of lactobacillus for children suffering from diarrhea. It can be given to children as a supplement, either in capsule form or mixed into a rehydration drink.

[You can find liquid *Lactobacillus acidophilus* – my favorite form – in the refrigerated section of health food stores. This treatment is totally safe, and a cherry-flavored version for children is available.]

In addition, children who receive probiotics (such as *acidophilus*) along with broad-spectrum antibiotics have fewer occurrences of the diarrhea that these drugs often initiate.

Sources: *Pediatrics* **2002;309:678-684;** *Journal of the Medical Association of Thailand* **2002; 85(Suppl2):S739-S742.**

WANT TO KNOW MORE?
[People in most countries use some form of fermented food containing friendly bacteria, with the US being an exception. That's why it is a good idea to use *Lactobacillus acidophilus* routinely to improve your overall gastrointestinal health. See hint #1,063 for more information.]

EAR/HEARING DISORDERS

While many adults are generally resistant to wearing hearing aids, emotional and social-situational problems may even be experienced by those with *minimal* hearing loss. Ear infections in children are commonplace, and may be initiated by allergies (usually to cow's milk) and poor dietary habits. Yet it is difficult to identify factors that are independently predictive of the development of progressive hearing loss.

418. NATUROPATHIC EARDROPS RELIEVE EAR PAIN

Otikon, a naturopathic herbal extract containing garlic, mullein, calendula and St. John's wort in olive oil, is as effective as anesthetic eardrops for reducing ear pain. Children suffering from ear pain (and who are diagnosed with acute otitis media) given this natural preparation – five drops three times a day into the affected ear canal – experience pain relief similar to those given regular anesthetic eardrops.

Source: *Archives of Pediatric & Adolescent Medicine* **2001;155:796-799.**

419. AVOIDING TINNITUS IN YOUR EARS

Short-term exposure to amplified music puts you at risk for tinnitus, which can result in a noise in the ears such as a ringing, buzzing, roaring, or clicking. The risk of permanent hearing loss resulting from short-term exposure to amplified music is low compared to the risk of continuous tinnitus. Your can reduce your risk of acute hearing damage by avoiding close proximity to music speakers.

Woodwind players are more likely to report tinnitus than other orchestral musicians. Brass players state that their hearing feels "duller" or "less sensitive," which may indicate a loss of hearing at the higher frequencies, whereas woodwind players report an over-sensitivity to some noises.

Both Ginkgo biloba and biofeedback have been known to be helpful in treating tinnitus.

Sources: *British Medical Journal* **2001;323:418;** *BMC Complementary Alternative Medicine* **2001;1(1):5; HNO 2001;49(1):29-35.**

420. TRY EMU OIL FOR EAR INFLAMMATION

Application of emu oil may be a helpful alternative remedy for treating ear inflammation. In test animals, topically applied emu oil *significantly* reduces the severity of acute ear inflammation. The greatest reduction in swelling is detected with high-dose emu oil after six hours.

The inner ear is capable of rapidly mounting an autoimmune response that can ultimately lead to permanent hearing loss. So ear inflammation should not be neglected.

Sources: *American Journal of Veterinary Research* Dec 1999;60(12):1558-1561; *Journal of the Association for Research in Otolaryngology* 2002.

EATING DISORDERS

Classifications of eating disorders usually include anorexia nervosa, bulimia nervosa, and binge-eating disorder. The identification and treatment of eating disorders in adolescents is a challenging and time-consuming commitment. (*American Journal of Psychiatry* 2000;157(6):851-3)
!
Some personality traits, such as perfectionism, and weight and shape concerns often cluster in families of those who have eating disorders. (*International Journal of Eating Disorders* 2002;31(3):290-9)

An increasing body of research literature suggests a seasonal pattern of mood fluctuations and eating behavior in bulimic patients. (*General Hospital Psychiatry* 1999;21(5):354-9)

421. ZINC DEFICIENCY & ANOREXIA

Supplementing with zinc may be helpful for people who are suffering from the eating disorder anorexia nervosa. There is a relationship seen between zinc deficiency and the regulation of food intake, particularly as an initiating cause of anorexia.

This also applies to children who are "non-eaters." If not the initiating cause, zinc deficiency can be an accelerating or exacerbating factor that may deepen the pathology of this eating disorder. Food intake in childhood can influence the expression of the genetic potential.

Childhood zinc deficiency, aggravated in puberty by high energy/low zinc ratio of the diet and stresses of various kinds, can influence both mental and physical development and ultimately lead to the development of anorexia nervosa.

[Unfortunately, zinc is becoming less available in our soil, and therefore less available in our food chain. It is generally not easy for most people, even on healthful diets, to get enough zinc. Zinc deficiency is not uncommon among infants, adolescents, and seniors.

Zinc deficiency has also been linked to diarrhea disease.]

Source: *Journal of Nutrition* 2000;130:1493S-1499S; *International Journal of Adolescent Medicine and Health* .

EDEMA

Edema (swelling) is associated with microcirculatory disorders. (*International Journal of Obesity* **2000;24:126-130;** *Journal of Wound Care* **1998;7(7 Supple):suppl 10-3)** Flavonoid extracts are a new direction for the treatment of fluid retention. Diuretics have side effects and fail to address the underlying cause of the problem. (*Phytotherapy Research* **2001;15(6):467-75)**

422. TURMERIC AS AN ANTI-INFLAMMATORY

If you are suffering from edema (bloating), the common curry spice turmeric may bring some relief. Turmeric has anti-inflammatory effects to counteract edema, a rare attribute for an herb. In fact, among a variety of herbal preparations, only turmeric shows any anti-inflammatory effects for edema,. (The amount used that elicited the positive results was 100 milligrams per kg of body weight. If you weighed 100 pounds, that would be about 45 kilograms, so you would need 4500 milligrams.) In contrast to nonsteroidal anti-inflammatory drugs (NSAIDs), turmeric does no harm to gastric function.

.[Turmeric is also helpful against diseases such as Alzheimer's disease and cancer. See Hints #76 and #153 for more information.]

Source: 9th Asia Pacific League of Associations for Rheumatology Congress, Beijing, China, Jun 2000.

EMPHYSEMA

The association between emphysema and smoking is well established. But there are other causes. Among them, extreme weight loss and surgical tooth removal of the lower third molar. And the next hint, reveals a not-so-surprising link. (*Anesthesia Intensive Care* **2001;29(6):638-41)**

423. MARIJUANA MAY LEAD TO EMPHYSEMA

Be warned: Smoking marijuana, even in the absence of tobacco, may lead to emphysema. The pathology seen in emphysema as a result of marijuana use is different from that caused by a lifetime of smoking tobacco. Based on the young age of the men who participated in this research project and the fact that their level of tobacco exposure was relatively low compared with the amount normally associated with emphysema, a possible causal role for marijuana is suspected in the development of an unusual pattern of this disease.

Source: *Thorax* **Apr 2000.**

EPILEPSY

As remarkable as the advances have been in the past century, it is hoped that the accelerating pace of our understanding of the fundamental mechanisms responsible for brain development will lead to even greater achievements in the clinical care of those with neurological disorders in the 21st century. This, in turn, could have the potential for resolving the mysteries and cure of epilepsy. (*Pediatric Research* 2003;53(2):345-361)

John Hall, a physician in the early 17th century (and William Shakespeare's son-in-law), offered treatments for epilepsy. His recommendations included extracts of the herb peony. We now know that peony root extract and its component, *gallotannin*, have excellent protective effects against neuron damage in epileptics. A few other natural helpers follow.

424. NATURAL HELPERS FOR EPILEPSY

Melatonin has been shown to be of low toxicity in both children and adults, and may be used in high-risk epileptic persons. As is the case with other neurodegenerative diseases, tissue damage in epileptics is the result of oxidative stress. Therefore, anti-oxidative therapy may be very beneficial. [A supplemental drink made from powdered young barley leaf is an excellent source of antioxidants.]

A warning: If you have epilepsy, stay away from the common herbal supplement ginkgo biloba. Even though it is attaining worldwide popularity as a potential treatment for dementia, it may precipitate seizures in epileptic patients.

Sources: *European Journal of Pediatric Neurology* Sep 2002;6(5):243; *Review of Neurology* Sep 2002;35(Suppl1):S51-S58; *Seizure* Oct 1998;7(5):411-414; *Experimental Neurology* Aug 1997;146(2):518-525.

425. EPILEPSY? EXERCISE MAY BE HELPFUL

If you are living with epilepsy, a basic exercise program may improve your life quality considerably. Regular exercise (a minimum of one hour each session, three times a week) may go far to influence mood, thus improving the quality of life. By the end of 12 weeks, physical function and health perception are *significantly* improved.

Not only does mood improve, but health improves, too. Less body fat, better oxygen capacity, and increased endurance and strength are part of the rewards.

Source: 56th Annual American Epilepsy Society meeting, Seattle, WA, Dec 2002.

EYE & VISION PROBLEMS

Is the increased visual acuity failure among primary school-age children in recent years caused by increased access to display screens (television, computers, hand-held computer games)? Combined with poor diet, these habits definitely show a causal link. (***British Journal of Community Nursing** 2002;7(2):80-9*) And what about adults? Needless to say, regardless of how we spend our time, nutrients have a major impact on vision and the visual system. This involves vitamin A deficiency, antioxidants and their role in age-related visual problems, and nutritional optic neuropathies. (***Current Opinions on Ophthalmology** 1999;10(6):464-73*)

IN THIS SECTION:
- CATARACTS
- BETTER CONTACT LENSES
- LASER EYE SURGERY CAVEATS
- NUTRITIONAL UV PROTECTION

- MACULAR DEGENERATION
- MYOPIA
- EYE STRAIN
- NIGHT BLINDNESS

EYE PROBLEMS: CATARACTS

426. HIGH-SODIUM DIET LINKED TO CATARACTS

A high-sodium diet may do more than put you at risk of developing hypertension, it may also increase your risk of cataracts. In order for the lenses of the eye to remain transparent, they must maintain low levels of intracellular sodium. Higher levels of extracellular sodium might make it more difficult for sodium pumps [in the cells] to maintain these low levels. Research shows that those with the highest sodium intake have approximately *twice* the risk of developing cataracts as do those with the lowest levels of sodium intake.

Therefore, a reduced sodium diet may have the added benefit of preventing cataracts in adults. [Be aware that most of the sodium you ingest comes from processed food, with bread having the highest amount.]

Source: *American Journal of Epidemiology* 2000;151:624-626.

427. VITAMIN SUPPLEMENTS AGAINST CATARACTS

Supplementing with multivitamins and certain vitamins may help to prevent the development of cataracts. The use of multivitamin supplements is associated with a reduced prevalence of cataracts, and this applies to both nuclear and cortical types of cataracts. Thiamin use is also associated with a reduced prevalence of both of these two cataract types. Vitamin A supplements are protective against nuclear cataracts only, and folate [a form of B] and vitamin B12 supplements are *strongly* protective against cortical cataracts.

Researchers conclude that long-term use of multivitamins, B group vitamins, and vitamin A supplements may reduce the prevalence of cataracts. (The strong protective influence of folate and vitamin B12 on cortical cataracts is a relatively new finding.)

Source: *American Journal of Ophthalmology* **Jul 2001;132(1):19-26.**

428. VITAMIN C AGAINST CATARACTS

Supplementing with vitamin C may help reduce your risk of developing cataracts.
Women who take vitamin C supplements for 10 years or more reduce their risk for developing cortical cataracts by 60 percent, compared with women who do not take vitamin C supplements. In women under 60 years of age, vitamin C appears to decrease cortical cataract risk: those with daily vitamin C intakes of 362 mg or more have a 57 percent lower chance of developing cortical cataracts, compared with women who have daily vitamin C intakes of less than 140 mg.

Additionally, carotenoids [such as lutein] reduce the risk of cataracts in women who have never smoked.

Research such as this adds more weight to the accumulating evidence that antioxidant nutrients can alter the rates of cataract development, as well as provides indirect evidence that smoking lessens the benefits of antioxidants.

Source: *American Journal of Clinical Nutrition* **2002;75:540-549.**

WANT TO KNOW MORE?
[To learn more about the role of lutein in preventing cataracts, see Hint #429.]

429. LUTEIN FOR CATARACT PROTECTION

Increasing your intake of lutein may be protective against age-related eye diseases.
Lutein supplements can maintain or improve visual function in people with age-related eye diseases, such as cataracts and macular degeneration. Patients with these eyes problems are found to have low blood and eye levels of lutein, an antioxidant carotenoid found in spinach, broccoli, corn, and other vegetables. [Carotenoids are a class of phytochemicals that also include beta-carotene and lycopene.]

Supplements of lutein *esters* (natural lutein compounds found in vegetables and fruit) can increase the density of the macular pigment, one sign of healthy eyes.

All of the patients taking lutein ester supplements reported improvements in vision. In fact, visual acuity in the cataract patients improved by an average of 40 to 50 percent, approaching normal. Tolerance of glare was also improved significantly, and none of the patients experienced any side effects.

Source: *Journal of the Science of Food & Agriculture* **2001;81:904-909.**

WANT TO KNOW MORE?
[See Hint #202 for information on lutein's protective properties against colon cancer.]

430. GERMANIUM SLOWS CATARACT PROGRESSION

If you have cataracts, germanium supplementation may help to slow their progression. Organic germanium (also referred to as Ge-132, and not to be confused with germanium dioxide) can be protective against the progression of cataracts. Organic germanium has been shown to be effective in preventing a process called *glycation*, which results in the development of cataracts. By preventing glycation, cataract progression can be delayed.

Sources: Department of Biological Sciences, Oakland University, Rochester, MI; *Experimental Eye Research*, **1995..**

WANT TO KNOW MORE?
Organic germanium has many other advantages, as well. Among them: When administered to test animals with normal blood pressure, the use of organic germanium shows no change. When given to test animals with high blood pressure, the animals return to normal within seven to 10 days.

In true adaptogenic style, it has lasting effects for a considerably long period after it is discontinued.

[An adaptogen is a substance with the ability to activate natural healing or immune responses, but that stops its action when no longer needed (in contrast to drugs, which continue their appointed job without stopping, leading to unwanted side effects).]

431. CATARACT EXTRACTION & HEART DISEASE

If you have cataracts, you should be aware of the [likely unexpected] risks associated with their removal. Among women, cataract extraction is *significantly* associated with an increased risk of coronary heart disease, as well as with overall mortality.

It is probable that cataract formation, rather than having a cause-effect relationship with coronary heart disease, rather is more reflective of general tissue damage due to oxidative stress, associated with the aging process.

But among over 60,000 women studied since 1984 by the Harvard School of Public Health in Boston, more than 2,000 reported cataract extractions by 1992. Ten years of follow-up showed a significant increase in coronary heart disease among these women, even after adjustment for smoking, diabetes, and other factors. (The association was even stronger among women with a history of diabetes.)

Source: *American Journal of Epidemiology* **2001;153:875-888.**

432. DON'T MIX ANTIBIOTICS WITH STATINS!

Be careful about mixing cholesterol-lowering drugs with antibiotics – such a combination can lead to the development of cataracts. Taking statins (cholesterol-lowering drugs) in combination with agents that slow the metabolism of these drugs in your body, such as erythromycin, could increase the risk of cataract development. The antibiotic increases the bioavailability of the statins, thereby increasing the risk of cataract development by as much as *three-fold*!

Statins are commonly prescribed cholesterol-lowering agents that inhibit an enzyme necessary for your body to produce cholesterol. Certain statins, including lovastatin, produce cataracts in test animals, even without the presence of antibiotics. Myopathy, or muscle weakness, is one of the most prevalent side effects of statins.

Sources: *British Medical Journal* **2002;325:1194;** *Medical Science Monitor* **2002;8(5):CR384-388;** *Archives of Internal Medicine* **2001;161(16):2021-22026;** *Journal of Lipid Research* **2002;** *Experimental Eye Research* **2002;75(5):603-609.**

EYE PROBLEMS: BETTER CONTACT LENSES

433. SELENIUM COATING FOR CONTACTS

An inexpensive coating made from the mineral selenium can keep contact lenses virtually bacteria-free without irritating your eyes or interfering with the lenses' corrective powers. Bacteria, which can adhere to the lens surface, can form stubborn coatings called "biofilms" on lenses, and infection can damage the cornea and even lead to blindness.

Source: Annual Meeting of the American Chemical Society, Boston, MA, Aug 2002.

EYE PROBLEMS: EYE STRAIN

434. STRESS CAN LEAD TO EYE STRAIN

Tired eyes at work? It could actually be from emotional or psychological stress. Previous studies have implicated psychological factors (such as job demands) in worker complaints of neck, shoulder, wrist and back pain, though few have examined complaints of eye strain. But psychological factors such as work satisfaction, self-esteem, and conflicts with coworkers are found to be *significant* contributors to complaints of eye strain, even in the absence of any vision problems.

In one group of workers studied, factors such as work satisfaction, self-esteem and coworker support were strongly correlated with complaints of eye troubles. In fact, only four percent of the participants' eye strain was due to environmental factors such as smoke and noise, and lighting played no role at all.

But we should not overlook prior research concluding that smoking, lighting, and even the exact placement of the computer screen can have a large effect on eye problems, too.

Source: *Journal of Occupational & Environmental Medicine* **2001;58:267-271.**

WANT TO KNOW MORE?
[The office environment can be extremely taxing on your health. See the *On-the-Job Health Concerns* section for helpful hints on reducing health risks while at work.]

EYE PROBLEMS: LASER EYE SURGERY CAVEATS

435. DRY EYE SYNDROME & LASER EYE SURGERY

Dry eye, a common problem – especially among patients considering laser eye surgery – may increase following such surgery, but normal production of lubrication can be restored with a natural formula of antioxidants and other special nutrients called BioTears Plus. Dry eye is the most frequent patient complaint heard by eye doctors. Causes include extended contact lens wear, bacterial infection, diseases such as diabetes, asthma, and rheumatoid arthritis, medications, computer use, and the natural aging process.

For those considering laser surgery, preoperative dry eye appears to be a risk factor for more severe postoperative dry eye. (The condition is associated with contact lens intolerance, a major reason why patients decide to undergo laser surgery in the first place).

Artificial tears sold over the counter may relieve symptoms, but never get to the causes, and may even aggravate the condition. Scientists have created an oral dietary supplement to restore the production of eye lubricants. The product is available from Biosyntrx Inc. in California.

Source: *Archives of Ophthalmology* **2002;120:1024-1028; BioSyntrx Inc.**

436. LASER SURGERY? TAKE YOUR VITAMINS!

If you are considering corrective laser eye surgery, supplementing with vitamins A and E may speed healing and greatly improve the outcome.
Supplements of vitamins A and E appear to reduce the risk of complications after laser eye surgery, as well as improve visual acuity in some patients.

These vitamins may also reduce levels of damaging free radicals and may help promote the growth of new cornea cells in the eyes. (Laser surgery likely generates free radicals, which could impair recovery and account for such complications as hazy vision and a regression of myopia.)

Patients taking these vitamin supplements heal substantially faster, experience significantly less hazy vision, and report much better visual acuity following surgery.

Source: *British Journal of Ophthalmology* 2001;85:537-539.

EYE PROBLEMS: MACULAR DEGENERATION

437. CAROTENOIDS & MACULAR DEGENERATION

Protect yourself from macular degeneration by increasing your intake of two important carotenoids. The carotenoids lutein and zeaxanthin may help protect your eyes against age-related macular degeneration. (Average levels of these two nutrients can be 32 percent lower in those with age-related macular degeneration.)

Retinal zeaxanthin actually prevents light-induced cell death, and the effect is dose-dependent (so the higher the carotenoid levels, the greater protection).

But ingestion of lutein isn't enough! These other factors also play a very substantial role in preventing or initiating this disease: age, race, education, body mass index, cholesterol level, exercise, sun exposure, smoking, and alcohol consumption.

Every 10 percent increase in dietary lutein [kale is a good source] plus zeaxanthin intake is associated with a 2.4 percent increase in serum lutein concentrations.
Sources: *Investigative Ophthalmology & Visual Science* 2002;43(11):3538-3549; *Journal of Epidemiology* 2002;12(5):357-366; *Ophthalmology* 2002;109(10):1780-1787; *American Journal of Clinical Nutrition* 2002;76(4):818-827; *Journal of Nutrition* 2002;132:525S-530S.

WANT TO KNOW MORE?
Intake of vegetables and fruits rich in lutein and zeaxanthin (carrot and pumpkin specifically) might also help to prevent high blood sugar, a relationship not observed with other fruits and vegetables. Lutein and zeaxanthin may also reduce the risk of several other chronic conditions, including diabetes.

438. WOMEN MAY NEED MORE LUTEIN

Another important point regarding lutein and eye health: Women may need higher levels of it than men. The greater storage of lutein in body fat may limit the amount of lutein available to the eye (where it might protect against macular degeneration), so women (especially overweight women) may need more lutein because they have a relatively higher percentage of body fat compared to men.

Macular degeneration is the leading cause of blindness among the elderly. Lutein [found in spinach] and zeaxanthin [found in corn] are associated with a decreased risk of macular degeneration.

In women, lutein levels found in fat tissue are inversely related to levels found in eyes (that is, the more found in fat, the less found in eyes). This is not seen in men, however.

Source: *American Journal of Clinical Nutrition* **2000;71:1555-1562.**

439. MACULAR DEGENERATION & FAT INTAKE

Reducing your intake of unhealthy fats while increasing intake of "healthy" fats (such as those found in fish) may protect you from macular degeneration.
Specific types of fat influence your risk of macular degeneration more than total fat intake. Foods that are high in harmful fats tend to be highly processed store-bought snack foods. Such foods might contain products that adversely affect blood vessels supplying the choroids (middle layer of the eye, between the retina and sclera) or the retina. These and other similar foods might also increase oxidative damage in the macula [as in "macular" degeneration].

In contrast, intake of omega-3 fatty acids and fish seems to have a protective effect.

As the incidence of macular degeneration in our older population is rising, finding a means of prevention is of utmost importance.

Source: *Archives of Ophthalmology* **2001;119:1191-1199.**

440. BUTTER YOUR BREAD FOR BETTER EYES

Go ahead and butter your bread – it will increase lutein availability, helping to protect you from age-related vision problems. Lutein has been shown to be protective against age-related macular degeneration, an increasing problem in this country.

Conflicting results on the use of lutein for macular degeneration may be due to the fact that this nutrient requires fat in the diet for optimal absorption. The lutein response is higher when lutein is consumed with a high-fat spread (207 percent increase) than with a low-fat spread (88 percent increase).

Source: *American Journal of Clinical Nutrition* **May 2000;71(5)1187-1193.**

WANT TO KNOW MORE?
[Real butter is also a good source of vitamin E, a nutrient found in very few foods.]

EYE PROBLEMS: MYOPIA

441. GOOD AGAINST MONSTERS, BAD FOR EYES

Encourage your young children to sleep with the lights out, as nighttime light in a child's bedroom can lead to near-sightedness. The absence of a daily period of darkness during early childhood is a potential precipitating factor in the development of myopia [near-sightedness].

Children who sleep in darkness during the first two years of life are at lower risk of developing this vision problem than are children who sleep in the presence of artificial light [such as a night-light].

Source: *Nature* 1999;399:112-113.

EYE PROBLEMS: NUTRITIONAL EYE PROTECTION

442. LACTOFERRIN: THE CORNEA PROTECTOR

Protect your eyes against damage with lactoferrin (a natural protein component of cow's milk). Lactoferrin supplementation protects against ultraviolet light-induced oxidation in the human cornea.

If damage has already occurred, lactoferrin will *not* inhibit the damage or affect wound healing. However, pretreatment by topical application of lactoferrin does suppress the development of a corneal defect induced by UV irradiation.

The presence of lactoferrin in human tears may also help to inhibit this kind of damage.

Source: *Cornea* Mar 2000;19(2):207-211.

WANT TO KNOW MORE?
[Lactoferrin can also help with athlete's foot. See Hint #125 for more details.]

443. LUTEIN, ZEAXANTHIN FOR HEALTHY EYES

Protect your eyes by increasing your intake of lutein and zeaxanthin. The antioxidant carotenoids lutein and zeaxanthin play crucial roles in maintaining the health of your eyes. Both are stored in the macula region of the retina (together comprising the macular pigment), where they filter out harmful blue light and trap hazardous free radicals.

Both lutein and zeaxanthin offer the greatest protection when combined with vitamins E, C, and other antioxidants, which protect the carotenoids themselves against free radical damage. (One good example of how a network of antioxidants can work together.)

[Spinach is a rich source of lutein, while corn is a rich source of zeaxanthin.]

Source: *Investigative Ophthalmology & Visual Science* 2000;41(4Suppl):S601.

EYE PROBLEMS: NIGHT BLINDNESS

444. VITAMIN A & ZINC FOR NIGHT BLINDNESS

If you suffer from night blindness, a combination of vitamin A and zinc may help (but either alone will not). Zinc deficiency can result in abnormal dark adaptation or night blindness, a symptom primarily of vitamin A deficiency.

Pregnant women who had developed night blindness were given various combinations of nutrients. Zinc treatment increased zinc concentrations in their blood, but by itself failed to restore night vision. But women with low serum zinc levels who were given vitamin A *plus* zinc were four times more likely to have their night vision restored, compared with women given a placebo.

So it appears that zinc was able to help the effect of vitamin A in restoring night vision.

Sources: Johns Hopkins University, Baltimore, MD; Society for the Prevention of Blindness, Kathmandu, Nepal, Jun 2001.

WANT TO KNOW MORE?
People with degenerative retinal diseases (such as retinitis pigmentosa), may have adequate day vision but suffer from poor night vision.. Night vision goggles have the ability to improve poor night vision in those with visual acuity. (*Optometry & Visual Science* 2002;79(1):39-45)

Night blindness during pregnancy caused by vitamin A deficiency is associated with serious increased risks among women. (*Journal of Nutrition* 2002;132(9suppl):2884S-2888S)

FATIGUE

Fatigue is one of the most common complaints heard by the primary care physician. Factors that contribute to fatigue include poor health status, psychological stress, poor nutrition, and pregnancy. Less well understood are factors that contribute to fatigue among healthy, nonpregnant individuals. But there are some very specific nutrients and herbs that can help to lessen any degree of fatigue. (*Biological Research In Nursing* 2002;3(4):222-33)

445. YOU SAY POTATO, I SAY POTASSIUM...

If you are experiencing fatigue or a lack of energy, you may be deficient in potassium, an important mineral. Here's a simple solution for potassium deficiency: Slice an organic potato with the skin intact and soak overnight in water. When you wake the next morning, drink the juice.

To keep the maximum amount of potassium in cooked potatoes, cook them whole — steaming is best. Fifty percent of potassium in potatoes may be lost during the boiling process.

Most of us are potassium deficient because our intake of sodium is too high. Even if you don't salt your foods, you are not home free: high intakes of sodium come from processed foods, restaurant foods, and many unexpected sources [such as bread]. If you are interested in the relationship between potassium deficiency and lack of energy, see my book, *Everything You Always Wanted to Know About Potassium But Were Too Tired to Ask.*

446. SMOKING: FATIGUE RISK FACTOR

Situational factors, including smoking, are key predictors for fatigue. Reports of fatigue do not correlate with body mass, inflammatory or immune status, or blood pressure. Positive psychological and situational predictors of fatigue include depression, state of anxiety, sleep quality, and sleep quantity. For men, smoking is a significant risk factor.

Source: *Biological Research In Nursing* 2002;3(4):222-33)

447. SIBERIAN GINSENG FOR AN ENERGY BOOST

Here's another great natural energy booster: Siberian ginseng! My favorite energy boost is Siberian ginseng, shown to enhance physical performance. It has been used in Asia for restoring energy for thousands of years. It is unlikely to have stood the test of time if it didn't work!

Source: *American Journal of Chinese Medicine* 2000;28(1):97-104; *American Journal of Clinical Nutrition* 2000;72(2 Suppl):624S-36S.

FEMALE SEXUAL PROBLEMS

The list for the causes of discontent among women and their sexuality is surprisingly long, with the most frequently reported concerns being decreased libido and vaginal dryness. More than 87 percent of women in the US complain of lack of interest in sex. A very frank discussion of this problem (with easy solutions) can be found in my book, *She's Gotta Have It!* A few solutions follow.

IN THIS SECTION:
- NATURAL LIBIDO ENHANCERS
- SEXUAL DYSFUNCTION
- VIAGRA FOR WOMEN

FEMALE SEXUAL PROBLEMS: NATURAL LIBIDO ENHANCERS

448. TOCOTRIENOLS FOR SEXUAL IMPROVEMENTS

Supplementing with vitamin E, especially the tocotrienol form of the vitamin, may help to improve your sexual life. Vitamin E is essential for the release of estrogen from cells, can improve the activity of nitric oxide, and plays an important role in the signaling aspects of smooth muscle cells – all of which helps to enhance sexual function.

Tocotrienols are a preferred, more complete form of vitamin E, highly absorbable and safe. Palm tocotrienols are removed from crude palm oil without toxic solvents and without adverse environmental impact. An added BIG bonus: Tocotrienols also have the power to inhibit or destroy tumors. The delta faction of tocotrienols may prevent and reverse breast cancer, both hormone- and nonhormone-initiated.

Source: *Journal of Surgery Research* **2000;91(1):9-14; B. Kamen, *She's Gotta Have It!***

449. GINSENG: A NATURAL APHRODISIAC?

Ginseng may not only protect your heart, but it may also help to maintain your sexuality. An active constituent in ginseng (ginsenoside) offers cardiovascular protection and has a nitric oxide-releasing action. Ginsenoside helps to reduce lipid peroxidation [that is, it helps to reduce free radicals in your body that can damage healthy cells].

It is postulated that ginseng's cardiovascular protection may be partly mediated through the release of the nitric oxide, which is also a potent antioxidant. This enhanced release of the nitric oxide is believed to account for the aphrodisiac effect of ginseng used in traditional Chinese medicine. [My favorite ginseng is Siberian ginseng.]

Source: *Clinical & Experimental Pharmacology & Physiology* **1996;23(8):728-732.**

450. NUTRITIONAL CREAM STIMULATES AROUSAL

If you experience decreased libido and/or decreased sexual enjoyment, you may want to try a specially prepared vaginal stimulant cream that contains several safe herbs. When applied vaginally, the transdermal absorption of the cream's consitituents stimulates blood flow, leading to a very satisfying sexual experience. The cream is comprised of the amino acids arginine and ornithine, and the herbs Siberian ginseng, Gingko biloba, tocotrienols, and velvet antler.

The optimum arousal effect may occur within ten to thirty minutes after applicaiton, bur for some women, it may take longer to reach that pinnacle. The more you use a gel-cream like this, however, the less time it usually takes for peak results, and the more potent the reactions.

The cream has been reported to resolve the problem of vaginal dryness, too.

Source: B. Kamen, *She's Gotta Have It!*

451. GINKGO BILOBA FOR LAGGING LIBIDO

Ginkgo can increase sexual responsiveness in those whose libido has been lost to antidepressive drugs. Derived from the leaf of the Chinese ginkgo tree, ginkgo is noted for its cerebral enhancing effects. It has been shown to relieve the sexual dysfunction caused by antidepressant drugs. Woman are more responsive to the enhancing effects of ginkgo biloba than men (91 percent effective for women; 76 percent effective for men.).

Ginkgo generally has a positive effect on all four phases of the sexual response cycle. It can be effective in dosages from 60 mgs daily to 120 mgs twice a day.

Source: *Journal of Sex & Marital Therapy* **1998;24(2):139-43.**

FEMALE SEXUAL PROBLEMS: SEXUAL DYSFUNCTION

452. GLUTEN, CELIAC DISEASE & LOW LIBIDO

If you experience decreased libido and sexual enjoyment, you may simply be suffering from a gluten [wheat] allergy. In celiac disease, the intestinal lining is inflamed in response to the ingestion of a protein known as gluten, present in many grains including wheat, rye, oats, barley, and triticale. It is now believed that the disease is rarely *diagnosed*, rather than rarely occurring.

Sexual dysfunction is more frequently observed in those with this gluten sensitivity. Patients with untreated celiac disease have a *significantly* lower frequency of sexual desire and a lower prevalence of satisfaction with their sex life. Sexual difficulties are even rampant in those with subclinical celiac disease (a problem more common than most people realize). But after one year of dietary treatment [that is, removal of all gluten from the diet], celiac patients show improvements in sexual behavior.

Source: *European Journal of Obstetrics & Gynecological Reproductive Biology* **2001;96(2):146.**

WANT TO KNOW MORE?
Sexual dysfunction is not the only negative result of celiac disease. Celiac patients consuming a normal diet [that is, one still containing gluten] have a shortened reproductive period with delayed menstrual cycles and early menopause.

Many studies have shown that celiac women are susceptible to reproductive difficulties such as infertility and miscarriages. The disease is also associated with low birth weight in babies and a short duration of breastfeeding.

Many of the symptoms of celiac disease are partly due to the malnourished state caused by the malabsorption of nutrients. Ingesting gluten can result in inflammatory damage of the small-intestinal mucosa, and the consequences are varied and far-reaching.

FEMALE SEXUAL PROBLEMS: VIAGRA FOR WOMEN

453. VIAGRA FOR WOMEN? FORGET ABOUT IT...

Women, forget about Viagra: Not only does the drug NOT improve sexual response in women, at higher doses there are significant increases of both headaches and flushing [hot flashes]. Women ages 18 to 55 with some type of sexual disorder were given Viagra and studied for six months. In the end, a placebo was found to be more effective than the drug for female sexual dysfunction.

In addition, 31 percent of the women taking 50 mg of Viagra complained of headaches and 35 percent experienced flushing. At 100 mg (the standard dose for men), 33 percent complained of headaches and 38 percent had flushing.

In a prepared statement, Pfizer Pharmaceuticals, manufacturer of Viagra, said that it is proceeding with a trial of Viagra in postmenopausal women taking hormone replacement therapy. (Since sexual disorders can be a common side effect of hormone replacement therapy, wouldn't it be wiser to remove the HRT rather than add *another* drug?)

Source: 48th Annual Clinical Meeting of the American College of Obstetricians & Gynecologists, San Francisco, CA.

FEMININE DISORDERS

Although we have always been a male-oriented medical community (with most of the studies conducted on men), the one area that deviated from that practice was the treatment of female hormonal balance. Ironically, results of that particular research led to the use of synthetic hormones and many procedures for women that are now considered harmful.

IN THIS SECTION:
- BACTERIAL VAGINOSIS
- ENDOMETRIOSIS
- MENSTRUAL PAIN OR IRREGULARITY
- PELVIC PAIN SYNDROME
- PERIMENSTRUAL ASTHMA
- POLYCYSTIC OVARIAN SYNDROME
- PREMENSTRUAL SYNDROME (PMS)
- VAGINAL & VULVAR DISEASE
- YEAST INFECTIONS (CANDIDA)

FEMININE DISORDERS: BACTERIAL VAGINOSIS

454. DOUCHING LEADS TO BACTERIAL VAGINOSIS

Avoid vaginal douching: It can increase your risk of developing bacterial vaginosis by almost *three-fold*! Frequent douching (once or more per month in the past year) and recent douching (within the past two months) are all associated with the *significant* increase in the prevalence of bacterial vaginosis.

Many women with bacterial vaginosis do not experience vaginal symptoms, so lack of symptoms is not a guarantee of safety.

Many women report that their reasons for douching are unrelated to vaginal symptoms and vaginal infections. A better plan is to apply a healthful vaginal cream.

[At least one vaginal cream has been developed containing nutrients that are easily absorbed by vaginal tissue and can increase the integrity of this sensitive area. In addition, the insertion of a vitamin E capsule vaginally helps to improve the health of the vaginal tissue.]

Source: *American Journal of Public Health* 2001;91:1664-1670.

WANT TO KNOW MORE?
[For more detailed information on these vaginal creams, and how they can also help increase your sexual function, see Hint #450, and see my book, *She's Gotta Have It!*]

FEMININE DISORDERS: ENDOMETRIOSIS

455. THE HEALTH RISKS OF ENDOMETRIOSIS

Adolescent girls and young women who have persistent pelvic pain should be screened for endometriosis, as there is typically a 10-year delay between the onset of pelvic pain and the diagnosis of this disease. Endometriosis is a condition characterized by the abnormal occurrence of tissue outside the uterus, causing pain. Women with endometriosis have high rates of autoimmune, endocrine and allergic disorders, as well as chronic pain and fatigue.

Ninety-nine percent of women with endometriosis experience pain, 41 percent are infertile, 61 percent have allergies, and 12 percent have asthma. (Normal rates for allergies and asthma are only 18 and 5 percent, respectively.)

Compared with rates in the general US female population, women with endometriosis have higher rates of many serious diseases and conditions as well: hypothyroidism (9.6 percent vs. 1.5 percent), fibromyalgia (5.9 vs. 3.4), chronic fatigue (4.6 vs. 0.03), rheumatoid arthritis (1.8 vs. 1.2), lupus (0.8 vs. 0.04), Sjögren's syndrome (0.6 vs. 0.03), and multiple sclerosis (0.5 vs. 0.07).

Source: *Human Reproduction* 2002;17:2715-2724.

FEMININE DISORDERS: MENSTRUAL PAIN OR IRREGULARITY

456. FISH OIL & B12 FOR MENSTRUAL PAIN

Have you tried everything but still suffer from menstrual problems? Try a combination of omega-3 fatty acids (in the form of fish oil) and vitamin B12. Women with low omega-3 and vitamin B12 intakes have a higher incidence of menstrual discomfort. But supplementation with fish oil (which contains omega-3 fatty acids in their free form) and vitamin B12 *significantly* reduce abdominal and loin pain, as well as such concurrent symptoms as bloating, headaches, nervousness, and irritability.

The omega-3 fatty acids are converted into *prostaglandins* (hormone-like substances that control pain, contraction of smooth muscle such as the uterus, vasoconstriction and dilation, and blood coagulation). Why vitamin B12 works is not fully understood, but it is believed to have something to do with its antioxidant properties. After about three months of treatment, there is a significant reduction in the number of menstrual symptoms.

Source: *Nutrition Research* 2000;20:621-632.

457. IRREGULAR PERIODS & HEART DISEASE

If your periods are irregular, embark on a program NOW to encourage regularity as this can indicate a predisposition to coronary heart disease. The Nurses' Health Study looked at 82,000 women and found that 61.9 percent had very regular cycles, 22.9 percent had usually regular cycles, 10.9 percent had usually *irregular* cycles, and 4.3 percent had *very irregular* cycles. Irregular periods did not appear to increase the risk of stroke. However, women who reported usually irregular or very irregular cycles were more likely to develop heart disease.

The association between irregular menses and heart disease is stronger among women who are heavier. Obese women with irregular menses have nearly twice the risk of fatal heart disease.

Source: *Journal of Clinical Endocrinology & Metabolism* 2002;87:2013-2017.

WANT TO KNOW MORE?
[For more in-depth information on normalizing female cycles, see the new 2002 edition of my book, *Hormone Replacement Therapy: Yes or No? How to Make an Informed Decision*.]

458. IRREGULARITY: IS IT EARLY MENOPAUSE?

If you are experience irregular menstruation, you may be experiencing early menopause. Disturbances in the usual menstrual pattern (such as missed periods) are the most common symptoms of premature menopause in women under forty. So if you are not "regular" then it is time to starting looking at your nutrition.

Loss of menstrual regularity can be a sign of ovarian insufficiency, and the associated imbalance is a well-established risk factor for osteoporosis and increased risk of bone fractures [as well as menopausal discomfort].

Source: *Obstetrics & Gynecology* 2002;99(5Pt1):720-725.

459. IRREGULAR MENSTRUATION & HIP FRACTURE

If you have irregular periods, be warned: Women with menstrual irregularities are at increased risk for hip fracture later in life. Women who report always having had irregular menstrual cycles have a 36 percent increased risk of hip fracture compared with women who never have irregular cycles. Those with an irregular menstrual bleeding duration have a 40 percent increased risk of hip fracture compared with women who have a regular bleeding duration. And women with both irregular menstrual cycles and irregular menstrual bleeding have an 82 percent increased risk compared with women who have neither irregularity.

But the good new is that it's never too late to turn things around! Regardless of age, your body will respond to exercise, better dietary habits, and good supplementation.

Source: *American Journal of Epidemiology* **2001;153:251-255.**

WANT TO KNOW MORE?
[One of the best nutritional supplements around is young barley leaf powder, stirred into water or juice and taken once a day. See Hint #1,109 for more details.]

460. CAFFEINE CAN AFFECT MENSTRUAL CYCLE

Watch your daily intake of caffeine, which can negatively affect your menstrual cycles. If you are female and drink three cups of coffee, nine cups of tea, or six caffeinated sodas daily, you are more likely to have menstrual cycles every 24 days or less instead of every 28 days.

Women who are heavy caffeine drinkers are *twice* as likely as caffeine abstainers to have short menstrual cycles.

Needless to say, these findings have implications for women's long-term health.

Source: *American Journal of Epidemiology* **1999;149:550-557.**

FEMININE DISORDERS: PELVIC PAIN SYNDROME
461. MAGNET THERAPY FOR PELVIC PAIN

Magnet therapy may be effective for chronic pelvic pain syndrome, a problem that affects at least one in eight women. Magnets are placed on two regions of the abdomen that are particularly painful when pressed.

As high as 60 percent of women treated with this procedure report a reduction in pelvic pain, and they report more pain relief when the magnets are used for longer periods of time.

This condition can be very frustrating, because its cause is often elusive. But magnet therapy may be one helpful solution.

Source: Meeting of the American College of Obstetrics & Gynecology, May 2000.

FEMININE DISORDERS: PERIMENSTRUAL ASTHMA

462. PROGESTERONE FOR PERIMENSTRUAL ASTHMA

If you suffer from symptoms of asthma during the premenstrual cycle (perimenstrual asthma), the natural hormone progesterone may be helpful. A drop in progesterone appears to be a major determinant in the exacerbation of asthma symptoms during the premenstrual cycle.

[Progesterone is one of the three principal sex hormones, along with estrogen and testosterone.]

The deeper we study, the more benefits for progesterone seem to surface. New studies confirm progesterone's role in fertility, not only for women, but for men, too. (It's sperm related.)

Source: Annual Scientific Meeting of the Thoracic Society of Australia & New Zealand, Brisbane, Australia, May 2001.

FEMININE DISORDERS: POLYCYSTIC OVARIAN SYNDROME

463. IDENTIFYING POS

You may have polycystic ovarian syndrome disorder if you have a menstrual cycle that ranges from more than 35 days or less than eight cycles a year to the complete absence of periods (*amenorrhea*). Polycystic ovarian syndrome disorder may be a major factor in infertility, and cardiovascular risk factors, insulin resistance, diabetes, and uterine diseases – all of which appear to be increased in women suffering from this condition.

Polycystic ovarian syndrome is a common but complex disorder, influenced by environmental factors such as obesity (particularly *abdominal*). It is characterized by the following: evidence of excess androgen (the male hormone) such as acne, hirsutism (heavy growth of hair, often in abnormal distribution), alopecia (loss of hair, baldness), or dark, wart-like patches on the skin. (It is, in fact, the most common cause of menstrual irregularity and female hirsutism.)

The syndrome frequently appears during adolescence, and may have its origins in childhood or even during fetal development.

Sources: *Journal of Nutrition* 2001;131:354S-360S; *Clinical Obstetrics & Gynecology* 2002;16(5): 685-702; *Journal of Endocrinology* 2002;174(1):1-5.

464. INSULIN RESISTANCE & CYSTIC OVARIES

If you have polycystic ovarian syndrome, take steps NOW to protect yourself from insulin resistance, which could eventually lead to diabetes. Insulin resistance is a common abnormality of polycystic ovarian syndrome. Insulin resistance refers to a condition in which insulin is present in the body to escort glucose into your cells, but your cells refuse to admit the glucose. (Pigmentation of the skin typically found at the nape of the neck and armpit may indicate insulin resistance.) Even women who are lean and not overweight can develop this condition.

Because insulin resistance can be a precursor to diabetes, taking steps to prevent and reverse it – such as supplementing with chromium polynicotinate or zinc – should be part of your daily regimen. [See the *Diabetes* section for more suggestions on how to correct insulin resistance.]

Sources: *Advance for Nurse Practitioners* 2000;8(11):38-43; *Investigacion Clinica* 2002;43(3):205-213; *Obstetrical & Gynecological Survey* 2002;57(9):587-597; *Journal of Nutrition* 2001;131:354S-360S; *Fertility & Sterility* 2002;78:1234-1239.

WANT TO KNOW MORE?
The most common abnormalities found in overweight women with polycystic ovarian syndrome are decreased high-density lipoprotein (HDL, the "good" cholesterol) and elevated triglycerides.

465. PROGESTERONE HELPS POLYCYSTIC SYNDROME

If you have polycystic ovarian syndrome, supplementing with the hormone progesterone may help to protect you from developing diabetes. Polycystic ovarian syndrome is known to place women at increased risk of developing type 2 diabetes. But short-term oral progesterone (the natural variety of this hormone) can improve insulin sensitivity, and may be protective for women with this syndrome.

Although vaginal application of progesterone doesn't have this effect, the oral form also helps to normalize lipid profiles and total testosterone.

[Too much testosterone is another risk factor for this condition.]

Sources: *Journal of Clinical Endocrinology Metabolism* Oct 2002;87(10):4536-4540; *Journal of Nutrition* 2001;131:354S-360S; *Current Drug Targets in Immune Endocrinology Metabolic Disorders* 2002;2(1):97-102.

WANT TO KNOW MORE?
Depression often accompanies polycystic ovarian syndrome too, but normalizing insulin resistance can help to relieve these depressive symptoms.

466. EXERCISE & POLYCYSTIC OVARIAN SYNDROME

If you have polycystic ovarian syndrome, exercise can be highly protective against your increased risk of cardiovascular disease. Cardiac risk factors are observed more frequently in those with polycystic ovarian syndrome. But exercise can help to decrease a serious side effect of this condition by decreasing homocysteine levels, thereby lowering the incidence of cardiac events.

An elevation in blood homocysteine is a risk factor for cardiovascular disease.

Sources: *Journal of Clinical Endocrinology & Metabolism* **2002;87(10):4496-4501;** *Japan Heart Journal* **2002;43(5):487-493.**

WANT TO KNOW MORE?
[To learn more about homocysteine and its link to cardiovascular disease, see the *Heart & Cardiovascular Disease* section.]

FEMININE DISORDERS: PREMENSTRUAL SYNDROME
467. CHASTE BERRY FOR PMS RELIEF

If you are suffering from PMS, the herb chaste berry may be helpful. Newly validated by the medical community, but known in the alternative nutrition arena for years, chaste berry [also known as chaste tree] can improve irritability, mood alteration, anger, headache, and breast fullness caused by the monthly cycle.

Bloating, however, is unaffected by the use of this herb.

Chaste berry stimulates the pituitary and helps the body produce progesterone. Women using an extract of chaste berry experience at least a 50 percent reduction in most symptoms of PMS.

Women should especially consider chaste berry when no causal origin for PMS can be established.

Sources: *British Medical Journal* **2001;322:134-137; B. Kamen,** *Hormone Replacement Therapy: Yes or No? How to Make an Informed Decision.*

WANT TO KNOW MORE?
[Chaste berry is helpful for relieving menopausal symptoms as well. See Hint #724 in the *Menopause & Hormone Replacement Therapy* section for more details.]

468. BALANCE YOUR HORMONES WITH VITAMIN B6

If you suffer from PMS or premenstrual depression, try increasing your intake of vitamin B6, which may help relieve symptoms. As we search for substitutes for dangerous synthetic hormones, let's not forget that vitamin B6 can be effective for treating premenstrual symptoms (PMS) as well as premenstrual depression. Studies show that up to 100 milligrams a day of vitamin B6 is likely to be of benefit. This vitamin appears to be connected to hormone and water balance.

We don't get enough B6 in our modern diets because this fragile nutrient is easily destroyed by light, heat, food processing, cooking, and storage. (For example, whole grains contain B6, but processed flour and even whole wheat bread does not.)

Dieting also depletes this vitamin, so B6 should always be supplemented when you are attempting to lose weight.

In addition, when estrogen levels increase, more B6 is required. So women on birth control pills and those still on HRT should also be supplementing with vitamin B6. The best natural sources of vitamin B6 are organ meats [such as liver], egg yolk, fish, dried peas and beans, and walnuts.

Sources: *British Medical Journal* **1999;318:1375-1381; E. Hass, MD,** *Staying Healthy With Nutrition* **(Berkeley: Celestial Arts, 1992), 122.**

WANT TO KNOW MORE?
[If you are one of those women who is still undergoing hormone replacement therapy, you need to learn more about its risks and dangers. See the extensive *Menopause & Hormone Replacement Therapy* section for lots of helpful information, including better, *natural* ways to balance female hormones at menopause.]

469. LOW FAT: ANTI-PMS SOLUTION

A diet consisting of grains, vegetables, legumes, and fruit, and free of animal products, fried foods, olives, nuts, nut butters, and seeds results in reductions in menstrual pain duration, pain intensity, and duration of PMS symptoms. In addition to increasing a beneficial hormone-binding substance, this diet is usually high in omega-3 fatty acids that are precursors of prostaglandins – the kind that have anti-inflammatory actions.

Diets high in seed oils are richer in omega-6 fatty acids, which break down into inflammatory prostaglandins. Research shows a link between a higher ratio of omega-3 fatty acid to omega-6 fatty acid intake with reduced menstrual pain.

Source: *Obstetrics & Gynecology* **95(2):245-250, 2000.**

FEMININE DISORDERS: VAGINAL & VULVAR DISEASE

470. PERSONAL CARE & VULVAR DISEASE LINKED

Women, take note: Vulvar disease persists longer in those who use excessive personal hygiene practices, as well as in those who self-medicate. The skin of the vulva is particularly sensitive. In one group of women treated for persistent vulvar disease symptoms, over two-thirds reported engaging in damaging hygienic practices, such as cleaning with irritating agents or using excessive friction.

Adverse self-treatment (including the use of previously prescribed or over-the-counter drugs without physician knowledge) was reported by 63 percent.

Source: *American Journal of Obstetrics & Gynecology* **2000;183:34-38.**

471. TAMPONS OVER SWABS FOR DIAGNOSIS

If your physician needs to test for a vaginal discharge disease, suggest the use of a tampon – a method that works better than the traditional swab method. Specimens collected during invasive examinations are necessary for laboratory diagnosis of vaginal discharge diseases. Tampons absorb fluid in the vagina that can later be tested for several diseases, including chlamydia and gonorrhea.

In one study done on 1,000 women, the tampon method proved to be more effective than the traditional one at identifying women with one of the most common sexually transmitted diseases that is often accompanied by vaginal discharge.

The tampon method detected 247 cases compared with only 191 cases detected by the traditional swab method. Tampon-collected specimens may also potentially be used for other diagnostic methods.

Source: Meeting of the American Society for Microbiology, Toronto, Canada, Oct 2000.

472. PAP TESTS: EVERY 3 YEARS MAY BE ENOUGH

If you (like most women) have a Pap screening every year, you should be aware that being tested once every *three* years may be often enough. Problems exist with annual Pap screenings that can result in potentially harmful treatment and stress (including the many false-positives, a common problem with these tests). For this reason, one group of experts suggests screening only once every three years.

Severe abnormalities are uncommon within three years of a normal Pap test, and the incidence of severe abnormalities is similar among women screened one, two, or three years following a normal Pap test.

In an analysis of over 128,000 women, no differences were found in the incidence of threatening lesions when comparing women tested within nine months of a normal Pap test result and those who had waited three years between tests.

Source: The Centers for Disease Control and Prevention (CDC), *Morbidity and Mortality Weekly Report* **2000;49:1001-1003.**

FEMININE DISORDERS: YEAST INFECTIONS
473. PROBIOTICS AGAINST YEAST INFECTIONS

Help protect yourself from vaginal yeast infections with the use of probiotics.
[Probiotics are food supplements that *promote* the growth and proliferation of healthful bacteria in your body, such as the *Lactobacillus acidophilus* found in viable, cultured yogurt.] Some strains of lactobacilli can help to prevent Candida, and may even prevent some sexually transmitted diseases.

The depletion of vaginal lactobacilli can lead to increased risk of urogenital [vaginal or urinary tract] infections and human immunodeficiency virus (HIV). The potent antiviral activity seen in some strains of lactobacilli may partly explain some women's reduced risk of acquiring sexually transmitted diseases – including HIV – when colonized by them.

Given that women may have abnormal vaginal flora at many points during their menstrual cycle, the ability to restore a healthy flora using self-care products such as selected probiotics could prove helpful.

Important note: Not all probiotic strains of lactobacilli, even of the same species, necessarily act similarly at the same site.

Source: *Journal of the American Medical Association* **2002;287(15).**

WANT TO KNOW MORE?
[The yeast responsible for those unpleasant "yeast infections" is known as *Candida albicans*, and an overgrowth of this yeast is referred to as Candida (or candidiasis). Candida of the vagina is known as vaginitis, while Candida of the mucous membranes of the mouth is known as thrush.]

FIBROMYALGIA

Because fibromyalgia was considered a psychogenic [mental rather than physical] condition, many people have gone for years without a correct diagnosis, with only sporadic, but largely ineffective treatment. However, it is now firmly established as a "real" disease. (*Arthritis & Rheumatism* **1997;40(4):752-60**) It is associated with disability of a magnitude comparable to that of other chronic pain conditions. Fibromyalgia has become increasingly common. As usual, antibiotics are of no help, but boosting your immune system can be extremely beneficial. (*NeuroRehabilitation* **2002;17(1):33-9**)

IN THIS SECTION:
- ALTERNATIVE THERAPIES
- DIETARY TACTICS
- EXERCISE THERAPY
- NATURAL REMEDIES & SUPPLEMENTS
- TREATMENT PROGRAM

474. FIBROMYALGIA — A REAL DISEASE

Studies confirm that fibromyalgia is a real disease, and that the altered responses to pain and exercise are *physiologically* based. Fibromyalgia patients are more tender and experience more pain at a much lower pressure level than those without the condition. In fact, fibromyalgia patients report pain at about *half* the level of pressure.

When healthy people receive the same level of mild pressure (which is painful to fibromyalgia patients) only two brain areas are activated, compared to 12 activated areas in those with fibromyalgia. In addition, such pain activates regions of the brain that are not activated in those with the disease – indicating that something is awry with the way the central nervous system processes painful stimuli in fibromyalgia patients, resulting in a lowered pain threshold. Purely behavioral or psychological factors are not primarily responsible for the pain and tenderness seen in fibromyalgia [as was previously believed].

Source: *Arthritis & Rheumatism* **2002;46:1136-1138,1333-1350.**

FIBROMYALGIA: ALTERNATIVE THERAPIES

475. ACUPUNCTURE CAN HELP FIBROMYALGIA

If you suffer from the chronic pain disorder fibromyalgia, acupuncture may provide some temporary relief of symptoms, including both pain and depression. Women who underwent 30-minute acupuncture sessions once a week showed *significant* improvements after the first month, compared to women who were given sham-acupuncture sessions. These women showed statistically significant improvement on measures of pain, depression, and mental health. The results lasted for up to 16 weeks, at which time the patients needed reinforcement acupuncture sessions.

Source: Annual Meeting of the American College of Rheumatology, San Francisco, CA, Nov 2001.

FIBROMYALGIA: DIETARY TACTICS

476. VEGAN DIET AGAINST FIBROMYALGIA

If you suffer from fibromyalgia or any rheumatic disorder, consider switching to a raw vegan diet, which may greatly improve your condition. Fibromyalgia pain and joint stiffness are greatly relieved by switching to a raw vegan diet, which consists of berries, fruits, vegetables and roots, nuts, germinated seeds, and sprouts (but no cooked foods).

Plants are rich natural sources of antioxidants, in addition to other nutrients. Referred to as living food, the uncooked vegan diet greatly relieves disease caused by inflammation, as in rheumatoid diseases. Foods eaten on this diet are rich sources of carotenoids, vitamins C and E, plus compounds like quercetin, myricetin and kaempherol. The shift of fibromyalgia sufferers to such a diet results in a significant decrease in joint stiffness and pain, as well as an overall improvement in health.

Source: *Toxicology* 2000;155(1-3):45-53.

[A vegan diet may also help to decrease symptoms of rheumatoid arthritis. See Hint #105 for more details.]

FIBROMYALGIA: EXERCISE THERAPY

477. EXERCISE FOR FIBROMYALGIA RELIEF

Fibromyalgia sufferers, take note: Exercise is more effective in alleviating symptoms of this disease than any other mode of treatment, helping to reduce pain and improve strength and overall activity. Women who exercised for three years experienced a *significant* decline in average pain, the biggest changes being seen at the one-year mark. (All of these women had experienced fibromyalgia symptoms for about 11 years prior to beginning the program.) Over time, these patients were able to reduce their medications such as acetaminophen, nonsteroidal anti-inflammatory agents, antidepressants, and tranquilizers. Alternative treatments were used increasingly during the second and third years, but physical exercise was considered to be the most helpful intervention.

In another compelling study, both patients with fibromyalgia and healthy individuals were put on a twice-weekly exercise program for 12 weeks. Those with fibromyalgia experienced clinically significant changes in muscle strength, flexibility, weight, body fat, tender point count, and disease and symptom severity. (The healthy study subjects, in comparison, demonstrated changes in only half these areas.)

Sources: *Arthritis Care Research* **2001;45:355-361;** *Journal of Rheumatology* **2002;29:1041-1048**

FIBROMYALGIA: NATURAL REMEDIES & SUPPLEMENTS
478. CHLORELLA FOR FIBROMYALGIA

If you suffer from symptoms of fibromyalgia, dietary supplementation with the alga Chlorella may be helpful. The "tender point index" of fibromyalgia patients declines *significantly* after only two months of chlorella supplementation (10 grams of chlorella tablets and one dose of the liquid form taken daily). The substances found in Chlorella that contribute to its health effects include chlorophyll, dietary fiber, amino acids, and nucleic acids. [Chlorella is one of the few supplements that contains beneficial nucleic acids.]

Source: *Phytotherapy Research* **2000;14:167-173.**

FIBROMYALGIA: TREATMENT PROGRAM
479. THE ANTI-FIBROMYALGIA PROGRAM

A specialized physician program is available to help sufferers of the chronic pain condition fibromyalgia. Dr. Garry Gordon, MD, offers an excellent treatment plan for fibromyalgia using supplements. He explains that the protocol must deal with three aspects of the problem: Thick blood, detoxification, and control of infections, which can all be controlled with the right supplementation. Antibiotics are not the answer; results can only be accomplished by bringing YOUR own immune system up to the level that enables YOU to handle the infection.

Dr. Gordon suggests that we must deal with hypercoagulability, among other factors, and take nutrients that help to heal the painful tissues. He makes suggestions for the kind of supplements that will assist in making this happen.

Source: Click on www.bettykamen.com; then click on the Fibromyalgia button to see Dr.Garry Gordon's thorough report on the subject.

GALLBLADDER DISEASE

A sedentary lifestyle, excess weight, a diet rich in animal fats (especially from red meat) and refined sugars, and a diet poor in vegetable fats and fibers are all significant risk factors directly related to the formation of gallstone, a highly prevalent condition. (*European Journal of Cancer Prevention* **2002;11(4):365-8**) Another very significant risk factor is synthetic hormone replacement therapy. (*Annals of Epidemiology* **2002;12(2):131-40**) There is also an increased prevalence among type 2 diabetics. (*Journal of Associate Physicians of India* **2002;50:887-90**) Now here's the good news:

480. VITAMIN C FOR GALLBLADDER HEALTH

Vitamin C – either from food or supplements – can reduce your chances of developing gallstones as well as other types of gallbladder diseases. Vitamin C (ascorbic acid) levels are associated with a decreased risk of gallbladder disease in women because this vitamin aids in the breakdown of cholesterol into bile acids, thereby helping to avoid cholesterol gallstones. Among women, ascorbic acid levels are inversely related to both clinical and asymptomatic gallbladder disease [that is, higher vitamin C levels = lower incidence of this disease].

Source: *Archives of Internal Medicine* **2000;160:931-936.**

481. EXERCISE, DIET, & GALLSTONE FORMATION

Physical activity, dietary monounsaturated fats, dietary cholesterol, and dietary fibers from cellulose are protective against the risk of gallstone formation. Saturated fats are a risk factor for gallstone formation and this association appears to be stronger for men than for women. [Keep in mind that many of these studies don't consider the kind of saturated fat involved. Some saturated fats are harmful, while others may actually be beneficial.]

Source: *American Journal of Clinical Nutrition* **1999;69(1):120-126.**

482. APPLE JUICE & OLIVE OIL FOR GALLSTONES

A simple program of apple juice and olive oil can be helpful for those suffering from gallstones. To help in the dissolution of gallstones, drink one liter (just a bit more than a quart) of apple juice daily for one week, and then one cup of olive oil on the seventh day just before going to bed. On that last day, lie on your left side during the night. In comparison with chemical prescriptions, apple juice and olive oil therapy is kinder to your body and has only minor untasty side effects.

Source: *Lancet* **1999;354:2171.**

GASTROINTESTINAL DISEASES & CONDITIONS

Gastrointestinal disorders are among the most common for which women seek medical attention. Most gastrointestinal diseases in women are not very different from those that occur in men, but several occur more frequently in women, or manifest themselves differently. Among the gastrointestinal diseases for concern are gastroesophageal reflux disease (GERD), peptic ulcers, irritable bowel syndrome, and inflammatory bowel disease. (*Medical Clinics of North America* **1998;82(1):21-50**) These diseases can have a huge impact on the quality of life, especially for those who are immune-compromised.

Advanced technology has led to noninvasive imaging devices that facilitate evaluation of the different facets of gastrointestinal disorders. (*Cancer Journal of Gastroenterology* **2000;14 Suppl D:163D-180D**)

IN THIS SECTION:
- ACID REFLUX
- COLITIS & CROHN'S DISEASE
- FRUCTOSE INTOLERANCE
- IRRITABLE BOWEL SYNDROME
- NATURAL REMEDIES & SUPPLEMENTS

GASTROINTESTINAL DISEASES: ACID REFLUX

483. CHEW ON THIS: RELIEF FROM REFLUX

If you suffer from acid reflux disease, relief may be as simple as a stick of chewing gum. Reflux disease (GERD) is a common problem that affects a substantial proportion of the American population. It is estimated that the symptoms of GERD may afflict 40 to 45 percent of Americans each month. The diagnosis of GERD can be difficult, as its symptoms vary from typical symptoms like heartburn to atypical symptoms such as hoarseness, coughing, and chest pain.

The only test that directly measures whether acid is refluxing into the esophagus is the pH probe, but this test is uncomfortable for the patient, difficult to interpret, and may not be necessary in all cases.

But studies show that the simple act of chewing regular sugarless gum appears to be *significantly* helpful in reducing symptoms of this disease.

Sources: *Journal of Clinical Gastroenterology* **2002;34(3):200-206;** *Annals of Otology, Rhinology, & Laryngology* **2001;110(12):1117-1119.**

484. ANTIOXIDANTS ARE ANTI-REFLUX DISEASE

If you suffer from acid reflux disease, increasing your intake of antioxidants might prove beneficial. Because free radicals produced by gastric acid may be more important than the acid itself in the development of reflux disease, supplementation of antioxidants could improve both treatment and prevention of this problem.

Antioxidant therapy significantly reduces the activation of a certain oxidative stress factor that is present at high levels in those with reflux. Pretreatment with antioxidants helps to lessen reflux in test animals, dose-dependently (the higher the dose, the better the results.)

Such new findings prove the hypothesis that free radical damage, rather than gastric acid, is the major cause of the tissue damage that leads to this condition. Antioxidant therapy might prove particularly beneficial for the many patients who have continued symptoms or complications caused by acid reflux.

Source: *Gut* **2001;49:364-371.**

485. SMOKING CONTRIBUTES TO REFLUX

Yet another reason to quit: Smoking may dull the closure reflex thought to protect the airways from gastric reflux. Smoking is already thought to increase the risk of acid reflux disease (GERD). Now we know that smokers exhibit a slower pharyngoglossal closure reflex, which momentarily closes off the vocal cords when fluid enters the pharynx. This reflex is much slower in smokers than nonsmokers, and damage to nerve endings in the pharynx or to tissue lining the pharynx or esophagus could be to blame.

Acids that reach the pharynx may over time harm the airways. If smokers' airway defenses are weakened, this could increase their risk of reflux-related respiratory problems.

Source: *Gut* **2002;51:771-775.**

GASTROINTESTINAL DISEASES: COLITIS & CROHN'S DISEASE

486. VITAMIN A AGAINST COLITIS & CROHN'S

Supplementation with vitamin A may be protective against inflammatory bowel diseases such as colitis, Crohn's disease, and irritable bowel disease. Inflammatory bowel diseases are characterized by oxidative stress, inflammation, and tissue damage. A depletion of antioxidants plays a large role in the development of irritable bowel disease, colitis [an inflammation of the colon], and Crohn's disease [an inflammation of the ileum, the lower portion of the small intestine]. Vitamin A is a potent antioxidant and vital to immune function. A deficiency in this vitamin has been linked to the development of colitis, while supplementation has been shown to improve the disease. (Vitamin A supplementation has even been shown to protect test animals from *induced* colitis.)

[Vitamin A can be found in liver, fish liver oil, and green and yellow vegetables and fruits.]

Sources: *Journal of Nutrition* 2002;132:2131-2136;2743-2747;2845S-2850S;2902S-2906S; *Scandinavian Journal of Gastroenterology* 2001;36(12):1289-1294; *Neoplasma* 2000;47(1):37-40.

WANT TO KNOW MORE?
It is difficult to achieve normal vitamin A status from plant diets alone. Fortification, supplementation, or other means of increasing vitamin A intake are needed to correct widespread deficiency.

487. DRINKING GREEN TEA HELPS COLITIS

Colitis sufferers, take note: Drinking green tea may be helpful in reducing symptoms of this disease. Green tea helps to inhibit inflammatory responses, and may therefore be helpful in the treatment of colitis. Test animals treated with green tea for six weeks have *significantly* less severe colitis symptoms. **We know that green tea can reduce toxicity, and now we can add the inhibition of inflammation to its list of benefits. This anti-inflammatory action may be useful in treating chronic inflammatory states, such as inflammatory bowel disease.**

Source: *Journal of Nutrition* 2001;131:2034-2039.

WANT TO KNOW MORE?
[Green tea may also have potent anti-cancer properties. See Hint #156 for more information.]

488. FIBER & INFLAMMATORY BOWEL DISEASE

Increasing your intake of dietary fiber can be protective against diseases such as colitis and Crohn's disease. A fiber-supplemented diet can help reverse the intestinal damage of inflammatory bowel disease (which includes ulcerative colitis and Crohn's disease) by reducing toxic activity and restoring protective levels of important nutrients.

Inflammatory bowel disease is a chronic disease of the digestive tract, and an exaggerated intestinal immune response plays a key role. Fiber helps restore this immune response back to normal. (One example: Oxidative stress can cause a depletion of glutathione, an important substance that normally helps the body to rid itself of toxins. But fiber both increases glutathione and helps with tissue healing.)

Source: *Journal of Nutrition* 2002;132:3263-3271.

489. OMEGA-3 FATTY ACIDS IMPROVE COLITIS

Increasing your dietary intake of omega-3 fatty acids can be helpful if you suffer from colitis. The polyunsaturated fatty acid omega-3 can improve the biochemical changes that occur in ulcerative colitis, and a balanced diet containing omega-3 fatty acids can help to ameliorate the inflammation and mucosal damage caused by this disease.

[Omega -3 fatty acids can be found in flaxseed, walnuts, fatty fish, berries, broccoli, and cabbage.]

Source: *Journal of Nutrition* 2002;132:11-19.

490. PROBIOTICS FOR COLITIS & CROHN'S

A combination of probiotics may aid the remission of ulcerative colitis and may prevent the postoperative recurrence of Crohn's disease. [Probiotics are food supplements that *promote* the growth and proliferation of healthful bacteria in your body, such as the *Lactobacillus acidophilus* found in viable, cultured yogurt.]

Probiotic compounds are shown to be beneficial in a wide range of gastrointestinal diseases. Bifidobacterium, *Lactobacillus*, and *Streptococcus* probiotics are the microorganisms which, when combined, may result in the remission of ulcerative colitis and the prevention of Crohn's disease.

Probiotic compounds are shown to be safe and very well tolerated.

Source: *Canadian Journal of Gastroenterology* 2001;15(12):817-822.

WANT TO KNOW MORE?
The administration of either *Lactobacillus* or *Saccharomyces boulardii* has also been shown to prevent the diarrhea that occurs when taking antibiotics. The most successful studies involve the use of *Lactobacillus* at a dose of 1x1010 viable organisms per day and the yeast *boulardii* at a dose of one gram per day. [See the *Diarrhea* section for further details.]

491. TOMATOES AGAINST COLITIS

Consuming more lycopene-rich foods such as tomato paste and tomato juice may help to protect against colitis. [Lycopene is a carotenoid, a class of compounds related to vitamin A. It is the red pigment that gives tomatoes their color, and can also be found in fruits such as pink grapefruit and watermelon.] Absorption of lycopene, which is protective against colitis, is actually *higher* from processed tomato-based foods such as tomato paste and tomato juice than from fresh and unprocessed tomatoes. (The precursor of lycopene, phytofluene, is better absorbed than lycopene itself.)

Since lycopene supplementation reduces the inflammation linked to colitis, a diet rich in this nutrient may be an effective measure against this disease.

Sources: *Journal of Nutrition* **2002;132:404-408;** *American Heart Journal* **Mar 2002;143(3):467.**

WANT TO KNOW MORE?
[Lycopene may also be preventive against lung cancer and atherosclerosis. See Hints #217 and #520 for more details.]

GASTROINTESTINAL DISEASE: FRUCTOSE INTOLERANCE

492. UNRECOGNIZED FRUCTOSE INTOLERANCE

If you have unexplained gastrointestinal symptoms – such as unexplained bloating, flatulence, and distention – you may have fructose intolerance. While much attention has been paid to lactose intolerance as a potential cause of these symptoms, fructose intolerance has received relatively little attention. But there is a surprisingly high prevalence of this condition, and extensive research indicates that many people with irritable bowel syndrome have an underlying fructose intolerance.

[Fructose can be found in most fruits and fruit juices, as well as honey. Avoiding these foods may help.]

Source: 66th Annual Scientific Meeting of the American College of Gastroenterology, Oct 2001.

GASTROINTESTINAL DISEASES: IRRITABLE BOWEL SYNDROME

493. HYPNOSIS FOR IRRITABLE BOWELS

Hypnotherapy may be a helpful treatment option for sufferers of various gastrointestinal disorders. Mounting evidence suggests that hypnotherapy is effective in reducing symptoms of gastrointestinal disorders such as irritable bowel syndrome and dyspepsia (heartburn, flatulence, and nausea). Used short-term, hypnotherapy helps people to improve by about 60 percent, and after one year the average reduction in symptom severity is higher than 73 percent.

Although not a cure, hypnotherapy also improves both short- and long-term quality of life. After hypnotherapy treatment, patients do not usually resume any form of drug therapy.

Source: *Gastroenterology* **2002;123:1778-1785,2132-2135.**

494. DIAGNOSING IBS WITH BOWEL GAS VOLUME

If you frequently pass excessive gas or have a bloated or distended stomach, you may have irritable bowel syndrome (IBS). If the quantity of bowel gas is reduced with treatment for IBS, it's a good sign that the treatment is working, and that gastrointestinal function is improving. Improvements may be possible by changes in diet (including the elimination of junk foods, processed dairy products, and all wheat products. Also, the addition of liquid acidophilus, soluble rice bran, or peppermint agents may also be helpful solutions.

Source: *American Journal of Gastroenterology* **2000;95:1618-1619,1735-1741.**

495. IBS? YOU COULD BE LACTOSE INTOLERANT

If you suffer from irritable bowel syndrome, you may be lactose intolerant and not realize it. Many patients with irritable bowel syndrome (IBS) have undiagnosed lactose intolerance, and eliminating all milk products markedly improves their symptoms. [Because of the some similarities between the protein molecules in milk and wheat, elimination of wheat products may also be beneficial. This is not an easy diet to follow, but the consequences are remarkable. It means no milk, no cheese, no bread, cake, pizza, crackers, biscuits, etc. And it means reading labels carefully, too, because casein (milk protein) is often added to many processed foods.]

Not only does lactose restriction improve IBS symptoms, it is also extremely cost- and time-saving. The average number of annual doctor visits per patient decreases significantly from 2.4, in the five years before diagnosis of lactose intolerance, to 0.6 in the five years following diagnosis. [See the *Lactose Intolerance* section for more helpful information.]

Source: *European Journal of Gastroenterology & Hepatology* **2001;13:941-944.**

496. GUAR GUM FOR IRRITABLE BOWELS

If you have irritable bowel syndrome and have trouble with high fiber, try guar gum, which is equally helpful but better tolerated. High fiber diets are commonly recommended for irritable bowel syndrome, although many people are not able to tolerate fiber. Guar gum is water soluble, but extremely difficult to incorporate into food. So it must be used as a partially hydrolyzed guar gum in beverage form, and has proved effective in softening and improving fecal output. Hydrolyzed guar gum is preferred by more people suffering with irritable bowel syndrome than other fibers, and should be considered for those who can't tolerate fiber or who report a worsening of their symptoms with fiber.

Source: *British Medical Journal* **2002;325.**

WANT TO KNOW MORE?
[As described in my book, *New Facts About Fiber,* guar also prevents blood sugar from rising after the ingestion of sweetened foods, so it is helpful for non-insulin-dependent diabetics. It also helps to control glucose and insulin responses in normal people. In fact, guar moderates sugar absorption better than any other fiber.]

GASTROINTESTINAL DISEASES: NATURAL REMEDIES & SUPPLEMENTS

497. LACTOFERRIN AGAINST GASTRO DISORDERS

Supplementing with lactoferrin, a natural protein component of milk, may be helpful in the treatment of intestinal disorders associated with oxidative stress and inflammation. Lactoferrin is found in high amounts in breast milk and other secretions. It is anti-microbial and immune-enhancing, and can exert a beneficial anti-inflammatory effect on colitis, the inflammatory bowel disease.

[Lactoferrin is a fairly new supplement, and has attracted attention because of its application to cancer therapy. It works by helping to regulate cellular immune responses. Normally, it is found in substances that help to protect our eyes, mouth, nose, and other openings of the body from infectious invasion. Lactoferrin may also be relevant for HIV and chronic viral infections, including chronic fatigue.]

Sources: *Journal of Nutrition* **2002;132:2597-2600;** *Journal of Immunology* **2002;168(8):3950-3957;** *American Journal of Physiology & Gastrointestinal Liver Physiology* **2002;283(1):G187-195;** *Nutricology In Focus* **newsletter 1997.**

WANT TO KNOW MORE?
[Bacteria require iron to do their harmful work. Lactoferrin binds with iron rendering it unavailable to bacteria. It does not, however, remove the iron, but releases it back into the body.]

498. "FRIENDLY" BACTERIA FOR BETTER HEALTH

Probiotics such as liquid *acidophilus* or the new high-bacterial yogurt are remarkable for alleviating stomach upsets and improving gastrointestinal health – for anyone at any age. Western civilization is facing a progressive increase in immune-mediated, gut-related health problems, such as allergies and autoimmune and inflammatory diseases. The experts tell us that genetic factors are an unlikely explanation for these rapid increases in disease incidence.

Probiotic bacteria reinforce the different lines of gut defense. They also stimulate resistance to microbial pathogens, thereby aiding in pathogen eradication and promoting defense mechanisms. By modifying the microflora in your gut, you can help to resist inflammatory responses that could otherwise lead to numerous health problems.

Source: *American Journal of Clinical Nutrition*;73(6):1142S-1146S.

499. PREBIOTICS FOR BETTER GASTRO HEALTH

Improve your health and reduce your risk of gastrointestinal disease by supplementing with prebiotics. You can change the composition and characteristics of the "healthy" bacteria that live in your gastrointestinal tract by consuming fermented dairy products or *prebiotics* such as oligofructose or inulin, substances that are preventive and therapeutic for many diseases.

[Prebiotics are non-digestible food ingredients that can stimulate the growth or activities of the bacteria that colonize the colon.] The presence or lack of these "good" microflora can affect how your body handles toxins, your immune status, and your colonic health. These microflora can even inhibit metabolic events that could potentially lead to colon cancer. Increasing lactobacilli in the gastrointestinal microflora can be beneficial to diseases of the gastrointestinal organs. Oligofructose is also able to counteract triglyceride and liver disorders.

Sources: *British Journal of Nutrition* 2002;87(Suppl2):S255-259; *Journal of Nutrition* 2002;132(3): 472-477;3721-3731; *International Journal of Food Microbiology* May 1998;41(2):127-131.

WANT TO KNOW MORE?
Supplementing with both fructooligosaccharides (FOS) and *acidophilus* together can help to improve your digestion and your nutrient absorption. FOS and *acidophilus* work synergistically, helping to decrease concentrations of fecal toxins to a greater extent than either supplement consumed alone. [To learn more about both probiotics and prebiotics, see my book, *Everything I Know About Nutrition I Learned From Barley*, for a good introduction to this important subject.]

500. BEWARE INTAKE OF DRUGS WITH ASPIRIN

Those who take serotonin reuptake inhibitors (SSRIs) and nonsteroidal inflammatory drugs (NSAIDs) are 12 times more likely to experience upper gastrointestinal bleeding than people who use neither. In agreement with previous reports, the current findings also indicate that even use of SSRIs alone is associated with an increased risk of gastrointestinal bleeding. The risk ratios are even higher when such drugs are taken in combination with low-dose aspirin. The findings indicate that SSRI therapy does increase the risk of bleeding and that the combined use of low-dose aspirin appears to potentiate this effect.

Source: *Archives of Internal Medicine* 2003;163:59-64.

HEADACHES & MIGRAINES

Headaches are common and the past decade has seen rapid growth in understanding headache disorders. (*British Journal of General Practice* 2002;52(480):569-73)

Most everyone has experienced a headache at one time or another. And most of us find some relief with current over-the-counter products available, or with some folklore cure. (My secret is six calcium tablets at one fell swoop, and six a half hour later, with a tablespoon of liquid *acidophilus* two or three times, also a half hour apart. Works every time for me!)

Our great advancement in medicine has been in diagnostics, so we have been taught to categorize the headache as a migraine, chronic tension headache, cluster headache, sinus headache, menstrual headache, hunger headache, hangover headache, and even substance-withdrawal headache. (*Cleveland Clinical Journal of Medicine* 2001;68(11):904, 906, 908, 910, 912)

But headache disorders deserve more attention, especially concerning strategies leading to adequate primary prevention and treatment. (*Cephalalgia* 2001;21(7):774-7)

It is no longer true that alternative or complementary modes of treatment lack scientific proof of efficacy. As with all the hints in this book, this section is also evidenced-based. Many complementary modes are inexpensive and harmless, and, we hope, also effective. Whether it's aerobic exercise; isometric neck exercise; biofeedback; a combination product containing magnesium, riboflavin, and feverfew; or acupuncture, you have the option for deciding which approach is the most appealing, affordable, and realistically doable. (*Medical Clinics of North America* 2001;85(4):1077-84)

IN THIS SECTION:
- ALTERNATIVE THERAPIES
- CAUSES & PRECURSORS

- NATURAL REMEDIES & SUPPLEMENTS

HEADACHES & MIGRAINES: ALTERNATIVE THERAPIES

501. BIOFEEDBACK WORKS AGAINST HEADACHES

If you suffer from headaches, you should be aware that biofeedback is a tool that helps many people. Biofeedback is an excellent treatment for the management of headaches — as effective as popular drugs commonly used for headaches, but without side effects. Literally hundreds of studies have shown support for this treatment.

[Many have probably heard of biofeedback without fully understanding what it is. Biofeedback is a technique that involves making involuntary or unconscious bodily processes (such a brain waves or heartbeats) perceptible to the senses.]

The National Headache Foundation reports that a National Institutes of Health Technology Assessment Panel found biofeedback to be more effective than a psychological placebo.

Source: *Biofeedback Newsmagazine* 2001.

502. MASSAGE AWAY TENSION HEADACHES

Tension headaches? Massage therapy make help considerably. Massage therapy directed to the neck and shoulder muscles can decrease the symptoms associated with tension headaches. Thirty minutes of massage therapy twice a week reduces the frequency of tension headaches significantly. In addition, the duration of headaches also tends to decrease. (Beneficial results are seen after only four total hours of treatment received over a one-month period.)

There may also be improvements in psychological factors associated with chronic pain: specifically, depression and anxiety.

Source: *American Journal of Public Health* 2002;92:1657-1661.

503. YES, TONIGHT, I HAVE A HEADACHE...

Here's a quickie: "YES, tonight, I have a headache," is a more appropriate response because women can get full or partial relief from a headache by having sex.

Source: **Research done at Southern Illinois University School of Medicine.**

WANT TO KNOW MORE?
Here's a hint for men: Certain sexual positions can help men who suffer from decreased blood flow. The recommendation is to try having sex standing up, because standing facilitates blood flow.

HEADACHES & MIGRAINES: CAUSES & PRECURSORS
504. MIGRAINE SUFFERERS: AVOID BRIGHT LIGHT

If you suffer from migraines, avoid bright light (even when not experiencing a headache) — it can reduce your pain tolerance *significantly*. After exposure to very bright light shined into the eyes, migraineurs demonstrate a marked reduction in the amount of pressure that can be tolerated. In healthy subject, no change at all is seen in pain tolerance after such bright light exposure.

The reason for this difference is not well understood, but it indicates that light plays an important role in the pain perception of certain nerves.

Source: 19th Brazilian Congress in Neurology, Salvador, Brazil, Oct 2000.

WANT TO KNOW MORE?
In women, the severity and frequency of migraines may vary with the phases of the menstrual cycle. Most migraines occur during the early follicular phase, fewer during the mid-cycle time period, and the least during the mid-luteal phase. The same pattern occurs for migraine headache severity, disability, and frequency. It has been suggested that migraines are less of a problem during the mid-luteal phase because of the abundance of progesterone [the "feel-good" hormone] in the body at that time.

Source: 44th Annual Scientific Meeting of the American Headache Society, Seattle, WA, Jun 2002.

505. GLUTEN & MIGRAINE-LIKE HEADACHES

If you experience migraine-like headaches, it may be due to gluten sensitivity. As much as one percent of the general population have this sensitivity to gluten, and the problem may be common but unrecognized. In one study, headaches completely disappeared in most of the patients after they went on a gluten-free diet. [Gluten is present in many grains including wheat, rye, oats, barley, and triticale.]

Source: *Neurology* 2001;56:385-388.

WANT TO KNOW MORE?
One of the most common neurological symptoms of gluten sensitivity is cerebellar ataxia [a disturbance in part of the brain that controls muscle function], followed by peripheral neuropathy. [For many helpful hints on gluten sensitivity, see the "Allergies" section.]

506. IS SINUS HEADACHE REALLY A MIGRAINE?

Many patients complaining of sinus headache may actually be experiencing a migraine, and would achieve better and faster relief if treated properly. Both sinus and migraine headaches can cause nasal drainage and may be brought on by changes in weather or season. And most migraine episodes are not preceded by visual sensations or an aura.

What may actually be happening is that the trigeminal nerve, which has branches in the forehead, cheeks, and jaw, may become inflamed. Consequently many people respond better to migraine-specific treatments than to treatments aimed at sinus relief.

Source: 10th Congress of the International Headache Society, New York, NY, Jul 2001.

HEADACHES & MIGRAINES: NATURAL REMEDIES & SUPPLEMENTS

507. MAGNESIUM AGAINST MIGRAINES

Supplementing with the mineral magnesium may bring relief to migraine sufferers. Magnesium deficiency contributes to migraine headaches both in children and adults. As high as 80 percent of migraineurs tested are found to have magnesium concentrations below the norm. However, only a small percentage of patients with tension-type headaches are found to be lacking in this mineral.

Oral magnesium supplementation may correct this magnesium deficiency and have a positive impact on migraine headaches.

Source: *Cephalalgia* **1999;19:802-809.**

WANT TO KNOW MORE?
[Magnesium supplementation may also be protective against heart disease. See Hint #561 in the *Heart & Cardiovascular Disease* section.]

508. COENZYME Q10 FOR MIGRAINE RELIEF

Supplementing with a natural substance known as coenzyme Q10 (CoQ10) may be beneficial against migraine headaches. Treatment with 150 milligrams of CoQ10 daily appears to be effective in preventing migraines, and unlike most other migraine preventives has no side effects.

After three months of treatment, patients with episodic migraines show a *significant* reduction in the average number of days with a migraine. Overall, 61.3 percent of patients have a greater than 50 percent reduction.

[Some dietary sources of CoQ10 are spinach, peanuts, beef, and fish such as mackerel and salmon.]

Source: *Cephalalgia* **2002;22:137-141.**

WANT TO KNOW MORE?
CoQ10 is the most extensively studied agent for the treatment of *mitochondrial* disorders, which includes migraines.

[Coenzyme Q10 may be also be beneficial for a variety of other health problems, including asthma (see Hint #119), diabetes (Hint #402), and hypertension (Hint #626).]

HEART & CARDIOVASCULAR DISEASE

Heart disease remains the number one cause of death in the US, even though very specific guidelines have been established for detection and treatment. We keep hearing about all the modifiable risk factors to control our blood pressure, to keep unfavorable fats out of our bloodstream, and to combat the tie-in with diabetes. We have also been told how harmful smoking is, how helpful exercise is, and how dangerous it is to be overweight. Obviously, these messages haven't been working. Perhaps reading some scary facts and learning a few doable lifestyle changes will help to turn the tide.

IN THIS SECTION:
- ALTERNATIVE THERAPIES
- ANGINA
- ARTERIAL DISEASE
- ASPIRIN CAVEATS
- ATHEROSCLEROSIS
- CAUSES & PRECURSOR
- DIETARY MISCONCEPTIONS
- DIETARY TACTICS
- HOMOCYSTEINE CONNECTION
- NATURAL REMEDIES & SUPPLEMENTS
- REDUCING RISK

HEART DISEASE: ALTERNATIVE THERAPIES

509. LOOK ON THE BRIGHT SIDE FOR YOUR HEART

To help avoid heart disease, learn to become more optimistic. Involvement in planning and problem solving is important. People who blame themselves for bad events and believe that things will never change are more likely to develop heart disease than their more optimistic peers. Of course, this is easier said than done. Sometimes, exercise and diet changes (as explained throughout this book) can help us to see that bright side.

Pessimism is linked with higher levels of anger, anxiety and depression – emotions that may be risk factors for heart disease. Because optimistic individuals actively engage in planning and problem solving, they may experience less stress, or they may have more resources with which to deal with it.

Optimists tend to be more social, a quality linked with better health. These individuals may also be more likely to adopt healthy behaviors such as exercising and not smoking. Pessimists are more likely to consume more than two alcoholic drinks per day.

Source: *Psychosomatic Medicine 2001;63:910-916.*

510. SAUNA VISITS GOOD FOR HEART HEALTH

If you suffer from heart problems, short visits to a hot sauna may help to improve your condition. Patients with chronic heart failure find that they experience *significant* improvements in vascular function after repeated sauna treatments. Patients with chronic heart failure lay on a bed in a 60° Celsius (140° Fahrenheit) sauna for 15 minutes and then remained on bed rest with a blanket to keep them warm for an additional 30 minutes, once daily, five days a week for a total of two weeks.

Because heat therapy improves vascular function, long-term, repeated sauna treatments may result in an improvement in cardiac function and clinical symptoms. This improvement is most likely due to improved nitric oxide production.

Source: *Journal of the American College of Cardiology* **2002;39:754-759.**

511. ACUPUNCTURE AGAINST HEART FAILURE

If you are suffering from heart failure, acupuncture may prove very beneficial. Acupuncture may be therapeutic for patients with heart failure because it effectively blocks life-threatening nerve activation that is *two to three times higher* in patients with heart failure. (In fact, the higher this nerve activity, the worse the prognosis.)

During mental stress testing, this dangerous activation increases 25 percent, with increases seen in heart rate and blood pressure. However, a single 20-minute acupuncture session completely blocks these increases. (No beneficial responses are seen in those receiving sham-acupuncture treatments, ruling out any placebo effect.) Acupuncture may therefore be a helpful complement to beta-blocker therapy for heart failure patients.

Source: Scientific Sessions of the American Heart Association, Anaheim, CA, 2001.

512. PRAYERS & MANTRAS HELP HEART RATE

Prayer *is* good medicine: The calming effect of saying prayers or mantras can improve your cardiovascular health. Reciting prayers such as the rosary or yoga mantras helps to slow respiration, thereby improving variations in heart rate in all cardiovascular rhythms. Such repetitive recitation is similar to regularity during controlled breathing, indicating that these methods could stabilize respiratory rate as effectively as precisely timed control. No surprises here! The history of the rosary can be traced back to Tibetan monks and Indian yogis. The practice introduced – consciously or not – a new and previously unrecognized element of Eastern health practice into Western culture.

Source: *British Medical Journal* **2001;323:1446-1449.**

HEART DISEASE: ANGINA

513. SELF-HELP PLAN WORKS FOR ANGINA

Angina sufferers, take note: A structured program of diet, exercise, and relaxation shows promise in helping to reduce many symptoms. A self-management plan, which includes eating a more healthful diet, increasing daily walking, and learning relaxation techniques, improves the psychological and physical functioning of those newly diagnosed with angina.

[Angina refers to a painful or "squeezing" sensation in the chest caused by insufficient oxygen reaching the heart, a result of coronary artery disease.]

After six months, participants experience *significant* reductions in anxiety, depression, frequency of angina, use of prescription drugs, and physical limitations.

Source: *British Journal of General Practice* **2002;52:194-201.**

514. SPECIAL FOOD BAR FOR ANGINA SUFFERERS

A special food bar containing the amino acid arginine may be very helpful for those with angina. In addition to traditional treatment, angina patients given a medical food bar enriched with L-arginine [the "L" simply denotes the chemical structure of the molecule] have improved vascular function and exercise capacity, as well as a better quality of life. (In addition to L-arginine, the bar contains folate, vitamins C, E, B6 and B12, niacin, and soy isoflavones.)

L-arginine enhances nitric oxide, which in turn increases the diameter of the arteries, helping to improve symptoms. Exercise time can improve 16 percent when compared to those given a placebo bar (which showed no beneficial changes). In addition, scores for quality of life also increased in those given the L-arginine bar.

Source: *Journal of the American College of Cardiology* **2002;39:37-48.**

WANT TO KNOW MORE?
[Long-term treatment with L-arginine also improves insulin sensitivity in patients with type 2 diabetes.

See Hint #400 in the *Diabetes Type 2* section for more details. And a vaginal cream containing L-arginine can help to increase sexual enhancement in women with libido problems. For more details, see my book on female sexuality, *She's Gotta Have It!*]

HEART DISEASE: ARTERIAL DISEASE

515. LEG PAIN & WEAKNESS? UP YOUR VITAMIN C

Increasing your intake of vitamin C may help to reduce the leg pain and weakness associated with peripheral arterial disease, a condition know as *intermittent claudication*. Vitamin C is *significantly* lower in those with peripheral arterial disease, a condition that produces symptoms of pain, aches, cramps, or severe fatigue in one or both legs when walking.

Essentially a problem of blood flow, peripheral arterial disease may affect up to 20 million people in the US. Arteries carry blood to the muscles and organs in your body, but when you have disease in your arteries, they become narrow or blocked. The most common cause of narrow or blocked arteries is fatty deposits, a condition also known as *atherosclerosis*. Less blood flows through the arteries, which affects the heart, brain, and legs. Those afflicted often describe symptoms of intermittent claudication.

[Some good dietary sources of vitamin C are (fresh and unprocessed) citrus fruits, kiwi, sprouts, broccoli, and cabbage.]

Source: *Circulation* 2001;103:1863-186.

516. DIALING FOR ARTERIAL DISEASE

Stay on the phone long enough and you may encounter problems worse than your phone bill. Everyday activities with a prolonged distortion of the neck can have unpredictable consequences for some people – including arterial disease. [If you must spend long hours on the phone, look into buying a telephone headset, and avoid squeezing the receiver between your head and shoulder for any length of time.]

Source: *Neurology* 1999;53:1886.

HEART DISEASE: ASPIRIN CAVEATS

517. ASPIRIN UNSAFE FOR THOSE AT LOW RISK

In healthy people at low risk for coronary heart disease, daily aspirin is of little value, and may be harmful. Aspirin is not right for everyone. Given the risk of aspirin's side effects (such as potentially serious bleeding) people who have a low risk of myocardial infarction might be better off without a daily dose. Low-risk individuals are defined as having no more than one of the common risk factors, including high blood pressure, family history of the disease, or diabetes. Aspirin therapy does not seem to reduce the mortality rate in low-risk subjects. In fact, findings suggest that low-risk individuals who take aspirin might be at increased risk for death!

In people with a one percent risk, aspirin is safe, but it is unlikely to be of much therapeutic value. However, in people with a 0.5 percent coronary event risk per year, aspirin therapy is actually unsafe. In this group, the bleeding risks of aspirin are likely to outweigh any beneficial effects.

Sources: *Heart* 2001;85:265-271; *Journal of Family Practice* 2002;51:700-704.

518. NO ASPIRIN FOR HIGH PRESSURE EITHER

If you have high blood pressure, daily doses of aspirin may do little to protect you from heart attacks or strokes, and may in fact be harmful. The use of aspirin for cardiovascular protection or stroke prevention is often self-prescribed by those who have not yet experienced heart attacks. But in those with high blood pressure, the use of aspirin has little if any benefit for heart health or stroke prevention, and even low doses of aspirin may carry an appreciable risk of potentially serious bleeding.

Research shows that only a few episodes will be prevented with aspirin use anyway. The US Physicians' trial indicated that older men and those with low cholesterol concentrations would benefit most.

British researchers also conclude that men with higher pressures may be exposed to the risks of bleeding with aspirin use, while deriving no beneficial reductions in coronary heart disease and stroke.

Source: *British Medical Journal* 2000;321:13-17.

HEART DISEASE: ATHEROSCLEROSIS
519. REVERSING ATHEROSCLEROSIS

To reverse atherosclerosis, a multi-faceted program focusing on diet, exercise, and stress control can be extremely effective. [Atherosclerosis is a disease in which fatty material gets deposited on the walls of the arteries, creating dangerous narrowing and risk of blockages.]

Atherosclerosis can be reversed in one year in older people through a combined program of meditation, antioxidant herbal supplements, a diet low in fat and high in fruits and vegetables, yoga exercises, and walking. (Yoga and walking both help to reduce stress.)

This multi-modality approach is shown to be more effective than more traditional approaches. The improvement has been medically measured, and leads to greater benefit than reported in previous studies of single interventions – even those that include beta-blockers, statins [cholesterol-lowering drugs], high dose antioxidants, and meditation.

This approach also appears to be more acceptable to patients because its dietary restrictions are not radical and the level of exercise is one with which people can easily comply.

Source: *American Journal of Cardiology* 2002;89.

520. TOMATOES AGAINST ATHEROSCLEROSIS

Increasing your consumption of lycopene-rich foods such as tomatoes may help to reduce your risk of atherosclerosis. [Lycopene is a carotenoid, a class of compounds related to vitamin A. It is the red pigment that gives tomatoes their color, and can also be found in fruits such as pink grapefruit and watermelon.]

Absorption of lycopene, which is protective against atherosclerosis, is higher from processed tomato-based foods such as tomato paste and tomato juice than from fresh and unprocessed tomatoes. (The precursor of lycopene, phytofluene, is better absorbed than lycopene itself.)

Sources: *Journal of Nutrition* 2002;132:404-408; *American Heart Journal* 2002;143(3):467-474.

WANT TO KNOW MORE?
[Lycopene may also be preventive against lung cancer and colitis. See Hints #217 and #491 for more details.]

521. RICE BRAN AGAINST ATHEROSCLEROSIS

Supplementing with the outer layer of rice can help to decrease plaque formation in your arteries, as well as improve your antioxidant status. The outer layer of rice [the rice bran] inhibits the formation of atherosclerotic plaque when given as a supplement to test animals, most likely due to its antioxidative or anti-inflammatory effects.

[Because these outer layers are chock-full of marvelous fatty acids, they get rancid very quickly. So the best source is *stabilized* rice bran, which has been stabilized to eliminate rancidity problems. In fact, this is one of my favorite supplements.]

Source: *Journal of Nutrition* 2001;131:2606-2618;2002;132:20-26.

522. AGED GARLIC AGAINST ATHEROSCLEROSIS

Aged garlic extract prevents the formation of plaque that can accumulate and cause atherosclerosis, and is even more effective than high-density cholesterol (HDL). Garlic extract even appears to dissolve, to some extent, the plaques that have already formed. This plaque formation occurs as the end result of LDL cholesterol (the "bad-guy" cholesterol) binding with molecules secreted from the inner lining of the arteries, forming tiny plaques that can accumulate and harden. HDL (the "good-guy" cholesterol) inhibits this process by absorbing excess plaque-forming molecules.

The good news is that garlic extract works exactly the same way, but more potently. In fact, garlic extract is *two and a half times* more effective in inhibiting plaque formation than HDL cholesterol. The positive benefits can actually occur within 30 minutes.

Sources: International Scientific Conference on Complementary, Alternative, and Integrative Medical Research, Boston, MA, Apr 2002; *Atherosclerosis* 1997;132:37-42; B. Kamen, *She's Gotta Have It!*

WANT TO KNOW MORE?
Many people report sensitivities to raw fresh garlic because it can irritate the digestive tract. Raw fresh garlic may also increase lipid oxidation (leading to free radicals that can damage cells), indicating that some compounds in raw garlic may actually act like oxidants rather than antioxidants. In addition, when raw fresh garlic kills certain organisms (*Candida*, for example), it creates a "die-off reaction," which means that the yeast organisms release toxic chemicals. This does not occur with the use of aged garlic.

[The heart-protective value of garlic extract is also discussed in my newest book, *Everything I Know About Nutrition I Learned From Barley.*]

523. VITAMIN E AGAINST ATHEROSCLEROSIS

Because heart disease takes many years to develop, long-term intake of vitamin E supplements may play a role in its prevention. Vitamin E has been shown to prevent the free-radical oxidation [damage] of cholesterol, considered to be an early step in the development of coronary artery disease. The development of atherosclerosis [fatty deposits] in the carotid artery is a very early sign of cardiovascular disease, and it can be detected years before any other symptoms appear.

Women with either a low intake or low blood levels of vitamin E are far more likely to have atherosclerotic plaques, while those with the highest intake or blood levels of this vitamin are the least likely.

Source: *American Journal of Clinical Nutrition* 2002;76:582-587.

WANT TO KNOW MORE?
Besides vitamin E, no associations are found between the intake or blood levels of other antioxidants studied and the presence of atherosclerotic plaques.

524. POMEGRANATE JUICE FOR ATHEROSCLEROSIS

Drinking pomegranate juice may help to reduce your risk of developing athero-sclerosis. Dietary supplementation with nutrients rich in polyphenol antioxidants, as found in pomegranate juice, can help reduce atherosclerosis [the progressive narrowing and hardening of the arteries over time].

Pomegranate juice helps to keep cells from clumping together, and increases the activity of a substance that protects against lipid peroxidation in humans. In test animals, pomegranate juice supplementation reduces the size of atherosclerotic lesions by as much as 44 percent.

These beneficial effects are believed to be due to the antioxidative properties of pomegranates.

Source: *American Journal of Clinical Nutrition* **May 2000;71(5):1062-1076.**

525. ELEVATED HOMOCYSTEINE INCREASES RISK

Elevated homocysteine levels increase risk of atherosclerosis, but aged garlic extract helps to reduce it. Homocysteine is a strong independent risk factor for the disease. Researchers found that as the levels of plasma total homocysteine increase in both men and women, there is a strong inverse association of thickened walls and plaque. Reducing homocysteine could reduce the risk of cardiovascular disease. Aged garlic extract (Kyolic) may help to lower homocysteine levels.

Source: *Circulation* **1999;99:2383-2388;2361-2363;** *FASEB (Federation of American Societies for Experimental Biology* **13(4):A232,#209.12.**

WANT TO KNOW MORE?
High levels of atherosclerosis are linked to cognitive decline in older people. This conclusion was reached after following 5,999-randomly selected people aged 65 or older for up to seven years. (*Journal of the American Medical Association* **1999;282:40-46**)

Dr. Fred A. Kummerow of the University of Illinois, Urbana, one of my favorite researchers, concludes that higher levels of toxins are found in those with heart disease than in those with healthy coronary arteries. Cholesterol levels alone do not always indicate the degree of heart disease present in one individual. "Coronary heart disease is more complex than a plasma cholesterol level indicates," says Dr. Kummerow. (*Atherosclerosis* **2000;149**)

HEART DISEASE: CAUSES & PRECURSORS

526. INFECTED GUMS & HEART DISEASE LINKED

Make that dentist appointment NOW: There is connection seen between periodontal disease and coronary artery disease and stroke. When periodontitis is present, oral bacteria and toxins may enter your bloodstream, causing inflammation and the acceleration of atheroma formation. (Atheroma refers to the thickening and fatty degeneration of the inner coat of your arteries.) Those with severe periodontal disease are nearly *four times as likely* to have significant levels of endotoxins than those with healthy gums.

Significant associations have also been identified between poor periodontal status and increased levels of C-reactive protein and fibrinogen, two risk factors for cardiovascular disease. Oral bacteria may also cause platelet aggregation, leading to a thrombotic event [obstruction in your arteries].

Periodontitis is almost universally present in patients with severe, end-stage coronary heart disease, and there is also a strong association seen between periodontitis and stroke.

Sources: *American Journal of Epidemiology* **2000;151:273-282;** *Reuter's Health Report* **Jun 2000;** *Journal of Periodontology* **2002;73:73-78.**

WANT TO KNOW MORE?
Periodontal status is also associated with LDL cholesterol levels [the "bad" variety]. These relationships are consistent regardless of age. It makes sense, because periodontal disease could result in repeated exposures to bacteria and bacterial products that may influence lipid metabolism and homeostasis. The association between bacterial infection and heart disease is an established fact.

527. TOO MUCH WORK, TOO LITTLE SLEEP...

Workaholics, be warned: Too much work and too little sleep are both linked to heart problems in men and women. Thirty-one percent of the population gets less than six hours of sleep a night, and this chronic sleep deprivation is associated with an increased risk of coronary heart disease in women. (Factors that affect length of sleep can be diabetes, snoring, hypertension, depression, shift work, alcohol, smoking, and the use of aspirin.) Men who frequently work long hours or get little sleep are *twice as likely* as other men to experience a non-fatal myocardial infarction [irreversible damage to the heart muscle], and frequent lack of rest enhances this risk.

Only about one third of the population (37 percent) gets at least eight hours of sleep each night.

Sources: 16th Annual Meeting of the Associated Professional Sleep Societies, Jun 2002; *Occupational Environmental Medicine* **2002;59:447-451.**

WANT TO KNOW MORE?
[Drinking coffee after lunch can wreak havoc with sleep patterns because (in addition to being a stimulant) caffeine interrupts the flow of melatonin, the hormone that sends us to sleep at night. For more details, see Hint #933 in the *Sleep Disorders & Deprivation* section.]

528. MORNING COFFEE CAN LAST UNTIL 10 PM

A few cups of coffee in the morning can raise your blood pressure and adrenaline levels well into the evening, increasing your risk for heart disease and stroke. Caffeine intake in the morning, in an amount equivalent to about four cups of coffee, puts your body into a state of sustained stress. Increased blood pressure and adrenaline excretion lasts into the late evening, with effects on both blood pressure and heart rate seen up until as late as 10 PM.

This blood pressure increase is enough to *significantly* amplify the risk of stroke and heart disease. In addition, the adrenaline increase can make your day feel more stressful. Cutting back on caffeine could be one way to reduce hypertension and heart disease. (If you drink fewer than four cups of coffee, you will still be affected, although perhaps with somewhat less severity – depending on your overall health status.)

[Important note: Decaffeinated coffee may not be a good alternative, as it has been associated with increased risk of rheumatoid arthritis. See Hint #102 in the *Rheumatoid Arthritis* section for more details.]

Sources: *Reuter's Medical Report* Mar 1999; Duke University Report, Meeting of the Society of Behavioral Medicine.

WANT TO KNOW MORE?
[Drinking paper-filtered coffee also contributes to heart disease by raising homocysteine levels. See the "Homocysteine Connection" section that follows shortly for more details.]

529. THE RISK OF MID-THIGH MUSCLE FAT

Since fat in mid-thigh muscle is associated with risk for cardiovascular disease as women age, GET OUT AND WALK if this is your problem! Fat deposits in the mid-thigh muscle increase with lack of exercise and obesity, but walking three times a week for six months can turn things around. With a weight loss and walking program, body weight can decrease by 8 percent and aerobic capacity can *increase* by 8 percent.

Increased physical fitness and weight loss can therefore be very helpful in reducing risk for cardiovascular disease in overweight postmenopausal women.

Source: *American Journal of Clinical Nutrition* 2000;72(3):708-713.

530. CARPET SHAMPOO AND HEART DISEASE

Keep children safe from exposure to carpet shampoo – it can lead to an infectious form of heart disease. A leading cause of acquired heart disease among children (Kawasaki syndrome), which can cause abnormalities that include coronary aneurysms, is associated with exposure to rug and carpet shampoo.

Carpet shampoo has been repeatedly associated with an increased risk of this disease. The time of exposure to shampooed or spot-cleaned rugs or carpets for Kawasaki syndrome patients who have a single exposure, and for all those who have multiple exposures, is between 13 to 30 days before the onset of illness.

Sources: Proceedings of the Fourth International Symposium on Kawasaki Disease, Dallas, TX, American Heart Association 1993:21-26; *Monatsschr Kinderheilkd* **1992;140(5):273-276;** *Pediatrics* **1991;87(5):663-669.**

531. NO-NO FOODS FOR HEALTHY HEARTS

Eating certain kinds of foods such as pastries and fried foods put you at serious risk of developing heart disease. Trans fatty acids, which are found in pastry, fried foods, foods containing shortening, salad oils, cooking oils, dairy products, meats, margarines, and anything labeled "hydrogenated" or even "partially hydrogenated," raise the negative kind of cholesterol and reduce good cholesterol – placing you at risk for heart disease.

Although bakery foods are the main source, many researchers declare that there is no safe level. Studies have shown that trans fatty acids also increase the risk of diabetes and colon cancer. The problem is so serious and widespread, the FDA is planning to have manufactures disclose the trans fatty acid content of foods on all food labels.

[Those of us who have doing our homework and our research have been exposing these facts for more than 30 years! We have been particularly concerned about the use of trans fats – especially for pregnant women and those already at high risk for any degenerative disease.]

Sources: *Journal of the American Dietetic Association* **2002;102(1):46-51;** *Current Opinions on Lipidology* **2000;11(1):37-42;** *Nutrition & Cancer* **2001;39(2):170-175.**

532. FOLATE DEFICIENCY = HEART DISEASE RISK

A deficiency in folate can greatly increase your risk of death from cardiovascular disease. Low blood levels of folate [also known as folic acid] appear to increase the risk of cardiovascular disease mortality, so be sure your multivitamin includes this important nutrient (400 micrograms). Those with the lowest folate levels have almost *three times* more cardiovascular disease, and in patients with diabetes the risk is increased even further.

[Some good dietary sources of folate are spinach, kale, beet greens, beets, chard, asparagus, broccoli, liver, and brewer's yeast. But cooking destroys the nutrient, as does storage at room temperature.]

Source: *Archives of Internal Medicine* 2000;160:3258-3262.

533. *ABDOMINAL OBESITY PUTS YOU AT RISK*

Warning: Abdominal obesity puts you at increased risk for developing coronary artery disease. We all know that generalized obesity is one of the major causes of ill health. However, abdominal obesity, which is closely associated with intra-abdominal fat and measured either by waist circumference or waist:hip ratio, predicts future coronary artery disease better than body mass index [that is, total body mass].

Abdominal obesity is also associated with insulin resistance, a sign of high triglyceride levels (and a common precursor to diabetes). High triglyceride levels are strongly and inversely related to HDL "good" cholesterol [meaning the higher the triglyceride levels, the lower the levels of protective HDL].

Of course, most folks who are overweight know that they are and know that this carries health risks. But perhaps an occasional reminder about the dangers involved can help to inspire changes in diet, especially for those with large waists and abdominal fat who are at greater risk for coronary heart disease.

Source: *British Medical Journal* 2001;322:687-689.

534. EXERCISE & HEART DISEASE MORTALITY

Men: If you have a low tolerance for exercise, you are at increased risk of death from cardiovascular disease. In men, low exercise *capacity* [ability] is a strong predictor of death from cardiovascular disease. More deaths occur among men with lower maximal heart rate, lower maximal systolic and diastolic blood pressure, and lower exercise capacity.

The strongest predictor of mortality among normal men and men with cardiovascular disease is their *peak* exercise capacity, and everyone should therefore be encouraged to increase it. Improving exercise tolerance warrants at least as much attention as other major risk factors, such as blood pressure and cholesterol levels.

Source: *New England Journal of Medicine* 2002;346:793-801,852-853.

535. RUNNING TOWARDS CARDIAC RISK

Intense physical exertion (such as running a marathon) can put your body at serious risk for *ischemia* – especially if you are already at risk. In marathon runners, inflammatory and blood markers of cardiac risk appear to increase the risk of acute ischemic events [meaning dangerous blockages of the arteries]. *Significant* increases in risk are observed in men (averaging 47.6 years of age) within four hours after completing a marathon race.

Some factors return to normal by next morning, but coagulation factors remain high and platelet aggregation increases.

[It is this blood platelet aggregation or "clumping" that can lead to dangerous blood clots.] There is evidence that some clotting takes place, although the athletes do not experience any symptoms.

For people who already have serious cardiac risk factors – high blood pressure, diabetes, high cholesterol, or early family history of heart disease – marathon running is probably compounding their risk.

Source: *American Journal of Cardiology* **2001;88:35-40.**

WANT TO KNOW MORE?
Even healthy people can decrease their risk from such intensive physical exertion by taking products to prevent platelets from getting "sticky" following a race. [Natural products with these properties would include Ginkgo biloba or fish oil.]

536. FREE FATTY ACID LEVELS TOO HIGH?

If your diet is high in meat and dairy foods, but lacking in fatty fish, you could be at increased risk for a dangerous cardiac event. High blood levels of free fatty acid molecules that come from meat and dairy foods can trigger abnormal heartbeats, and are predictors of sudden death from heart disease in otherwise healthy men.

Free fatty acids are released from the body's fat cells and serve as fuel for heart cells. When blood levels of fatty acids become too high, they can cause *arrhythmia*, an irregular heartbeat that can stop the heart and cause death. Men with the highest levels of fatty acids have a 30 percent increased risk.

Arrhythmia triggered by high levels of fatty acids can turn an otherwise survivable heart attack into a fatal one. It is more likely to occur if blood levels of omega-6 fatty acids are not in balance with blood levels of omega-3 fatty acids (which come from sources such as fish). When people eat fish rich in omega-3 fatty acids (such as salmon, tuna, and mackerel), they have a lower risk of sudden death. Blood levels of fatty acids can be why one person will survive a heart attack that is fatal to another.

Source: *Circulation* **2001.**

537. HIGH IRON STORES & HEART DISEASE RISK

lead to elevated iron stores in the body, Beware excessive iron intake, as it can be putting you at risk for heart disease. High iron intake from more than 21 servings of fruit juice a week, or more than four servings of red meat a week, or more than 30 milligrams of supplemental iron daily, can elevate your body's stores of iron. And even *moderately* elevated iron stores may increase your risk of heart disease (as well as diabetes and cancer).

Fruit and fruit juices are rich dietary sources of organic acids such as ascorbic (vitamin C), citric, malic, and tartaric acids. A positive association with high iron from fruit may be due to the combined effects of vitamin C and these other organic acids in enhancing iron bioavailability [meaning the degree to which iron can be used by the body].

Although red meat increases the risk, poultry and seafood do not.

Source: *American Journal of Clinical Nutrition* **2002;76(6):1375-1384.**

WANT TO KNOW MORE?
Your body has a considerable capacity to store iron. Among older people especially, intakes of highly bioavailable forms of iron promote high iron stores, whereas foods containing phytate (whole grains) decrease these stores. (Phytate and calcium, as found in flour used in sweet baked products, inhibit iron absorption.)

538. LOW VITAMIN E = SENIOR HEART RISK

Seniors, be advised: A low level of vitamin E is a predictor of cardiovascular events in healthy older people. Those with the lowest vitamin E levels have *six times* the risk of cardiovascular events compared to those with the highest vitamin E levels. (But no similar association is seen for vitamin C, beta-carotene, or total cholesterol.)

[Some dietary sources of vitamin E are butter, egg yolks, and liver. Tocotrienols, a superior form of vitamin E, are natural compounds found in various foods and oils such as palm oil, rice bran oil, wheat germ, barley, saw palmetto, and certain types of nuts and grains.]

Source: *Journal of the American Geriatric Society* **May 2001;49(5):533-537.**

WANT TO KNOW MORE?
[Vitamin C is one of the least stable vitamins, and cooking can destroy much of it. Some good dietary sources of vitamin C are citrus fruits, strawberries, green peppers, broccoli, dark leafy greens, and tomatoes.]

HEART DISEASE: DIETARY MISCONCEPTIONS

539. AN EGG (OR MORE) A DAY IS OKAY

Consumption of one egg per day is not a risk factor for coronary heart disease.
More than a decade of studies show that dietary cholesterol is *not* a contributor to heart disease risk – which means, folks, that it's okay to eat eggs (a concept I have been advocating for many decades!). The myth that egg restriction can reduce the risk of heart disease is just that: a myth!

No studies in the past decade have reported a significant relation between either egg consumption or dietary cholesterol intakes and heart disease risk.

The hypothesis that dietary cholesterol is a risk factor for heart disease should be dismissed.

A small, statistically significant increase in the ratio of total to HDL cholesterol has little biological importance concerning heart disease risk when compared with those dietary and lifestyle factors that do contribute to heart disease risk.

Eggs contain hard-to-come-by sulfur amino acids, and they make a very important contribution to the diet. [And they are relatively inexpensive and versatile!]

The best way to eat an egg is raw, Rocky style. Next best is to lightly steam the egg so that the yolk is still runny. Don't cook or fry that egg to death. An egg really is the almost perfect food! There's little else you can buy that offers the same nutritional value.

Sources: *American Journal of Clinical Nutrition* **2002;75(2):333-334;** *American Journal of Clinical Nutrition* **2001;73(5):885-891;** *Journal of the American College of Nutrition* **2000;19(5Suppl):549S-555S;** *Journal of the American Medical Association* **1999;281:1387-1394.**

540. JACK SPRAT *COULD* EAT FAT!

It's finally official: Low-fat diets do NOT improve your heart health. Despite decades of effort and many thousands of people studied, there is still only limited and inconclusive evidence of the effects of modification of total, saturated, monounsaturated, or polyunsaturated fats on cardiovascular morbidity and mortality.

Twenty-seven different studies indicate that alteration of dietary fat intake has a small effect. More importantly, it's the *quality* of the fat consumed that is significant.

Source: *British Medical Journal* **2002;322:757-763.**

HEART DISEASE: DIETARY TACTICS

541. VEGGIES, FRUITS & HEART DISEASE

Protect yourself from heart disease and stroke by making sure to get several servings of fresh fruits and vegetables daily. There is an inverse association between fruit and vegetable intake and cardiovascular disease, meaning the more you eat, the lower your risk.

These numbers speak for themselves: Consuming fruits and vegetables more than three times a day (compared with less than once a day) is associated with a 27 percent lower stroke incidence, a 42 percent lower stroke mortality, a 24 percent lower ischemic heart disease mortality, a 27 percent lower cardiovascular disease mortality, and a 15 percent lower all-cause mortality [that is, death from any cause].

[Too many of us cannot tolerate large amounts of fruit because of their high carbohydrate content. An excellent rule of thumb is: One portion of fruit for every three portions of vegetables.]

Source: *American Journal of Clinical Nutrition 2002;76(1): 93-99.*

542. WALNUT POWER AGAINST HEART DISEASE

There is now scientific evidence for a beneficial health relationship between the intake of walnuts and the reduction and prevention of coronary heart disease. Compared to most other nuts, which contain monounsaturated fatty acids, walnuts are unique because they are rich in omega-6 (linoleate) and omega-3 (linolenate) polyunsaturated fatty acids.

Walnuts also contain multiple health-beneficial components, such as having a low lysine:arginine ratio and high levels of arginine, folate, fiber, tannins, and polyphenols.

Walnuts in particular can decrease LDL cholesterol (the negative variety).

Though walnuts are energy rich, studies show that walnut consumption does not cause body weight gain when eaten as a replacement food.

[A quick and easy lunch: mixed organic greens, a handful of organic walnut pieces, a light dusting of garlic grapeseed oil, and a tablespoon of freshly ground flaxseed. Delicious! Just make sure the walnuts are organic and fresh.]

Sources: *American Journal of Clinical Nutrition 2001;74(1):72-79; Journal of Nutrition 2002;132(5): 1062S-1101S.*

WANT TO KNOW MORE?

Walnut supplementation may beneficially alter fat distribution even when total plasma lipids do not change. This may be an additional mechanism underlying the protective properties of nut intake.

543. ALMONDS PROTECT AGAINST HEART DISEASE

Adding almonds to you diet can help to protect you from heart disease, especially if you already have high cholesterol. Risk factors for coronary heart disease are *significantly* reduced when whole almonds are added to the diet, especially for those with high blood fat (high cholesterol, triglycerides, etc), and they should therefore be included in lipid-lowering diets.

Just 73 grams of almonds daily can lower LDL (the "bad" cholesterol) and other blood fats. [100 grams of a food is usually an amount equal to the size of your fist.] Half that amount of almonds will also be effective, but not as strongly. (Note: Low-fat whole-wheat muffins have no such effect.)

[Be sure you purchase untreated, organic nuts, preferably in the shell. Very strong free radical scavenging is found in almond skins, so you don't want to blanch or scald the almonds.]

Source: *Circulation* 2002;106; *Journal of Agricultural Food Chemistry* 2002;50(8):2459-2463; *Journal of Nutrition* 2002;132(4):703-707; **Department of Nutrition, Harvard School of Public Health, Boston, MA.**

WANT TO KNOW MORE?

Results of a 14-year study show that women who eat more than five ounces of nuts a week have a significantly lower risk of total coronary heart disease than women who never eat nuts or who eat less than one ounce a month. Potentially protective constituents in nuts include vegetable protein, magnesium, vitamin E, fiber, and potassium.

544. EAT PECANS FOR HEART PROTECTION

Frequent consumption of pecans can decrease your risk of cardiovascular disease.
Pecans were studied as an alternative to the Step 1 diet (a diet that helps to normalize cholesterol levels). A pecan-enriched diet is shown to *significantly* decrease both total cholesterol and LDL cholesterol, as well as triglyceride levels – all without increasing body weight.

Nuts such as pecans that are rich in monounsaturated fat may therefore be recommended as part of the prescribed cholesterol-lowering diet of patients or as part of the habitual diet of healthy individuals.

[Note: The higher the oil content of any food, the more quickly it will go rancid. Buy organic pecans in the shell, and crack them open as needed. This not only prevents rancidity, but also helps to limit the amount you consume.]

Sources: *Journal of Nutrition* 2001;131:2275-2279; *Archives of Internal Medicine* 2002;162(12): 1382-1387; *American Journal of Clinical Nutrition* 2002;76(5):1000-1006; *Archives of Internal Medicine* 2002;162:1382-1387.

WANT TO KNOW MORE?

The monounsaturated fat contained in most nuts also helps to prevent blood clots that lead to heart attack or stroke. Components of nuts may even have an anti-arrhythmic property. So if you have any arrhythmia, consider adding a daily handful of nuts to your diet.

545. COD LIVER OIL AGAINST HEART ATTACKS

Supplementing daily with cod liver oil may be preventive against heart attacks. Research recently conducted at Southampton University in England shows that cod liver oil capsules taken for seven weeks help to fend off heart attacks.

The oil stabilizes plaque structure in those waiting for surgery to unclog the inner lining of the heart arteries.

Source: *Advances In Therapy* 2002;19(2):101-107.

WANT TO KNOW MORE?

[See Hint #774 in the *Osteoporosis & Other Skeletal Problems* section for information on how cod liver oil can protect women from the risk of hip fractures.]

546. FIBER AGAINST CARDIOVASCULAR DISEASE

High intake of dietary fiber reduces the risk of cardiovascular disease in women. When investigators compare those people with the highest fiber intake and those with the lowest, their findings support current dietary recommendations to increase the consumption of fiber-rich whole grains, fruits, and vegetables as a primary preventive measure against coronary artery disease.

[Unfortunately, the American diet is sorely lacking in fiber. In addition to efforts to include high fiber vegetables and grains (most fruits are actually rather low in fiber), a good fiber supplement has become a necessity for optimal health. Look for one in your local health food store, and make sure it includes an assortment of fibers rather than just one.]

Source: *Journal of the American College of Cardiology* 2002;39:49-59.

WANT TO KNOW MORE?

[As discussed in my book, *New Facts About Fiber*, bulk-forming fiber supplements are also a first-line therapy for one of the most common ailments, hemorrhoids. And they may prevent or delay the vascular complications usually associated with diabetes.]

547. WHOLE GRAIN CEREALS & HEART DISEASE

Eating oat fiber, rice bran, and barley tends to lower total and LDL cholesterol, but eating wheat fiber does not. Several nutrients found in cereals are known to help reduce the risk of coronary heart disease: linoleic acid (LA), fiber, vitamin E, selenium, and folate. Cereals also contain phytoestrogens of the lignan family and several phenolic acids with antioxidant properties. Consuming whole grain cereal foods may therefore reduce your risk of coronary heart disease.

[Important note: Beware the processed varieties, including the quick-cook stuff, as processing generally reduces these nutrients. Processed cereal foods (such as bread and some breakfast cereals) are also high-sodium foods, and can contribute to high blood pressure.]

Source: *European Journal of Clinical Nutrition* **2002;56(1):1-14.**

548. MAKE HIGH-FAT MEALS LESS DAMAGING

If you are eating a meal high in fat, make sure to eat either oats or a good source of vitamin E at the same time. Nutrient distribution and meal composition may have important implications for cardiovascular health. Heart problems induced by a high-fat meal can be prevented if you consume either oats or vitamin E at the same meal – but not wheat.

Unlike the results observed in those who eat a high-fat meal along with oats or vitamin E, detrimental effects *are* seen in those who eat a high-fat meal along with wheat cereal only.

Source: *Yale Prevention Research Center* **2001;20(2):124-129.**

549. FISH FOR HEART DISEASE PREVENTION

Eating more fish can help lower your risk of developing heart disease. We've known for a long time that higher consumption of fish and omega-3 fatty acids is associated with a lower risk of coronary heart disease (CHD) in men, and now we know that this also applies to women. Among women, a higher consumption of fish and omega-3 fatty acids is associated with a lower risk of coronary heart disease, as well as particularly lower incidence of CHD-related deaths.

Compared to women who rarely eat fish (less than one portion per month), those with a higher intake of fish (five times per week) have a lower risk of CHD. Add omega-3 fatty acids and the risk of death drops even lower. [In addition to fatty fish, omega-3 fatty acids can be found in flaxseed, walnuts, berries, broccoli, and cabbage.]

Source: *Journal of the American Medical Association* **2002;287:1815-1821.**

HEART DISEASE: HOMOCYSTEINE CONNECTION

550. B VITAMINS HELP LOWER HOMOCYSTEINE

Increasing your intake of vitamins B6, B12, and folic acid helps to decrease your homocysteine levels, which in turn helps lower your risk for heart disease. [Homocysteine is an amino acid produced naturally in your body, but high levels in the blood are associated with many health problems, including heart disease.] Higher intakes of B6, B12, and folic acid [also a B-complex vitamin] have been shown to lower homocysteine levels, thereby decreasing cardiovascular risk. The recommended doses of these three nutrients are: folic acid (1 mg daily), vitamin B12 (400 micrograms daily), and vitamin B6 (10 mg daily).

[The best natural sources of vitamin B6 are organ meats (such as liver), egg yolk, fish, dried peas and beans, walnuts, and brewer's yeast. Vitamin B12 can also be found in organ meats, eggs, and brewer's yeast, as well as dairy products and seafood.

As for folic acid (also known as folate), some good dietary sources are spinach, kale, beet greens, beets, chard, asparagus, broccoli, liver, and brewer's yeast. It's not difficult to be deficient in folic acid. In fact, folic acid deficiency surpasses even iron deficiency. The average diet has only marginal amounts, and absorption is yet another problem. Cooking destroys this nutrient, as does storage at room temperature.]

Source: *American Journal of Public Health* **2000;90:1636-1638;** *Journal of the American College of Cardiology* **2001;37:1858-1863;** *Lancet* **2002;359:227-228;** *Reuter's Medical Health Report* **Apr 2001;** *Journal of the American Medical Association* **2002;288(8):973-979.**

WANT TO KNOW MORE?
Following a turnaround by the FDA, consumers can expect to see this new claim on some dietary supplement labels touting the ability of vitamin B to reduce the risk of vascular disease: "As part of a well-balanced diet that is low in saturated fat and cholesterol, Folic Acid, Vitamin B6 and Vitamin B12 may reduce the risk of vascular disease." [High homocysteine levels have also been linked to Alzheimer's disease. See Hint #73 in the *Alzheimer's* section for more details.]

551. FOLIC ACID: A YEAR MAKES A DIFFERENCE

Just one year of folic acid therapy can make a big difference in terms of your cardiovascular health. The beneficial effects of 10 milligrams of folic acid a day in reducing homocysteine levels persist after a year of such supplementation. Folic acid use for one year is associated with a significant increase in plasma folate levels and a significant decrease in homocysteine levels.

Just as most people know their cholesterol levels, we should also know our homocysteine levels, especially if we have heart disease or have had or are at risk for stroke. Folic acid is a safe and cost-effective vitamin therapy.

Source: *American Journal of Medicine* 2002;112:535-539.

552.   COFFEE, TEA, OR HEART DISEASE?

Watch your coffee (and black tea) intake – it can raise your homocysteine levels, putting you at increased risk for heart disease. Drinking large quantities of paper-filtered coffee raises concentrations of homocysteine in healthy individuals, creating a strong risk factor for cardiovascular disease. But abstaining from coffee for six weeks can decrease unwanted homocysteine and total cholesterol in those who drink an average of four cups of filtered coffee daily.

Out of 26 subjects given one liter of paper-filtered coffee daily, nearly all (24 out of 26) had increased homocysteine concentrations after four weeks. (As mentioned previously, vitamins B6, B12, and folic acid are known to prevent homocysteine development, but even though these nutrients were unaffected in the coffee drinkers, they still accumulated the homocysteine.)

In another study, filtered-coffee drinkers aged 24 to 69 who abstained from coffee for six weeks had lowered levels of both homocysteine and cholesterol.

In addition to coffee, high intake of black tea (the most commonly consumed tea in the world) also has this homocysteine-raising effect. And there is also an association seen between high homocysteine levels and high intake of alcohol (60 drinks a month).

Source: *American Journal of Clinical Nutrition* 2000;72(5):1107-1110;2001;73(3):532-538;628-637;74(3):302-307.

WANT TO KNOW MORE?
It remains unclear whether a high homocysteine concentration is causally related to cardiovascular disease or is merely an indicator of another process that causes cardiovascular disease.

553.   RIBOFLAVIN MAY ALSO LOWER HOMOCYSTEINE

In addition to folic acid, increased intake of riboflavin may also help reduce homocysteine levels, thereby reducing your heart disease risk. We know that homocysteine can be reduced with supplemental folic acid [folate], vitamin B6, and vitamin B12, but the benefit of riboflavin [vitamin B2] is a relatively new concept. [Both of folic acid and riboflavin can be found in the sprouted barley leaf.]

There is a widespread opinion that maintaining homocysteine at relatively low concentrations is advisable. Many people have higher folate requirements than others, and the lower the folate, the higher the homocysteine levels. But it has also been shown that the combined influence of folate and riboflavin appears to be beneficial.

Source: *American Journal of Clinical Nutrition* 2002;76(2):301-302; B. Kamen, *Everything I Know About Nutrition I Learned from Barley.*

WANT TO KNOW MORE?
Researchers are discovering that large percentages of the population may have higher requirements for specific vitamins, making it more difficult to determine who exactly is "deficient" or not. The previously recommended daily intake of riboflavin was certainly not generated with homocysteine in mind.

HEART DISEASE: NATURAL REMEDIES & SUPPLEMENTS

554. VITAMIN C AGAINST HEART ATTACKS

Vitamin C may help improve blood flow and possibly prevent heart attacks in those with coronary artery disease. Coronary artery disease is characterized by both inadequate blood flow to the arteries leading to the heart, and an inability of blood vessels to open up when the heart demands increased blood flow during work or exercise. This abnormality in blood vessel function can impede blood flow to the heart, eventually causing a heart attack.

But blood vessels widen in heart-disease patients who take two grams of vitamin C (while no effect is seen in those who take a placebo). Even short-term treatment may be beneficial.

This beneficial effect may be due to the antioxidant properties of vitamin C. Antioxidants mop up free radicals and other unstable compounds that damage blood vessel linings, causing them to constrict, thereby preventing the normal flow of oxygen-rich blood.

Source: Medical Tribune News Service, 1996; *Circulation* **1999;99(25):3234-3240.**

WANT TO KNOW MORE?
The notion that vitamin C deficiency may play a role in heart disease actually dates back to the early 1900s.

555. VITAMIN C AND E FOR HEART HEALTH

In addition to taking supplemental vitamin C, adding E to the mix is an even better protective tactic against heart disease. Higher dietary and supplemental intakes of vitamins C and E are associated with increased levels of an enzyme that allows HDL (the "good" cholesterol) to protect against damaging heart oxidation.

It appears that these dietary antioxidants protect or preserve this enzyme (called *paraoxonase*). The activity of this enzyme is a better predictor of vascular disease than inherited genetic factors. (Note: Smoking can decrease paraoxonase activity.)

[Some good dietary sources of vitamin C are citrus fruits, strawberries, green peppers, broccoli, dark leafy greens, and tomatoes. Vitamin E can be found in butter, egg yolks, liver, palm oil, rice bran oil, wheat germ, barley, saw palmetto, and certain types of nuts and grains.]

Source: *Arteriosclerosis, Thrombosis, & Vascular Biology* 2002;22:1248-1250,1329-1333.

556. VITAMIN D REDUCES CARDIOVASCULAR RISK

Supplementing with vitamin D may be protective against coronary artery disease. Low serum [blood] levels of vitamin D are associated with high levels of coronary artery calcium and coronary artery disease, so it's no surprise that women who take vitamin D supplements have a 31 percent lower risk of death from heart disease compared with women who do not take vitamin D supplements. (Even past use of the vitamin may have some protective effect.)

Calcium supplementation or the lack of it has no effect on the protective effect of vitamin D. But since most women get their vitamin D as part of a multivitamin, vitamin C, vitamin E, and folic acid and vitamin B12 (which lower homocysteine levels) could have some influence.

[Some good dietary sources of vitamin D are dairy products, eggs, and fish liver oils. Exposure to sunlight also allows the body to produce vitamin D.]

Source: 42nd Annual Conference on Cardiovascular Disease and Epidemiology Prevention, Honolulu, HI, Apr 2002.

557. TEA CATECHINS AGAINST HEART DISEASE

Consumption of catechins, a type of flavonoid found in some teas and in apples, can reduce your risk of death from heart disease. Results of a 10-year study show that men who consume the greatest amount of catechins are 51 percent less likely to die of ischemic heart disease compared with men who consume the lowest amount. (The average amount of catechins in the study was 72 mg. which can be obtained by drinking two cups of black tea daily.)

Catechins are part of the group of antioxidant plant compounds called flavonoids that have also been linked to a lower risk of lung disease and certain cancers. They are a major component of tea, accounting for roughly 30 percent of the dry weight of green tea and nine percent of the dry weight of black tea.

It is suggested that catechins may work by preventing LDL cholesterol (the "bad" cholesterol) from damaging cells, by recycling other antioxidants such as vitamin E, or by reducing the risk of inflammation.

Sources: *American Journal of Clinical Nutrition* **2001;74:227-232;** *Circulation* **2002.**

WANT TO KNOW MORE?
[Catechins found in green tea may also be preventive against arthritis. See Hint #86 in the *Arthritis* section for more details.]

558. GAMMA-ORYZANOL FOR HEART HEALTH

Gamma-oryzanol, a powerful antioxidant, can protect your heart in many ways, and is found in significant quantities only in stabilized rice bran. Gamma-oryzanol inhibits platelet aggregation (the "sticking together" of cells), protecting you from cardiovascular problems. It can also inhibit LDL oxidation, which leads to the harmful effects of cholesterol.

In addition, gamma-oryzanol has been shown to be anti-mutagenic and anti-carcinogenic. Hard to come by, gamma-oryzanol is found in significant quantities in soluble rice bran.

Source: R. Cheruvanky, "Bioactives In Rice Bran and Rice Bran Oil," *Phytochemicals as Bioactive Agents*, **(Lancaster, PA: Technomic Publications, 2000) 227-228.**

WANT TO KNOW MORE?
In addition to protecting you from heart disease and cancer, gamma-oryzanol also prevents lipid peroxidation in the retina, helping to protect your vision.

559. ESSENTIAL FATTY ACIDS FOR YOUR HEART

Consuming more foods rich in both linolenic and linoleic acids can help protect your from heart disease. A higher intake of either linolenic (LNA) or linoleic acid (LA) is protective against coronary artery disease, and these two fatty acids together have a synergistic effect (meaning the combined effect of linoleic and linolenic acids is stronger than the individual effect of either fatty acid alone.)

[Linoleic (omega-6) and alpha-linolenic (omega-3) acids are the two essential fatty acids we cannot manufacture, so they need to be on your plate. Omega-6 is found in evening primrose oil and borage oil, and omega-3 is found in fish oil and flaxseed oil. Nuts and seeds are good sources, too.]

Source: *American Journal of Clinical Nutrition* **Nov 2001;74(5):612-619.**

560. AMINO ACID ARGININE FOR HEALTHY HEARTS

Dietary arginine supplementation may help to both prevent and treat cardiovascular disease. Because arginine [an amino acid] is necessary for the production of nitric oxide, it is believed to be helpful for heart disease prevention. Nitric oxide helps to prevent platelet aggregation (the "sticking together" of cells, a common precursor to heart disease).

Compelling evidence shows that administration of arginine reverses the kind of dysfunction associated with high cholesterol, smoking, hypertension, diabetes, obesity, insulin resistance, and aging. It also ameliorates coronary and peripheral arterial disease, ischemia injury, and heart failure.

Source: *Journal of Nutrition* 2000;130:2626-2629.

WANT TO KNOW MORE?
[Since arginine is necessary for good sexual function, which in turn has been demonstrated to reduce heart disease risk, the puzzle pieces begin to fall into place. See my book, *She's Gotta Have It!*, for more information on this topic.]

561. MAGNESIUM & HEART HEALTH

Increasing your intake of the mineral magnesium may be protective against heart disease. Magnesium is beneficial in counteracting all of the processes that lead to ischemic heart disease, including terminal events such as arrhythmia and sudden death. Because magnesium is considered nature's physiological calcium blocker, it protects the cells against calcium overload. In addition, this mineral also helps to decrease blood pressure.

Oral magnesium taken for six months by those with coronary artery disease results in *significant* improvement in artery function and exercise tolerance, as well as fewer arrhythmias.

Magnesium concentrations in important body cells are significantly lower when dietary magnesium is lower. The recommended dietary allowance of 320 milligrams a day seems correct. [Some rich dietary sources of magnesium include meat, fish and seafood, dairy products, brewer's yeast, and green leafy vegetables.]

Sources: *Circulation* 2000;102(19):2353-2358; *American Journal of Clinical Nutrition* 2002;75(3): 550-554.

WANT TO KNOW MORE?
Evidence that links magnesium deficiency to coronary artery disease has been investigated for more than 30 years. Those who live in soft water areas, who use diuretics, or who are predisposed to heartbeats out of the normal range may require more dietary magnesium than others.

[For those who tend to get diarrhea with large doses of magnesium, try magnesium glyconate. This form of magnesium is known to be protective against this problem.]

562. HAWTHORN EXTRACT IS HEART PROTECTIVE

Extract of hawthorn fruit protects against cardiovascular disease, lowers blood pressure, and helps prevent the oxidation of low-density lipoprotein (the "bad" cholesterol). Hawthorn fruit contains many compounds that are protective against human LDL oxidation (such as quercetin and rutin), and the effect is dose-dependent (so the higher your intake, the higher your protection).

Hawthorn may also be beneficial to patients with mild heart failure without the risk of common or serious adverse effects. After taking 1800 milligrams of hawthorn extract for 16 weeks, those with heart failure show *significant* improvements in exercise tolerance, which may in turn improve heart function. The low incidence of adverse effects indicates that hawthorn is safe and well tolerated, even among ill patients. This treatment is effective even in those with advanced degrees of heart failure.

Sources: *Journal of Nutritional Biochemistry* Mar 2001;12(3):144-152; *American Heart Journal* 2002;143(5):910-915.

WANT TO KNOW MORE?
Part of the mechanism for the cardiovascular protective effects of hawthorn fruit might involve either the *direct* protection to LDL from oxidation or *indirect* protection by maintaining the concentration of alpha-tocopherol in LDL.

HEART DISEASE: REDUCING RISK

563. AEROBIC EXERCISE AGAINST HEART DISEASE

Vigorous aerobic exercise can improve coronary function in those with coronary artery disease (if there are no exercise risk factors involved). Improvements in vascular-wall function are observed after four weeks in patients exercising under supervision for 10 minutes a session, six times a day. (There is a growing understanding that changes in vascular-wall function have important implications for cardiovascular disease.)

If, however, you have risk factors that could be affected by exercise, such as diabetes, hypertension, high cholesterol, or smoking, this does NOT apply to you.

Source: *New England Journal of Medicine* 2000;342:454-460,503-504.

564. REDUCE INFLAMMATION WITH EXERCISE

Physical activity may lower your risk for coronary heart disease by reducing inflammation. Inflammation plays an important role in the development of atherosclerosis, but exercise helps to reduce inflammation. Those who participate in light, moderate, or vigorous physical activity have lower levels of elevated C-reactive protein. C-reactive protein plays a key role in heart disease: The higher the level, the greater the disease risk.

Omega-3 fatty acids also have anti-inflammatory properties. They are found in:
~ fish oil
~ flaxseed oil
~ walnuts
~ organ meats

Sources: *Epidemiology* 2002;13:561-568; *Journal of the American College of Nutrition* 2002;21(6): 495-505.

565. WALKING PROTECTS WOMEN FROM CHD

Women who walk as little as one hour a week, regardless of pace, have a *significantly* lower risk of coronary heart disease compared with sedentary women. Women 45 or older who walk at least one hour a week have about *half* the risk of coronary heart disease compared with women who do not walk regularly. Time spent walking seems more important in predicting the lower risk than the pace of walking.

Women who spend at least 2.5 hours per week walking briskly or engaging in intense exercise are 30 percent less likely to develop cardiovascular disease.

Adopting a brisk pace appears to be most beneficial for walkers, but even women who cover one mile in 15 to 20 minutes are protected.

Limited physical activity also benefits women who are overweight, who smoke, or who have high cholesterol. It's not always this easy, is it?

Source: *Journal of the American Medical Association* 2001;285:1447-1453; *New England Journal of Medicine* 2002;347:716-725,755-756.

WANT TO KNOW MORE?

Important note: Prolonged sitting appears to counteract the benefits of exercise — among women who engage in the same amount and levels of exercise, those who spend more time sitting during the day are more likely than others to develop cardiovascular disease.

566 EXERCISE IMPROVES BLOOD FAT PROFILES

Physical activity can help protect your heart by beneficially altering your blood-fat profiles, an important predictor for heart disease. Increased physical activity is related to reduced risk of heart disease, possibly because it leads to improvement in blood-fat profiles (such as cholesterol, etc.), and the highest amount of weekly exercise has the greatest beneficial effects.

Those who engage in higher amounts of exercise experience greater lipid-profile improvements than do those who engage only in lower amounts of exercise. At the same time, however, lower amounts of exercise *always* result in better results than no exercise at all.

Source: *New England Journal of Medicine* 2002;347(19):1483-92.

567. DRINK TO A HEALTHIER HEART!

To protect your heart, make sure to drink several glasses of water daily. Many of the risk conditions directly related to coronary heart disease are known to increase with dehydration. People who drink five or more glasses of water per day are less likely to experience a fatal heart disease event than those who drink no more than two glasses per day.

Those with a high intake of non-water fluids (such as juice, coffee, tea, or soft drinks) are more likely to experience a fatal event than those with low intakes of these fluids. This may be because the higher intake of diuretic and high-energy beverages could result in more frequent and larger exposure to conditions that increase the risk of thrombosis and atherosclerosis.

Source: *American Journal of Epidemiology* 2002;155:827-833.

568. HAVE MORE SEX TO PROTECT YOUR HEART

Middle-aged men can halve their risk of heart attack or stroke by having sex three or four times a week. The results of a study of 2,400 healthy men followed over 10 years showed that those who had three or more orgasms a week were half as likely to have had a heart attack or a stroke. Mild to moderate exercise [such as sexual intercourse] can have cardiovascular protective effects.

Sources: Fourth World Stroke Congress, Melbourne, Australia, Nov 2000; *Journal of Epidemiology & Community Health* **2002;56:99-102.**

WANT TO KNOW MORE?
[This information is explored in my book, *She's Gotta Have It!*, with clear explanations of the pathways involved and the reasons for the protection.]

569. HEART ATTACK? GET CHECKED FOR DIABETES

If you have suffered a heart attack, there is a chance that you could also have undiagnosed diabetes. People admitted to the hospital with a heart attack have an increased risk of having undiagnosed diabetes, so checking glucose levels should be standard procedure before dismissal.

The presence of disturbed glucose levels will compound the risk of a patient already afflicted by heart attacks, but checking glucose levels immediately following a heart attack can help determine who is at risk for future cardiovascular problems.

Although glucose tests are seldom done in coronary care units, these tests are quick and inexpensive and should be standard before discharge.

[One supplement that has been shown to help modulate blood sugar is *stabilized rice bran*. See Hint #376 in the *Diabetes* section for more information.

Another supplement is the mineral *chromium*. For more information, see my book, ***The Chromium Connection: A Lesson In Nutrition.***]

Source: *Lancet* 2002;359:2140-2144.

WANT TO KNOW MORE?

[Too many people have undiagnosed diabetes, and many are also unaware of nutrient deficiencies. If you want to have extensive blood testing done (independent of your physician), call YFH at 877-468-6934 for information about their fees and their rather thorough blood testing and diagnostic services. See Hint #1000 for more detailed information about this service.]

Men with osteoarthritis in their finger joints are 42 percent more likely to die of cardiovascular disease than men without this form of arthritis. This link was discovered by following 8,000 Finns for 14 years. Many explanations could account for the link between arthritis and cardiovascular disease. For example, high serum fat levels, which can boost cardiovascular disease risks, can also degrade the body's cartilage. Systemic inflammation could also increase the risks for both arthritis and heart disease. (***Annals of Rheumatic Disease* 2003;62:151-158**)

In one study, it was shown that men with heart disease had mercury levels that were15 percent higher than those of control subjects. The mercury level was directly related to the risk of myocardial infarction. Patients with the highest levels were 2.16 times more likely to experience myocardial infarction than those with the lowest levels.(***New England Journal of Medicine* 2002;347:1747-1760**)

HEARTBURN

Chronic heartburn has been linked to esophageal cancer, which makes treatment of such digestion problems all the more important. Acid suppression medications have become one of the most commonly prescribed classes of therapeutic agents. (*American Journal of Gastroenterology* **2003;98(1):51-8**) And of course, acid is not always the cause of heartburn. (*Gastroenterology Clinics of North America* **2002;31(4 Suppl):S45-58**) The mechanisms responsible for pain, clinical characteristics, and the optimal therapeutic approach for heartburn remain poorly understood. (*Gut* **2002;51(6):885-92**)

570. HERBAL TEA FOR HEARTBURN & FLATULENCE

For a healthful digestive and antiflatulent remedy, try sipping a cup of herbal tea containing fennel, anise, and caraway. In addition to relieving flatulence, this tea also prevent heartburn. Some added bonuses: The essential oils that fennel, anise and caraway release into hot tea are superior antioxidants, and both fennel and anise contain a substance that has been shown to block both inflammation and carcinogenesis.

Source: *International Journal of Food Science & Nutrition* **1998.**

WANT TO KNOW MORE?
[Everyone in my family uses liquid acidophiluse to relieve heartburn. Works every time!]

HEAT EXHAUSTION

The medical complications of heat exhaustion include cardiovascular, neurological, and renal damage. (*Occupational Medicine* **2000;50(4):259-63**) Heat-related stress affects memory and performance. (*Journal of School Nursing* **2002;18(4):237-43**)

571. HOT WEATHER TACTICS: BEAT THE HEAT

Outdoors on a brutally hot day? Going bare-chested makes you more susceptible to heat exhaustion because you pick up more radiant heat exposure with your shirt off. And stay away from beer! Once you start perspiring, a shirt can act like a cooling device when the wind goes through it. (Don't forget to replace fluids, vitamins, and minerals lost in sweating by drinking lots of water.) As for beer, it can actually promote heat exhaustion by accelerating dehydration. Since beer is a diuretic causing excessive urination, it should be avoided even before going out into the hot sun. Pedialyte, an infant rehydrating formula, is effective for heat exhaustion in adults as well as kids.

Source: *Doctors Book of Home Remedies*, (Emmaus, PA: Rodale Press, 1990), 276-278.

HEMORRHOIDS

Hemorrhoids are masses of dilated and swollen veins that can appear at the anus or within the rectum. They are often painful and can sometimes even bleed. Like so many other diseases of the modern age, hemorrhoids are common in Western societies but rare in the Third World. Despite the frequent occurrence of hemorrhoidal disease, its underlying cause remains controversial.

572. FIBER CAN HELP WITH HEMORRHOIDS

Increase your intake of dietary fiber with a supplement to protect yourself from hemorrhoids. A deficiency of dietary fiber increases your risk of developing hemorrhoids, but a high-fiber diet, or including a good fiber supplement, can be helpful. High-fiber stools, being soft and pliable, are readily molded and propelled by the colon, decreasing transit time. The passage of small, firm stools has been implicated in this condition.

[Transit time is the time it takes for your food to travel through your system. Transit time averages only about one and a half days in rural communities in the Third World. In Western countries, it's three days in young healthy adults, ten or more among the constipated, and two weeks for the elderly. It is virtually impossible to get enough fiber from the Western diet without supplementation.

Once hemorrhoids are already in place, drinking lots of water and taking sitz baths can help. Stool softening is a first step in the management of chronic constipation, a major cause of hemorrhoids. Chronic constipation and painful elimination frequently contribute to malnutrition.

Sources: Journal of Nutrition 1999;129:1431S-1433S; Alimentary Pharmacology Therapeutics 1998;12(5):491-497; Romanian Journal of Gastroenterology 2002;11(3):191-195; B. Kamen, New Facts About Fiber.

WANT TO KNOW MORE?
[See the *Constipation* section for useful tips on how to deal with that condition, which can in turn help prevent hemorrhoids in the first place.]

573. NATURAL HEMORRHOID RELIEVERS

Large doses of the enzyme trypsin, ground and mixed into a skin cream and applied topically, may help to relieve inflamed hemorrhoids. As constipation can be a possible cause of hemorrhoids, natural remedies to soften stools are also helpful. Drinking six mugs of black tea daily can act as a stool softener, helping to relieve constipation.

Sources: Romanian Journal of Gastroenterology 2002;11(3):191-195; Disease of the Colon & Rectum 1997;40(2):215-219; British Journal of Nutrition 1997;78(1):41-55.

HEPATITIS

Hepatitis is an inflammation of the liver, causing damage or death to liver cells, usually caused by a viral infection. Toxins, usually filtered out by the liver, build up instead. Hepatitis is classified according to the virus that causes the condition.

574. LACTOFERRIN FOR HEPATITIS PROTECTION

Lactoferrin, a protein component of milk, has been shown to inhibit the hepatitis C virus, one of the most common causes of chronic hepatitis. [We have long known about the antiviral activity of lactoferrin, an iron-binding substance excreted in bodily fluids, including breast milk. It has the unique ability to trigger our sophisticated immune-system mechanisms. It does this by binding iron in the blood, keeping it away from cancer cells, bacteria, viruses, and any other pathogens requiring iron to grow. Remarkably, not only does the lactoferrin protein make iron unavailable to harmful pathogen, it actually transports the iron to areas of the body where it *is* needed.] Lactoferrin as a supplement is safe and well tolerated. It is available in health food stores.

Sources: *Japanese Journal of Cancer Research* **2002;93(9):1063-1069;** *Journal of Dairy Science* **2002;85(9):2065-2074;** *Hepatology Research* **2002:24(3):228.**

WANT TO KNOW MORE?
[Lactoferrin is a fairly new supplement, and has attracted attention because of its application to cancer therapy (it has been shown to inhibit the growth of leukemia cells). Normally, it is found in substances that help to protect our eyes, mouth, nose, and other openings of the body from infectious invasion. Lactoferrin may also be relevant for HIV and chronic viral infections, including chronic fatigue.]

HERPES

Genital herpes remains one of the most prevalent sexually transmitted diseases. The problem is increasing, affecting more women than men, but an equal number in the most prevalant age group, those from 20 to 29. (*Sexually Transmitted Disease* **1997;24(3):149-55**)

575. AMINO ACID LYSINE FOR HERPES INFECTION

The essential amino acid lysine may be helpful in the prevention and treatment of herpes. Supplementing with 936 milligrams of lysine daily may help to prevent the recurrence or decrease the frequency of herpes infection. Without lysine, healing may take six to 15 days. With lysine, lesions may heal in five days or less.

Source: *Journal of Antimicrobial Chemotherapy* **1983;12(5):489-496.**

HIGH CHOLESTEROL

Along with eggs, cholesterol has been unfairly maligned. Hardly the villain, cholesterol is necessary for life itself. In fact, it is so important, that your body will manufacture more of it when and if it recognizes a deficit. It's that *oxidized* cholesterol that can do us in. How do we prevent the bad-guy cholesterol from interfering with our health? Let me count the ways.

IN THIS SECTION:
- CAUSES & PRECURSORS
- DIETARY TACTICS
- DRUG WARNINGS
- NATURAL REMEDIES & SUPPLEMENTS
- REDUCING RISK

HIGH CHOLESTEROL: CAUSES & PRECURSORS

576. BEWARE HYDROGENATED FOODS!

WARNING: No level of trans fatty acids (found in all hydrogenated foods) is safe to consume, so the FDA is recommending that you consume as little as possible. Industrial hydrogenation of vegetable or fish oils (even partial hydrogenation) is the main source of trans fatty acids in our diet. They are common in foods containing shortening, including pastries and fried foods, margarines, salad oils, cooking oils, frying fats used in industrial food preparation, and other spreads.

Trans fatty acids are known to increase blood levels of low-density lipoprotein (LDL, the "bad-guy" cholesterol), while lowering levels of high-density lipoprotein (HDL, the "good-guy" cholesterol). One study showed a 50 percent greater risk of developing colon cancer when high levels of trans fatty acids are consumed. There is also an association of stores of trans fatty acids with postmenopausal breast cancer. The negative effect of these fats appears to be unmatched by any other natural fatty acid.

In some countries the content of trans fatty acids in margarines has long since been decreased as a result of the continuous discussions about their negative effects.

Sources: *Journal of Nutrition* **1997;127(3):514S-520S;** *Cancer Epidemiology Biomarkers Prevention* **1997;6(9):705-710;** *Nahrung* **2000;44(4):222-228;** *Nutrition & Cancer* **2001;39(2):170-175; Institute of Medicine Report, Washington, DC, Jul 2002.**

WANT TO KNOW MORE?
[Hydrogenation is widely used to deal with the spoilage problem of oils. This also increases the melting point of the fat, thereby hardening many products that would otherwise be liquid. Beware partially hydrogenated foods, too. Partial hydrogenation is like being a little bit pregnant. The resulting oils are in a totally unnatural form, causing high cholesterol and even carcinogenesis.]

577. FRUCTOSE CAN RAISE TRIGLYCERIDES

Men: Watch your consumption of fructose, which can raise your triglyceride levels.
Research done at Fairview-University of Minnesota Medical Center showed that (in men) dietary fructose is associated with increased fasting, as well as increased triglyceride levels in the blood following a meal, and may therefore be undesirable.

About nine percent of the average American dietary energy intake comes from fructose [found in most fruits and fruit juices, as well as honey]. Such a high consumption is cause for concern about the metabolic effects of this sugar.

Source: *American Journal of Clinical Nutrition* **2000;72(5):1128-1134.**

WANT TO KNOW MORE?

[Many people suffering from irritable bowel syndrome may have an underlying fructose intolerance, which can cause bloating, flatulence, and distension. See Hint #492 in the *Gastrointestinal Diseases & Conditions* section for more details.]

578. BREASTFEEDING & ADULT CHOLESTEROL

Adults who were bottle-fed as infants have higher total cholesterol and LDL cholesterol levels [a well-known risk factor for heart disease] than do their breastfed peers.
Although these levels are often measured for the first time in adulthood, recent reports suggest that early life factors may play a role in determining adult cholesterol levels. What may be confusing is that during infancy these levels are higher among breastfed infants than among bottle-fed infants. However, in adulthood, just the opposite is true, with lower levels noted among those who were breastfed during infancy.

Breast milk typically contains more cholesterol than formula does. But high cholesterol intake during infancy reduces the body's production of cholesterol, which may persist into adulthood.

Source: *Pediatrics* **2002;110:597-608.**

WANT TO KNOW MORE?

[As I wrote in my book, *Total Nutrition for Breast-Feeding Mothers*, published in 1986 by Little, Brown: "We should use breast milk as a model. It is, after all, the most primal of all foods – the only food we know for certain was meant for human consumption. The lesson is: Don't be concerned about eating natural or primal foods containing cholesterol (foods like eggs or shellfish). Processed foods, stress, and lack of exercise are major contributors to raised cholesterol levels – not the ingestion of primal foods, even those high in cholesterol."

(Although out of print, this book is available through online, out-of-print book-finding services.)]

HIGH CHOLESTEROL: DIETARY TACTICS

579. WALNUTS CAN LOWER CHOLESTEROL

Increase your consumption of walnuts to help protect yourself from high cholesterol.
Walnuts can help to reduce both total and low-density lipoprotein (LDL) cholesterol levels in those whose cholesterol levels are too high.

When walnuts are partially substituted for olive oil and other fatty foods, cholesterol levels decrease. The average drop is about nine percent for total cholesterol, and 11.2 percent for LDL (the "bad-guy" cholesterol). So great benefits might be obtained by partially substituting walnuts for traditional western dietary fats.

Source: *Annals of Internal Medicine* **2000;132:538-546.**

WANT TO KNOW MORE?
[For more information on the beneficial effects of walnuts on cholesterol levels, and the relation to heart disease prevention, see Hint #542 in the *Heart & Cardiovascular Disease* section.]

580. MACADAMIA NUTS & IMPROVED CHOLESTEROL

In addition to walnuts, eating macadamia nuts can also help improve your cholesterol levels. Macadamia nuts are high in oleic acid, a monounsaturated fatty acid also found in olive and canola oils, believed to be beneficial in reducing cholesterol. These nuts are the only food that also contains significant amounts of palmitoleic acid, another monounsaturated fatty acid.

(Monounsaturated fats may help to make blood platelets less "sticky" and less likely to form clots in blood vessels, helping to prevent heart attacks and strokes.)

A macadamia-nut diet consisting of 37 percent fat produces lower levels of triglycerides than do diets with the same amount of fat derived from other foods. Despite an increase in the proportion of fat in their diets, volunteers studied show no significant changes in weight or cholesterol levels. In fact, no negative side effects from eating macadamia nuts are seen.

[One note of warning: Beware rancidity, as the higher the oil content of any food, the quicker the oxidation. So purchase organic macadamia nuts in the shell and crack them as you eat them.]

Source: *Circulation* **1999;** *Archives of Internal Medicine* **2000.**

581. SMALLER MEALS LOWER CHOLESTEROL

If you want to lower your cholesterol, eating smaller meals may be helpful. Consuming large meals, especially in the evening, can raise your cholesterol levels. So try dividing your dinner and eating each half several hours apart. (Even if your divided meal equals the same amount of food, it has a different effect on your cholesterol levels when eaten in this way.)

Source: *American Journal of Clinical Nutrition* **1993;57(3):446-51.**

582. EGGS DON'T RAISE CHOLESTEROL LEVELS

Eat eggs! They are good for you and do NOT raise your cholesterol levels, despite what many people still think. A fatty acid in egg yolk (phosphatidyl choline) decreases the absorption of cholesterol, confirming my view that consuming eggs does NOT increase cholesterol levels – and that eggs are, in fact, a food in your best health interest.

The first experiments that maligned eggs as a cholesterol threat were conducted years ago with dried egg yolk. Many studies since then have demonstrated that eating whole, fresh eggs does not have the same effect. Not only does the phosphatidyl choline in eggs work to prevent the absorption of cholesterol, it also prevents age-related memory loss.

Source: *Journal of Nutrition* **2001;131:2358-2363**

583. SOY PROTEIN LOWERS CHOLESTEROL

Eating soy protein may help to lower cholesterol levels in the blood. Dietary intake of soy protein (but not necessarily isolated soy isoflavones) is associated with reductions in plasma cholesterol. The cholesterol-lowering effect of soy protein occurs in part because it is responsible for decreased cholesterol absorption, an effect not attributed to soy isoflavones. [Once again we see the advantage of a whole food, rather than its isolated parts.]

Other components of soy such as saponins, phytic acid, or the amino acid composition may instead be involved in the cholesterol-lowering effects.

Source: *Journal of Nutrition* **2000;130:820-826.**

WANT TO KNOW MORE?
[Isoflavones are unique to soybeans, and have structures very similar to the body's natural estrogens. Research shows that isoflavone dietary supplements may actually be harmful and *promote* breast tumor growth. See Hint #179 in the "Cancer, Breast" section for more details.]

584. BARLEY LOWERS CHOLESTEROL

Eating a high-fiber meal containing barley can help to lower your cholesterol. Fiber regulates the rate and site of fat and carbohydrate digestion and absorption. When fiber sources are included in a meal, a slower rate of carbohydrate and fat absorption modifies the hormone and fat responses.

Consumption of barley-containing meals with a fiber content of 15.7 grams (in this study, pasta partially made from barley flour) can help to lower cholesterol.

In addition, plasma glucose and insulin concentrations increase significantly after meals, but the insulin response is more blunted after a barley-containing meal.

Source: *American Journal of Clinical Nutrition* 1999;69(1):55-63.

585. OATS, NOT WHEAT, FOR LOWER CHOLESTEROL

Not all grains are created equal – eating oatmeal can help you to reduce your cholesterol levels, but eating wheat can actually raise it. The addition of large servings of oat cereal to the diet produces several favorable changes in cholesterol and triglycerides levels, whereas unfavorable changes occur with the addition of wheat cereal.

Oatmeal results in lower concentrations of LDL cholesterol (the bad kind) and triglycerides, without producing adverse changes in HDL cholesterol concentrations (the good variety). These beneficial alterations may contribute to the heart-protective effect of oat fiber. Wheat cereal, however, increases triglycerides, along with other unfavorable lipid changes.

A diet high in fiber has been linked to a decreased risk of mortality from cardiovascular disease, independent of energy intake, dietary fat intake, and other dietary factors. But the type of dietary fiber is important – oat is rich in *soluble* fiber, while wheat is rich in *insoluble* fiber. High fiber wheat consumption can cause an increase in total cholesterol.

[So beware wheat bran, and perhaps even whole grain wheat breads.]

Source: *American Journal of Clinical Nutrition* 2002;76(2):351-358.

586. VEGETARIAN DIETS BEST FOR CHOLESTEROL

If you are trying to lower your cholesterol through dietary changes, only a vegetarian diet – and not a lean-meat diet – will yield significant improvements. The cholesterol-lowering effect of lean-meat diets falls far short of that of vegetarian diets. In fact, lean-meat diets have virtually no lipid-lowering effect at all. The reduction in serum cholesterol concentration of a group consuming "lean" red meat did not reach statistical significance, and a white-meat diet yielded similarly dismal results.

Vegetarian diets, by and large, are met with better adherence than non-vegetarian diets. The reason, presumably, is that effective diets reward compliance with important clinical improvements, while ineffective diets do not.

A low-fat vegetarian diet can reduce the need for cholesterol-lowering drugs and cardiac surgery. Unlike drugs or surgery, its side effects are entirely desirable, including weight loss, blood pressure reduction, and better diabetic control.

Fat-modified meat diets condemn most heart patients to the progression of their illness, and the clinical use of such diets can no longer be justified. Diets that set aside all meats are much more effective in the long run.

Source: *Archives of Internal Medicine* 2000;160:3.

587. FERMENTED DAIRY INCREASES HDL

Consuming fermented dairy products can help to increase your HDL ("good-guy") cholesterol levels. Long-term consumption of 300 grams of probiotic yogurt (over a period of 21 weeks, or about five months) can increase high-density lipoprotein (HDL) levels, leading to an improvement of the LDL/HDL cholesterol ratio.

Source: *European Journal of Clinical Nutrition* 2002;56(9):843-849.

HIGH CHOLESTEROL: DRUG WARNINGS
588. CHOLESTEROL DRUGS OVER-PRESCRIBED

If your doctor has prescribed a "statin" to help lower your cholesterol, consider a second opinion – statins are shown to be prescribed needlessly for as high as 69 percent of patients receiving them as a primary prevention! Instead of following the guidelines of the National Cholesterol Education Program, doctors are using this more aggressive approach in attempts to lower cholesterol in their patients.

Source: *Archives of Internal Medicine* 2001;161:53-58.

589. STATINS & MUSCLE DISEASE RISK

Be warned: People who use cholesterol-lowering drugs (statins) are much more likely to develop muscle disease than are those who don't use these drugs. The link between the use of cholesterol-lowering drugs and muscle disease has now been validated. For some drugs, the risk is as high as 42.4 percent.

According to the advocacy group Public Citizen, many of these drugs have been associated with hundred of recent reports of *rhabdomyolysis* (a muscle-destroying disease). The group has filed a petition with the FDA, urging "black-box" warnings on all statin cholesterol-lowering drugs. (A black box warning is the strongest labeling caution that can be mandated by the FDA.)

Statins are especially dangerous when combined with certain other drugs, particularly fibrates, which are cholesterol-lowering drugs that lower triglycerides and increase HDL levels. A combined therapy of statins and fibrates is commonly prescribed.

Sources: *Reuters Medical Report* 2001; *Clinical Cardiology* 2001;24(7Suppl):II-6-9; *Annals of Pharmacotherapy* 2001;35(7-8):908-917; *Epidemiology* 2001;12:565-569.

WANT TO KNOW MORE?
One healthful alternative to statins could be barley. Glucans, found in significant concentrations in barley, can help to reduce cholesterol safely.

590. CHOLESTEROL DRUGS & FATIGUE

If you are taking cholesterol-lowering drugs, other serious side effects you may face can include muscle aches and fatigue. All cholesterol-lowering drugs (statins) have the potential for muscle damage. Weakness in stair-stepping and hip-strength tests is not unusual among those taking these drugs. When patients go off their statins, they feel better, they feel stronger, and their tissue samples look normal again – indicating that the problem can be reversed.

Switching to different cholesterol-lowering drugs does not eliminate the muscle symptoms. (Statin drugs include Lipitor, Lescol, Mevacor, Pravachol, and Zocor.)

We also know that statins are not beneficial to those with cerebrovascular disease (stroke).

Sources: *Annals of Internal Medicine* 2002;137:581-585; **Cochrane Database System Review** 2002;(3):CD002091; *Alternative Medicine: The Definitive Guide*, 2nd ed, (Berleley,CA: 2002)

WANT TO KNOW MORE?
[Safer ways to lower cholesterol include exercise, the use of probiotics (such as *acidophilus*), soluble rice bran, colostrum, ginseng, ginger, or taking up yoga, Qigong, or Tai Chi.]

HIGH CHOLESTEROL: NATURAL REMEDIES & SUPPLEMENTS

591. REDUCE YOUR CHOLESTEROL WITH GINGER

Consuming ginger extract can help reduce triglycerides and cholesterol levels, as well as prevent atherosclerosis. High doses of ginger extract given to test animals results in a 76 percent reduction in cholesterol after 10 weeks. Consumption of 250 micrograms of ginger extract a day also reduces the level of LDL-associated lipid peroxides by 62 percent. (LDL acts as a carrier for cholesterol and fats in the bloodstream.)

The dietary consumption of ginger extract may also significantly decreases the development of atherosclerotic lesions, due to a reduction of cholesterol levels, as well as reduced susceptibility to oxidation [free radical damage] and aggregation [the "sticking" together of cells].

Source: *Journal of Nutrition* **2000;130:1124-1131.**

WANT TO KNOW MORE?
[For more helpful tips on preventing atherosclerosis, see the "Heart & Cardiovascular Disease" section.]

592. RICE BRAN HELPS REDUCE CHOLESTEROL

Supplementing with rice bran, rich in tocotrienols, can be effective in reducing cholesterol. [Tocotrienols are the best form of vitamin E, containing not only the alpha form, but other important factions, too.] Studies done at the USDA demonstrate that a tocotrienol-rich component of rice bran significantly lowers serum, low-density lipoprotein (LDL) cholesterol, and fatty acids in test animals. These lower concentrations persist for 10 weeks! Other factors that place people at risk for heart disease are also reduced.

In addition, glucose and triglyceride levels are lowered, and insulin is 100 percent greater in the treatment group compared to the non-treatment group. [So rice bran can play an important role in diabetes prevention as well.]

Sources: *American Journal of Clinical Nutrition* **2000;72(6):1510-1515;** *Journal of Nutrition* **2001;131:223-230.**

WANT TO KNOW MORE?
[Because soluble rice bran helps so many people with so many conditions, including diabetes and gastrointestinal problems, it is on my short list of must-take supplements. See Hint #376 for more information on this remarkable supplement.]

593. AGED GARLIC EXTRACT FIGHTS CHOLESTEROL

Not only does aged garlic extract lower cholesterol, but it supports healthy heart function through several other mechanisms, too. Aged garlic extract reduced total cholesterol 6.1 percent compared to placebo in one double-blind, controlled six-month study done at Brown University. Another study, conducted at Penn State University, showed reduction in total cholesterol by 7 percent, and LDL cholesterol by 10 percent.

A study conducted at Loma Linda University noted a 10 to 31 percent drop in cholesterol in those taking liquid Kyolic (aged garlic extract) for six months.

That high levels of LDL pose a risk for heart disease is well known. But oxidized LDL can be more damaging. It affects blood vessels by directly damaging cells lining the vessels. Aged garlic extract not only prevents the oxidation of LDL, but also prevents oxidezed LDL from damaging membranes, oxidizing lipids (fats), and damaging or killing cells.

Sources: *American Journal of Clinical Nutrition* **1996;64:866-70**; Y. Yee et al, *Food Factors for Cancer Prevention* (Tokyo: Springer Verlag, 1997); *Planta Medicine* **1997;63:263-264**; *Pharmacology* **1997;49:908-911**; *Annals of Internal Medicine* **1993;119:599-605.**

594. LOWER CHOLESTEROL WITH GROUND FLAXSEED

Consumption of 40 grams of ground flaxseed daily for three months can lower your cholesterol and triglyceride levels significantly. [For reference, 100 grams of food is usually equal to about the size of your fist.] Most physicians recommend one to two tablespoons of ground flaxseed daily. Since flaxseed oil goes rancid easily (even in capsules and in dark glass bottles), it's best to simply grind it daily – easily done with an inexpensive small coffee bean grinder. Ground flaxseed has a light, nutty taste and can be sprinkled over salads and cereals.]

Flaxseed is also useful for inflamed, irritated mucous membranes in the mouth, throat, stomach, bowels, bladder and kidneys. It can enlarge and soften bowel content, helping to prevent constipation. In addition, flaxseed is helpful for a wide variety of other health problems, including breast cancer (see Hint #XXX), colitis (Hint #XXX), and kidney disease (Hint #XXX).]

Source: *Journal of Clinical Endocrinology & Metabolism* **2002;87:1527-1532.**

595. THE HEALTH BENEFITS OF LICORICE

Licorice-root extract can lower your cholesterol and increase your resistance to LDL cholesterol (as well as protect your heart and decrease your blood pressure). Just one month of licorice consumption results in many positive changes: Susceptibility to oxidation (free radical damage) is reduced by 19 percent. Resistance to aggregation (blood cells "sticking" together) is reduced by 28 percent. Blood cholesterol levels are reduced by five percent, LDL levels by nine percent, and triglyceride levels by 14 percent. Finally, systolic blood pressure is reduced by 10 percent. But when participants in this study were then given a placebo, these parameters went back to their previous levels in just one month (except for the blood pressure, which was sustained throughout).

So dietary consumption of licorice-root extract may act as a moderate cholesterol-lowering nutrient and a potent antioxidant, protecting against high cholesterol and cardiovascular disease.

Source: *Nutrition* 2002;18(3):268-273.

596. HAWTHORN LOWERS CHOLESTEROL

The natural supplement hawthorn fruit can help to lower your cholesterol. Consumption of hawthorn fruit powder for 12 weeks can help to lower cholesterol by as much as 23.4 percent, and triglycerides by as much as 22.2 percent. In test animals, hawthorn supplementation results in 50.6 percent less cholesterol accumulation in the aorta, and 23 to 95 percent greater excretion of substances that normally cause high cholesterol levels.

The mechanism by which hawthorn fruit decreases blood cholesterol levels involves the inhibition of cholesterol absorption.

Source: *Journal of Nutrition* 2002;132:5-10.
WANT TO KNOW MORE?
[For more related information on how hawthorn can help protect against cardiovascular disease, see Hint #562 in the *Heart & Cardiovascular Disease* section.]

HIGH CHOLESTEROL: REDUCING RISK

597. NIACIN TAKEN ALONE CAN BE HAZARDOUS

If you are taking niacin to lower your cholesterol (or for any other reason) be sure to take a good B-complex supplement to protect yourself. The serious risk of large doses of niacin (vitamin B3, often taken to reduce cholesterol) is minimized when taken with other B vitamins, namely vitamin B6. Niacin causes an increase in plasma homocysteine levels in patients with peripheral arterial disease, which could increase their risk of arterial occlusive disease. But B-complex vitamin supplementation can reverse this effect while retaining niacin's beneficial effects on lipoproteins.

Sources: *Journal of Nutrition* 1997;127(1):117-121; *American Heart Journal* 1999;138:1082-1087.

HIGH TRIGLYCERIDES

Triglycerides are naturally occurring fatty acids found in animal and vegetable tissues. They are an important energy source forming much of the fat stored by your body. But when levels are too high, you are at risk for heart disease. Triglycerides elevate your blood viscosity (thickness), and this is a predictor of cardiovascular disease. (*Atherosclerosis* **2002;161(2):433-9**)

598. EXERCISE LOWERS TRIGLYCERIDES

Triglyceride reductions are often observed after exercise training regimens. Thresholds established from training studies indicate that 15 to 20 miles a week of brisk walking or jogging is associated with triglyceride reductions of 5 to 38 milligrams, and HDL (the favorable cholesterol) increases by two to eight milligrams.

Exercise training seldom alters total cholesterol and LDL cholesterol unless dietary fat intake is reduced and body weight loss is associated with the exercise training programs, or both.

Source: *Journal of Cardiopulmonary Rehabilitation* 2002;22(6):385-98.

599. FISH OIL HELPS LOWER TRIGLYCERIDES

If your triglyceride level is high, fish oil supplementation will help to bring it down. Moderate intake of omega-3 fatty acids (found in fish oil) is associated with cell resistance to oxidative stress in those with high triglyceride levels. [Oxidative stress can lead to the production of damaging free radicals in the body.]

When individuals with either normal or high triglyceride levels are given six grams of fish oil daily for eight weeks, the fish oil supplementation induces omega-3 fatty acid incorporation into cells. And in the normal-level group, it also enhances the effectiveness of vitamin E.

(Although they exhibit a high susceptibility to oxidation, omega-3 fatty acids may protect cell membranes and are of great benefit in the treatment of those with high triglyceride levels.)

Source: *American Journal of Clinical Nutrition* 2001;74(4)449-456.

WANT TO KNOW MORE?
[Omega-6 fatty acid – found in oils such as evening primrose and borage oil – lowers cholesterol, but in large amounts it can lower HDL (the "good" cholesterol) and cause inflammatory problems.]

600. FIBER CAN LOWER TRIGLYCERIDE LEVELS

Take note: The higher your dietary fiber intake, the lower your cholesterol and triglyceride levels. High triglycerides also impair glucose tolerance and are the main risk factors of insulin sensitivity. A good fiber complex can favorably affect insulin resistance, and decrease high blood fats.

So fiber supplementation should be considered to offset type 2 diabetes, because insulin resistance is this disease's best prediction factor.

Keep in mind that there is an association between fiber intake, exercise, and triglyceride levels. And don't forget the fermentable fibers in supplemental form, as in fructooligosaccharides.

[It is very difficult, however, to get an adequate amount of fiber, given the high rate of processed and restaurant foods we tend to consume. Salads are not usually a large source of fiber: an entire head of lettuce, for example, contains only 1.6 grams! (Physicians recommend a minimum of 30 grams daily.) That's why it is important to add a good supplemental fiber mix to your daily regime. Look for one with a mix of several types of fibers.]

Sources: *Journal of the American College of Nutrition* **2001;20(6):649-655;** *Zhonghua Yu Fang Yi Xue Za Zhi* **(China) 2002, 36(3):184-6;** *Diabetes* **1999:48(8):1600-6.**

HOSPITAL VISIT CAVEATS

Anyone who has spent any time in a hospital as a patient knows it's no exaggeration to be awakened to take a sleeping pill.

Nor is it unusual to conclude that you have just helped put your doctors' kids through college when you see your bill.

Medicalization, over which you have no control during your hospital stay, is not always in your best health interest. Shah Ebrahim, a professor of the epidemiology of aging, says: "Legitimate concerns exist about the risks of infection, over-prescribing, inappropriate use of tranquillizers, and the hazards of pressure sores."

If it's surgery, you want to select a physician with experience. Before accepting a drug, ask your nurse to check your chart to be sure the one she is offering is actually intended for you. Know how to use your call button, and that it is within reach. And after your discharge, find out how you can stay in touch with your doctor for follow-up questions.

Have a close friend or family member check on you frequently, and, best of all, do everything you can to shorten your hosptial stay.

601. NUTRIENT "COCKTAIL" FOR A SHORTER STAY

Consuming a nutrient cocktail before and after surgery can help you to shorten your hospital stay considerably. A "cocktail" of omega-3, arginine [an amino acid], and nucleotides – started one to two weeks prior to major surgery, and continued three to five days postoperatively – can maximize immune function and speed recovery.

[Nucleotides can be found in chlorella, a supplemental alga.]

This mix of nutrients can help patients reduce their stay in an intensive care by 4.5 days, and reduce hospital costs by $5,000.

Source: Studies conducted at Guys Hospital, London, as reported at the European Society for Intensive Care Medicine, Berlin.

602. DON'T LIE DOWN WITH PNEUMONIA!

If you are sleeping in a hospital bed, don't lie completely flat – it could increase your risk of pneumonia. The risk of developing pneumonia in hospital patients can be reduced by a semi-recumbent position; that is, leaning, or partially reclining, rather than a supine position.

The recumbent posture of the Romans at their meals is the one recommended for patients today in an effort to avoid hospital-caused pneumonia.

Source: *Lancet* 1999;354:1858.

603. TOO MUCH BED REST DELAYS RECOVERY

Beware bed rest: It can delay recovery from lower back pain, labor, hypertension, myocardial infarction [heart attack], and acute infectious hepatitis. In 1944, Australian researchers concluded: "The physician must always consider complete bed rest as a highly unphysiologic and definitely hazardous form of therapy, to be ordered only for specific indications and discontinued as early as possible."

Our modern medical community, however, has had a very difficult time accepting and recommending this advice, despite the fact that many studies show that bed rest can delay recovery for many illnesses.

Source: *Lancet* 1999;354:1229-33.

604. DRAW BLOOD FROM THE EARLOBE INSTEAD

If you require your blood to be drawn for a glucose check, ask that your blood be taken from your earlobe rather than your finger – you will experience far less pain. Taking blood for a glucose concentration check is one of the most commonly performed procedures in clinical practice. Fingers are sensitive, and many patients experience pain as their blood is drawn. Studies show that taking blood from the side of the thumb is less painful than from a finger or at the elbow, but taking blood from the earlobe is even less painful. The earlobe is both accessible and vascular. The reason for the difference in pain is unclear. It may have to do with the thickness of certain cells (less in the earlobe) or perhaps it's because you can't see your ear being lanced.

Source: *British Medical Journal* **2000;321:20.**

605. NO FASTING BEFORE ELECTIVE SURGERY

If you are preparing to undergo elective surgery, fasting is not necessary beforehand. Most elective surgery patients no longer need to follow the old-fashioned rule of "nothing by mouth after midnight" on the day of surgery because of newer anesthesiology techniques, as well as the unnecessary and unpleasant side effects of fasting. There is a growing body of evidence that pulmonary aspiration [the entry of gastric contents into the respiratory tract] rarely occurs with modern anesthesia. Prolonged preoperative fasting can lead to irritability, headaches, dehydration, and hypoglycemia, and serves little purpose. New guidelines permit clear liquids up to two hours before elective surgery, a light breakfast such as toast and tea six hours before surgery, and a heavier meal eight hours beforehand.

Source: *American Journal of Nursing* **2002;102:36-44.**

606. EAT SOON TO SHORTEN HOSPITAL STAY

Here's another food-related hospital hint: Eating soon after surgery is safe and may help to speed your recovery. Women should be fed the first day after major abdominal surgery (gynecologic oncology or urogynecologic surgery) to reduce the length of their hospital stay, rather than waiting for bowel function to return.

Early feeding is safe, with no increased adverse effects. Feeding can begin with clear fluids on the first postoperative day, and once 500 milliliters of clear fluids are tolerated, a regular diet can be started.

This cuts the length of the hospital stay from six days to four days. Benefits of early postoperative feeding may include improved nutritional status (which promotes wound healing), decreased risk of infection, and an improved sense of well-being.

Source: *American Journal of Obstetrics & Gynecology* **2002;186:861-865.**

HYPERTENSION

Hypertension is recognized as the most common chronic condition. About sixty million Americans suffer from hypertension, and two-thirds are under 65 years of age. We've heard the risk factors time and again: smoking, alcohol, obesity, lack of exercise, eating too much fat, stress, salt. And we know that the diabetic is more susceptible. The high prevalence of hypertension in seniors (nearly one out of every two people aged 60 and older), and its high risk of cardiovascular disease, suggests that we should pay attention to safe, easy remedies to reduce the problem.

An interesting article in the *Archives of Internal Medicine* (2002;162:2204-2208), states that "for more than 25 years, the medical literature has mostly blamed patients for poor blood pressure control and argued that patients need to receive more education for better compliance. While patient compliance is an important factor, physician education and behavior is perhaps a bigger problem responsible for the continuing lack of appropriate blood pressure control in millions of patients."

"Even those with borderline systolic hypertenion are at serious risk for serious disease," continues the article. "Blood pressure is defined as hypertension when the pressure is higher than 140/90 mm Hg in all adults, including the elderly. Since hypertension is largely a disease with no noticeable symptoms, inadequate treatment is often the result. And too many physicians continue to use the wrong classes of medications (eg, calcium channel blockers). Dietary changes, low salt intake, and weight loss and stress reduction techniques are often not emphasized enough by physicians."

IN THIS SECTION:

- ALTERNATIVE THERAPIES
- BLOOD PRESSURE CAVEATS
- CAUSES & PRECURSORS
- DIETARY TACTICS
- DRUG WARNINGS

- NATURAL REMEDIES & SUPPLEMENTS
- REDUCING RISK
- SODIUM REDUCTION
- STROKE CONNECTION

HYPERTENSION: ALTERNATIVE THERAPIES
607. YOGA FOR HYPERTENSION

If you have hypertension, taking up yoga may be helpful. One-hour sessions of yoga, practiced in the morning and in the evening, can *significantly* lower blood pressure after just 11 days. In fact, this treatment is comparable in effectiveness to taking blood pressure medication.

[Yoga classes are popular and easy to find nowadays. Many gyms offer yoga courses in addition to their more traditional aerobic exercise classes.]

Source: *Indian Journal of Physiological Pharmacology* 2000;44(2):207-210.

HYPERTENSION: BLOOD PRESSURE CAVEATS

608. DON'T FOLLOW "100 + AGE" RULE

The clinical folklore that an appropriate systolic blood pressure is "100 + age" is just that: folklore, and it should be abandoned. Less than one in four Americans has blood pressure values at or below the recommendation of 140/90 mm Hg.

Source: *Journal of Hypertension* 2000;2:132-133.

WANT TO KNOW MORE?
[The designation mm Hg refers to "millimeters of mercury."]

609. MEASURE BLOOD PRESSURE IN *BOTH* ARMS

When having your blood pressure taken, make sure to check both arms, since differences in pressure between your arms could suggest a problem. The identification of any difference in blood pressure between arms is a vital part of the assessment of hypertensive patients. Although the difference could be a normal characteristic, it may also be an indication of vascular problems, so further testing in the case of a variation is advisable.

The importance of blood pressure differences between the arm and the leg has been known for a long time.

Source: *British Medical Journal* 2001;323:399.

610. "WHITE-COAT *NORMO*TENSION" EXISTS TOO

Since up to one quarter of patients who have normal blood pressure when measured in their doctor's office may have high blood pressure outside of the office, it's a good idea to check your blood pressure at home. The phenomenon of white-coat syndrome has received a great deal of attention: those with normal blood pressure show high levels in the doctor's office. But what about the opposite? The phenomenon of "white-coat normotension" has received little study, but it turns out that 23 percent of patients checked had white-coat normotension for systolic blood pressure, and 24 percent had white-coat normotension for diastolic blood pressure.

It may a good idea to monitor your blood pressure at home in order to get a more accurate reading.

Source: *Archives of Family Medicine* 2000;9:533-540.

611. BEWARE "HIGH-NORMAL" BLOOD PRESSURE

Because high-normal blood pressure often quickly progresses to hypertension, it's important to start practicing natural ways to normalize blood pressure now! Adults with high-normal blood pressure often develop hypertension within four years or less. In fact, nearly half of adults 65 and older with high-normal blood pressure develop hypertension within this time frame.

Over a four-year period, 5.3 percent, 17.6 percent, and 37.3 percent of those younger than 65 with optimum, normal, and high-normal blood pressure, respectively, develop hypertension. The same distribution for those over 65 years is 16 percent, 25.5 percent, and 49.5 percent.

The likelihood of developing hypertension is increased an additional 20 to 30 percent for subjects who experience a five percent weight gain, so weight control is of prime importance for all groups.

[In addition to weight control, measures for preventing or lowering high blood pressure include aerobic exercise, consumption of stabilized, stabilized rice bran, aged garlic supplements, essential fatty acids, increased fiber, decreased caffeine, avoidance of aspartame [Nutrasweet], and supplementing with vitamin C and zinc.]

Source: *Lancet* **2001;358:1682-1686.**

WANT TO KNOW MORE?
Optimum, normal, and high-normal blood pressure is defined as lower than 120/80 mm Hg., 120-129/80-84, and 130-139/85-89, respectively. Hypertension is defined as 140/90 or greater.

HYPERTENSION: CAUSES & PRECURSORS

612. HEADACHES LINKED TO HYPERTENSION

Suffer from headaches? Get your blood pressure checked. Headaches are not only a problem for those with severe hypertension — they may also be symptomatic of mild to moderate hypertension.

In hypertensive patients treated for headaches, the incidence of headache was found to correlate with increased diastolic blood pressure.

(Those younger than 50 years of age had more headaches than those older than 50.)

Source: *Archives of Internal Medicine* **2000;160:1645-1658.**

WANT TO KNOW MORE?
[Here's a quick headache cure: Try taking six calcium tablets at once; repeat 30 minutes later.]

613. SYSTOLIC, NOT DIASTOLIC, REVEALS RISK

Uncontrolled systolic blood pressure in hypertensive men is *significantly* associated with the risk of death from cardiovascular and coronary heart disease — but the diastolic level has little relevance. Those with a systolic blood pressure of 160 or higher exhibit a 2.2-times increased rate of death from cardiovascular disease than do those with pressures below 140.

Even for those with intermediate elevations of systolic pressure, there is an elevated risk. But no association is seen, however, between *diastolic* blood pressure and cardiovascular or coronary heart disease mortality.

Source: *Archives of Internal Medicine 2002;162:506-508,577-581.*

HYPERTENSION: DIETARY TACTICS
614. OLIVE OIL AGAINST HYPERTENSION

If you have high blood pressure, increased consumption of olive oil may help reduce your need for hypertension medication. A diet rich in monounsaturated fatty acids from extra virgin olive oil reduces the required daily dosage for anti-hypertensives in those with mild-to-moderate hypertension.

The use of olive oil may even enable some patients to get off medication completely.

Patients using olive oil can reduce their daily anti-hypertensive drug dosage by 48 percent compared with a reduction of only 4 percent while on a polyunsaturated fatty acid diet of sunflower oil.

This effect may be due to enhanced nitric oxide levels stimulated by the polyphenols found in olive oil (but not found in sunflower oil).

[Important note: This research was done in Italy, where olive oil is available in its purest form. By the time the olive oil crosses the ocean, it no longer retains its original quality. Try to buy your olive oil from a source that does not store it on shelves for too long, and does not allow the temperature of the storage room to reach undesirable levels.]

Source: *Archives of Internal Medicine 2000;160:837-842.*

615. REVERSING HYPERTENSION THROUGH DIET

A diet high in fat and refined carbohydrates causes oxidative stress that can lead to hypertension – but this can be reversed with a change in diet. When test animals were fed a diet that simulated the average American diet (high in fat and refined carbohydrates), they exhibited a gradual rise in arterial blood pressure and were hypertensive within 18 months.

When after two years this diet was discontinued and the animals were given a more normal diet, much of the abnormalities reversed.

[Once again it is demonstrated that it is never too late to reverse the effects of a bad diet! Start today.]

Source: *Hypertension: Journal of the American Heart Association* **2000;36:423-429.**

WANT TO KNOW MORE?
Hypertension is not a single event but is generally packaged with a series of other risk factors.

616. GARLIC LOWERS BLOOD PRESSURE

Garlic can help to normalize blood pressure, and has been proven to be beneficial when taken as a supplement. In one group studied, those with blood pressure on the normal side were found to consume more garlic in their diets, either in cooked, raw, or pickled form. (The results were statistically significant for systolic blood pressure only.)

Garlic appears to have the potential for the prevention and control of cardiovascular disorders.

Sources: *Journal of Pakistan Medical Association* **2000;50(6):204-207;** *Journal of Nutrition* **2001;131(3s):1020S-1026S;1016S-1019S;977S-979S.**

WANT TO KNOW MORE?
Garlic may also be useful for the prevention of atherosclerosis because it can protect against oxidized LDL, the process that causes injury to epithelial cells, leading to heart disease.

Aged garlic serves as an antioxidant, preventing lipid peroxide damage in a dose-dependent manner (meaning the more you take, the less the damage).

[For more information on how garlic extract is preventive against atherosclerosis, see Hint #522 in the *Heart & Cardiovascular Disease* section.]

617. THE IMPORTANT POTASSIUM:SODIUM RATIO

Protect yourself from hypertension (and stroke) by eating foods with the proper potassium/sodium ratio, which translates to natural foods, rather than processed foods. Foods high in potassium and low in sodium may reduce your risk of high blood pressure and stroke, but such foods are hard to come by unless you consume lots of raw green peas, raw green lima beans, raw parsley, raw asparagus, avocados, bananas, or walnuts.

Although containers of orange juice will soon be allowed to make the low-risk health claim, the ratio of potassium to sodium in an orange is not as good as that in the foods mentioned above. And because orange juice is a processed food, there are nutrient depletions (vitamin C, for example, is diminished – another nutrient that lowers blood pressure), plus it has an unnaturally high concentration of carbohydrates. No processed food can ever offer the benefits of whole foods. There are many other foods with high potassium content, but their sodium content sends them to the back of the line in terms of life-and-death disease risk. (Juice the oranges yourself!)

Sources: *Reuter's Medical Report* Oct 2000; B. Kamen, *Everything You Always Wanted to Know About Potassium But Were Too Tired to Ask*.

618. HIGH FIBER + PROTEIN = LOW PRESSURE

Increasing dietary fiber and protein *significantly* reduces blood pressure in those being medically treated for hypertension. Those who consume high-fiber, high-protein diets experience the greatest decreases in blood pressure, with their average systolic blood pressure dropping by 10.5 mm Hg compared with control subjects. (The diet consisting of 12.5 percent of energy from protein, and 15 grams of fiber daily.) Adequate intake of protein and fiber, particularly with fruits and vegetables as sources of soluble fiber, should be considered as part of an optimal diet to reduce of cardiovascular risk.

Source: *Hypertension* 2001;38:821-826.

619. LOWER BLOOD PRESSURE WITH OATMEAL

A low-calorie diet containing oats consumed over a six-week period can result in great improvements in blood pressure. One of the most effective methods for improving high blood pressure and lipid profiles is the loss of excess weight. Including oats in a weight-loss diet can help lower blood pressure, lower cholesterol, and improve the pattern of fat in your blood.
It's the fiber content that initiates the benefits. [Consider a fiber supplement — one to two tablespoons of a good, organic fiber mix daily.]

Source: *Journal of Nutrition* 2001;12(1):49-53;131:1465-1470.

HYPERTENSION: DRUG WARNINGS

620. BLOOD PRESSURE DRUGS & HEART PROBLEMS

If you are among the millions taking a calcium channel blocker for your high blood pressure, ask your doctor about the possibility of changing your medication because of very serious side effects. These drugs are so widespread that even a small increase in ill effects associated with them may be responsible for 85,000 excess heart-related events.

Although the drugs control blood pressure, an increase in heart attacks and episodes of heart failure comes without any particular advantage.

Patients taking calcium channel blockers have a 27 percent increased risk of heart attack, and a 26 percent increased risk of having an episode of heart failure. The risk of people on calcium channel blockers having a major coronary event increases by 11 percent. Will this be front page news ten years from now like the HRT hadlines of today?

Source: 22nd Congress of the European Society of Cardiology, Amsterdam, the Netherlands, Aug 2000.

HYPERTENSION: NATURAL REMEDIES & SUPPLEMENTS

621. VITAMIN C FOR BLOOD PRESSURE CONTROL

For those with hypertension, supplementing with vitamin C daily is useful for blood pressure control. Experimental research on hypertension suggests that increased production of reactive oxygen may play a role in the development of high blood pressure.

But supplementing with 500 milligrams of ascorbic acid (vitamin C) daily can lower blood pressure [perhaps due to its antioxidative properties]. You must remain on the treatment for one month before results can be noticed.

[Vitamin C is one of the least stable vitamins, and cooking can destroy much of it. Some good dietary sources of vitamin C are citrus fruits, strawberries, green peppers, broccoli, dark leafy greens, and tomatoes.]

Source: *Lancet* 1999;354(9195):2048-9.

622. VITAMIN D AGAINST HYPERTENSION

Vitamin D3 may play a large role in the prevention and treatment of high blood pressure. Factors that lead to hypertension, cardiac problems, and increased water intake may be controlled with vitamin D3 [cholecalciferol, produced in the skin in response to sunlight exposure]. Studies show an inverse relationship between circulating vitamin D levels and blood pressure (meaning, the higher the vitamin D levels, the lower the pressure). Although the relationship between vitamin D3 and blood pressure is complex and not fully understood, the results are positive.

So it's a half hour in the sun daily, or a good D3 supplement.

Source: *Journal of Clinical Investigation* **2002;110:229-238.**

623. OMEGA-3 FATTY ACIDS & BLOOD PRESSURE

Try omega-3 fatty acids, commonly found in fish oil, to help reduce high blood pressure. According to the American Heart Association, there is evidence that omega-3 fatty acids may have beneficial effects on blood pressure, endothelial function, and platelet function. Omega-3 fatty acids may have a dose-dependent response in reducing blood pressure in hypertensive individuals (that is, the more you take, the more the effect), and dietary supplementation (three grams per day) may help untreated hypertensives lower their blood pressure.

[Omega-3 fatty acids can be found in fatty fish and fish oils, as well as in flaxseed and walnuts.]

Source: *Reuter's Health Report* **May 2000.**

624. MAGNESIUM LOWERS BLOOD PRESSURE

Supplementing with magnesium may be helpful in reducing high blood pressure. Findings from extensive studies provide evidence that increased magnesium supplementation is associated with reductions in blood pressure, and the effect is dose-related. In over 1,200 subjects studied, for each 10 mmol increase in daily magnesium intake, systolic and diastolic blood pressure decreased by 4.3 and 2.3 mm Hg, respectively.

Higher blood pressure is associated with obesity and lack of regular physical activity. It is also associated with a higher sodium, alcohol, and protein intake, and *inversely* with potassium, calcium, and magnesium intake. [Some good dietary sources of magnesium include dairy products, meat, fish, seafood, bananas, garlic, green leafy vegetables, and nuts.]

Sources: *American Journal of Hypertension* **2002;15:691-696;** *Nutrition & Clinical Care* **2002;5(1):9-19.**

625. ALPHA-LIPOIC ACID FOR HYPERTENSION

The antioxidant alpha-lipoic acid (ALA) may be helpful in preventing hypertension. Alpha-lipoic acid prevents the rise of systolic blood pressure when given to test animals. The antihypertensive effects of alpha-lipoic acid seem to be associated with its antioxidative properties.

[There are not many dietary sources of alpha-lipoic acid, but it can be found in broccoli, spinach, and organ meats.]

Source: *Hypertension: Journal of the American Heart Association* 2002;39:303-307.

WANT TO KNOW MORE?
[Alpha-lipoic acid also prevents insulin resistance and can be used to treat diabetes. See Hint #404 in the *Diabetes* section for more details.]

626. COENZYME Q10 CAN HELP HYPERTENSION

Supplementing with a natural substance known as coenzyme Q10 (CoQ10) may be beneficial in treating hypertension. Daily supplementation with 200 milligrams of CoQ10 results in a threefold increase in plasma CoQ10 concentration.

[Some dietary sources of CoQ10 are spinach, peanuts, beef, and fish such as mackerel and salmon.]

Source: *European Journal of Clinical Nutrition* 2002;56:1137-1142.

WANT TO KNOW MORE?
[CoQ10 may be also be beneficial for a variety of other health problems, including asthma (see Hint #119), diabetes (Hint #402), and migraines (Hint #508).]

HYPERTENSION: REDUCING RISK
627. EXERCISE HELPS HIGH BLOOD PRESSURE

Exercise is important both for treating high blood pressure and in preventing the condition from developing in the first place, so the message to one and all is: GET MOVING! Even if your blood pressure is normal, walking, cycling, jogging, or swimming can help reduce any subsequent risk of heart attack and stroke later on. This has been confirmed again and again, by countless studies.

A variety of aerobic exercises at all frequencies are beneficial to those who were previously sedentary – in other words, some activity is better than none. The goal should be at least 30 minutes of moderate exercise, five or more days a week.

Sources: *Annals of Internal Medicine* **2002;136:493-503;** *Hypertension* **2000;36:171-176.**

WANT TO KNOW MORE?
In addition to the cardiovascular risks, high blood pressure can damage kidneys, eyes, and brain.

628. EXERCISE BENEFITS LAST A LONG TIME

A little exercise goes a long way: *Significant* **reductions in blood pressure persist for up to 16 hours in hypertensive patients after a single, 45-minute exercise session.** The effects of exercise on blood pressure were studied in a group of obese, sedentary men (aged 49 to 67, with an average blood pressure of 153/96). Blood pressure was recorded on one day when subjects engaged in three 15-minute bouts of treadmill exercise testing and on a second day when they did not exercise. Systolic blood pressure remained lower for 16 hours after exercise.

If similar reductions in blood pressure are achieved after only 10 minutes of exercise, a hypertensive person could go for a vigorous 10-minute walk at breakfast, lunch, and dinner, and they would experience significant reductions in blood pressure for nearly every hour of the day. Knowing that a single exercise session helps reduce blood pressure might keep hypertensive patients motivated to exercise regularly.

Source: *American Journal of Hypertension* **2000;13:44-51.**

629. A LITTLE WEIGHT LOSS GOES A LONG WAY

Even modest weight loss can help to normalize blood pressure in those with hypertension. Weight gain in adult life seems to be an especially important risk factor for the development of hypertension, while weight loss has been shown to be the most effective non-drug hypertension treatment approach. Modest weight loss has also been shown to lower or even *discontinue* the need for anti-hypertensive medication.

Source: *Obesity Research* **May 2000;8(3):270-278.**

630. WALK AWAY FROM HIGH BLOOD PRESSURE

Just 30 minutes of daily moderate-intensity physical activity (such as walking) can help to lower your blood pressure. Postmenopausal women with hypertension who increase their daily walking show blood pressure improvements after 12 weeks, and even greater improvements after 24 weeks. Body mass is also moderately reduced.

In addition to blood pressure, there are also positive benefits seen between walking and triglyceride levels, bone mass, aging, cognitive decline, breast cancer, diabetes, and more.

Source: *Medical Science of Sports & Exercise* 2001;33(11):1825-1831.

631. FIT WOMEN & BLOOD PRESSURE CONTROL

If you are female, the more fit you are, the less likely it is that your blood pressure will rise when under physical stress. Increases in systolic pressure are inversely related to fitness among women when under physical stress (meaning the fitter a woman is, the less likely her systolic pressure will rise when under stress). However, this is NOT true for men.

Source: *Psychophysiology* 2002;39(5):568-76.

632. HYPERTENSION? LEARN STRESS MANAGEMENT

Learning stress management techniques can result in *significant* blood pressure reductions in those with hypertension, helping to avoid the need for drugs and their side effects. In a study involving over 60 hypertensive men and women (with blood pressures greater than 140/90 mm Hg), those who received 10 hours of stress management training showed significant reductions in blood pressure, compared with no reductions observed in those who received no training. When those in the no-treatment group eventually received stress management training, their blood pressures were also reduced.

Source: *Archives of Internal Medicine* 2001;161:1071-1080.

633. HYPERTENSION & RISK OF MEMORY PROBLEMS

Did you know that hypertension causes changes in brain blood flow that could affect your short-term memory? Hypertensive patients with memory impairment have less blood flow in specific brain areas compared to those with normal blood pressure. To compensate, there is an increase in left hemisphere blood flow, which may explain the memory loss. Memory changes are similar to the type of difference you might see between a healthy 45-year-old person and a 55-year-old person. [Eating apples and asparagus can be protective against hypertension: Apples contain potassium (helps compensate for salt in processed foods) and pectin (an excellent fiber source that can bind water and quickly eliminate it, helping to avoid water retention). Asparagus, also high in potassium, contains asperagin, which helps stimulate kidney function.]

Sources: **American Heart Association's 55th Annual Fall Conference of the Council for High Blood Pressure Research, Chicago, IL, Sep 2001;** B. Kamen, *Everything You Always Wanted to Know About Potassium But Were Too Tired to Ask.*

634. HAVE BOTH HYPERTENSION & DIABETES?

If you have hypertension and are also diabetic, exercise may help you to reduce your increased risk of cardiovascular disease. The benefits of exercise for cardiovascular health, as well as for preventing and treating type 2 diabetes and hypertension, are well known. Exercise reduces overall body fat, as well as abdominal fat, which may lower the risks of both cardiovascular disease and type 2 diabetes.

One important note: Patients with diabetes and hypertension should first undergo an exercise stress test to rule out severe cardiovascular disease.

Source: *Journal of the American Medical Association* **2002;288:1622-1631.**

WANT TO KNOW MORE?
[See the extensive "Diabetes" section for helpful hints on preventing and treating this disease through diet, exercise, and nutritional supplementation.]

HYPERTENSION: SODIUM REDUCTION
635. LESS SODIUM: GOOD FOR EVERYONE

A diet low in salt and rich in vegetables and fruits is the way to go for *everyone*, no matter what your blood pressure. The advice to lower sodium only if you have high blood pressure has been misleading. As usual, it takes a "new" study to bring the facts to our attention. According to the National Heart, Lung, and Blood Institute, salt affects blood pressure, and the lower your salt intake, the lower your blood pressure — no matter what diet you are on. In addition, they find that lowering sodium intake enhances the beneficial effects of a fruit and vegetable diet.

Source: Meeting of the American Society of Hypertension, New York, NY, as reported by CBS Health Watch, May 2000.

WANT TO KNOW MORE?
[Of the 10 pounds of salt ingested by each American every year, over eight pounds are already added to your food before it is purchased.

The conclusion that lowering salt intake is good for everyone *You Always* (including the reasons why) was stated in my book, ***Everything Wanted to Know About Potassium But Were Too Tired to Ask,* published back in 1992.]**

636. SALT & INCREASED MORTALITY

You don't need to have hypertension to suffer deleterious effects from too much salt. Results of a study started 27 years ago show a link between salt sensitivity and death in people with normal blood pressure. There have been other studies that link high salt intake to organ damage. So even if it doesn't affect your blood pressure, sodium can cause the development of other very serious medical problems.

The recommended amount is 2,400 milligrams of sodium per day, which is approximately half of that consumed in the typical American diet.

Source: *Hypertension* 2001;37:429-432.

637. REDUCING SODIUM MAKES A BIG DIFFERENCE

Restricting sodium and eating whole foods is as effective as taking hypertension medication for lowering blood pressure. In those with hypertension, the combination of reducing dietary sodium and eating unprocessed foods can decrease systolic blood pressure by as much as 11.5 mm Hg and diastolic by 7.1 mm Hg. Among persons with normal blood pressures, the reductions are 8.9 mm Hg systolic and 4.5 mm Hg diastolic.

Reductions of that magnitude would reduce the prevalence of heart disease by 20 percent and stroke by 35 percent!

Source: DASH (Dietary Approach to Stop Hypertension) study.

WANT TO KNOW MORE?
[One gram of sodium in 3.5 ounces of fresh peas compares with 115 grams in frozen peas and 236 grams in canned peas, and that jumps to 374 total grams of sodium when 1/2 ounce of salted butter is added.

More importantly, the ratio of sodium to potassium often gets reversed when foods are processed. For an excellent understanding of the sodium/potassium ratio and how this impacts your health, plus charts on the sodium content of commonly consumed foods, see my book, *Everything You Always Wanted to Know About Potassium But Were Too Tired to Ask*.]

638. THE SINGLE LARGEST SOURCE OF SALT

Did you know that three-quarters of dietary salt comes from processed foods, and bread is the single largest source? Participants fed three types of whole meal bread (identical in all respects except for salt content) were unable to guess which bread contained the most salt.

Recommendations could be made to food manufacturers that small reductions in salt content would not reduce sales. As well as eventually reducing the taste for salt, reductions in the salt content of processed foods would shift population blood pressures downward, with considerable health benefits.

Source: *Lancet* 1999;353:1332.

639. LESS SALT DOESN'T AFFECT NUTRIENTS

Salt restriction does not lead to other nutrient deficiencies, and should be the first-line treatment for high blood pressure. Subjects in one study were shown how to reduce salt intake, and they were provided with low-salt bread during the salt-restriction period. It was concluded that salt restriction does not affect any other nutrients, as was previously believed.

[One of the problems with trying to restrict salt is that it pervades almost all restaurant, catered, and store-bought processed foods. Again – it's the ratio between the sodium and potassium that is important.

Because nature has supplied us with foods that are high in potassium and low in sodium, our bodies retain sodium and easily get rid of potassium. However, the ratio in the foods we eat today is unfortunately reversed.]

Sources: *American Journal of Clinical Nutrition* 2000;72(2):414-420; **B. Kamen**, *Everything You Always Wanted to Know About Potassium But Were Too Tired to Ask.*

HYPERTENSION: STROKE CONNECTION

640. HYPERTENSION NOW, STROKE LATER?

Be warned: Hypertension in your adult life *significantly* increases your risk of stroke later on. Men and women who were stroke-free when they enrolled in The Framingham Heart Study, but who had hypertension, experienced strokes years later.

This suggests that blood pressure levels in midlife affect the future risk of stoke, not only over a short span, but up to prolonged periods of 30 years or more.

To achieve optimal reductions in the risk of ischemic stroke when you are older, it is necessary to prevent, diagnose, and manage blood pressure elevations throughout adulthood.

Source: *Archives of Internal Medicine* 2001;161:2343-2350.

WANT TO KNOW MORE?
[See the "Stroke" section for lots of helpful information on reducing your stroke risk.]

HYSTERECTOMY

You have to wonder about the fact that we perform more hysterectomies in this country than any other modern nation. Interesting, isn't it, that women with *more* education are more likely to undergo hysterectory. Miscarriages, especially if caused by uterine prolapse, also increases the probability of hysterectomy. Women who have their first child before the age of twenty are at increased risk because of endometriosis. (*Journal of Womens Health* **1997;6(3):309-16)**

There is also great variation in hysterectomy procedure in the US .The surgery can done vaginally, abdominally, or laparoscopically. The large variations in practice indicate that the route of surgery is more dependent on the clinical prefence of the gynecologist than the medical condition of the patient. (*Journal of Obstetrics & Gynecology* **2001;21(2):166-170)**

The important thing to remember about a hysterectomy is that the surgery eliminates the symptoms, but does not address the cause. Since the confirmation about the harm of synthetic hormones has been released, many women who have had hysterectomies (and their physicians) are confused about what to do next. The use of a natural progesterone cream has been one safe solution, highly recommended by nutrition-aware physicians.

Most women are told by their physcians that they MUST be on estrogen therapy if they've had hysterectomies. Just think of why the hysterectomy was performed in the first place. Large fibroids? Cysts? Endometriosis? Cancer? Wasn't too much estrogen responsible for these problems to begin with?

641. HYSTERECTOMY & CHRONIC CONSTIPATION

A high-fiber diet plan is an inexpensive and effective way of alleviating the constipation that is a common result of hysterectomy. After having had a hysterectomy, women on a high-fiber diet find that they have fewer painful bowel movements, have less abdominal pain and cramps, take a shorter time to defecate, need to strain less, and also need to rely on medications for irregularity less often.

On this high-fiber diet, women find their changes in bowel function to be generally positive, compared with the negative changes reported by those who did not start such a diet after their hysterectomies.

Source: *Gynecology & Oncology* **1997;66(3):417-424.**

WANT TO KNOW MORE?
[Fiber is essential for optimum health, but it is very difficult to get an adequate amount in the American diet without adding a good fiber supplemental mix. See my book, *New Facts About Fiber,* for a good introduction to this subject. Also, see the *Constipation* section for other natural remedies to bowel irregularity. For those women who experience a declining libido after hysterectomy, a vaginal stimulant cream, as described in my book, *She's Gotta Have It!* happily resolves that problem.]

IMMUNE SYSTEM DISORDERS

The word immunity and its theories were first proposed in the late 1800s. The notion of using immunity against cancer and other debilitating diseases has a long history. But the proposals and the products and those who initiated them were mostly ridiculed – until very recently. Those who understood the concepts and proposed the intake of naturally derived elixirs were cast aside and even humiliated

Before holistic immunotherapy took hold, the more astute and perceptive doctors sought information to help them design the correct studies. In their efforts to discover what helps and what doesn't, they began to ask: *Why do some die and others get well from the same illness?* The answer is: *the integrity of the immune system!*

IN THIS SECTION:
I. HIV & AIDS
- DIETARY TACTICS
- NATURAL REMEDIES & SUPPLEMENTS

II. IMMUNE SYSTEM DYSFUNCTION (NON-HIV)
- CAUSES & PRECURSORS
- NATURAL REMEDIES & SUPPLEMENTS
- REDUCING RISK

HIV & AIDS

HIV & AIDS: DIETARY TACTICS

642. NUTRITIONAL SUPPORT FOR AIDS

If you are suffering from AIDS, paying closer attention to your diet can have a significant beneficial effect on your health. Because weight gain is an issue for all AIDS patients on antiretroviral therapy, nutritionists advise patients to cut fat and calories, but not to eliminate the good fats, such as monounsaturated fats [found in olive and avocado oils] and omega-3 polyunsaturated fats [found in fatty fish such as salmon and mackerel].

Because AIDS-related illnesses can cause loss of lean body mass and wasting, people with AIDS need to consume more protein. It is also important to maintain calcium in the diet for bone health, blood clotting, nerve transmission, and regulation of heartbeat. Carbohydrates [as in fruit and whole grains] round out the healthy diet by lowering cholesterol, lowering glucose absorption, alleviating constipation, and facilitating movement through the bowel. It is also important to prepare food safely [for example, no deep frying or charcoal grilling], and to know the source of any drinking water.

Source: *The Body Positive* 1998;11(9):24-27,30-31.

HIV & AIDS: NATURAL REMEDIES & SUPPLEMENTS

643. LACTOFERRIN SUPPRESSES HIV-1

If you are HIV+, you should know that a supplement known as lactoferrin (a protein component of milk) can help to suppress HIV-1 infection. Lactoferrin interferes with the replication of HIV-1 in a dose-dependent manner [so the more you take, the greater your protection]. Lactoferrin enhances the manufacture and transmission of a substance that suppresses HIV-1 infection, and may have implications for other interactions between the human body and the HIV virus.

Lactoferrin as a supplement is perfectly safe, stable in powder or capsule form, and is effective against a number of microbes, including HIV and bacteria. Both recombinant [genetically manipulated] human and bovine lactoferrin prove to be equally effective.

Source: *Journal of Immunology* 2001;166:4231-4236.

644. ANTIOXIDANTS AGAINST HIV

Large doses of antioxidants, particularly vitamin E, may be protective against the HIV virus. The role of nutrition in the management of HIV infection and AIDS is now widely recognized, and a healthy immune system may account for the lack of HIV-1 infection in some highly exposed men. Supplemental antioxidants can improve the health of those infected with HIV, but doses well above recommended daily amounts are needed to achieve "normal" blood levels.

Vitamin E is of particular interest because its antioxidant action inhibits the activity of a protein that the virus needs in order to reproduce. (The amount of vitamin E recommended is 800 milligrams daily.) This vitamin also destroys free radicals, which are increased in HIV-infected people and can stimulate HIV replication. The use of vitamin E supplements may enhance the therapeutic effects of anti-viral treatment. It may also help restore higher levels of immune cells and red blood cells, possibly because the vitamin helps protect the membranes of red blood cells from free radical damage. In addition, deficiencies of vitamins A, B6, B12, riboflavin, zinc, and copper may be linked to HIV progression. Glutathione and glutamine supplementation may also improve immunity.

Sources: *Clinical Chemistry & Laboratory Medicine* 2002;40:456-459; *AIDS Research & Human Retrovirus* 2002;18:1051-1065; *European Journal of Immunology* 2002;32(10):2711-2720; *European Journal of Medical Research* 2000;5(6):263-267; *HIV Hotline* 1998;8(2):11-12.

WANT TO KNOW MORE?
See Hint #651 for information about a successful study on AIDS patients using aged garlic extract.

IMMUNE SYSTEM DYSFUNCTION (NON-HIV)

IMMUNE SYSTEM DYSFUNCTION: CAUSES & PRECURSORS

645. LACK OF SLEEP = WEAKENED IMMUNITY

Sleep deprivation can mean more than just drowsiness in the morning – it can also lead to a weakened immune system that is more susceptible to illness. Chronic partial sleep loss (as experienced by millions of Americans today) has an adverse effect on immune function, even making you more prone to colds and other illnesses.

Sleep deprivation may actually lower your immune response. It can elevate stress hormones and reduce your circulating thyroid hormones without giving your body the message to produce more. It affects your subsequent response to stress, and also affects body temperature. In fact, it is believed that chronic sleep deprivation may have many as yet unknown health consequences.

Physical signs of sleep deprivation are dark rings under the eye and muscle stiffness in the shoulders. (These signs, by the way, are present in a large number of children who are excessive video-game players.)

Sources: *Journal of the American Medical Association* 2002;288;1471-1472; *Journal of Neurophysiology* 2002;88(2):1073-1076; *American Journal of Physiology & Endocrinology Metabolism* 2002;283(1):E85-93.

WANT TO KNOW MORE?
[Coffee can wreak havoc with sleep patterns, and not just because caffeine is a stimulant. To learn more, see Hint #933 in the *Sleep Disorders & Deprivation* section.]

646. SOY HORMONE MAY HARM IMMUNE SYSTEM

A natural component of soy may actually be harmful to your immune health. Genistein is a phytoestrogen [a plant estrogen] found in soy-based infant formulas and also used by adults in supplemental form. When given to test animals, genistein reduces the weight of the thymus gland by up to 80 percent. [The thymus is an organ that plays an important role in the production of immune cells.] In addition, genistein also reduces other important immune cells, all of which can lead to impaired immune function.

Estrogens are known to decrease the size of the thymus and interfere with immune function if given in high levels, but this is the first time that a phytoestrogen has been shown to do this.

There is now a concern that genistein may have harmful effects in humans. [This is in accordance with my view that active isolated substances extracted from foods are not usually in your best health interest. Whole food-type supplements are a better way to go.]

Source: Proceedings of the National Academy of Science 2002;99:7616-7621.

IMMUNE SYSTEM DYSFUNCTION: NATURAL REMEDIES & SUPPLEMENTS

647. VITAMIN B6 FOR BETTER IMMUNITY

Supplementing with vitamin B6 increases the production of important immune cells in your body, strengthening your immune system. In American women aged 20 to 40, the average vitamin B6 intake is only 1.3 to 1.6 milligrams a day. But women who consume 2.1 milligrams of vitamin B6 daily show a 35 percent improvement in immune cell proliferation after just seven days. (The form of vitamin B6 that does the job is known as PLP, or pyridoxal 5'-phosphate.)

[B6 is found in brewer's yeast, liver, cabbage, eggs, peas, walnuts, and whole grains. Heating destroys its bioavailability, and also affects the quality of this vitamin.]

Source: *Journal of Nutrition* 2002;132:3308-3313.

648. VITAMIN C STRENGTHENS IMMUNITY

Increasing your intake of vitamin C can help to strengthen your immune system. Vitamin C increases glutathione (a powerful antioxidant) in immune cells, thereby increasing your immune power and disease protection. In a four-year study of more than 30,000 men and women, the risk of mortality due to all causes was about one-half among those who had the highest blood concentrations of vitamin C.

Ascorbate (vitamin C) and glutathione play key roles in the defense against free radicals and oxidants implicated in many chronic diseases. Supplementing with 500 to 1,000 milligrams of vitamin C daily for 13 weeks increases both ascorbate and glutathione in immune cells. Ascorbate and glutathione appear to mutually protect each other, perhaps because of overlapping antioxidant functions.

Source: *American Journal of Clinical Nutrition* 2003;77(1):189-195.

WANT TO KNOW MORE?
Diseases that have been associated with mild vitamin C deficiency include cardiovascular diseases, cancer, and cataracts. Most studies of vitamin C and cancer point to an inverse association (that is, the lower the vitamin C levels, the higher the cancer risk) – particularly for cancer of the oral cavity, pharynx, esophagus, stomach, colon, and lungs.

649. VITAMIN E FOR A STRONGER IMMUNE SYSTEM

Vitamin E supplementation protects immune cells against oxidative stress, thereby strengthening your immune system. Vitamin E is not only an efficient antioxidant, but it is also a modulator of the immune system. This vitamin is necessary for T-helper cell proliferation. (T-cells are the cells that you produce in response to foreign invaders attempting to take up residence in your body.)

[It is no wonder so many people are immune-deficient. Vitamin E is essential for the production of immune-protective cells, yet we hardly get any of this nutrient in today's diet.

Some sources of vitamin E are butter, egg yolks, and liver.

Tocotrienols, a superior form of vitamin E, are natural compounds found in various foods and oils such as palm oil, rice bran oil, wheat germ, barley, saw palmetto, and certain types of nuts and grains.]

Source: *Journal of Nutrition* **2000;130:2932-2937.**

650. PROBIOTICS FOR IMMUNE ENHANCEMENT

Consuming specific strains of "friendly" bacteria can help to enhance your immune system as you age. [Probiotics are food supplements that promote the growth and proliferation of healthful bacteria in your body, such as the Lactobacillus acidophilus found in viable, cultured yogurt. Other strains of friendly bacteria are also finally being recognized as having special immune benefits.]

Bifidobacterium lactis is a safe and effective probiotic supplement for enhancing immunity. After consuming *Bifidobacterium* for nine weeks, there is a *significant* increase in the proportion of important immune-protective cells.

As is so often the case, the greatest improvements in immunity are seen in those who have poor immune response before treatment.

Source: *American Journal of Clinical Nutrition* **2001;74(6):833-839;** *Journal of Nutrition* **1999;129:1492S-1495S.**

651. AGED GARLIC EXTRACT AND IMMUNITY

Aged garlic extract has been shown to lessen infectious diseases through enhancement of the immune system. It has been found to do this by having a beneficial effect on:

~ killer cell activity
~ immune macrophages (large protective immune cells)
~ T-lymphocyte activity (white blood cells that coordinate the immune system)
~ natural killer cell activity (cells that go after toxins)
~ production of protective antibodies

It has also demonstrated antiviral and antifungal activities and has been shown to modify, both directly and indirectly, the function of immune cells – particularly those that play a leading role in allergic cascade reactions including inflammation. Aged garlic extract has also been shown to improve age-related deterioration of the immune response.

In test animals, aged garlic extract stimulated an increase in spleen cells.It doubled the ability of natural killer cells to destroy a particular cancer cell line.

In one study with AIDS patients, *remarkable* results were seen after six weeks. Natural killer cell activity was within normal range for all subjects. Many patients noted improvements in diarrhea, candidiasis [thrush], and interruption of recurrent cycles of genital herpes.

Sources: *Onkolgie* **1989;21:52-53;** *Phytomedicine* **1998;5(4):259-267;** *Molecular Biotherapy* **1991;3:103-107.**

IMMUNE SYSTEM DYSFUNCTION: REDUCING RISK

652. WEAK IMMUNITY? AVOID PREPARED SHRIMP!

Ready-to-eat shrimp can contain antibiotic-resistant bacteria, and should be avoided by anyone with a weak immune system. Researchers recovered bacteria from all shrimp samples tested, and 42 percent of the strains were found to be resistant to antibiotics. It is suspected that the bacteria come from both the water in which the shrimp grow, as well as contamination during packaging.

While these bacteria do not pose a danger to healthy people, those with weakened immune systems should stay away from such prepared food. [That would include anyone with a degenerative disease such as diabetes or heart problems, as well as those who are older.]

Source: Annual Meeting of the American Society for Microbiology, May 2002.

INCONTINENCE

Large numbers of perimenopausal women experience urinary incontinence with 25 percent wearing protection or changing undergarments on several days per week. Mutable factors predicting severity include body mass index and current smoking. (*Obstetrics & Gynecology* **2002;100(6):1230-8**)

The average age of those with an overactive bladder is 64. (*Journal of Urology* **2003;169:529-534**) At least 50 percent of nursing home residents in Britain and North America suffer from urinary incontinence. It is associated with resident and staff morbidity. In these cases, behavioral strategies are more likely to be beneficial than drug treatment. (*Age Ageing* **2003;32(1):12-18**)

653. LESS WEIGHT = LESS INCONTINENCE

To help solve a problem with urinary incontinence, consider starting an exercise program to lose weight. People who are overweight are at risk for incontinence, but a successful weight loss program (including exercise) can be very effective in alleviating this embarrassing problem. Women suffering from urinary incontinence who lose weight have fewer episodes of urine loss, even 9 months after having lost the weight.

Weekly episodes of incontinence can be as reduced by as much as 50 to 60 percent!

Source: 23rd Annual Meeting of the American Urogynecologic Society, San Francisco, CA, Oct 2002.

WANT TO KNOW MORE?
[To learn how doing simple "kegel" exercises can help to improve urinary incontinence, see Hint #26 in the *Aging* section.]

654. NUTRITION & INCONTINENCE

Fecal incontinent subjects may improve their nutritional patterns by lowering sodium and protein intake and increasing dietary fiber and monounsaturated fat intake. Calcium and vitamin D supplementation may improve dietary deficiencies and lower disease risks. Diets are generally similar to those with normal bowel function.

Improved oral care also has its effect on incontinence.

Source: *Journal of Wound Ostomy Continence in Nursing* 2000;27(2):90-1, 93-7; 1997;24(2):79-85.

KIDNEY DISEASES & CONDITIONS

Chronic kidney disease is a major public health problem that has been insufficiently studied. There is little published information on outcomes among chronic kidney disease patients, specifically, data on quality of life. (*Seminars In Dialysis* 2002;15(5):366-9) The high prevalence of cardiovascular disease in those with kidney disease is well described.

Low protein diets are known to slow the decline in renal function. Albeit controversial, evidence also suggests that dietary protein restriction can slow the rate of progression of renal failure. But when low-protein diets are prescribed, patients should be closely monitored to assess dietary compliance and to ensure nutritional adequacy. (*American Journal of Clinical Nutrition* 2001;20(4):291-9) Needless to say, the protein that is consumed should be of high biologic value. (*American Journal of Kidney Diseases* 2001;37(1 Suppl 2):S66-70)

IN THIS SECTION:
- KIDNEY STONES
- NATURAL REMEDIES & SUPPLEMENTS

- REDUCING RISK

KIDNEY DISEASE & CONDITIONS: KIDNEY STONES

655. FLUIDS REDUCE KIDNEY STONE RISK

Protect yourself from painful kidney stones by making sure to drink enough fluids (preferably water) daily. Those who drink about two quarts of fluid daily have a 38 percent lower risk of developing kidney stones than those who drink less than one quart daily.

What you drink is as important as how much liquid you consume. Grapefruit juice increases the risk, while both coffee and tea decrease it. Cola drinks are implicated as a possible kidney stone culprit in men. The safest liquid? Filtered or bottled pure water!

Risk for stone formation decreases by the following amount for each eight-ounce serving consumed daily: 10 percent for caffeinated coffee, nine percent for decaffeinated coffee, and eight percent for tea. In contrast, a 44 percent increase in risk is seen for each serving of grapefruit juice consumed daily.

Source: *Annals of Internal Medicine* 1998;128(7):534-40.

WANT TO KNOW MORE?
[Concentrated cranberry supplements (but not cranberry juice) have also been implicated in kidney stone formation in some susceptible women. See Hint #994 in the *Urinary Tract Infection* section.]

656. KIDNEY STONES: DIETARY PROTECTION

The most important dietary actions for protection from kidney stones: increase intake of fluids and leafy greens, reduce intake of refined sugar, and supplement with soluble rice bran. In addition, large doses of vitamin B6 may reduce the risk of kidney stone formation in women, although there is no association between ascorbic acid (vitamin C) levels and the prevalence of kidney stones in either women or men.

High intake of dietary calcium appears to decrease risk, whereas intake of supplemental calcium may *increase* risk.

Kidney stone formation may be a bacterial disease, similar to the relationship seen between *H. pylori* infection and peptic ulcer disease. Both diseases are initiated by bacterial infection, and dietary factors influence their progression. Improving your diet can therefore be an important protective measure.

Sources: *Alternative Medicine: The Definitive Guide*, **2nd ed, (Berkeley, CA: Celestial Arts, 2002), p. 1038;** *Kidney International* **1999;56(5):1893-1898;** *Journal of Hypertension* **1999;17(7):1017-1022;** *Journal of the American Society of Nephrology* **1999;10(4):840-845;** *Archives of Internal Medicine* **1999;159(6):619-624;** *Annals of Internal Medicine* **1997;126(7):497-504.**

WANT TO KNOW MORE?
Hypertension in middle-aged men is a significant predictor of kidney stone disease.

KIDNEY DISEASES & CONDITIONS: NATURAL REMEDIES & SUPPLEMENTS

657. VITAMIN E & IMPROVED KIDNEY FUNCTION

Kidney function appears to be improved with vitamin E supplementation. Many studies show that vitamin E decreases lipid peroxidation [causing those nasty free radical problems], platelet aggregation [the clumping together of cells], and functions as a potent anti-inflammatory agent. Now we can add improved kidney function to the list of benefits.

[Some dietary sources of vitamin E are butter, egg yolks, and liver. Tocotrienols, a superior form of vitamin E, are natural compounds found in various foods and oils such as palm oil, rice bran oil, wheat germ, barley, saw palmetto, and certain types of nuts and grains.]

2001; Sources: *Journal of Nutrition* **2001;131:1297-130;** *Current Opinions in Lipidology.*

WANT TO KNOW MORE?
Some of the reasons for our rampant vitamin E deficiency:
> ~ ordinary cooking removes most of the vitamin E content of whole foods
> ~ our consumption of fried foods
> ~ the chlorine in tap water
> ~ the use of estrogen hormone therapy.

658. FLAXSEED CAN IMPROVE KIDNEY DISEASE

Consuming phytoestrogens like those found in flaxseed appears to have a beneficial role in chronic kidney disease. Phytoestrogens are naturally occurring plant compounds that are present in flaxseed and have an estrogen-like effect without any harmful side effects.

Flaxseed lessens structural damage in those with various forms of kidney disease.

It remains unclear which component of flaxseed is responsible for its protective effects, but vegetable protein in general has been shown to have a beneficial effect on kidney disease in both humans and animals.

[Because flaxseed oil turns rancid quickly, I recommend purchasing whole flaxseed and grinding it as needed. A small, inexpensive coffee grinder works well. Ground flaxseed has a light, nutty flavor and can be sprinkled over salads or cereal.]

Source: *Journal of Renal Nutrition* **2001;11(4):PAGE.**

KIDNEY DISEASES & CONDITIONS: REDUCING RISK

659. EXERCISE RISK OF KIDNEY DISEASE AWAY

Being physically active is the single most important preventive measure you can take against chronic kidney disease. In one group of adults (aged 30 to 74) studied, those with low physical activity had a 2.2-fold greater risk of developing chronic renal disease when compared to those with high physical activity. This increased risk was not explained by diabetes, blood pressure, or serum cholesterol.

Although smoking and obesity are also risk factors, they are not nearly as significant as a lack of exercise.

Source: 33rd Annual Meeting of the American Society of Nephrology, Toronto, Ontario, Oct 2000.

LACTOSE INTOLERANCE

Lactose intolerance, a congenital condition suffered by people throughout the world, is caused by an enzyme deficiency resulting in an inability to digest and absorb lactose, a protein commonly found in dairy foods.

Symptoms of lactose intolerance can include bloating, abdominal pain, flatulence, and diarrhea following the consumption of lactose-containing foods.

Although cow's milk *allergy* and cow's milk *intolerance* are two different terms, they are often used interchangeably, resulting in confusion. Cow's milk allergy is an immune reaction to cow-milk proteins. Its prevalence is probably one to three percent, being highest in infants and lowest in adults. Cow's milk intolerance does not involve an immune response. It is linked to race, being highest in dark-skinned populations and lowest in northern Europeans. (In fact, about two thirds of the world's adult population has some form of the condition.)

While milk allergy is often outgrown, lactase deficiency lasts a lifetime.

Sources: *Annals of Allergy & Asthma Immunology* **2002;89(6Suppl1):56-60;** *Journal of the American College of Nutrition* **2000;19:165S-175S.**

660. PROBIOTICS FOR LACTOSE INTOLERANCE

If you are lactose intolerant, consuming probiotic bacteria may be helpful. Lactose intolerance can be relieved with the ingestion of the so-called "friendly" probiotic strains of Lactobacillus, Bifidobacterium, and Streptococcus bacteria. The addition of these bacteria is helpful for two reasons: One is that when added to dairy foods, they reduce the lactose content by promoting fermentation. In addition, the probiotics increase in your gastrointestinal tract, thereby releasing lactase [the enzyme needed to break down lactose]. It is the deficiency of lactase that is causing the problem to begin with!

Newest research shows that symptoms of lactose intolerance – bloating, abdominal pain, and diarrhea – are caused by how your body processes the maldigested lactose in your colon.

Sources: *European Journal of Clinical Investigation* **2003;33(1):70-75;** *Journal of Nutrition* **2000;130:396S-402S;** *Annals of Italian Internal Medicine* **2002;17(3):157-165.**

WANT TO KNOW MORE?
Probiotics can also protect you from pathogens, so they are useful in the prevention of antibiotic-induced and traveler's diarrhea, and may play a role in the management of *H. Pylori* infection [ulcers]. Their efficacy in inflammatory bowel diseases and in food allergy has also been shown. Probiotics may even play a role in the prevention of cancer and of tumor growth.

661. LACTOSE INTOLERANT? TRY YOGURT INSTEAD

Problems digesting dairy products? Even if you are lactose intolerant, you don't necessarily need to avoid yogurt. Those deficient in the enzyme lactase generally tolerate lactose better from yogurt than from milk. The contribution of lactase by the bacterial cultures in the yogurt is thought to enhance lactose digestion. In addition, the slower gastric emptying of yogurt compared with milk may also play a role.

Good results are more dependent on the *quantity* of the "friendly" bacteria in the yogurt, rather than the particular strain of bacteria.

(Important note: Keep in mind that, like so many other enzymes, total intestinal lactase activity decreases with age.)

Source: Journal of Nutrition 1997;127(7):1382-1387; 2000;130:384S-390S.

WANT TO KNOW MORE?
In the US, yogurt is not required to contain any viable cultures. An industry group, the National Yogurt Association, allows yogurt manufacturers use of its "Live Active Culture Seal" on products that contain 10^8 viable cultures per gram at time of manufacture. However, no distinction is made between yogurt starter cultures used primarily for acid production (*S. thermophilus* and *L. delbreuckii bulgaricus*) and probiotic species (*L. acidophilus, L. casei, L. reuteri, Bifidobacterium* species, among others). Therefore, this seal is of little value in assuring consumers of effective probiotic levels. Probiotic-containing dietary supplements frequently indicate a viable count per dose contained in the product at time of manufacture, not at the end of shelf life.

662. DO'S AND DON'TS OF LACTOSE INTOLERANCE

One of the main reasons to avoid foods with lactose is because they are almost always highly processed. Milk products, cheese, creams – are usually in that high-tech, over-processed category. Here are some additional facts: Lactose intolerance is increased in those with irritable bowel syndrome; lactase enzyme supplements may be helpful; most with lactose intolerance can ingest up to 12 ounces of milk daily without symptoms; those with lactose intolerance must ensure adequate calcium intake; some persons with normal lactase activity may become symptomatic on consumption of products containing lactose; lactose maldigestion may coexist in children with recurrent abdominal pain; a few individuals with severe lactose intolerance may have a large number of vertebral fractures; the best management of lactose intolerance consists primarily of dietary changes.

Sources: Journal of Gastroenterology 2002;37:1014-9; Postgraduate Medicine 1998;104(3):109-11,115-6,122-3; Comprehensive Therapy 2000;26(4):246-50; Tropical Gastroenterology 2001;22(4):202-4; American Family Physician 2002;65(9):1845-50.

LIVER DISEASE & CIRRHOSIS

Chronic liver disease is the 10th leading cause of death in the US, and hepatitis C virus infection is the most frequent cause of it. Patients with hepatitis C infection should also be careful to abstain from alcohol.

The three most widely recognized forms of alcoholic liver disease are:
> ~ *alcoholic fatty liver* (steatosis)
> ~ *acute alcoholic hepatitis*
> ~ *alcoholic cirrhosis.*

The exact ways in which alcohol abuse leads to cirrhosis are still not fully understood, but the immune system and free radical injury are both thought to play a large role. Abstinence from alcohol is the most important aspect of treatment.

IN THIS SECTION:
- CAUSES & PRECURSORS
- NATURAL REMEDIES & SUPPLEMENTS

LIVER DISEASE: CAUSES & PRECURSORS
663 . LIVER DISEASE, ALCOHOL, & HEPATITIS C

Vitamin supplements and good nutrition are vital to help combat liver disease, as malnutrition is a frequent complication of cirrhosis, but improved nutritional habits can help. Alcohol consumption is one of the major causes of liver cirrhosis in the Western world.

Alcohol is the most commonly abused substance in the US, and alcohol abuse leads to alcoholic liver disease, a long recognized major public health concern. The high prevalence of chronic hepatitis C virus (HCV) infection, along with the clinical observation that HCV infection is common in alcoholic patients presenting with liver disease, has directed attention to the interaction between alcohol and HCV infection.

The prevalence of liver diseases is increasing in the United States, particularly as a result of the recent hepatitis C epidemic.

Sources: *Journal of Gastroenterology & Hepatology* 2002;17(4):462-466; *Nutrition Reviews* Aug 2000;58(8):242-247; *Postgraduate Medical Journal* 2000;76(895):280-286; *Journal of the American College of Nutrition* 1999;18(5):434-441; *Metabolism* 1998;47(7):792-798.

LIVER DISEASE: NATURAL REMEDIES & SUPPLEMENTS

664. MILK THISTLE AGAINST LIVER DISEASE

Those suffering from chronic liver disease should supplement with the herb milk thistle, which protects both the liver and kidneys from toxins and pollutants, as well as stimulates the production of new liver cells. Because many herbal remedies can in fact be toxic to the liver, milk thistle [also known as wild artichoke], proves to be the only herb that those with chronic liver disease can safely use. In addition to milk thistle, weight loss and exercise can also improve liver function in those with fatty liver [*steatosis*].

Source: *American Family Physician* 2001;64(9):1555-1560.

665. PC & OMEGA-3s AGAINST LIVER DISEASE

If you are suffering from liver disease, supplementing with both phosphatidyl choline and omega-3 fatty acids may be helpful. Phosphatidyl choline [a component of lecithin, also known as PC] is helpful in preventing numerous health conditions, including liver problems. [Lecithin can be found in eggs, brewer's yeast, fish, legumes, wheat germ, and grains.]

Omega-3 fatty acids have anti-inflammatory effects, and as a dietary supplement are beneficial for those with chronic liver disease who are susceptible to fibrosis. [Good dietary sources of omega-3 fatty acids are fatty fish, fish oil, and vegetable oils such as canola, flaxseed, and walnut.] Salmon roe also proves to be especially beneficial.

Source: *Current Medical Research Opinion* 1999;15(3):177-184.

666. VITAMIN E FOR CIRRHOSIS

If you have cirrhosis of the liver, start supplementing with vitamin E. Supplementing with vitamin E may help reduce both lipid peroxidation and the formation of blood clots. (Lipid peroxidation is usually the result of free radicals, which damages the cells.)

[Some good dietary sources of vitamin E are grains, nuts, and egg yolk. Tocotrienols, a superior form of vitamin E, are natural compounds found in various foods and oils such as palm oil, rice bran oil, wheat germ, barley, saw palmetto, and certain types of nuts and grains.]

Source: *Blood* May 1999;93(9):2945-2950.

667. PROBIOTICS FOR FATTY LIVER

If you have a nonalcoholic fatty liver disease, you no doubt have developed intestinal bacterial overgrowth, so consumption of probiotics is advised. The probiotics will help to modify the intestinal flora.

Sources: *Current Gastroenterology Report* **2003;5(1):86-92;** *Hepatology* **2003;37(2):86-92.**

668. ZINC IS BENEFICIAL FOR CIRRHOSIS

If you are suffering from cirrhosis of the liver, supplementing with zinc can help to relieve a host of health problems.

Zinc deficiency is common in those with cirrhosis, and this deficiency can affect glucose metabolism. But long-term zinc treatment in patients with advanced cirrhosis improves glucose intolerance, thereby helping to prevent cirrhosis-related diabetes.

Cirrhosis can also cause muscle cramps, which, while not life threatening, can severely affect the quality of life in those suffering from them. Zinc supplementation can also help improve these muscle cramps and may even completely resolve the problem.

[Some good dietary sources of zinc include brewer's yeast, egg yolks, seafood, poultry, legumes, liver, soybeans, and whole grains.]

Source: *Journal of the American College of Nutrition* **2000;19(1):13-15.**

WANT TO KNOW MORE?
[One of the reasons liver disease is so serious is because all the nutrients coming from your intestinal tract, with minor exceptions, go to your liver, where they are processed before they are released into your bloodstream. Your liver also filters out wastes and toxins. It is critical for your liver to be functioning at its optimum.

The treatment of liver disease requires a major shift in eating habits. Every time you consume trans fatty acids, processed foods, or fatty meats, you are abusing your liver because it must work harder to detoxify the junk you are forcing it to deal with. Only a diet of natural, whole foods – preferably vegetarian – can help to mend a sick liver.

Beans, peas, potatoes, and tofu are good vegetable sources of protein. Supplemental enzymes and fiber can help liver detoxification. Apples and rolled oats are particularly beneficial for your liver because they stimulate bile secretion. Sulphur-containing foods like eggs, turnips, onions, and garlic also have a cleansing effect on the liver.]

LUPUS

Systemic lupus erythematosus (SLE) is a serious autoimmune disorder, affecting many body systems, and without a known cure. This autoimmune disease is characterized by high levels of inflammatory cells produced by your own body. Conventional medicine typically approaches the disease with a treatment plan that includes the use of corticosteroids, non-steroidal anti-inflammatory drugs (NSAIDs), antimalarial drugs, and chemotherapeutic agents. The results vary and safety is questionable. this is one disorder that has compelled the traditional medical community to look at alternative therapies for help.

The rate of lupus is higher in people of west African descent than in Europeans.

669. NUTRITIONAL TACTICS FOR LUPUS

The use of vitamins, minerals, and fatty acids have been shown to have an impact on the activity of lupus. Alternative treatments may include Chinese medicines, such as Tripterygium wiifordii Hook F (TwHF), have also gained interest recently.

There have been a number of clinical trials assessing the benefits of dietary supplementation with fish oils in autoimmune diseases, including lupus. The results reveal significant benefit, including decreased disease activity.

Sources: *Alternative Medicine Review* 2001;6(5):460-71; *Journal of the American College of Nutrition* 2002;21(6):495-505

670. MORE NUTRITIONAL TACTICS FOR LUPUS

Making certain specific changes to your diet and supplement regimen may help to relieve symptoms of Lupus. Factors that aggravate Lupus include excess calories, excess protein, high fat (especially saturated and omega-6 polyunsaturated fatty acids), zinc, and iron, whereas beneficial compounds include vitamin E, A, selenium, fish oils, flaxseed, and DHA.

In addition to the factors stated above, L-canavanine found in alfalfa tablets has a negative effect (but fresh alfalfa sprouts do not). Some people placed on food allergy elimination diets report an improvement in Lupus symptoms. Others report that bromelain [an enzyme extracted from pineapple] or a vegetarian diet that includes fish is beneficial.

Source: *Journal of Renal Nutrition* 2000;10(4):170-83.

[An autoimmune disease relates to a disease caused by an immune reponse by the body against one of its own tissues, cells, or molecules.]

MALE SEXUAL PROBLEMS

Male sexuality is affected by normal physiologic aging changes. These problems may be vascular, and they may also be influenced by medications, neurologic conditions, or any other metabolic functions. Penile sensitivity and erectile responses may be altered as part of those changes, and men may have concerns about ejaculatory disorders and erectile dysfunction. It took the promotion of the drug Viagra to emphasize the extent of the problem American men were having with sexual dysfunction. (*Geriatrics* **1997 ;52(9):76-8, 84-6)**

The high frequency of self-reported sexual disorders and the hesitancy of family physicians to deal with this topic signals a neglected area in primary health care. (*Journal of Family Practice* **2001 ;50(9):773-8)**

IN THIS SECTION:
- ERECTILE DYSFUNCTION & VIAGRA
- MALE HORMONE SWINGS
- NATURAL REMEDIES & SUPPLEMENTS
- PENILE DERMATOSES
- PROSTATITIS
- SPERM VIABILITY

MALE SEXUAL PROBLEMS: ERECTILE DYSFUNCTION & VIAGRA

671. ERECTILE DYSFUNCTION COULD MEAN WORSE

Men with erectile dysfunction could be at risk for more serious health problems, such as cardiovascular disease. Erectile dysfunction very commonly signals more extensive vascular disease, and so the use of a drug that allows a man with erectile dysfunction to suddenly perform vigorous exercise (in the form of sexual intercourse) could have an adverse effect on his cardiac status.

Cardiologists and other physicians are now seeing men with erectile dysfunction who may not demonstrate any overt symptoms, but who are actually at high risk for heart disease. It is believed that if there is vascular disease in one area, then there is a much higher risk of vascular disease in other areas.

Source: 72nd Scientific Sessions of the American Heart Association.

WANT TO KNOW MORE?
[There are safer alternatives to drugs such as Viagra. The natural supplement velvet antler, for example, has been known for millennia to relieve erectile dysfunction without any side effects. For more information, see my book, *The Remarkable Healing Power of Velvet Antler*. There are also topical creams available containing small amounts of herbs that work synergistically, used by Asians for centuries. These are described in *She's Gotta Have It!*]

672. IMPOTENCY & UNDIAGNOSED DIABETES

If you are a man with erectile dysfunction, get tested for diabetes. Men with erectile dysfunction are more likely than men who are not impotent to have undiagnosed diabetes, and these men should therefore be screened for the disease. Fasting blood glucose testing should be the standard test to screen for diabetes in men with erectile dysfunction. (Urine glucose measurement is a very insensitive and unreliable test for diabetes, and it fails to diagnose four out of five men with the disease).

If impotent men are not properly screened for diabetes, the disease could remain undiagnosed for several years.

Source: *British Journal of Urology* 2001;88:68-71.

673. VIAGRA & THE RISK OF HEART ATTACKS

If you are a man with erectile dysfunction taking the drug sildenafil (Viagra), you could be at risk for a heart attack. As mentioned in Hint #671, erectile dysfunction is often a symptom of underlying cardiovascular disease, which means that many men taking Viagra may be at very serious risk for death from a cardiovascular event.

The German Health Ministry reports that 616 people worldwide have died after using Viagra, and according to the Swedish Drug Monitoring Center, there may not be adequate systems to prevent unnecessary harm from globally marketed drugs.

Sources: Swedish-based Uppsala Monitoring Center, Sep 2001; German Institute for Pharmaceutical and Medical Products; *Herz* Aug 2001;26(5):353-359.

WANT TO KNOW MORE?
According to the Massachusetts Male Aging Study, the prevalence of erectile dysfunction in 40-year-old men is 39 percent, while in 69-year-old men it is as high as 67 percent.

674. DOES VIAGRA LEAD TO VIOLENT BEHAVIOR?

The drug sildenafil (Viagra) is now associated with instances of aggressive behavior and sexual violence (although this conclusion is being debated). More than 270 reports collected and archived by the US Food and Drug Administration detail psychological side effects with Viagra use, including dizziness, disorientation, and amnesia.

The drug is also listed as a suspect in 22 reports involving aggression, 13 involving rape, and 6 involving murder. (An Israeli court mentioned in a 1999 ruling against a rapist that the drug had played a role in the attack.)

The FDA overview has a lot of information that hasn't been pulled together in one place before. Among those contesting the aggressive behavior conclusion is Pfizer, the manufacturer of Viagra. Adverse-event reports are often used as a way to flag side effects in the general population that may have been missed during clinical studies.

Effects that fail to show up in several thousand test subjects have a better chance of being noticed when millions of people are taking a drug.

Source: *Reuter's Medical Health Report*, Washington, DC, Dec 2002.

675. VIAGRA & HEAVY NOSEBLEED DANGER

Those taking sildenafil [Viagra], be warned: This drug has required hospitalization to treat prolonged, heavy nosebleeds in some men. One man in his late 50s who took a standard 50-mg dose of sildenafil to boost his sexual performance required hospitalization for six days. He had suffered several short-lived but heavy nosebleeds for a few days after taking the medication, and on the day of admission bleeding had continued for six hours without stopping.

Another case involved a man in his 70s who was admitted to the emergency room after five hours of nosebleeds after taking sildenafil in the morning. Both men had high blood pressure.

It was surmised that the drug led to engorgement of certain nasal tissues. ("Honeymoon rhinitis," in which both men and women can experience nasal stuffiness during sexual intercourse, is listed as a possible side effect of Viagra.)

Source: *Journal of the Royal Society of Medicine* 2002;95:402-403.

676. WHEN VIAGRA FAILS...

n men in whom sildenafil (Viagra) fails, arterial insufficiency is often the cause — so it's time to check things out under these circumstances. Researchers found that men with arterial insufficiency comprised the largest group of Viagra failures (54 percent). Those with mixed vascular insufficiency made up 22 percent of the group and 24 percent were diagnosed with venous leak.

Other possible causes for Viagra failure:
~ taking the drug with a high-fat meal
~ taking the drug without any sexual stimulation.

Source: **Society for the Study of Impotence, as reported in** *Reuter's* **Sep 2000.**

677. VIAGRA LESS EFFECTIVE OVER TIME

Because the efficacy of Viagra is reduced or lost over time, men should instead consider more natural substances [such as velvet antler] to increase their libido. Those who initially respond to Viagra may begin responding to it less, or even stop responding completely. Forty-three patients interviewed reported their need to increase the dosage by 50 mg to achieve the desired results. This loss of the treatment's efficacy had taken between one to 18 months, and there was no relationship between the need to increase the dose and the frequency of use. (Among the reasons cited for discontinuing Viagra: lack of efficacy and the drug's side effects.)

Source: *Journal of Urology* 2001;166:927-931.

678. NO GRAPEFRUIT JUICE WITH VIAGRA

If you are taking Viagra to treat erectile dysfunction, avoid drinking grapefruit juice at the same time. Consumption of grapefruit juice along with the use of the drug sildenafil (Viagra), although not dangerous, is not advisable because grapefruit juice tends to delay the absorption of the drug. Oral bioavailability of Viagra reaches only 40 percent, but when taken with grapefruit juice, the absorption becomes less predictable.

In one study, volunteers received single 50-mg doses of Viagra. Two 250-ml doses of either grapefruit juice or water were administered one hour before and together with the drug. In those who were given the grapefruit juice, a prolonged time to reach blood concentration of the drug was observed.

Source: *Clinical & Pharmacological Therapy* 2002;71(1):21-29.

MALE SEXUAL PROBLEMS: MALE HORMONE SWINGS

679. MEN CAN HAVE HORMONE SWINGS TOO!

Hormone swings don't discriminate – men can also have hormone variations that can affect their mood and behavior. It's even called Irritable Male Syndrome, initiated by lowered testosterone levels. But here's a major difference: It can affect men at any age. It happens when stress causes reductions in testosterone. The symptoms may resemble those of the so-called "male menopause." Among the stresses that can have this effect are bereavement, divorce, or life-threatening illness. So does this mean Hormone Replacement Therapy for men? No! As with women, HRT is equally dangerous for men, increasing the risk of heart disease.

Source: *Reproduction, Fertility & Development* 2002;13:567.

MALE SEXUAL PROBLEMS: NATURAL REMEDIES & SUPPLEMENTS

680. "NATURAL VIAGRA": VELVET ANTLER!

Men: In place of drugs to enhance your sexual potency, why not give the natural supplement velvet antler a try? Chinese traditional medicine has long considered velvet antler to possess sexual-reinforcing and anti-aging properties. [In fact, velvet antler is sometimes referred to as "natural Viagra."]

Although there aren't many well-defined studies demonstrating the effectiveness of velvet antler in bringing back male sexual potency, personal testimonials abound.

Test animals show an increase in plasma testosterone levels when given velvet antler. The active components of antler might be effective in counteracting physiological alterations of the long-term aging process.

Sources: *Chemical & Pharmacology Bulletin* 1988;36(7):2587-2592; B. Kamen, *Everything I Know About Nutrition I Learned from Barley*.

WANT TO KNOW MORE?
[For those who want to know more about velvet antler, especially for arthritis and bone integrity (with extensive scientific research cited), see my book, *The Remarkable Healing Power of Velvet Antler*.]

681. AGED GARLIC CAN HELP LAGGING LIBIDOS

In the presence of a high protein diet, aged garlic extract supplements can increase the production of testosterone, and may help to improve low libidos (in women too!).
A specific hormone (luteinizing hormone) secreted by the pituitary gland helps to regulate testosterone production. The concentration of this hormone increases with increased garlic supplementation.

One reason why this is of interest is because testosterone production is important for sexual desire (in both men and women). In addition, this increase is needed due to the excess estrogen in our environment, which can contribute to curtailing testosterone production.

Garlic also helps bring blood to tissues, so this adds to its benefit for achieving optimum sexuality. It) can widen the blood vessels on the outer edges of your body, so those of you with cold feet or hands should be especially interested.

Sources: *Journal of Nutrition* 2001;131:2150-2156; B. Kamen, *She's Gotta Have It!*

MALE SEXUAL PROBLEMS: PENILE DERMATOSES

682. CIRCUMCISION & PENILE DERMATOSES

Circumcision protects men against common infective penile dermatoses, extending the known benefits of circumcision in protecting men against penile cancer as well as sexually transmitted diseases. The presence of the foreskin may promote inflammation due to an infectious agents. Men who have not been circumcised have a more than threefold increased risk of genital dermatoses compared with circumcised men. In addition, the majority of patients diagnosed with psoriasis, lichen planus, and seborrheic eczema are also uncircumcised.

Source: *Archives of Dermatology* 2000;136:350-354.

MALE SEXUAL PROBLEMS: PROSTATITIS

683. ONIONS & GREEN TEA FOR PROSTATITIS

A substance found in onions and green tea can *significantly* alleviate symptoms of nonbacterial chronic prostatitis [an inflammation of the prostate]. Quercetin, a bioflavonoid, is a naturally occurring substance found in high concentrations in onions and green tea. After taking 500 mg of quercetin twice daily, chronic prostatitis patients show significant improvements. In addition, when bromelain and papain are added to the quercetin, even greater improvements are seen. [Bromelain is an enzyme that comes from pineapples, while papain comes from papayas.]

Source: *Urology* 1999;54:960-963.

684. SUNLIGHT PROTECTS AGAINST PROSTATITIS

Getting adequate daily exposure to sunlight may help reduce your risk of developing chronic prostatitis-like symptoms. Of over 16,000 twenty-year-old men studied (six percent having significant chronic prostatitis-like symptoms) the average duration of sunlight exposure was inversely linked to the risk of developing prostatitis-like symptoms – that is, the longer the exposure, the less the risk. [I have long been an advocate of a half hour of sunlight daily, which can be preventive against many other diseases, including cancer, multiple sclerosis, and osteoporosis. See Hints #163, #730, and #800 for more details.]

Source: *Urology* 2001;58:853-858.

MALE SEXUAL PROBLEMS: SPERM VIABILITY

685. ZINC & FOLIC ACID INCREASE SPERM COUNT

For infertile men (and even those who are fertile), supplemental zinc sulfate and folic acid (folate) can *significantly* increase sperm count. A daily dose of folic acid (5 mg) and zinc sulfate (66 mg) increases sperm count in men with inadequate fertility by as much as 74 percent. (However, it is yet to be determined whether these improvements in sperm concentration would lead to an increase in pregnancy rates.)

Source: *Fertility & Sterility* 2002;77:491-498.

686. VITAMIN C IMPROVES SEMEN QUALITY

Ascorbic acid (vitamin C) may be helpful in improving the quality of semen. Treatment with ascorbic acid helps to increase testosterone concentrations, improve semen characteristics, and alleviate the negative effects caused by toxins (specifically, *aflatoxins*, contaminants found in peanuts, cotton seed meal, corn, and other grains).

When test animals are given two lethal doses of aflatoxins, serum testosterone is significantly reduced, and an increase is seen in the number of abnormal and dead sperm cells (in a dose-dependent manner). But ascorbic acid appears to have a beneficial influence against the negative effects of these toxins on production and reproduction.

Source: *Toxicology* 2001;162(3):209-218.

687. SPERM ANOMALIES INCREASE WITH AGE

Men in their 60s and 70s have a greater number of chromosome abnormalities in their sperm compared with men in their 20s and 30s. Comparing semen samples from men ages 59 to 74 with those of men ages 23 to 39, the older group show significantly more abnormalities in terms of chromosome number and structure.

Structural abnormalities in sperm increase once men hit their 40s and 50s. And a higher rate of such anomalies has been found in men 25 to 50 years old whose female partners have had recurrent miscarriages.

Source: *Fertility & Sterility* 2001;76:1119-1123.

MEMORY & COGNITIVE DYSFUNCTION

Cognitive vitality is essential to quality of life, but its decline is one of the greatest concerns among those approaching senior years, mainly because it is so common. It doesn't have to happen, and it can even be reversed if it has already taken hold. (Be sure to see the *Aging: Cognitive Decline* section to learn more NOW, no matter your current age. There is no question about the association between lifestyle factors and mental acuity. (***Mayo Clinic Proceedings* 2002;77(7):681-96)**

IN THIS SECTION:
- CAUSES & PRECURSORS
- NATURAL REMEDIES & SUPPLEMENTS
- REDUCING RISK

MEMORY & COGNITIVE DYSFUNCTION: CAUSES & PRECURSORS

688. HIGH-FAT, LOW-CARBS = IMPAIRED BRAINS

A high-fat, low-carbohydrate diet may impair your brain function over time. High-fat diets may hinder brain function by promoting insulin resistance. Test animals fed high-fat diets are slower in learning new tasks and perform more poorly on tests of learning and memory.

There is also evidence that carbohydrates may boost memory. In a small study of older adults, a "breakfast" of mashed potatoes or barley was found to increase participants' performance on memory tests. (Note: Needless to say, the quality of the carbohydrates is important.)

Diets lacking in carbohydrates reduce the supply of glucose, which can impede the acetylcholine synthesis, necessary for memory. (We have known about the connection between memory and choline for a long time.)

Source: *Neurobiology of Learning & Memory* 2001;75.

689. LDL CHOLESTEROL & COGNITIVE IMPAIRMENT

In addition to clogging your arteries, high cholesterol is also associated with cognitive impairment. Women with high levels of LDL ("bad-guy" cholesterol) score worse on cognitive tests and are more likely to have cognitive impairment than are women with lower LDL levels. (HDL levels and normal triglyceride levels, however, show no connection to cognitive impairment.)

So lowering these LDL lipoprotein levels may be one strategy for preventing cognitive impairment. [Among the many ways to lower cholesterol are daily aerobic walking, supplemental soluble rice bran, high-fiber diets, garlic supplementation, grapeseed oil, and supplemental tocotrienols. See the *High Cholesterol* section for more information.]

Source: *Archives of Neurology* 2002;59:378-38.

690. PESTICIDES & COGNITIVE DYSFUNCTION

Think twice before spraying your house for pests on a regular basis because exposure to pesticides appears to increase the risk of mild cognitive dysfunction. The relationship between pesticide exposure and cognitive dysfunction remains even after adjusting for alcohol consumption, smoking, drugs, and relevant diseases or family history. (In addition to pesticides, subjects studied were questioned about any exposure to organic solvents, metals, and other chemicals – but no relationship was observed between exposure to these substances and cognitive dysfunction.)

Because the results seen are similar between both currently employed and retired individuals, it is believed that pesticide exposure may have long-term adverse effects.

Source: *Lancet* 2000;356:912-913.

691. NO MSG, PLEASE...

This is a reminder to ask for food *without* MSG (monosodium glutamate) when ordering in Asian restaurants, because of the mounting evidence that excitatory amino acid neurotransmitters (primarily glutamate) are *neurotoxic*, and may contribute to cognitive decline.

692.. MARIJUANA, MEMORY & ATTENTION SPAN

Long-term use of marijuana is associated with impaired memory and attention, which lasts beyond intoxication and becomes worse with continued use. Long-term marijuana users perform significantly worse on memory and attention tests compared with those who have never used marijuana.

It is interesting to note that NO difference is observed between short-term users and those who have never used marijuana.

Source: *Journal of the American Medical Association* 2002;287:1123-1131,1172-1174.

693. COGNITIVE IMPAIRMENT & YOUR EYES

Retinopathy (the inflammation of the light-sensitive layer of the eye) may lead to a decline in cognitive thinking. Because diabetes and hypertension are known to influence retinopathy and cognitive function, researchers studied those with and without these two conditions. The results of the cognitive tests were similar in both groups, suggesting that cerebral microvascular disease may play an important role in cognitive impairment. [At the very least, we should all be making efforts to keep our blood sugar and blood pressure levels under control.]

Source: *Stroke* **2002;33:1487-1492.**

MEMORY & COGNITIVE DYSFUNCTION: NATURAL REMEDIES & SUPPLEMENTS

694. B VITAMINS AGAINST COGNITIVE DECLINE

Increased intake of folate, vitamin B12, and vitamin B6 can help memory performance in women of any age, even if taken for a short period of time. 750 micrograms of folate (folic acid), 15 microgram of B12, and 75 milligrams of B6 taken daily help to increase some aspects of memory performance, including speed of processing, recall, recognition, and verbal ability. These positive effects are noted after just one month. (No effect is seen on mood, however.)

Source: *Journal of Nutrition* **2002;132:1345-1356.**

WANT TO KNOW MORE?
[The best dietary sources of folate are green leafy vegetables such as spinach, kale, and beet greens, as well as beets, chard, asparagus, broccoli, bean sprouts (lentil, mung, and soy), and brewer's yeast.

The best sources of vitamin B6 are organ meats, egg yolk, fish, dried peas and beans, walnuts, and brewer's yeast, while B12 is found mainly in animal protein foods such as eggs, dairy products, organ meats, and seafood.]

695. LONG-TERM VITAMINS C & E PROTECTIVE

Taking vitamin C and vitamin E supplements may help protect memory and mental decline as you age, especially if the supplements have been taken long-term. Older men who have taken vitamin C and E supplements at least once a week over a number of years are protected from dementia and actually show improvements in cognitive function – a catch-all term that includes memory, creativity, and mental acuity.

Long-term use is required to improve cognitive function in late life, so start now! Vitamin C and E may protect against brain damage because they are antioxidants and can mop up brain-damaging free radical particles.

Source: *Neurology* Mar 2000;54:1265-1272.

696. UP YOUR VITAMIN E FOR BRAIN PROTECTION

More good news about vitamin E: Increasing your intake of foods and supplements containing vitamin E (butter, egg yolk, liver, seeds, nuts, and tocotrienols) may help improve your cognitive abilities. Men and women with the highest vitamin E consumption make the fewest errors on tests involving thinking abilities, while those with the lowest vitamin E intake (less than half of the recommended dietary amount) make the most errors. (This pattern remains even when levels of vitamin E and the ratio of vitamin E to cholesterol are assessed. Higher blood levels of vitamin E alone or relative to cholesterol are associated with better cognitive function.)

High intake of this nutrient is also linked to a reduction in the risk of Alzheimer's disease.

Sources: *Journal of Nutrition* 2002;132:2065-2068.

WANT TO KNOW MORE?
[We consume very few foods today that contain vitamin E. The best vitamin E supplement is the nutraceutical, tocotrienol, from palm oil. Second best are formulas that contain all of the eight isomers of vitamin E or the d-mixed tocotrienols (not just the alpha-tocopherol varieties). The amount of vitamin E in our diets has declined 90 percent in the last 100 years, and very few people get all they need of this vitamin from food alone.

Frying oils, processing and milling of foods, the bleaching of flours, cooking, and purifying vegetable oils remove most vitamin E from whole foods.]

697. SIBERIAN VELVET ANTLER FOR YOUR MIND

Supplementing with velvet antler (specifically, Siberian red deer velvet antler) may help to improve your mental abilities. A preparation formulated from Siberian red deer shows that it has a positive influence on cognitive functions and helps promote adaptation to mentally stressful situations.
In test animals, this substance has been shown to improve learning ability, memory, and overall mental functioning.

Source: First International Symposium on Antler Science & Product Technology, Banff, Canada, Apr 2000, reported by the Research Institute of Pharmacology, Tomsk, Russia.

WANT TO KNOW MORE?

[Velvet antler has anti-inflammatory properties, and is useful in the treatment of diseases such as arthritis (see Hints #85 and #107) and diabetes (Hint #385). For a good introduction to this supplement, see my book, *The Remarkable Healing Power of Velvet Antler*.]

698. TAKE ALA & ALC FOR A MEMORY BOOST

Protect your memory by supplementing with alpha-lipoic acid (ALA) and acetyl-L-carnitine (ALC). The substances alpha-lipoic acid (an antioxidant) and acetyl-L-carnitine (which helps transport fats in cells) have been shown to potentially reverse certain aspects of aging, including age-related memory decline. Mitochondria, tiny structures found in every cell, break down sugar and fat and convert them into energy. Many researchers believe that aging, including the age-related decline in memory, is related to a decrease in mitochondrial activity.

The combination of ALA and ALC *significantly* improves and reverses age-related declines in the memories of older test animals, and the combination of supplements is more effective than either taken alone. Consumption of high levels of ALA and ALC may help to delay brain aging and age-related neurodegenerative diseases in humans as well.

[Dietary sources of alpha-lipoic acid are slim, but it can be found in broccoli, spinach, and organ meats. Acetyl-L-carnitine is produced naturally in the body, but is also available in supplemental forms.]

Source: *Proceedings of the National Academy of Sciences* 2002;99:2356-2361.

WANT TO KNOW MORE?

[Alpha-lipoic acid also prevents rises in systolic blood pressure and can be used to treat hypertension. See Hint #625 in the *Hypertension* section for more details. It can also help to prevent insulin resistance and may reduce your risk of diabetes, as discussed in Hint #404 in the *Diabetes 2* section.]

699. DHA, PC & ENHANCED BRAIN FUNCTION

Supplementation with two natural substances, docosahexaenoic acid (DHA) and egg-phosphatidyl choline (PC), may improve your cognitive abilities. Dietary docosahexaenoic acid and egg-phosphatidyl choline have been shown to enhance brain function in older test animals, suggesting that intake of these two products taken together may effectively enhance human learning ability and brain function.

[While fish oils are the most common source of DHA, it can also be found in egg yolks. An important note: DHA has a slight blood thinning effect, so those on heart medication should check with their physician before increasing doses of this substance.]

Source: *Journal of Nutrition* 2000.

WANT TO KNOW MORE?
[DHA may also be protective against many health problems, including asthma (see Hint #118), diabetes (Hint #403), and lupus (Hint #670).. In addition, a mixture of DHA and another substance found in fish oils, EPA (eicosapentoic acid) appears to be beneficial in treating unipolar depression (see Hint #351.]

MEMORY & COGNITIVE DYSFUNCTION: REDUCING RISK

700. EXERCISE PREVENTS COGNITIVE DECLINE

Exercise is not just important for your body – it also helps to protect your mind. At least 10 percent of persons older than 65, and 50 percent older than 85, have some form of cognitive impairment, ranging from mild deficits to dementia, but those with higher levels of physical activity are less likely to experience this decline.

There are several possible mechanisms by which physical activity could affect cognitive function, including increasing blood flow to the brain, reducing the risk of cardiovascular disease, and stimulating nerve growth and survival.

[If you are relatively inactive, no matter your age, changing your habit now can reduce your risk of cognitive dysfunction down the road.]

Source: *Archives of Internal Medicine* **2001;161:1703-1708.**

701. BOTANICALS PREVENT COGNITIVE DECLINE

Specific botanicals, when used as an early intervention program, have proven degrees of efficacy and generally favorable benefit-to-risk profiles. They are: phosphatidylserine, vinpocetine, Ginkgo biloba extract, and Bacopa monniera (Bacopa). Phosphatidylserine is a phospholipid enriched in the brain, validated through double-blind trials for improving memory, learning, concentration, word recall, and mood. It has an excellent benefit-to-risk profile.

Vinpocetine is an excellent vasodilator and cerebral metabolic enhancer with proven benefits for vascular-based cognitive dysfunction. Ginkgo and vinpocetine may be incompatible with blood-thinning drugs. Bacopa is an Ayurvedic botanical with apparent anti-anxiety, anti-fatigue, and memory-strengthening effects. These substances offer interesting contributions to a personalized approach for restoring cognitive function.

Source: *Alternative Medicine Review* **1999;4(3):144-61.**

MENOPAUSE & HORMONE REPLACEMENT THERAPY

I wrote the book on menopause. And I don't mean that figuratively! In 1992, I became aware of the very serious dangers of synthetic hormones. I also learned about the benefits of natural progesterone, applied topically.

My book, *Hormone Replacement Therapy: Yes or No? How To Make An Informed Decision* was the first to address these issues for lay people. and of course you know the REST OF THE STORY: It took more than a decade for the "powers that be" to announce to the world that the doctors had made a mistake.

IN THIS SECTION:

- HORMONE REPLACEMENT THERAPY
- HRT & CANCER RISK
- HRT & CARDIOVASCULAR PROBLEMS

- HRT & OTHER HEALTH CONCERNS
- HOT FLASHES
- NATURAL HRT ALTERNATIVES

MENOPAUSE: HORMONE REPLACEMENT THERAPY
702. HRT CRITICIZED - AT LAST!

At long last, hormone replacement therapy (HRT) for women is finally being criticized by the medical community at large. According to members of the Heart and Estrogen/Progestin Replacement Study (HERS) Research Group, women without symptoms related to postmenopause actually experience greater declines in physical function when treated with hormone replacement therapy. This study, the largest one ever conducted on the subject, only strengthens the clinical recommendations that hormone therapy should generally be avoided.

[The only reason women with symptoms benefit is because the symptoms are suppressed. HRT does not address the *cause*.]

Source: *Journal of the American Medical Association* 2002;287:591-597,641-642.

WANT TO KNOW MORE?
[This study did not investigate the correlation between HRT and other negative health effects, of which there are many.

To understand all of this, I encourage you to read the latest edition of my book, *Hormone Replacement Therapy: Yes Or No? How to Make an Informed Decision.*]

703. MORE & MORE HRT PROMISES INVALIDATED

More negative news about HRT: Hormone replacement therapy does not slow down a decline in cognitive functioning in postmenopausal women, nor does it reduce the risk of death or recurrence of stroke in women with cerebrovascular disease. No consistent change in cognition is detected with the use of estrogen replacement therapy. This is true for current estrogen use and for the duration of estrogen use, for women of all ages.

Nor does estrogen therapy reduce a woman's risk of death alone or the risk of a nonfatal stroke. Results show that estrogen therapy should NOT be initiated for the purpose of secondary prevention of cerebrovascular disease.

In addition, there is an evolving body of evidence from clinical trials that show no benefit of estrogen for women with established vascular disease.

[The deeper we study, the more we find that so many of the original promises for HRT cannot be validated.]

Sources: *New England Journal of Medicine* 2001;345:1243-1249; *American Journal of Epidemiology* 2001;154:733-739.

MENOPAUSE: HRT & CANCER RISK

704. HRT & BREAST CANCER RISK

Women still considering HRT, be warned: Such hormone replacement therapy has a myriad of negative effects on your breasts that can lead to breast cancer. Hormone replacement therapy increases breast pain, increases the frequency of benign cysts and fibroids in the breast, and results in the growth of some already established benign lesions.

Breast density increases in 17 to 73 percent of women who use hormone replacement therapy, falsely affecting mammography readings. Combinations of estrogen and progestins increase breast density more than estrogen alone does.

Increasing numbers of women in their 50s and 60s are using hormone replacement therapy to alleviate menopausal symptoms, and the effects of long-term use of these agents is only now becoming apparent.

Source: *British Medical Journal* 2001;323:1381-1382.

705. HRT & BREAST CANCER: FROM PROGESTINS?

A woman's increased risk of breast cancer while undergoing HRT is most likely related to the use of *progestins* [synthetic progesterone]. New findings help explain the increased risk of breast cancer in women who use hormone replacement therapy, and it relates to the use of progestins.

The effects of progestins are dose-dependent, and the target is normal tissue as well as different types of tumors, including those that are initiated by estrogens. [Years ago I cited research in the first edition of my book on hormone replacement therapy about the increased risk of cancer with the addition of progestins. And now, once again, that conclusion has been validated!]

Source: *International Journal of Cancer* 2001;92:469-473.

WANT TO KNOW MORE?
[The terms progestin and progesterone are still being confused. Progestin is the synthetic variety, the mischief-maker. Progesterone is the natural stuff. When applied transdermally in a very low-dose cream formula that includes small quantities of tried-and-true herbs, the mix can very beneficial to the health of menopausal women.]

706. HRT & RISK OF ENDOMETRIAL CANCER

If you insist on synthetic estrogen therapy, consider the use of natural progesterone as well, because the greatest risk for endometrial cancer occurs from the use of unopposed estrogens. Extended use of hormone replacement therapy (HRT) has been confirmed to increase the risk of endometrial cancer. A research team found that users of any type of HRT were at greater risk of endometrial cancer than were nonusers. (This confirms earlier studies done on long-term use. Women using HRT for three years or more have an increased risk.)

The use of progestin, the synthetic form of progesterone, increases the risk of breast cancer. Be sure to use *progesterone*, the natural form.

Source: *Journal of Clinical Epidemiology* 2000;53:385-391.

707. HRT & RISK OF OVARIAN CANCER

You've heard it before, but here it is again: yet another study demonstrates that hormone replacement therapy may increase your risk of developing epithelial ovarian cancer. Swedish researches have found that, compared with women who had never used estrogen replacement, women who use unopposed estrogen replacement therapy are at increased risk of serous, mucinous, and endometrioid types of ovarian cancer.

Women who use estrogen with sequentially added progestins [synthetic progesterone] are at an increased risk of epithelial ovarian cancer, especially if used for more than 10 years. This is especially significant because of the poor prognosis of this form of cancer.

Source: *Journal of the National Cancer Institute* 2002;94:497-504.

708. HRT & RISK OF GALLBLADDER CANCER

More bad news about HRT: The use of hormone replacement therapy in menopause is associated with an increased risk of gallbladder cancer. This is the first direct epidemiological evidence of an association between HRT and gallbladder cancer. Conclusions were confirmed after a 12-year study of digestive tract cancers in women aged 45 to 79.

The risk for gallbladder cancer increases with increasing duration of HRT use.

[Yet another reason to stop HRT now if you are still taking it, and start learning about safer, natural alternatives.]

Source: *International Journal of Cancer* 2002;99:762-763.

WANT TO KNOW MORE?
[I referred to an association between HRT and gallbladder disease in the first edition of my book on hormone replacement therapy, 10 years ago.]

709. ESTROGEN: A CARCINOGEN?

In a very controversial move, the National Institute of Environmental Health Sciences wants to list *estrogen* as a known human carcinogen. At the 12th Annual Menopause Meeting, the case for listing estrogen as a carcinogen was presented. The group making the proposal came to this conclusion after careful analysis of all published epidemiological studies.

The speaker making the proposal said that the cancer risk associated with estrogen is similar to the "risk of environmental tobacco smoke."

Needless to say, there was heated opposition. The opposing group would only concede that more than five years of HRT can modestly increase the risk of breast cancer.

Source: **12th Annual Meeting of the North American Menopause Society, New Orleans, LA, Oct 2001.**

MENOPAUSE:
HRT & CARDIOVASCULAR PROBLEMS

710. HRT & HEART DISEASE: OPINIONS CHANGING

Britain's Medicines Control Agency is advising that hormone replacement therapy has _not_ been shown to prevent heart disease, and may even increase the risk in women with existing coronary disease. Proponents of HRT have argued that while the treatment may slightly increase the risk of breast cancer, this is offset by the protection it offers against coronary heart disease and osteoporosis. But initial results from a large ongoing trial suggest that, in women who already have heart disease, HRT does _not_ have a beneficial effect. In fact, your risk of heart disease may be slightly increased in the first year of use (see Hint #711 following this one).

Women should stop taking HRT and see their doctor _immediately_ if they experience centralized crushing chest pain with sweating, breathlessness, or dizziness.

Source: _Reuter's Medical Report_ **May 2002.**

WANT TO KNOW MORE?
The American Heart Association also advised last year that HRT should not be initiated solely for its potential protective effects against cardiovascular disease.

711. SHORT-TERM HRT & CARDIOVASCULAR EVENTS

Even short-term HRT can have serious health consequences: Using postmenopausal hormones for less than a year seems to increase a woman's risk of recurrent major coronary events. Compared with women who have never used hormones, women who have used hormones for less than a year have a far greater risk for a major coronary event [such as a heart attack]. After the one-year mark, the relative risk decreases, but is still present.

Such finding also suggest that, in addition to putting a woman at risk for coronary events, HRT should _not_ be initiated solely for the prevention of recurrent heart diseases.

Source: _Annals of Internal Medicine_ **2001;135:1-8.**

712. HRT & VENOUS THROMBOEMBOLISM DANGER

Postmenopausal women on HRT, be warned: You are at increased risk of dangerous blood vessel blockages due to _venous thromboembolism._ Venous thromboembolism refers to blood vessel obstruction with clotting material carried by the bloodstream. Studies of over 2,700 women across the country indicate that hormone replacement therapy increase the risk of venous thromboembolism by *three times or more*. Even after adjusting for other risk factors, HRT remains a *significant* predictor of venous thromboembolism.

In addition, women already at high risk for this condition (due to a previous history of venous thromboembolism, as well as a history of cancer, lower-extremity fracture, or immobilization) are especially advised to avoid postmenopausal HRT.

Source: *Annals of Internal Medicine* 2000;132:689-696.

713. HRT & RISK OF VENTRICAL ARRHYTHMIA

One more link between HRT and potential cardiovascular problems — this time it's the risk of dangerous heart *arrhythmia*. Yet another study points to a possible risk of hormone replacement therapy (which prolongs the interval of a measure of heart rhythm) with risk for ventricular arrhythmia, or rapid heartbeat. In athletes, this arrhythmia is often associated with sudden death.

This research targeted women between the ages of 45 and 64 who were free of heart disease at the onset of the study. When women who used HRT were compared to those who had never used HRT, the risk of the prolonged interval of heart rhythm was *significant*.

Source: Stanford Study, presented at the American Heart Association's Scientific Session, Nov 2001.

WANT TO KNOW MORE?
One interesting point of this study was that women who use HRT generally are healthier overall than women not on HRT, and on average this held true for the women in this particular study. This indicates that these women started out healthier overall but after initiating HRT their risk for this arrhythmia problem *doubled*.

714. HRT & MICROALBUMINURIA RISK

Here's another negative to add to the growing list for HRT: It is associated with an increased risk of microalbuminuria (early stages of albumin in the urine), which in turn increases the risk of cardiovascular disease. In postmenopausal women, HRT use is more prevalent in those with microalbuminuria than in those without. In fact, HRT use doubles the risk of microalbuminuria in postmenopausal women, and those who have used HRT for more than five years face an even higher risk.

Source: *Archives of Internal Medicine* 2001;161:2000-2005.

WANT TO KNOW MORE?

[In premenopausal women, the use of oral contraceptives is also associated with an increased risk of microalbuminuria. See Hint #332 in the *Contraceptive Caveats* section for more details.]

MENOPAUSE: HRT & OTHER HEALTH CONCERNS
715. HRT ALSO LINKED TO ASTHMA

More bad press for hormone replacement therapy: In addition to cancer and cardiovascular problems, HRT has also been linked to an increased risk of asthma. Information about the association between HRT and asthma comes from Harvard Medical School, which analyzed data collected from the Nurses' Health Study (which studied over 121,000 female nurses). Conclusion: current users of estrogen have an increased risk of asthma when compared with women who have never undergone HRT (after adjustment for age and smoking), and this risk increases with the dose and length of estrogen use. Even past users have a similarly elevated risk of asthma.

[So the obvious hint, ladies, is to get off those synthetics and learn about the use of progesterone cream to help balance your hormones.]

Source: Annual Meeting of the American College of Chest Physicians, San Francisco, CA, Oct 2000.

716. DRY-EYE SYNDROME, A SIDE EFFECT OF HRT

Women on HRT, take note: You are at a significantly increased risk of dry-eye syndrome. Dry-eye syndrome is a very common condition affecting millions of middle-aged and older women. It should be recognized that the prevalence of dry-eye syndrome is extensively related to the use of HRT, and the longer a woman is on HRT, the higher her risk.

Women who use estrogen alone have the highest prevalence, while those who have never used HRT at all have the lowest. The prevalence in women who use estrogen plus progesterone/progestin runs a close second to those who use estrogen alone. Each three-year increase in the duration of HRT use is associated with a significant 15 percent elevation in risk of clinically diagnosed dry-eye syndrome or severe symptoms. Dry-eye syndrome can have a serious impact on a woman's quality of life and can also increase her risk of ocular infection.

[Once again I want to stress the benefit of using a low-dose progesterone cream with tried-and-true herbs, and reading *Hormone Replacement Therapy: Yes Or No?*, to learn about balancing hormones without side effects.]

Source: *Journal of the American Medical Association* 2001;286:2114-2119.

717. HRT & GALLSTONE DEVELOPMENT

Hormone replacement therapy (HRT) appears to increase a woman's risk of developing gallstones. Women who take HRT have a much higher risk of developing gallstones than do non-HRT users, and the effect is dose-dependent (so the more HRT administered, the more your risk climbs). Women who have taken HRT for less than three years are two and a half times more likely to develop gallstones, while those who have used HRT for more than three years have *four times* the risk of gallstones.

Because gallstones are composed primarily of cholesterol, the use of estrogen may promote an increase in cholesterol in bile that leads to gallstone formation.

Source: 103rd Annual Meeting of the American Gastroenterological Association, San Francisco, CA, May 2002.

WANT TO KNOW MORE?
[In addition to gallstones, HRT is also linked to much more serious gallbladder problems such as gallbladder cancer. See Hint #708 earlier in this section for more information.]

MENOPAUSE: HOT FLASHES

718. PROGESTERONE CREAM ABSORPTION TIPS

If you have not had success with the progesterone/herbal creams for hot-flash relief, try applying a hot cloth to your skin before application of the cream to increase absorption. Most women report total relief of hot flashes and improved skin conditions with the application of progesterone creams. But occasionally someone does not experience a positive result. Opening pores with a hot cloth helps to increase absorption.

Some women find that using more cream than is recommended also works (provided the cream is a low-dose progesterone product), and others find that applying the cream vaginally increases absorption.

Source: B. Kamen, *Hormone Replacement Therapy: Yes or No? How to Make an Informed Decision*.

719 EXERCISING AWAY HOT FLASHES

Inactive women, take note: Hot flashes and night sweats are only *half* as common among physically active postmenopausal women as among benchwarmers.

Endorphins, those "feel-good" hormones, affect your thermoregulatory centers (your body's thermostat). Exercising increases these endorphins, helping to decrease hot flashes.

Estrogen is actually manufactured in body fat from other hormones after menopause, so a very thin woman may have less natural estrogen in her system, which may give her more problems with hot flashes.

Source: B. Kamen, *Hormone Replacement Therapy: Yes or No? How to Make an Informed Decision*.

MENOPAUSE: NATURAL HRT ALTERNATIVES

720. HOW TO SWITCH TO NATURAL ALTERNATIVES

Menopausal women, take note: Stopping your hormone replacement therapy NOW and replacing it with a natural progesterone cream not only reduces your risk of many serious health problems, it can also reduce bloating, weight gain, depression – and even increase your sex drive! We all know now about the long-term study on HRT being curtailed because of the increased risk of stroke, thrombosis, coronary heart disease events, and invasive breast cancer. Those of you involved in alternative therapies already knew this.

For those women who want to get off their synthetic hormone drugs, my recommendation is the use of a topically applied cream containing small amounts of tried-and-true herbs, including Siberian ginseng, Dong quai, black cohosh, burdock root, Mexican yam extract, and a small amount of the hormone progesterone. The cream must be formulated for optimal absorption.

To avoid temporary symptoms that are likely to occur when you suddenly stop using hormone drugs, you may want to reduce the drug slowly, while starting the application of the cream. Start by skipping the use of the drug every fifth day for a week or two; then skip every fourth day, etc.

Switching from an oral HRT synthetic estrogen-progestin combination to the transdermal application of this safe cream decreases the sex hormone binding globulin, thereby increasing free androgens, which increases libido. You may also get rid of bloating, weight gain, and depression when you stop using those harmful drugs.

This same cream can also relieve symptoms of PMS, usually caused by the same problems that initiate menopausal symptoms. In other words, if you suffer from PMS, you can look forward to problems with menopause – unless you decide to change your ways now. The cream is safe, and any amount can be used.

Sources: *Journal of the American Medical Association* 2002;288:366-368; B. Kamen, *Hormone Replacement Therapy: Yes or No? How to Make an Informed Decision*.

721. THE BENEFITS OF PROGESTERONE CREAM

Transdermal (topical) natural progesterone cream has become a popular alternative to hormone replacement therapy. The cream, which can be applied vaginally or topically, provides an excellent delivery system for the hormone progesterone. Progesterone cream can protect the cells of the endometrium from proliferating [whereas, as discussed earlier, HRT *increases* a woman's risk of developing endometrial cancer]. In one study of menopausal women with an average age of 55.2 years, all routes and concentrations of progesterone cream (topical and vaginal) resulted in *significant* decreases in the proliferation of endometrial cells, while both topical and vaginal placebo groups showed no change.

The cream also helps to prevent spontaneous abortions (miscarriages), improving the prognosis of women who suffer from multiple miscarriages.

Sources: *Obstetrics & Gynecology* 2001;97(4Suppl1):S10; *Minerva Gynecology* 2000;52(9):367-374; *Fertility & Sterility* 1991;56(5):995-996.

WANT TO KNOW MORE?
[Ten years ago I wrote that natural progesterone cream offered an improved delivery method to achieve sustained physiological progesterone levels with a single daily application. Now new studies confirm this.]

722. RED CLOVER FOR MENOPAUSAL SYMPTOMS

Extract of the herb red clover can be an effective natural HRT alternative for menopausal women. Red clover extract is weakly estrogenic, and should be considered as a possible candidate for safe, natural hormone replacement therapy. And although red clover has estrogenic effects, it does not stimulate breast cell proliferation, making it an ideal phytoestrogen (or plant "estrogen"). Studies demonstrate red clover as useful in the treatment of menopausal symptoms.

Red clover also has powerful antioxidant potential. It can reduce the inflammatory edema reaction and the suppression of sensitivity induced by the sun's radiation. Because of this quality, it may have an additional role as a sun-protective cosmetic ingredient.

Sources: *Journal of Nutrition* 2002;132:27-30; *Journal of Agricultural Food Chemistry* May 2001;49(5):2472-2479; *Photochemical Photobiology* Sep 2001;74(3):465-470.

WANT TO KNOW MORE?
[I have been sprouting red clover seeds for many years. A tablespoon of the sprouted seeds (grown from an eighth of a teaspoon of seeds) per family member added to salads is an easy way to increase the nutritional value of any meal.]

723. FLAXSEED FOR MENOPAUSAL SYMPTOMS

Flaxseed is another effective natural HRT alternative for menopausal women. Because of their structural similarity to the estrogens we make in our body, the kind of phytoestrogens found in flaxseed exert estrogen-like effects.

(Phytoestrogens are naturally occurring plant compounds present in flaxseed as lignans.)

[A small coffee grinder makes it easy to grind a tablespoon of flaxseed daily, to be sprinkled over salads. Use one tablespoon for each family member on a daily basis.]

Source: *Journal of Renal Nutrition* **2001;11(4);PAGE.**

WANT TO KNOW MORE?
There is increasing evidence that dietary phytoestrogens have a beneficial role in chronic renal (kidney) disease. Lignans are readily absorbed from the gut and converted to active metabolites, which may be partly responsible for the beneficial renal effects of flaxseed.

[See Hint #658 in the *Kidney Diseases & Conditions* section for more information.]

724. CHASTE BERRY FOR MENOPAUSAL SYMPTOMS

Women using an extract of the herb chaste berry experience *significant* relief from menopausal symptoms. Known in the alternative nutrition arena for years, but newly validated by the medical community, chaste berry can improve irritability, mood alteration, anger, headache, and breast fullness caused by the monthly cycle. (Bloating, however, is unaffected.) This herb stimulates the pituitary and helps the body produce progesterone.

Sources: *British Medical Journal* **2001;322:134-137;** B. Kamen, *Hormone Replacement Therapy: Yes or No? How to Make an Informed Decision.*

WANT TO KNOW MORE?
[Chaste berry is also helpful for relieving symptoms of PMS. See Hint #467 in the *Feminine Disorders* section for more details.]

725. BLACK COHOSH FOR MENOPAUSAL SYMPTOMS

Yet another effective natural HRT alternative for menopausal women is the herb black cohosh. Considered a phytoestrogen, black cohosh has favorable estrogenic effects on both bone and blood lipids.

[Benefits of black cohosh include anti-inflammatory and gentle sedation effects. As explained in my book, *Hormone Replacement Therapy: Yes Or No?*, black cohosh is useful for menstrual pains and for reducing hot flashes. It also lowers blood pressure and relaxes muscles.]

Source: 84th annual meeting of The Endocrine Society, June 24, 2002.

WANT TO KNOW MORE?
[Black cohosh is also sometimes known as "black snakeroot."]

726. SOY HORMONES, HOWEVER, NOT MUCH HELP

The long-term effects of soy protein on your hormone levels, even if the soy is high in various concentrations of isoflavones, prove to be *ineffective*. Isoflavones are unique to soybeans, and have structures very similar to the body's natural estrogens (hence the name plant estrogens or phytoestrogens). Postmenopausal women consuming soy protein with 56 milligrams of isoflavones were checked after three months and again at six months, but no significant differences were found for levels of estrogens, cortisol, DHEA, insulin, glucagon, or even follicle-stimulating hormones.

There appears to be no altering of steroid hormone values with long-term ingestion of soy protein.

Soy protein may have small effects on thyroid hormone values, but they are unlikely to be clinically important.

Source: *American Journal of Clinical Nutrition* **2002;75(1)145-153.**

MOTION SICKNESS

727. GINGER ALLEVIATES MOTION SICKNESS

A simple hint: If you are you are subject to motion sickness while driving, take some ginger (or other decongestant) to help alleviate the problem. And if you suffer from middle-ear pain during air travel (which often occurs during takeoff and landing), ginger can also help. The efficacy of ginger rhizome for the prevention of nausea, dizziness, and vomiting as symptoms of motion sickness (kinetosis), as well as for postoperative vomiting and vomiting of pregnancy, has been well documented and proved beyond doubt in numerous high-quality clinical studies.

Source: *Advances In Therapy* **1998;15(1):25-44**

MULTIPLE SCLEROSIS (MS)

If you are a white male WWII veteran with an urban address, have nine or more years of education, uncorrected visual acuity less than 20/20, live in a more northern latitude, and a higher proportion of people in your state are of Swedish ancestry, you have an increased risk of developing multiple sclerosis.

In addition to geography, age, sex, and race, per se, and higher socioeconomic status is significantly associated with higher MS risk in black and white men and in white women in the United States. (*Neurology* **1997;48(1):204-13**)

The disease affects the central nervous system, and most often occurs in early adult life. The immune system attacks the myelin sheath that surrounds nerve cells. *Multiple* nerve sheaths then become hardened (hence the term *sclerosis*).

IN THIS SECTION:
- CAUSES & PRECURSORS
- DIETARY TACTICS
- NATURAL REMEDIES & SUPPLEMENTS
- REDUCING RISK

MS: CAUSES & PRECURSORS

728. SMOKED SAUSAGE & MULTIPLE SCLEROSIS

Reduce your risk of developing multiple sclerosis (MS) by avoiding smoked meats or fish, foods that have been linked to this disease. Studies point to an association between autoimmune problems – such as multiple sclerosis – and the nitrates used in meat and fish preparations plus the chemicals used in the smoking process. Eating these foods frequently in childhood seems to be linked to an increased risk of developing multiple sclerosis later in life.

There seems to be a link between the combination of nitrates and nitrites (used to prepare meat for production of smoked sausages) and the phenols from smoke with the production of *nitrophenols*, compounds connected with autoimmunity problems.

Communities in northern Europe have smoked their foods for many centuries without developing MS, but did not use nitrates or nitrites on the meat or fish before smoking. (MS emerged at the start of the 19th century.) Nitrogenous chemicals are generally used to ensure that the meat or fish does not lose its color during the smoking process.

Source: 12th Meeting of the European Neurological Society, Berlin, Germany, Jun 2002.

MS: DIETARY TACTICS

729. NUTRITION AGAINST MULTIPLE SCLEROSIS

Men and women whose main source of protein comes from vegetables have a 60 percent lower risk of developing multiple sclerosis. Other factors that might help delay or even prevent the onset of MS include low calorie intake, low saturated fats (true more for males than for females), high dietary fiber, and individual nutrients including vitamin C, thiamine, riboflavin, calcium and potassium.

These factors are *significantly* protective. For example, dietary fiber is associated with between a 30 to 36 percent lower risk of developing MS.

Source: Congress of Epidemiology, Toronto, Ontario, Jun 2001.

MS: NATURAL REMEDIES & SUPPLEMENTS

730. VITAMIN D & MULTIPLE SCLEROSIS

Taking vitamin D supplements may positively influence the immune systems of patients suffering from multiple sclerosis. Although most MS patients have a normal life span, this disease, which causes the immune system to attack the body's own cells as "foreign," causes vision changes and muscle weakness in its victims.

MS may progress steadily, or acute attacks may be followed by a temporary remission of symptoms.

Vitamin D status affects chemicals called *cytokines* that modulate the immune system, and these changes may benefit patients with this disease. The current recommended dietary allowance for vitamin D is 400 micrograms (units) per day. Sources of vitamin D include cod liver oil and adequate exposure to sunlight.

Source: Experimental Biology Conference, Orlando, FL, Apr 2001.

WANT TO KNOW MORE?
It's interesting to note that the number of cases of MS is nearly zero near the equator and increases with latitude in both hemispheres. The increased sunlight near the equator allows the body to produce more vitamin D, and may theoretically reduce the incidence of MS.

MS:
REDUCING RISK

731. THE TRUTH ABOUT CATS & BIRDS

Exposure to cats may actually decrease your risk of developing multiple sclerosis, while exposure to birds may *significantly increase* your risk. If you have had a cat for the last 10 years, the risk of MS is decreased by 50 percent, whereas if you have a bird, the risk of having this disease is more than *doubled*. Those individuals with either a family history of MS, or who already have had some signs of MS, are advised to consider these risk factors carefully.

Source: Congress of Epidemiology, Toronto, Ontario, Jun 2001.

MUSCULAR DYSTROPHY (MD)

Muscular dystrophy is a disease that progresses steadily, destroying muscle tissue on its way. It appears at a young age, and it can vary in severity. In spite of rapidly increasing insight into the molecular basis of neuromuscular diseases, treatment for this disease still relies on convention and clinical studies. However, the alternative physician knows that degenerative diseases do not have to be a death sentence, or even a lifestyle spoiler.

732. GREEN TEA SLOWS MUSCULAR DEGENERATION

Extract of green tea may be able to slow the progression of muscular dystrophy (MD). Daily doses of green tea extract appear to slow deterioration in some muscle tissue (possibly through its antioxidant effects), and this benefit is helpful for problems such as muscular dystrophy. The tea may have protective effects against oxidative stress in muscle tissue.

Previous studies have suggested that green tea might help prevent heart disease and certain cancers, possibly due to polyphenols, which are potent antioxidants. Oxidative stress may also contribute to muscle wasting.

The lowest effective dose in this study is equal to seven cups of green tea per day. [But be aware that green tea does contain caffeine.]

Source: *American Journal of Clinical Nutrition* 2002;75:749-753.

NASAL DRYNESS

Although dry nose is usually associated with age-related changes in nasal physiology and structure, air dust may cause physiological changes at any age. (*Geriatrics* **2002;57(10):29,32;** *Indoor Air* **2000;10(4):237-45)**

733. PURE SESAME OIL FOR NASAL DRYNESS

Pure sesame oil may be an effective remedy for the nasal dryness caused by low humidity during the winter. Dry nasal mucosa during the winter is a common problem experienced by many people. Normally, the standard treatment is the use of an isotonic sodium chloride solution (ISCS) administered either via a nasal spray, nose drops, or other application methods.

But patients with dry noses given pure sesame oil have significant improvements in nasal dryness, stuffiness, and crustiness compared to those given the standard ISCS. Sesame oil appears to be a much more effective remedy– just make sure it is pure, pharmaceutical-quality sesame oil.

Source: *Archives of Otolaryngology – Head & Neck Surgery* **2001;127:1353-1356.**

NASAL POLYPS

Despite the prevalence and long history of nasal polyps, many questions still exist with respect to incidence and pathogenesis, although allergy has been commonly thought to be a major cause. (*Otolaryngology – Head & Neck Surgery* **2000;122(2):298-301)** Epithelial cells may increase in an attempt to cover a defect, but the final result will be nasal polyps. (*China* **2002;101(3):227-9)**

734. WOODSTOVES CAN LEAD TO NASAL POLYPS

Using a woodstove to heat your home (rather than electricity or oil) may lead to nasal polyps and sinus disease. **Byproducts of woodstoves, which can include formaldehyde, can be a trigger for these diseases. A significant number of people with these medical problems report using wood stoves at some time in their lives. One third of those with nasal polyps report being exposed to woodstoves for many hours a day. (Formaldehyde can also be found in cosmetics, preservatives, and building insulation.)**

Individuals with on-the-job exposure to noxious inhalants –- such as wood dust and paint solvents — are *six times more likely* to be diagnosed with nasal polyps than are those without such exposures.

Source: *Archives of Otolaryngology – Head, & Neck Surgery*, **2002;128:682-686.**

NAUSEA

For most people, nausea and vomiting are simply unfortunate consequences of overindulgent college days or overenthusiastic amusement rides. We can experience nausea for psychological or physical factors, including expectations, beliefs, and conditioning. Regardless of the reason, we've all been there, and we all hope never to repeat the experience. (*Support Care Cancer* **2002;10(2):96-105**)

735. ACUPRESSURE FOR NAUSEA RELIEF

Nausea may be relieved through the traditional Chinese technique of acupressure, or a modern variation in which electrical stimulation is delivered to a pressure point. Stimulation of a point above the wrist on the inside of the forearm is thought to relieve nausea and vomiting related to morning sickness, chemotherapy, or motion sickness.

Wearing special wristbands also seems to be useful in reducing nausea during pregnancy. The bands are inexpensive, are not associated with any side effects, and deliver immediate benefits.

Symptoms of morning sickness also decline when women wear wristbands delivering electrical stimulation to a pressure point.

Women who reported nausea and vomiting in the early first trimester of pregnancy wore a wristband for an average of about two months. Most reported that they felt less nauseous, and nearly all said they would use the device during a future pregnancy or would recommend it to someone else.

Source: *Journal of Reproductive Medicine,* **2001;46:811-814,835-839.**

WANT TO KNOW MORE?
[For many more helpful hints on relieving pregnancy-related nausea, see the *Pregnancy & Childbirth* section.]

736. GINGER FOR NAUSEA

Ginger (*Zingiber officinale*) is often advocated as beneficial for nausea and vomiting. Whether the herb is truly efficacious for this condition is, however, still a matter of debate. However, one study was found for each of the following conditions: seasickness, morning sickness, and chemotherapy-induced nausea. These studies collectively favored ginger over placebo.

Source: *British Journal of Anesthesia* 2000;84(3):367-71.

OBESITY

So far, the fight against weight gain has been disappointing. The US Surgeon General said in his 2001 report on the subject that about 300,000 deaths annually are associated with overweight. In other words, the 2001 *Surgeon General's Call to Action to Prevent and Decrease Overweight and Obesity* is falling on deaf ears.

IN THIS SECTION:
- ALTERNATIVE STRATEGIES
- CAUSES
- DIETARY STRATEGIES
- NATURAL REMEDIES & SUPPLEMENTS
- REDUCING RISK
- WEIGHT LOSS & EXERCISE

OBESITY: ALTERNATIVE STRATEGIES

737. LOSE WEIGHT WITH YOUR THERMOSTAT

If you keep the temperature of your house at 68 degrees instead of 70 degrees, you may find yourself weighing a couple of pounds less after a short period of time. In its effort to keep your body temperature under control (98.6 degrees), you will burn more calories in a colder environment. Getting into a cold bed at night has the same effect.

738. MORE WATER = LESS HUNGER PANGS

Drink up! One glass of water shuts down midnight hunger pangs for almost 100 percent of dieters. In 37 percent of Americans, the thirst mechanism is so weak that it is often mistaken for hunger. Seventy-five percent of Americans are chronically dehydrated. Even *mild* dehydration will slow down your metabolism as much as three percent, so drinking more water may provide you with more energy. Lack of water is the number one trigger of daytime fatigue.

Source: University of Washington study, reported in *Integrated & Alternative Medicine Clinical Highlights* Aug 2002;1(16).

WANT TO KNOW MORE?
Help with weight loss is not the only benefit of increasing your water consumption: Preliminary research indicates that eight to 10 glasses of water a day could significantly ease back and joint pain for up to 80 percent of sufferers. A mere two-percent drop in body water can trigger fuzzy short-term memory, trouble with basic math, and difficulty focusing on the computer screen. And drinking five glasses of water daily may decrease your risk of colon cancer, breast cancer, and bladder cancer.

OBESITY: CAUSES

739. INFECTIOUS OBESITY?

Infection is now believed to be among the causes of obesity. There has been a 30 percent increase in obesity from 1980 to 1990, and this number continues to escalate. Although there are many causes for obesity, one overlooked possibility is obesity of an infectious origin.

Six pathogens are reported to cause obesity in animals, and two in humans. Although the exact mechanism isn't known, infection attributable to these organisms should be included in the long list of potential factors responsible for obesity. The possibility of a similar role for other pathogens is not unreasonable.

[So here's another reason to help protect ourselves against infection by shoring up our immune systems with smart food choices and nutritional supplementation.]

Source: *Journal of Nutrition* 2001;131:2794S-2797S.

740. WATCH OUT FOR ADDED FRUCTOSE

Watch those food labels for added fructose, which can unfavorably increase fat profiles. Fructose intake has increased steadily during the past two decades. One study done on the effect of fructose intake on lipid metabolism in test animals suggests that long-term fructose consumption has strong adverse effects, including an increase in triglycerides and cholesterol levels.

[Note that this study applies to fructose in an *isolated* form, added to foods, not fructose as it appears in foods naturally.]

Source: *Journal of Nutrition* 2002;132:918-923.

OBESITY: DIETARY STRATEGIES

741. LOW-STARCH MEALS CAN CONTROL HUNGER

Eating a low-starch meal can help prevent hunger more effectively than eating a high-starch one. Despite equal caloric content, instant oatmeal has a higher glycemic index than unprocessed oatmeal, causing a sharp rise in blood glucose followed by a sudden drop, thereby triggering hunger.

Twelve obese teenage boys were given unlimited snacks for five hours after consuming meals with low-, medium-, or high-glycemic indexes. (The low-glycemic index meal consisted of a vegetable omelet and fruit; the medium was unprocessed oatmeal; and the high-glycemic index meal was processed "instant" oatmeal. All meals contained an equal number of calories.)

The boys who had eaten the high-starch instant oatmeal ate 81 percent more snacks than those who had eaten the low-starch omelet and fruit.

Source: *Pediatrics* 1999;103:e26.

742. DIETERS: ADD AIR TO SHAKES

Consuming a shake a half hour before a meal – with lots of air mixed into it – can increase your satiety level and help decrease your appetite. Even though the caloric content and the weight of a shake may be identical, mixing lots of air into it has an effect on how much food you'll eat at mealtime. The volume of the shake can vary, depending on the amount of air mixed into it.

In one study, participants reported greater reductions in hunger and greater increases in fullness after consumption of yogurt-based shakes that had the most air mixed into them.

Source: *American Journal of Clinical Nutrition* 2000;72(2):361-368.

743. LOSE WEIGHT WITH A BIG BREAKFAST

Dieters, take note: When on a weight-loss regimen, you will lose slightly more weight if you have your larger meal in the morning. Change in fat mass and loss of body energy is affected by the order of meal pattern ingestion. Ingestion of larger breakfasts results in slightly greater weight loss. (Although ingestion of larger evening meals results in better maintenance of fat-free mass.)

Source: *Journal of Nutrition* 1997;127(1)75-82.

744. THE CHICKEN FAT MYTH

If you are dieting, it is not necessary to remove the skin on a piece of chicken during cooking. Transfer of fat from the skin to the meat of the chicken is a myth. It is the eating of the skin that adds the calories.

Source: Jane Kinderlehrer, *Prevention* magazine editor, personal interview on WMCA, New York, 1979.

OBESITY: NATURAL REMEDIES & SUPPLEMENTS

745. GREEN TEA FOR WEIGHT LOSS

Green tea extract can help you to lose weight – only it's not the caffeine in the tea, but rather the high amounts of catechin phenols. Green tea extract significantly increases 24-hour energy expenditure by 4 percent. And because green tea does not affect heart rate, it may also be appropriate as a weight-loss tool for those at risk for cardiovascular disease.

Source: *American Journal of Clinical Nutrition* **1999;70.**

WANT TO KNOW MORE?
[Green tea may be preventive against numerous diseases as well, including arthritis (See Hint #86, many forms of cancer (Hint #156, colitis (Hint #487), prostatitis (Hint #683), and muscular dystrophy (Hint #732).]

746. ADDING FIBER RESULTS IN WEIGHT LOSS

Increasing your intake of fiber (whether from food or fiber supplements) can help promote weight loss in several ways. Fiber helps weight loss because fiber causes a true alteration in digestion and absorption of fat. Part of the fat becomes associated with the fiber, making it unavailable for digestion — thereby increasing fat excretion. The greater your fiber consumption, the higher your caloric waste.

Fiber also slows transit time (the time it takes for your food to go through your system), which delays nutrient absorption and produces a sensation of satiety. Fiber supplementation is an attempt to return the carbohydrates in your diet to a more natural state. A good fiber supplement will increase the incidence of elimination without diminishing the metabolism of nutrients.

In view of the fact that the average American dietary fiber intake is currently only 15 grams a day (half the American Heart Association's recommendation of 25-30 grams a day), efforts to increase dietary fiber could help to decrease the high prevalence of obesity throughout the country.

Sources: *Nutrition Review* **May 2001;59(5):129-139; B. Kamen,** *New Facts About Fiber.*

WANT TO KNOW MORE?
[Some physicians recommend even higher doses of fiber for optimum health. Keep in mind that most fruits and vegetables are NOT high in fiber. See my book, *New Facts About Fiber*, to fully understand the correlation between fiber and disease, and to learn which foods can easily help you to increase your fiber intake.]

747. CALCIUM-RICH FOODS FOR WEIGHT LOSS

Given two diets of the same caloric content, more weight will be lost on the one that has more dietary calcium. Dietary calcium helps determine whether calories go to storage (in the form of fat) or get burned. Women on high-calcium diets lose significant amounts of body fat, even though calorie intake remains the same. It remains unclear why calcium from food (in this case, from dairy products) might stimulate fat loss any more efficiently than supplemental calcium, but it does!

Source: Experimental Biology 2000 Conference, University of Tennessee, Knoxville, Apr 2000.

WANT TO KNOW MORE?
[For those who are lactose intolerant, or consider the usual dairy products less than ideal, consider health-store yogurt or heaping teaspoons of colostrum powder mixed with water. The fermentation process used in making yogurt produces the lactase necessary to digest lactose; and colostrum is very low in lactose and rarely causes problems.]

748. EPHEDRA SAFE IN CONTROLLED DOSES

Ephedra (also known as ma huang) appears to be safe and effective for weight loss at 90 mg per day, divided into 30 mg doses. According to the Council for Responsible Nutrition, "consumers can feel confident that if they use ephedra according to labeling, they have an effective tool to aid their weight loss efforts." This conclusion was reached after a total of 19 clinical trials were reviewed, including data from a thorough Harvard and Columbia University study.

A temporary increase in blood pressure is associated with the initiation of ephedra and caffeine therapy, but there are no increases in cardiac irritability. Weight loss is statistically significant among those taking this supplement (and, in fact, only minimal adverse events occur with 150 mg/day).

Source: *Reuter's Medical Report*, Jan 2001.

749. GINSENG BERRY FOR WEIGHT LOSS

If you are overweight, taking ginseng berry may be a helpful, natural way to lose some pounds. An extract of the ginseng berry [as opposed to the root, the commonly consumed form] appears to help bring about weight loss. Test animals treated with this extract lost more than 10 percent of their body weight in just 12 days compared with untreated animals who gained five percent of their weight in the same period.

Source: University of Chicago study, Chicago, IL, as reported in *The Daily Mail*, UK, May 2002.

WANT TO KNOW MORE?
[Ginseng berry extract also helps to normalize blood glucose levels in diabetics. See Hint #375 in the *Diabetes* section for more details.]

OBESITY: REDUCING RISK

750. A LITTLE GOES A LONG WAY...

Even a small amount weight loss can have a positive impact on your health: Weight reduction of only one pound a year can *substantially* reduce the long-term risk of developing hypertension if the weight loss can be maintained. Regardless of age, persons who lose a pound or more a year and sustain that loss have a 25 to 30 percent reduction in risk of developing hypertension. Among younger people, losing more weight increases the benefit even more.

Source: *International Journal of Obesity & Related Metabolism* **2001;25(2):258.**

751. OVERWEIGHT? SUPPLEMENT WITH VITAMIN D

Since vitamin D absorption is decreased in those who are overweight, a good vitamin D3 supplement is advisable for the large percentage of Americans who fall into this category. When compared with non-overweight people of the same age, overweight subjects have 57 percent less vitamin D concentrations 24 hours after receiving a 1.25 mg oral dose of the vitamin. It is theorized that obesity-associated vitamin D insufficiency is likely due to the decreased bioavailability of vitamin D3 because of its deposition in body fat compartments. [Vitamin D deficiency can lead to many serious health problems, including osteoporosis.]

Source: *American Journal of Clinical Nutrition* **2000;72(3):690-693.**

752. LOSING WEIGHT CAN MEAN LOSING BONE TOO

Because weight loss is associated with bone loss, take steps to protect your bones if you are on a serious and extended weight-loss program. The risk of bone loss may be greater in lean individuals than in heavier ones. Although all the mechanisms involved are not clear, it is known that calcium absorption is reduced during weight loss.

[See the *Osteoporosis & Other Skeletal Problems* section for many hints on protecting your bones.]

Source: *Journal of Nutrition* **2002;132:2660-2666.**

OBESITY: WEIGHT LOSS & EXERCISE

753. TIPS FOR MAINTAINING WEIGHT LOSS

When dieting, the greater the weight loss, the more likely you are to keep the weight off, just as those who exercise the most are more likely to keep weight off than those who don't exercise as much. When people lose 45 to 50 pounds and are no longer obese — or have put a great deal of energy into exercising – they have more incentive to keep the weight off than those who lose 15 to 20 pounds or haven't exercised quite as much.

People who lose more weight have more time and energy invested in their weight success and may have learned more in the process than those who lose smaller amounts of weight.

Researchers conclude that a very low-calorie diet that includes shakes, energy bars and low-calorie entrees may be the key to long-term weight loss. Meal replacements make it easier for people to follow a restricted energy regimen.

After five years, a very low energy diet resulted in a six percent loss of body weight, compared with two percent for those who followed low-calorie diets with more usual foods.

Source: *American Journal of Clinical Nutrition* 2001;74:579-584.

754. SHORT EXERCISE BOUTS JUST AS EFFECTIVE

Exercisers, take note: Short bursts of activity daily are just as effective as one long session when it comes to burning calories, losing weight, and improving aerobic fitness. Working in shorter bouts (such as three 10-minute bouts or two 15-minute bouts) may be easier than trying to find time for one continuous 30-minute exercise session.

Ten minutes of moderate exercise daily can also improve mood and reduce fatigue.

Just two minutes of stair climbing several times a day can lower total cholesterol, raise HDL cholesterol (the "good-guy" variety), and improve the resting pulse rate in sedentary young women.

Source: *Journal of the American College of Nutrition* 2001;20:494-501.

755. MIDDLE-AGED MEN: WEIGHT LOSS SAFE

Weight loss and weight fluctuation in middle-aged men do not directly increase health risk, provided there are no preexisting diseases – so no excuses guys! The increased mortality in middle-aged men is determined to a major extent by disadvantageous lifestyle factors and preexisting disease, not from sustained weight loss and weight fluctuation (cycling) itself. Middle-aged men who are recent ex-smokers show the most marked increase in mortality associated with sustained weight loss.

Source: *Archives of Internal Medicine* **2002;162:2575-2580.**

ON-THE-JOB HEALTH CONCERNS

IN THIS SECTION:
- MOBILE PHONE DANGERS
- NIGHT SHIFTS
- OFFICE HAZARDS
- FERTILITY RISK JOBS
- CAR MECHANICS
- BUTCHER, BAKER

ON-THE-JOB HEALTH CONCERNS: MOBILE PHONE DANGERS

756. MOBILE PHONES: HEADACHES & MORE

If you experience headaches, warmth on your ear, or burning sensations on your face, consider reducing your mobile phone use. Users of mobile phones commonly report headaches, warmth on the ear, and burning sensations of facial skin. A study of 17,000 people in Sweden and Norway who use mobile phones as part of their job was conducted, and reported symptoms were similar for both groups:

The sensations of warmth were predominately experienced during the actual phone call. Other symptoms, like headaches, began during or within half an hour after the call and usually lasted for up to two hours. A large percentage reported that the symptoms developed only after phones calls lasting five minutes or longer. Other factors related to symptom onset were stress conditions and difficulty hearing. The most common strategies for symptom relief, according to the researchers, were reducing the duration of calls and using hands-free equipment.

Swedish research on people with brain cancer found that tumors are more likely to occur on the side of the head more often in contact with mobile phones.

Source: *Occupational Medicine* **2000;50:237-245;** *Reuter's Medical News* **Aug 2000.**

757. HANDS-FREE KIT CAN REDUCE RADIATION

If you talk often on a mobile phone, invest in a hands-free mobile phone kit. This can result in a *90 percent* reduction of the electromagnetic radiation that such phones give off. Analog phones, widely used in the US, transmit higher power and radiation levels, but hands-free kits reduce these levels. Britain recently urged parents to curb children's use of mobile phones after a government-backed report showed early evidence that mobile phone use had a "cooking" effect on the brain. And Japan recently announced its plans to impose new limits on mobile phone radio-wave emissions, in line with international safety recommendations that maximum exposure be less than two watts per kilogram (2.2 lb) of the user's weight.

Source: *Reuter's Medical News* Aug 2000.

WANT TO KNOW MORE?
[See Hint #288 in the *Childhood Illnesses & Health Problems* section for an informative hint on the risks cell phones pose to children.]

758. MOBILES PHONES, STUFFY NOSES & WORSE

Stuffed-up nose? Yet another reason to use an earpiece when talking on your mobile phone, which can cause a measurable increase in skin temperature and "stuffy nose." The use of mobile phones has been associated with headaches, increased blood pressure, and brain damage. Furthermore, people exposed to very low intensity microwave energy (as emitted by mobile phones) report hearing sounds such as buzzes, clicks, and tones. There are also reports of fatigue, sensation of burning skin, and hot ears. A significant increase in temperature is found after just two minutes of telephone conversation.

The increase in nasal resistance in the nostril on the same side as the phone may be due to the dilation of the arteries and veins in the nose caused by this temperature increase – resulting in the sensation of a stuffed-up nose. But such changes are *not* seen when an earpiece is used to avoid close exposure to the electromagnetic field.

Sources: World Congress on Lung Health; 10th European Respiratory Society Annual Congress, Florence, Italy, Sep 2000; *Reuter's Medical News* Aug 2000.

WANT TO KNOW MORE?
Some recommendations issued by Britain's Department of Trade and Industry: If you place your mobile phone in your pocket, place it with the keypad toward your body; let the earpiece cable of the hands-free kit hang down from your ear rather than making contact with your cheek; keep the cable away from the phone's antenna; don't place the phone directly against your body.

ON-THE-JOB HEALTH CONCERNS: NIGHT SHIFTS

759. SHIFT WORK & THE TOLL ON YOUR HEALTH

Working the night shift can throw off your body's natural rhythms, leading to chronic sleep disturbances, gastrointestinal problems – even heart disease. The modern world's move away from 9-to-5 jobs is taking a toll on the health of workers. Attempts to sleep at inappropriate phases of the circadian cycle can result in shorter sleep episodes and more awakenings. Short-term effects of shift work are similar to symptoms of jet lag: daytime sleepiness, disturbed sleep, gastrointestinal problems, and lowered alertness. The difference is that travelers will eventually adapt to their environment, while shift workers continue to live out of synch with their daily surroundings.

Shift workers also face a higher risk of developing heart disease – possibly due to the metabolic effects of working and sleeping unusual hours. Some things that can help lessen the negative effects of shift work include controlling your caffeine and alcohol intake, and sleeping in a dark, quiet environment.

Source: *Lancet* **2001;358:999-1005.**

WANT TO KNOW MORE?
[Night shifts have also been linked to breast cancer in women workers. See Hint #172 in the *Cancer, Breast* section for more information.]

ON-THE-JOB HEALTH CONCERNS: OFFICE HAZARDS

760. HEALTH HAZARDS OF THE OFFICE

The negatives aren't just low pay and annoying coworkers – the office environment can be bad for your health in many ways. Photocopying is associated with nasal irritation; working with self-copying paper is associated with eye, nose, skin, and respiratory problems (including wheezing, coughing, mucus production, and bronchitis), and lethargy; and working in front of a video display terminal is associated with headache, eye problems, and lethargy.

Specific office tasks appear to result in specific symptoms. Adverse symptoms from photocopying may be related to emission of volatile organic compounds. Symptoms associated with work at video display terminals may be related to eye strain and musculoskeletal strain, rather than exposure to electromagnetic fields. If you work under any of these conditions, consider a daily green supplement and a fiber mix powder to help detoxification and optimal health status.

Source: *American Journal of Epidemiology* **1999;150:1223-1228.**

761. COMPUTER FANS SHOULD BE CLEANED

Protect yourself from exposure to harmful microorganisms by having your computer fan cleaned on a regular basis. Cleaning the inside of your computer regularly, especially around the power supply fan, helps avoid accumulation of fungus.

Several types of yeast and mold were found in samples taken from computer fan screens.

When checked in a hospital setting, samples gathered from room air approximately six feet from computers revealed isolates of *Candida*, *Aspergillus niger*, *Phaeoannellomyces*, *Rhodotorula*, and *Rhizopus*.

Source: American Society for Microbiology meeting, Orlando, FL, May 2001.

762. BEWARE COMPUTER eTHROMBOSIS

Sitting in front of the computer for hours on end could increase your risk of thrombosis, referred to as "economy class syndrome" when it develops in passengers taking long plane trips. Just as you must get up and walk around in a plane on long-haul trips, so should you regularly stand up while sitting at your computer desk. Thromboemolism (blood clots) can form even if you have no other risk factors. Thrombosis caused this way is referred to as "eThrombosis."

In view of the widespread use of computers in relation to work, recreation, and personal communication, the potential burden of eThrombosis may be considerable.

It is advisable for anyone who commonly sits for prolonged periods at a computer to undertake frequent leg and foot exercises and take regular breaks for mobilization away from the computer.

It's very common for people sitting still for a few hours to get little tiny blood clots, that disappear when they get up and walk. But if they then sit there for long periods of time, you can see how the clot might grow and the leg might swell, and how a bit [of the clot] might break off and go to the lung [or the brain].

"If you add to that other risk factors, like somebody who perhaps in the past broke their leg, or somebody with some sort of co-existing illness, then you get to a point where you might develop a serious blood clot," conclude the researchers.

[You might also want to consider some anti-coagulation supplements such as aged garlic extract and nattokinase.]

Source: *European Respiratory Journal* 2003;21:374-376.

ON-THE-JOB HEALTH CONCERNS: FERTILITY RISKS

763. MISCARRIAGE RISK FOR FLIGHT ATTENDANTS

The risk of miscarriage may nearly double for female flight attendants who continue to work during pregnancy. Fifteen percent of women who continue to fly during pregnancy have a miscarriage (also called spontaneous abortion). Flight attendants who miscarry usually work an average of 74 hours per month, compared with 64 hours a week for those who deliver live babies.

Age, smoking, alcohol use, and previous miscarriages increase the risk.

Flight attendants have many potentially hazardous on-the-job exposures, including increased gravitational forces and increased radiation exposure.

Source: *American College of Occupational and Environmental Medicine* 1998;40(3):210-216.

764. WORK EXPOSURE & LOWERED MALE FERTILITY

Men exposed to pesticides and radiofrequency energy (including communication equipment, microwave ovens, and medical and industrial heating devices) have higher rates of fertility problems. These jobs lead to reduced sperm counts and other effects on semen quality. These subtle abnormalities can affect fertility.

Researchers estimate that nine million US workers are exposed to radiofrequency energy from sources such as communication equipment, microwave ovens, and medical or industrial heating devices.

These devices can emit high electromagnetic fields (though no radioactivity).

Workers exposed to pesticides have reductions in several measures of semen quality, including sperm concentration and percentage of sperm with normal motility (movement).

The higher the level of pesticide exposure, the greater the sperm abnormalities.

Organophosphate pesticides, including the widely used pesticides *ethylparathion* and *methamidophos*, have known toxic effects on the male reproductive system at high exposure levels. However, the men in this new study had low-level exposure, within recommended safety limits.

Source: *American College of Occupational and Environmental Medicine* 2000;42(10):993.

ON-THE-JOB HEALTH CONCERNS: AUTO MECHANICS

765. CAR MECHANICS AT RISK FOR NEUROPATHY

Car mechanics need to be wary of breathing in aerosol brake cleaner because of the potential for serious neurotoxic problems caused by its use, and water-based solutions should be considered in the future. Aerosol brake cleaner and certain other products used by car mechanics contain hexane, a known peripheral neurotoxin.

The neurotoxic effects of hexane can be intensified when it is used with other chemicals found in automotive degreasers. These products are sprayed on brakes, tools, small spills, and engine surfaces, and can cause *paresthesias* (a skin sensation, such as burning, prickling, itching, or tingling), in hands and feet, even if the aerosol products contain only one to five percent hexane and only two percent of the methyl ethyl ketone.

Even when levels meet government standards, deleterious effects can occur. Just breathing in the hexane can result in problems. Water-based rather than hexane-based cleaning solutions should be used instead.

Source: *Morbidity and Mortality Weekly Report* **2001;50:1011-1013.**

ON-THE-JOB HEALTH CONCERNS: BUTCHER, BAKER, CANDLE-STICK MAKER

766. BUTCHER, BAKER...TESTICULAR CANCER?

Meat and bakery workers are about three times more likely to develop a specific form of testicular cancer. Risk is also elevated in janitors, kitchen workers, and utility company employees, especially in the electrical power industry. Some of the groups at risk share common characteristics, such as exposure to cleaning agents, disinfectants, and insecticides.

Leather workers have a nearly fivefold increase in the risk of this cancer, called *nonseminoma testicular cancer.*

Source: *Journal of Occupational & Environmental Medicine* **2001.**

WANT TO KNOW MORE?
Seminoma type cancers are more common among doctors, dentists, and veterinarians.

OSTEOPOROSIS & OTHER SKELETAL PROBLEMS

Osteoporosis is epidemic in the US. One out of three women will demineralize her bones enough to cause fracture during her lifetime. Nor are men exempt! Measures to control or minimize the occurrence of osteoporosis have been leaping forward and spreading like wildfire. Too many are missing the boat. The most prominent advice has been the increased use of calcium. The application of calcium as an additive in foods and drugs, plus the excessive promotion of large doses of calcium supplementaion with disregard for othe important nutrients, is just one part of the misinformation.

IN THIS SECTION:
I. BONE FRACTURES
·   CAUSES & PRECURSORS
·   NATURAL REMEDIES & SUPPLEMENTS

II. HIP FRACTURES
·   CAUSES & PRECURSORS
·   NATURAL REMEDIES & SUPPLEMENTS
·   REDUCING RISK

III. OSTEOPOROSIS
·   CALCIUM CONNECTION
·   CAUSES & PRECURSORS
·   NATURAL REMEDIES & SUPPLEMENTS
·   DIETARY TACTICS
·   REDUCING RISK

I. BONE FRACTURES

BONE FRACTURES: CAUSES & PRECURSORS

767. SODA CAN LEAD TO BONE FRACTURES

Try to limit both your own and your children's consumption of carbonated beverages such as soda, which can increase the risk of bone fractures. Drinking any type of carbonated beverage is linked to an increased likelihood of having a bone fracture, with an even greater increase seen in those who drink cola and who are also very physically active. Active girls who drink cola are *five times* more likely to have bone fractures than girls who don't drink soda.

One reason for this may be that cola drinks contain phosphoric acid, which has been shown to affect calcium metabolism and bone mass. Since teen consumption of soft drinks is on the rise, and because adolescence is such a crucial time for bone development, parents should limit their children's intake of these beverages.

Activities such as walking, jumping, and hopping can help increase bone mass, but this benefit does not occur in the presence of cola consumption.

Sources: *Archives of Pediatric & Adolescent Medicine* 2002;154(6):610-613; *Adolescent Medicine* 2002;13(1):53-72; *Pennsylvania Dental Journal* 2000;67(5):29-32.

768. EARLY FRACTURES = LATER FRACTURE RISK

If you have already broken a bone (or bones) in the past, you have an increased risk for more bone fractures later in life – so NOW is the time to take preventive measures. A history of bone fractures between the ages of 20 and 50 (excluding those related to auto accidents) is a significant independent predictor for the risk of subsequent fractures after the age of 50.

[My favorite preventive measures for better bone health include the supplement velvet antler (for its chondroitin, glucosamine, and other amazing bone-protective substances), regular exercise, 20 minutes of sunshine daily (for vitamin D), silica (as found in rolled oats), figs (for their calcium, phosphorus, and magnesium content), fatty fish (such as salmon and mackerel), nuts and seeds (for boron), and green veggies (for calcium and the other minerals necessary for proper calcium absorption). In addition, avoiding red meat and sugar is also helpful.]

Source: *Archives of Internal Medicine* 2002;162:33-36.

BONE FRACTURES: NATURAL REMEDIES & SUPPLEMENTS

769. ANTLERS FOR FASTER BONE HEALING

Break a bone? The supplement velvet antler can help to speed up the healing process. Velvet antler accelerates fracture healing by stimulating the proliferation of chondrocytes and osteoblast precursors, cells that are essential for healthy bones. (Chondrocytes are the living cartilage cells of the collagen fibers that give cartilage its physical properties. Osteoblasts are cells that help to build bone.) Test animals given velvet antler have a healing rate 75 percent faster compared to those animals not given the supplement.

The fact that chondroitin sulfate and glucosamine sulfate are found together in velvet antler supports the notion that the whole natural velvet antler product will continue to outperform any one of its constituents used in isolation.

Sources: Research Center of New Drugs, Changchun College of Traditional Chinese Medicine, China; *Zhongguo Yao Li Xue Bao* 1999;20(3):279-282; **B. Kamen,** *The Remarkable Healing Power of Velvet Antler.*

WANT TO KNOW MORE?
[Velvet antler has anti-inflammatory properties, and is also useful in the treatment of diseases such as arthritis (see Hints #85 and #107). For a good introduction to this supplement, see my book, *The Remarkable Healing Power of Velvet Antler*.]

II. HIP FRACTURES

HIP FRACTURES: CAUSES & PRECURSORS

770. FLUORIDATED WATER & HIP-FRACTURE RISK

Make sure to drink bottled or filtered water both at home and when in restaurants, as the fluoride found in tap water increases the risk of hip fractures in women. The Environmental Protection Agency (EPA) has set a maximum contaminant level for fluoride at four parts per million (ppm), or four mg/liter, to prevent crippling skeletal fluorosis. However, crippling skeletal fluorosis has been reported even in areas naturally fluoridated at one ppm – the level a majority of Americans consume from their fluoridated water supply.

[Fluoride may make bones denser, but it also makes them more brittle. If a restaurant you frequent does not use bottled water for your tea, coffee, or soup, be sure to complain (and bring your own bottle to the table for your drinking water until they get the idea). And, of course, drink only bottled or filtered water at home.]

Source: *American Journal of Epidemiology* **Oct 1999.**

WANT TO KNOW MORE?
[See Hint #785 for a hint about how fluoride can lead to osteoporosis.]

771. WRIST FRACTURE NOW, HIP LATER?

f you have experienced a wrist fracture, you are at twice the risk of a future *hip* fracture – so take measures NOW to improve you bone health. Most women who fracture a wrist do not get nutritional advice from their doctors on how to protect their bone health in the future. But in the majority of cases, a wrist fracture should be a warning that osteoporosis is very likely.

As many as 350,000 hip fractures occur each year in the United States, and with the aging population that number could reach 650,000 by the year 2050.

Source: *Journal of Bone Joint Surgery* **2000;82:1063-1070.**

772. TOO MUCH VITAMIN A & HIP FRACTURES

Be advised: Long-term excessive vitamin A intake may contribute to an increased risk of hip fractures. [Retinol (another name for preformed vitamin A) is often added to breakfast cereals and meal replacement beverages – without the benefit of FDA regulation. Low-fat and nonfat milk is found to contain 624 micrograms of retinol per liter, margarine 55 micrograms per pat. So you can start to see where the excess retinol in our diets may be coming from.]

In an 18-year study of over 72,000 women, those with the highest vitamin A intake were found to have a *significantly* elevated relative risk of hip fracture compared with women with the lowest intake (less than 1,250 micrograms a day) – leading researchers to conclude that the amounts of retinol in fortified foods and vitamin supplements may need to be reassessed.

Source: *Journal of the American Medical Association* **2002;287:47-54.**

773. NOT HAVING CHILDREN INCREASES RISK

Women who have never given birth, be warned: You are at increased risk for postmenopausal hip fractures. Those women who have never had a child have an increased risk of both hip and spine fractures compared with women who have had children. However, it is the hip-fracture risk that is significant: such women have a 45 percent increased risk of postmenopausal hip fractures independent of bone mineral density. Each additional birth confers a protective effect against postmenopausal hip fracture. (For each additional birth, there is a 14 percent decreased risk.)

Source: 23rd Annual Meeting of the American Society for Bone and Mineral Research, Phoenix, AZ, Oct 2001.

HIP FRACTURES: NATURAL REMEDIES & SUPPLEMENTS

774. COD LIVER OIL FOR VITAMIN D PROTECTION

Because women who experience hip fractures are usually deficient in vitamin D, good old-fashioned cod liver oil is a simple and important solution to this ever-increasing problem. An estimated 26 to 38 million American adults have osteoporosis. This risk increases with age. Reductions in sun exposure contribute to low vitamin D levels. The National Institutes of Health recommend 400 IU of vitamin D supplement daily for individuals ages 51 to 70, and 600 IU daily for those older than 70 years of age.

Source: *Journal of the American Medical Association* **1999.**

775. VITAMIN K AGAINST HIP FRACTURES

Increasing your dietary intake of vitamin K can help reduce your risk of future hip fractures. Although vitamin K does not appear to increase bone mineral density, it does reduce the risk of hip fractures. Consumption of one or more daily servings of lettuce (the food that contributes the most to dietary vitamin K intakes) is associated with a lowered hip-fracture risk.

[Vitamin K, a fat-soluble vitamin (the others are A, D, and E) can be manufactured by your body. The natural form is found in plants such as alfalfa, dark leafy greens, and kelp. Animal foods that supply vitamin K are liver, egg yolk, and fish liver oils.

High intake of vitamin E or calcium (as in supplemental form) may reduce vitamin K absorption. Rancid oils (as in salad dressings) and fats, X-rays, radiation, aspirin, air pollution, and frozen foods all destroy vitamin K. *Acidophilus*, by increasing the functioning of intestinal bacterial flora, contributes to vitamin K production.]

Sources: *American Journal of Clinical Nutrition* **1999;69(1):74-79;2000;71(5):1201-1208.**

WANT TO KNOW MORE?
Studies such as these support the suggestion for a reassessment of the vitamin K requirements that are based on bone health and blood coagulation.

HIP FRACTURES: REDUCING RISK
776. HELP TEENS *NOW* TO AVOID HIP FRACTURES

Parents of young girls, take note: For women, *exercise* during the teenage years may be more important to future bone mineral density than calcium intake. Results from the Penn State Young Women's Health Study show an association between adult hipbone density and exercise patterns during the teenage years, but *not* teenage calcium consumption.

In healthy girls, an association is seen between participation in sports between the ages of 12 and 18 and eventual hipbone mineral density by age 18 (but not total body bone mineral gain).

However, daily calcium intake (ranging from 500 to 1,500 mg/day in the study) is not associated with either hipbone mineral density at 18 or total body bone mineral gain between the ages of 12 through 18.

The amount of physical activity that distinguishes a sedentary teenager from one who engages in some form of daily exercise is related to a *significant* increase in peak hipbone mineral density.

Source: *Pediatrics* **2000;106:40-44.**

WANT TO KNOW MORE?
[More exercise and play, and less sedentary activities such as television watching, is important for the bone mineral density of very young children. See Hint #293 in the *Childhood Illnesses & Health Problems* section for more details.]

777. ACTIVE MEN HAVE FEWER HIP FRACTURES

Get moving, guys: It has been confirmed that exercise reduces the risk of osteoporotic hip fractures in men 44 years of age or older. In a 21-year study of over 3,200 healthy men aged 44 years or older, it was found that even *moderate* levels of physical activity protect men from future hip fractures. (A greater improvement is seen in those men who go from being *completely* sedentary to being moderately active, compared with those who go from modest to moderate activity.)

One warning, however: Excessive athletic activity is tied to an increased likelihood of arthritic changes in the hips and the knees in both men *and* women. [Aerobic walking is the best exercise. It doesn't require any expensive equipment and you already know how to do it.]

Source: *Archives of Internal Medicine* 2000;160:705-708.

WANT TO KNOW MORE?
[Did you know that stroke patients are at increased risk of hip fractures? See Hint #981 in the *Stroke* section for more information.]

III. OSTEOPOROSIS
778. OSTEOPOROSIS IS *NOT* A DISEASE

Before learning how to prevent and treat osteoporosis, it is important to better understand what it is. Osteoporosis describes the bone mineral density when it falls below an *arbitrarily* defined threshold. It is not a disease in its own right. Like hypertension, it is a *risk factor* – one of several which may lead to a potential bone fracture.

Fracture prevention involves many factors; therefore, difficulties exist with simply measuring bone density and interpreting the results. Which means that bone-density screening should not be so widely promoted. [This has been my view for a long time, so it is gratifying to learn that it is shared by physicians who have spent time evaluating the problems involved.] While it is unfortunate that bone-density scanning is so popular, it is easy to see why: it appears to demonstrate graphically what is going on. But it's hardly the whole picture, or even the most important aspect. Treating a single risk factor is never in your best health interest. Treatment is almost always with drugs, and doctors cannot be sure that their advice is appropriate (as demonstrate with the use of hormone replacement therapy).

Source: *British Medical Journal* 2000;321:882-885;2001;322:862.

WANT TO KNOW MORE?
[A third of women and one in eight men will sustain an osteoporotic fracture at some time.]

OSTEOPOROSIS: CALCIUM CONNECTION

779. CHOOSING THE BEST CALCIUM SUPPLEMENT

When selecting your calcium supplement, choose calcium *citrate* over calcium carbonate, as it will provide your body with more available calcium. Although calcium carbonate supplements may contain more elemental calcium per pill than calcium citrate, studies confirm calcium citrate is 2.5 times more *bioavailable* than calcium carbonate. (In the case of calcium supplements, bioavailability refers to the amount of calcium a person actually absorbs from a supplement, rather than the amount of elemental calcium a supplement contains before it is taken.)

But be aware that calcium absorption from supplements does not necessarily confer bone protection.

Source: *American Journal of Therapeutics* 1999;6(6):313-21.

780. CALCIUM ABSORPTION & OSTEOPOROSIS

Did you know that the more calcium you consume, the *less* efficient you are at absorbing it? Low-calcium diets actually increase calcium absorption through complex mechanisms. Part of that process involves your vitamin D metabolism. Adequate intakes of vitamin D are needed to optimize calcium absorption and promote bone health.

Other factors that can influence calcium absorption include weight, smoking, and intestinal transit time. High-protein diets can increase urinary calcium excretion and result in a negative calcium balance.

But some of these factors explain only a small percent of the variation in calcium absorption efficiency. Reviews of studies focusing on the causes of osteoporosis often give little emphasis to the important role of calcium absorption. Although this omission reflects attention on bone mineral density (merely one parameter for judging your bone health), low calcium absorption *significantly* increases the risk of hip fracture in women.

Sources: *Annals of Internal Medicine* 2000;132(5):345-53; *American Journal of Clinical Nutrition* 2000;72(3):675-676.

WANT TO KNOW MORE?
[See my booklet, *Startling New Facts About Osteoporosis*, for a good introduction to this subject.]

781. DAIRY PRODUCTS ARE *NOT* BONE PROTECTIVE

Be advised: An extensive study shows no evidence that higher intakes of milk or calcium-rich foods can help reduce the incidence of bone fractures — and cottage cheese may even have a negative affect on bones! A 12-year study of over 77,000 women, aged 34 through 59, indicates that higher intakes of total dietary calcium or calcium from dairy foods is *not* associated with a decreased risk of hip or forearm fractures. So a higher consumption of calcium-rich foods by adult women may not be protective against broken bones.

Dairy foods vary widely in their content of those nutrients known to affect calcium excretion and skeletal mass. Cottage cheese may actually adversely affect bone health. (The few studies with evidence that dairy foods may be protective mostly had outcomes that were not significant.)

There are too few studies done on men to determine whether dairy foods promote male bone health. But the current body of evidence proves inadequate to support a recommendation for daily intake of dairy foods in the general population.

Sources: *American Journal of Clinical Nutrition* 2000;72(3):681-689; *American Journal of Public Health* Jun 1997;87(6):992-997.

782. ALUMINUM INHIBITS CALCIUM ABSORPTION

Aluminum – which can come from sources such as tap water, canned drinks, antacids, cooking utensils, and preservatives – can *inhibit* calcium absorption. Aluminum is a ubiquitous element found in especially significant amounts in corn, yellow cheese, salt, and tap water. Aluminum cookware can also be a major source. Too much aluminum can cause problems with metabolic processes, in particular those concerning calcium, phosphorus, and iron. So it's especially harmful to the skeleton and the nervous system.

Other sources of aluminum are canned drinks, cosmetics, and the water and utensils used in food preparation. Aluminum in the environment can be the result of acid rain leaching it from the soil. Common aluminum-containing food ingredients are used mainly as preservatives, coloring agents, leavening agents, and anti-caking agents (but the amount of aluminum in the diet is small, compared with the amount of aluminum in antacids and in some buffered analgesics.)

Sources: *Journal of Nutrition* 2001;131:2007-2013; Przegl Lek 2000;57(11):665-668; *Regulatory Toxicology & Pharmacology* 2001;33(1):66-79; *Toxicology Ind Health* 1997;13(5):649-654; 1998;14(1-2):209-221.

WANT TO KNOW MORE?
It's interesting to note that high concentrations of aluminum are found in cancer cells.

783. ALCOHOL, DRUGS & EFFECTS ON CALCIUM

Be advised: The consumption of alcohol (but not wine) can contribute to calcium loss. Other substances that can contribute to calcium loss include tetracycline, diuretics [such as caffeine], and aluminum-containing antacids, which can cause calcium loss through the kidneys.

On the other hand, supplementary calcium can decrease the antibiotic power of tetracycline. Excess calcium can also inhibit thyroid activity and can suppress levels of zinc, magnesium, and manganese. And even modest amounts of supplementary calcium can cause constipation.

Source: W.A. Heiby, *The Reverse Effect* (Mediscience Publishers), 576-578.

784. VEGGIES HELP REDUCE CALCIUM EXCRETION

Increasing your intake of vegetables and fruits can help reduce the amount of calcium excreted by the body. The average American diet contains a large amount of acid (in the form of phosphates and sulfates). On such a diet, the dietary acid causes urinary excretion of both the acid and calcium.

Reducing the acid load – by consuming a diet rich in fruits and vegetables – reduces the amount of acid and the associated amount of calcium excreted in the urine.

Source: *Lancet* 1997;337(9):637.

OSTEOPOROSIS: CAUSES & PRECURSORS

785. FLUORIDATED WATER & OSTEOPOROSIS

Make sure you are getting your water from bottled or filtered sources, as drinking fluoridated water (such as tap water) increases your likelihood of developing osteoporosis. There has always been a lingering doubt about the safety of water fluoridation in relation to the skeleton. Consumption of fluoridated water has increased in the US, and high concentrations can produce fluorosis, a crippling bone and joint disorder.

Unfortunately, as water fluoridation becomes more widespread, osteoporosis in the general population increases. [All the more reason to learn how to start protecting yourself!]

Source: *Lancet* 2000;355:247-248.

WANT TO KNOW MORE
[Not surprisingly, fluoride in our drinking water also increases the risk of hip fractures. Two studies in the US and several in Europe have provided ecological evidence that exposure to fluoridated water over a lifetime can increase the risk of hip fractures, despite causing increases in bone-mineral density. See Hint #770 for more information.]

786. STEROID DRUGS CAN CAUSE BONE LOSS

Be warned: When taken without adequate calcium and vitamin D supplementation, steroid drugs such as cortisone can cause rapid bone loss.
This kind of drug-induced osteoporosis may develop in as many as 50 percent of those who take steroid drugs (referred to as *glucocorticoids*) for six months or longer, including those inhaled by asthma patients. Initial bone loss during this time might be as much as 15 percent! Those taking high doses for longer periods are at even higher risk for fractures.

About half of asthmatic children who use inhaled steroids every other day have low bone mass (*osteopenia*). Maintaining adequate calcium and vitamin D intake, as well as engaging in physical activity, is essential – especially for children at risk for osteoporosis.

Source: *Clinician Reviews* 2002;12(4):75-82.

787. CAFFEINE & CALCIUM LOSS

Ladies, do you really need that second cup of coffee? Be warned that caffeine intake increases the rate of bone loss in women over 50. Osteoporotic fractures are, like coronary artery disease, largely a disease of Western societies. Increasing evidence validates that diets high in fruit and vegetables are beneficial in preventing fractures (while high calcium intake does *not* prevent them).

A long-standing question [something I have been exploring for years] is: Why do populations who consume low-calcium diets have fewer fractures than do Western societies who consume high-calcium diets?

New information shows that intakes of caffeine in amounts more than 300 milligrams a day (equivalent to about 18 ounces of brewed coffee) accelerate bone loss at the spine.

Source: *American Journal of Clinical Nutrition* Nov 2001;74(5)571-573;694-700.

WANT TO KNOW MORE?
[Did you know that the more calcium we consume, the less efficient we are at absorbing this mineral? This is explained in detail in my booklet, ***Startling New Facts About Osteoporosis***.]

788. LOW IGF-1 & OSTEOPOROTIC FRACTURES

Low levels of the hormone IGF-1 (*insulin-like growth factor*) and postmenopausal osteoporosis are strongly linked. Research shows that low IGF-1 concentrations, although not a strong determinant of bone mineral density, does predict the risk of fracture independently of bone mineral density. IGF-1 may have an important role to play in maintaining bone strength by other mechanisms not yet fully understood. [IGF-1 can be found in significant amounts in the supplements velvet antler and colostrum.

IGF-1 may also be beneficial for adolescent diabetics. See Hint #383 in the *Type 1 Diabetes* section for more information.]

Source: *Lancet* **2000;355:898-899.**

OSTEOPOROSIS: DIETARY TACTICS

789. LESS ANIMAL PROTEIN FOR BONE HEALTH

Increasing your intake of vegetable protein while decreasing your intake of animal protein may help to decrease bone loss and the risk of hip fracture. Different sources of dietary protein have different effects on bone metabolism. Animal foods provide predominantly acid precursors, whereas the protein in vegetable foods is accompanied by base precursors not found in animal foods.

A high dietary ratio of animal to vegetable protein results in more rapid bone loss and a greater risk of hip fracture than does a low ratio. (The associations are unaffected by age, weight, estrogen use, tobacco use, exercise, total calcium intake, or total protein intake.)

Source: *American Journal of Clinical Nutrition* **2001;73(1):118-122.**

790. VEGGIE POWER FOR HEALTHIER BONES

Increasing your dietary intake of vegetables is important for better bone health. After examining more than 3,000 women for markers of bone resorption, researchers conclude that a low intake of vegetables is associated with increased levels of substances that are *not* bone protective. These findings remain statistically significant for postmenopausal women and also for those on hormone replacement therapy. [So much for the theory that synthetic HRT helps to prevent osteoporosis!] And this relationship remains significant even after adjustment for important confounding factors – further evidence that a high consumption of alkaline-forming foods is positively linked to the skeleton.

The results of this study relate to vegetables specifically – no similar beneficial associations are seen with high fruit intake as are seen with high vegetable intake.

Source: **Aberdeen Prospective Osteoporosis Screening Study, UK, 2002.**

791. INCREASE CALCIUM IN SOUP WITH A BONE

Increase the calcium content of any soup or stew by adding a beef bone and cooking it for a prolonged period. Because low dietary calcium intake may accelerate bone loss, we are often advised to increase our dietary intake of calcium. However, many are unable to tolerate common calcium sources such as milk and dairy products. But experiments conducted on different soup preparation show that prolonged cooking of a bone in soup increases the calcium content of the soup.

Source: *Calciferous Tissue International* **1994:54(6):486-488.**

792. CANDY NOT SO DANDY (FOR YOUR BONES)

Here's yet another reason to limit candy and sweets: High candy consumption is associated with low bone mineral density. A high consumption of fruit and vegetables has a more positive effect on bone mineral density than do diets containing high amounts of meat, dairy, bread, a combination of meat and sweet baked products, sweet baked products alone, alcohol, candy, or cereal. Candy has the *most* negative effect among these groups of dietary patterns.

Here again is a demonstration that bone mineral density is the result of dietary patterns. The nutrients known to affect bone-mineral density are often found *together* in foods.

Source: *American Journal of Clinical Nutrition* **2002;76(1):245-252.**

OSTEOPOROSIS: NATURAL REMEDIES & SUPPLEMENTS
793. VITAMIN D: TAKING TOO LITTLE?

Be advised: The recommended daily dose of 400 IU of vitamin D is *not* sufficient for bone protection – but it is safe, easy, cheap, and effective to double the dose to 800 IU. Vitamin D is both a vitamin and a hormone. One study showed that 400 IU of vitamin D with a high amount of calcium produces no reduction in the rate of bone fractures. But increasing your daily intake to 800 IU produces no side effects, and should have an impact on the enormous problems and cost attributable to osteoporotic fractures, especially among older people.

Dietary sources of vitamin D are scarce [limited to mostly dairy products, eggs, and fish liver oils], yet it is *essential* for bone health. Widespread vitamin D deficiency continues to be neglected, despite its high prevalence. Deficiency is even seen in patients with vitamin-D intakes above recommended levels.

[The sun is effective for correcting the deficiency. I recommend about 30 minutes daily – but I also encourage you to take detoxifying supplements like chlorella to compensate for the ultraviolet rays.]

Source: *British Medical Journal* 1998;317:1466-1467.

794. SUNNY LOCALE? TAKE VITAMIN D ANYWAY

Even if you live in a sunny climate, supplementing with vitamin D may help preserve your bones and reduce your risk of fractures. Vitamin D has a significant seasonal variation, but levels are generally deficient in 27 percent of the population and borderline in 40 percent. Supplementation with vitamin D helps to normalize low vitamin D status, as well as increase bone mass.

Although vitamin-D deficiency is a major problem among older people, pubertal adolescent females with low vitamin D are at a significant risk of not reaching maximum peak bone mass, particularly in the lumbar (lower) region of the spine.

In addition to getting sufficient amounts of vitamin D, high intakes of vegetables and fruits (as much as nine portions per day), along with active participation in physical activities, are key to optimizing bone health – especially in postmenopausal women.

Source: World Congress on Osteoporosis, 2002.

795. VELVET ANTLER AGAINST OSTEOPOROSIS

The supplement velvet antler may help to stimulate bone formation, protecting you from osteoporosis and the risk of bone fractures. Current treatments for osteoporosis are based on maintaining bone mass by inhibiting bone resorption. But compounds have been identified in velvet antler that stimulate *bone formation* in test animals with osteoporosis.

Velvet antler appears to increase bone mass substantially, restoring the disrupted bone architecture common in those suffering from osteoporosis.

Source: First International Symposium on Antler Science and Product Technology, Banff, Canada, Apr 2000. Reported by G.R. Mundy, MD, UT health Science Center, San Antonio, TX.

WANT TO KNOW MORE?
[Velvet antler has anti-inflammatory properties, and is also useful in the treatment of diseases such as arthritis (see Hints #85 and #107). For a good introduction to this supplement, see my book, *The Remarkable Healing Power of Velvet Antler*.]

796. TAKE GINKGO FOR STRONGER BONES

The common herbal supplement ginkgo may help prevent bone loss and reduce your risk of osteoporosis-related fractures. The conventional recommendation is that strong bones (and a low risk of developing osteoporosis) depend on adequate calcium intake. However, a variety of other nutrients play roles in bone formation. The herb ginkgo (as in Ginkgo biloba) contains several antioxidant compounds, called *polyphenolics*, that may prevent bone loss and osteoporosis-related bone fractures. (Many of the antioxidant polyphenolics found in ginkgo are similar to those found in vegetables.)

Osteoblast cells are bone-building cells. When exposed to ginkgo, these cells have a nearly *fourfold* increase in proliferation, perhaps due to the herb's effect on cell-energy levels.

Source: *Nutrition Research* **2001;21:1275-1285.**

WANT TO KNOW MORE?
[Warning: As ginkgo is also a mild blood thinner, it should be avoided by those already on blood-thinning medications. And epileptics should also steer clear of ginkgo, as it may cause seizures in those with this condition.]

797. COFFEE, TEA, OR BONE DENSITY?

When given the choice, choose tea over coffee: Although caffeine may reduce bone-mineral density, tea contains other nutrients (such as flavonoids) that may actually improve bone mass. The majority of studies demonstrating reduced bone mass from caffeine are from populations in which coffee drinking predominates and is the major caffeine source. But an extensive study shows that women who drink tea have higher bone-mineral density than those who do not drink tea. Habitual tea consumption, especially for more than 10 years, has significant beneficial effects on bone-mineral density of the total body, lumbar spine, and hip regions in adults.

Bone-mineral density is influenced by compounds contained in tea extracts, including a variety of important phytochemicals – meaning that tea drinking may be protective against osteoporosis.

Sources: *American Journal of Clinical Nutrition* **2000;71(4):1003-1997;** *Archives of Internal Medicine* **2002;162:1001-1006.**

OSTEOPOROSIS: REDUCING RISK

798. LOW-IMPACT EXERCISE & BETTER BONES

Are you walking yet? Walking for about 30 minutes, a few days a week, is enough to improve bone mass. Aerobic exercise can increase bone density, and it need not be a high-impact exercise regimen. Because exercise improves balance and coordination, it could also reduce older women's odds of falling. The benefits are similar among premenopausal and postmenopausal women. The good news is that the most popular form of exercise in the US – walking – can give a lift to bone mass. Since strength training with weights also helps bone density, the ideal exercise plan includes aerobics *and* weights [see Hint #799 that follows for more information].

Source: Annual Meeting of the American Public Health Association, Atlanta, GA, Oct 2001.

799. WEIGHT-BEARING EXERCISES FOR BONES

Women, take note: In addition to aerobic exercise, weight-bearing exercise can help you to better maintain bone mineral density. In a five-year study done on postmenopausal women, those who participated in weight-bearing exercises (in this case, simple controlled jumping three times a week while wearing an 11-pound weighted vest) showed a three to five percent improvement in bone mineral density compared to the women who exercised but did not participate in the weighted-vest routine. This number is significant, as a five percent advantage in bone mass equals a *30 percent* reduction in fracture risk. (All of the women who participated had been walkers before but none were strong muscularly.) Long-term exercise combining weights with jumping are key to preserving bone mass. The earlier you start, the better. Consider buying an inexpensive mini-trampoline and some hand weights.

Source: *Reuter's Medical Report*, Jun 2000.

800. DON'T HIDE FROM THE SUN!

Walking at noon exposes you to more vitamin D from the sun than at any other time of the day – important for your bone health. Vitamin D is in short supply in our diets, and deficiency of this nutrient contributes to malabsorption of calcium. Twenty minutes of daily exposure to sunshine will be highly beneficial to your bones, and hardly detrimental to your skin (especially if you consume lots of fresh vegetables and fruits for their protective antioxidant content).

Sources: *Journal of Bone Mineral Research* 2000;15(9):1856-62; *Zhonghua Wai Ke Za Zhi* 1992; 30(8):454-7, 508.

WANT TO KNOW MORE?
[Daily sunlight is not just good for your bones. It can help prevent many serious health problems, including cancer. See Hint #163 in the *Cancer (General)* section for more details.]

801. YOUNG ADULTS & VITAMIN-D DEFICIENCY

Protect teens and young adults from osteoporosis down the road by making sure they are taking supplemental vitamin D and getting enough daily sunlight. Vitamin-D deficiency is extremely prevalent in seniors, but young adults aged 18 to 29 have an equal to greater risk of this nutrient deficiency. In fact, vitamin-D deficiency is increasing in young adults. And contrary to what many people believe, simply drinking vitamin D-fortified milk is of no help.

Vitamin D, which helps you to absorb calcium, is made by your body whenever your skin is exposed to sunlight. A deficiency of this vitamin places you at risk for osteoporosis, as well as chronic bone and muscle pains. In fact, muscle pain and fatigue can be the first signs of vitamin-D deficiency. But luckily, treatment is simple: 800 IU of vitamin D daily, and making sure to get out into the sun for about 30 minutes a day [even in the winter]. Many young adults who take daily multivitamin supplements during the summer and winter months have vitamin D levels 30 percent higher than those who do not take vitamin supplements.

Sources: *American Journal of Medicine* 2002;112:659-662; *Biogerontology* 2002:3(1-2):73-77.

WANT TO KNOW MORE?
[A deficiency in vitamin D may also increase your risk of developing certain cancers. See the *Cancer (General)* section for good advice on how to reduce your risk.]

802. DON'T LET OSTEOPOROSIS GO UNTREATED!

If you have been diagnosed with osteoporosis, take control of your health — learn about and begin bone-health therapies as soon as possible. Results of a study done by the University of Buffalo show that almost half of American women diagnosed with osteoporosis remain untreated even one year after diagnosis. After one year, of those women who had discussed the diagnosis with their doctor, only approximately 54 percent had started actual treatment. (In general, those starting treatment tended to have a more advance form of the disease, saw their physician more than once a year, and were better educated compared to the women who knew they had osteoporosis but did not begin treatment.)

The researchers conclude that there are many women with osteoporosis who are unaware of their condition – and a great deal of education about this disease is still needed.

Source: Annual Meeting of the Society for Epidemiological Research, Palm Desert, CA, reported in *Reuter's Health,* Jun 2002.

803. EAT NATTO FOR VITAMIN K

Increasing evidence indicates a significant role for vitamin K in bone metabolism and osteoporosis, and one of the best ways to get it is to consume natto, a fermented soybean food. Natto is eaten frequently in the eastern part of Japan, but seldom in western Japan. The women in the western part of Japan experience significantly more fracture risk. Concentrations of vitamin K are much higher in frequent natto eaters, resulting in increased serum vitamin K.

A statistically significant inverse correlation is found between incidence of hip fractures in women and natto consumption in each prefecture throughout Japan. These findings indicate that the large geographic difference in the vitamin K levels may be ascribed, at least in part, to natto intake and suggest that higher level resulting from natto consumption may contribute to the relatively lower fracture risk in Japanese women.

See Hint #775 for more information on vitamin K and fractures.

Source: *Nutrition* 2001;17(4):315-21.

804. MALABSORBERS: BETTER BONE UP!

One obstacle that likely interferes with calcium consumption among many ethnic groups is lactose *maldigestion*. Several investigators have observed a relationship between lactose maldigestion, dietary calcium, and osteoporosis in Caucasian populations. Dietary management strategies for lactose maldigesters is to include consumption of viable yogurt.

See Hint #224 and Hint #321, and the *Lactose Intolerance* section for more information.

Source: *Journal of the American College of Nutrition* 2001;20(2 Suppl):198S-207S.

805. EAT PRUNES FOR BONE HEALTH

Dried prunes are an important source of boron, which plays a role in the prevention of osteoporosis. A serving of prunes (100 grams, equivalent to about the size of a fist) fulfills the daily requirement for boron (two to three mg). Prunes are dried plums, cultivated and propagated since ancient times.

Dried prunes contain approximately 6.1 g of dietary fiber per 100 g, while prune juice is devoid of fiber due to filtration before bottling. The laxative action of both prune and prune juice could be explained by their high sorbitol content. Prunes are a good source of energy in the form of simple sugars, but do not mediate a rapid rise in blood sugar concentration, possibly because of their high fiber content.

Phenolic compounds (compounds with high antioxidant activity) in prunes had been found to inhibit human LDL oxidation and thus might serve as preventive agents against chronic diseases, such as heart disease and cancer. Additionally, the high potassium content of prunes (745 mg/100 g) might be beneficial for cardiovascular health.

Source: *Critical Reviews in Food Science & Nutrition* 2001;41(4):251-86.

806. SHAKE OUT THE SALT SHAKER

Salty foods and the addition of salt to food should be avoided. There is a direct correlation between salt intake and calcium excretion. Several studies have reported that high sodium intake increases not only urinary sodium but also urinary calcium .

Sources: *Medical Journal of Australia* 2000;173 Suppl:S106-7; *Mineral Electrolyte Metabolism* 1997;23(3-6):265-8.

807. NO BONES ABOUT IT: MEN AT RISK

Osteoporosis in older men typically causes greater morbidity and earlier mortality, so senior men should heed *all* the osteoporosis advice. High fruit and vegetable intake appears to be protective in men.

Sources: *American Journal of clinical Nutrition* 2002;76(1):245-52; *Geriatric Nursing* 2000;21(5):242-4.

WANT TO KNOW MORE?
Bone loss affects both men and women of all cultures and races. In spite of the universality of this phenomenon, variations in bone loss do exist. Women are more affected by this age-related bone loss than men; white women more so than black women; smaller women more than larger women; meat eaters more than vegetarians, those taking prescribed drugs more than those who are drug-free; the sedentary more than the active; malabsorbers more than those with excellent digestive systems, and smokers are more susceptible than nonsmokers.

To confuse the issue, the sex component varies in different cultures. For example, there is an equal incidence among men and women in Hong Kong, and more men than women get osteoporosis in Singapore. Obviously, factors other than whether you are male or female may be similarly influential. We've all seen toddlers take frequent falls while learning to walk. At this stage they rarely break their rubbery, still-underdeveloped bones. The grade-school child may get a hairline crack. The bones are as supple as young twigs, bending and breaking only partway through. And then there are the parents, who may break a bone if they fall heavily on it. Grandpa might even break a bone without falling at all. healthy bones are more resistant to fracture, and likely to heal more readily if a break occurs.

808. FAT BOOSTS CALCIUM ABSORPTION

The amount of dietary fat consumed has an important role to play in calcium absorption, so it's advisable to consume some food with natural fat in it with your meals. Among the factors influencing calcium absorption are the foods ingested in the same meal. Foods that enhance the absorption of calcium are fatty fish, eggs, butter, and liver. Foods that diminish the absorption of calcium are sodas, unleavened bread, and milk.

So two people with the same calcium intake will absorb different amounts of calcium if one is enjoying:
>   scrambled eggs for breakfast
>   salmon salad for lunch
>   liver and onions for dinner

while the other has:
>   cornflakes and milk for breakfast
>   drinks a Tab midmorning
>   has a hamburger and a Coke for lunch
>   another soft drink in the afternoon
>   a dinner of beef stew pita pouches or unleavened bread

Both diets offer calcium of about equal quantity, but the amount of calcium utilized can be very different.

Further evidence of the complexity of calcium absorption is demonstrated by the fact that despite the vast difference of calcium between cow's milk and mother's milk – cow's milk contains four times more calcium than human milk – the infant who is breastfed absorbs more calcium. The experts are still trying to sort out the mechanisms at work here.

809. GERMANIUM MAY HELP, TOO!

Germanium may be physiologically important, especially as it relates to bone DNA concentrations. [Although there isn't too much research on this element, I was pleased to find this one correlation. Plants and waters known to have special therapeutic properties have relatively high concentrations of germanium. These plants are garlic, aloe, comfrey, chlorella, ginseng, and watercress. Some additional plants have significant quantities of germanium, but they are herbals that are not familiar to most people. These include shelf fungus (a variety of Reishi mushroom), shiitake mushrooms, pearl barley, sanzukon, sushi, waternut, boxthorn seed, and wisteria knob.

Some of the first tests validating the safety of germanium in supplemental form were actually conducted in the US in the 1960s. For more information on germanium, see my booklet, *Germanium: A New Approach to Immunity.*]

Sources: *Biological Trace Element Research* 2002;89(1):239-50.

810. STAY AWAY FROM HIGH PHOSPHORUS FOODS

A correct calcium/phosphorus ratio is essential for good calcium absorption, but we get entirely too much phosphorus in our American diet. Phytic acid impairs calcium bioavailability. This can be prevented by using fructo-oligosaccharides. And the ratio becomes more in keeping with good health with physical exercise.

[Both calcium and phosphorus should be supplied by food in almost equal amounts. The average American diet, which is so high in phosphorus, is definitely not conducive to this one-to-one ratio. Consuming high calcium foods such as milk does not serve to correct the problem or alter the ratio. Milk and milk products are almost equal sources of both phosphorus and calcium, and sometimes contain even more phosphorus. Cottage cheese, for example, is considerably higher in phosphorus than calcium.

At high levels of ingestion, calcium absorption decreases sharply. (Remember – it's only a quicker picker-upper at low levels.) Therefore, even if the same quantities of calcium and phosphorus are absorbed the ratio shifts in favor of phosphorus.

Foods containing phosphorus are:
- almost all processed or canned meats (hotdogs, ham, bacon)
- processed cheeses
- baked products that use phosphate baking powder (commonly used)
- cola drinks and other soft drinks
- instant soups and puddings
- toppings and seasonings
- bread
- cereal
- meat
- potatoes
- phosphate food additives: phosphorus acid, pyrophosphate, polyphosphates, such as chelators, sequestering and emulsifying agents, acidulators, water binders, including sodium phosphate, potassium phospthate, or phosphoric acid.

Foods that contain calcium in abundance and are devoid of phosphorus are not exactly everyday fare. Seaweed, anyone? Foods that contain an excellent ratio of calcium and phosphorus are also limited.

Sprouts are on top of that short list. Corn on the cob is good, fresh halibut and chicken breast are not bad, peanuts are good if not salted, split-pea soup is excellent, whole eggs are right in the ball park, whole milk has too much phosphorus, and collard greens, although high in phosphorus, are so healthful, they should be eaten with a variety of other good foods anyway.

Sources: *Biological Trace Element Research* **2002;89(1):43-52;** *Nutrition Hospital* (**Nutricion Hospitalaria) Spain)2002;17(4):204-12.**

PAIN

In her inimitable style, Emily Dickenson wrote:about pain in 1863. Two of my favorites examples follow.

"Pain: cannot recollect when it begun – or if there were a time when it was not. It has no future – but itself."

"There is a pain – so utter – it swallows substance up. Then covers the abyss with trance, so memory can step around, across, upon it."

Many pharmaceutical companies are pursuing the "holy grail" of an effective pain relief drug that has no harmful side effects. A few natural herbs come close. But we must remember that pain is a signal that something somewhere in our body has gone askew.

811. ACUPUNCTURE *DOES* RELIEVE PAIN

If you are suffering from chronic pain, acupuncture may offer relief. There is scientific evidence that acupuncture is effective as a replacement for long-term use of painkillers for various chronic illnesses. Acupuncture has been found to relieve nausea, back pain, dental pain, and migraine headache.

(There is still debate, however, whether acupuncture is effective against osteoarthritis, and it is found to be *ineffective* in overcoming the urge to smoke or eat.)

Since more and more patients *and* doctors are now turning to acupuncture as a viable treatment, it is recommended that medical schools begin training their students about its safety and effectiveness.

Source: *Acupuncture: Efficacy, Safety & Practice***, report of the British Medical Association.**

812. HOT & COLD WATER FOR PAIN RELIEF

For relief from severe pain in your feet or legs, try this old-fashioned remedy: Alternate between applications of hot and cold water – a hot water soak for 10 minutes, followed by an icy water soak for 10 minutes, and repeat two or three times. Alternating hot and cold water is excellent for poor circulation and pain relief. The trick is to apply both the hot and cold for the same length of time. If ten minutes is not doable, start with three minutes for each application.

This suggestion belongs in the "Grandma knows best" department. But it works, and you don't have to buy or swallow anything!

813. DEVIL'S CLAW CHASES PAIN

The herb devil's claw appears to be an effective plant alternative for the treatment of chronic back pain. No serious side effects have been observed with its use, and it has an excellent compliance and tolerability record. An effective dose is two 480 mg tablets a day.

Source: *Phytotherapy Research* **2001;15(7):621-4.**

814. LAVENDER, THE "FEEL-GOOD" AROMA

Lavender oil aromatherapy has been shown to result in a positive change in blood pressure and pulse, pain, anxiety, depression, and sense of well-being in hospice cancer patients.

Source: *American Journal of Hospital Palliative Care* **2002;19(6):381-6.**

PARASITES

The competitive interactions between invading parasites and antibodies in your living being are incomparable. The awesome sophistication of the strategies involved are still being sort out by the scientists. *(Trends in Parasitology* **2002;18(9):387-90)**

815. FIBER AGAINST PARASITES & TOXINS

Protect yourself from intestinal parasites by adding a good supplemental fiber mix to your daily regimen. Low fiber diets encourage the attachment of parasites. A good fiber supplement is a necessity in the American diet because most of our foods do NOT supply enough fiber (and that includes most fruit and many vegetables).

If the intestinal contents move too slowly, toxic by-products of digestion and bacterial fermentation remain in the bowel too long, and get reabsorbed back into your body. Over time, this contributes to illness.

Source: B. Kamen, *New Facts About Fiber.*

WANT TO KNOW MORE?
[Your fiber supplement should contain several fiber sources, not just one or two. See my book, *New Facts About Fiber*, for a good introduction to this important subject.]

PARKINSON'S DISEASE

Diagnosis of Parkinson's Disease remains challenging because of variability of symptoms and signs. Tremors, loss of balance, shuffling gait, trouble with tasks such as turning a bed, opening jars [hey, isn't that all of us?], and difficulty walking heel to toe should be regarded as suspect for this disease. (*Journal of the American Medical Association* **2003;289:347-353**)

IN THIS SECTION:
- CAUSES & PRECURSORS
- NATURAL REMEDIES & SUPPLEMENTS

PARKINSON'S DISEASE: CAUSES & PRECURSORS

816. CONSTIPATION & PARKINSON'S DISEASE

Men with constipation are more likely to develop Parkinson's disease than are those with regular, daily bowel movements – another good reason to add a supplemental fiber mix to your daily regimen. An extensive 12-year study shows that men who do not have daily bowel movements are 2.7, 4.1, and 4.5 times more likely to develop Parkinson's than are men who have one, two, or more bowel movements per day, respectively. (This demonstrates that the pathology of Parkinson's involves more than just the brain.)

[Increasing your intake of dietary fiber is one good way to relieve constipation. Try eating a bowl of organic oatmeal for breakfast, along with a couple of tablespoons of a good multi-fiber supplement – every day! Although various fibers have similar characteristics, their differences outweigh the features they share. That's why I recommend supplements containing a variety of fibers.]

Sources: *Neurology* **2001;57:456-462**; B. Kamen, *New Facts About Fiber*.

PARKINSON'S DISEASE: NATURAL REMEDIES & SUPPLEMENTS

817. FOLATE DEFICIENCY & PARKINSON'S

If you have a family history of Parkinson's disease, you should be taking a supplement containing 400 micrograms of folate daily. Folate (folic acid) is a B vitamin that allows nerve cells to repair their damaged DNA and continue to function properly. A diet that contains inadequate amounts of folate may increase the risk of developing Parkinson's disease.

Cells in the brain are more susceptible to damage and death when animals consume a folate-deficient diet, which also elevates levels of homocysteine, which in turn exacerbates Parkinson's-like symptoms.

[Homocysteine is an amino acid produced naturally in your body, but high levels in the blood are associated with an increased risk of many health problems.] Animals fed a folate-deficient diet show more severe symptoms and have homocysteine levels *eight times higher* than those fed a diet with folate.

[Some good dietary sources of folate are spinach, kale, beet greens, beets, chard, asparagus, broccoli, liver, and brewer's yeast. But cooking destroys the nutrient, as does storage at room temperature.]

Source: *Journal of Neurochemistry* 2002;80:101-110.

818. VITAMIN E AGAINST PARKINSON'S DISEASE

Reduce your risk of Parkinson's disease by increasing your consumption of dietary vitamin E. Dietary intake of vitamin E from food and the consumption of nuts appears to reduce your risk of developing Parkinson's disease, but supplemental vitamin E does not have the same effect. [It is quite possible that the vitamin E used by most people is synthetic and/or of the alpha-tocopherol variety, rather than a total E-complex. E-complex vitamin E (tocotrienols) contain all the beneficial factions, not just the alpha faction.]

[Some dietary sources of vitamin E are butter, egg yolks, and liver. Tocotrienols can be found in foods and oils such as palm oil, rice bran oil, wheat germ, barley, saw palmetto, and certain types of nuts and grains.]

Source: *Neurology* 2002;59:1161-1169.

WANT TO KNOW MORE?
[Because frying oils, processing and milling of foods, bleaching of flours, and cooking remove much of the vitamin E content in foods, we are now consuming at least *90 percent less* vitamin E than we consumed 100 years ago!]

819. COENZYME Q10 AGAINST PARKINSON'S

Treatment with a natural substance known as coenzyme Q10 may help to slow the functional deterioration associated with Parkinson's disease. Treatment with 1200 milligrams of coenzyme Q10 (CoQ10) daily slows the progression of Parkinson's disease *significantly*. This high dose slows decline in all areas measured, including mental and motor skills, but the greatest effect is seen in the activities of daily living. Although lower doses of the drug also slow disease progression, the differences are not as dramatic as with the higher dose.

Researchers had originally started investigating whether CoQ10 would be useful in treating the disease because Parkinson's patients show reduced levels of this antioxidant. Treatment with CoQ10 appears to be safe and very well tolerated.

[Some dietary sources of CoQ10 are spinach, peanuts, beef, and fish such as mackerel and salmon.]

Source: Archives of Neurology 2002;59:1523,1541-1550.

WANT TO KNOW MORE?
[CoQ10 may be also be beneficial for a variety of other health problems, including asthma (see Hint #119), type 2 diabetes (Hint #402), hypertension (Hint #626), and migraines (Hint #508).]

PNEUMONIA

The first signs of classic pneumonia are a painful dry cough, intense fatigue, and a high fever. Among the risk factors are low body mass, smoking, respiratory infection, previous pneumonia, chronic lung disease, lung tuberculosis, asthma, treated diabetes, cronic liver disease, use of aerosols, smoking 20 cigarettes a day, and chronic bronchitis. (*European Respiratory Journal* **1999;13(2):349-55)** The next hint reveals another risk factor

820. PNEUMONIA & ORAL HYGIENE

Reduction of death rates from pneumonia, especially among older people, may come from a very unlikely place – your mouth. Oral care is much more effective in decreasing mortality rates for pneumonia than are medical treatments for the disease, especially among senior citizens.

Individuals suffering from pneumonia who do not have proper dental care have *twice* the rate of fever as do those pneumonia-sufferers who receive proper dental care. And patients receiving proper dental care have *half* the mortality rate due to pneumonia.

(These benefits are NOT restricted to seniors who retain their own teeth.)

Source: *Journal of the American Geriatric Society* 2002;50:430-433.

WANT TO KNOW MORE?
[Poor dental health, especially gum disease, has been linked to many serious diseases and health problems, such as rheumatoid arthritis (see Hint #103), heart disease (see Hint #526), and low birth weight (see Hint #851).]

POISONING

In cases of poisoning admitted to hospitals, there is a peak between the ages of 16 and 25. Analgesics are the most common agents among drugs incriminated in poisoning. (*Journal of Toxicology; Clinical Toxicology* **2002;40(7):833-7**)

821. KEEP ACTIVATED CHARCOAL HANDY

Make sure to keep activated charcoal on hand to be given in case of accidental poisoning. Activated charcoal is the preferred initial treatment for most poisons ingested by children. It is easily administered at home and significantly reduces the time it would take to otherwise be administered in the hospital. (The average time to activated charcoal treatment at home is 38 minutes compared with 73 minutes in the emergency room.) While parents are advised to have activated charcoal in the home, it is still a good idea to speak to either the poison center or a pediatrician before administration.

Source: *Pediatrics* **2001;108(6):100.**

POOR CIRCULATION

Serious interruptions in circulation can lead to strokes and heart attacks, but your clever body attempts to cope and compensate long before the fatal, final event. Symptoms such as a cold, pale complexion, or slow-healing cuts may be the harbinger of circulation problems to come.

822. AGED GARLIC FOR COLD HANDS & FEET

If you suffer from poor circulation, including cold or numb hands and feet, taking aged garlic extract may help. Available in most health stores, aged garlic extract can raise skin temperatures and improve numbness and chilling of the limbs. Aged garlic extract given to healthy subjects increases skin temperatures in the hands and feet, and after 14 days of daily administration even higher skin temperatures are seen in those same areas.

These results suggest that aged garlic extract can help improve blood flow and aid those suffering from poor circulation. [See Hint #812 for a pain-relief remedy that is also good for improving circulation.]

Source: *Japanese Pharmacology & Therapeutics* **1994;22(8):3695-3701.**

PREGNANCY & CHILDBIRTH

Rejecting traditional lore and often ignorant of scientific nutrition, many doctors chastise mothers-to-be if they gain weight beyond a magic number they have invented. Following this advice has resulted in the epidemic of premature, low-birth-weight infants in the US.

The period of reproduction imposes the greatest physiological stress. At no other time is there such an extemely altered process of biological mechanisms. Because of these demands and changes, nutritional requirements are of prime importance. Nutrition that might support an adult may not support a growing fetus. Actually, it may not support an older, frail adult either. Therefore, many of these recommendations also apply to our aging society!

It is interesting to note that some of the evidence-based results that follow demonstrate how modern science is rediscovering the value of the "natural way." There is no question about the correlation between good food intake during pregnancy and healthy babies, or the pregnancy diet and a child's ability to reach his or her intellectual potential.

IN THIS SECTION:
I. STAYING HEALTHY THROUGH YOUR PREGNANCY

II. MORNING SICKNESS & NAUSEA
- ALTERNATIVE THERAPIES
- NATURAL REMEDIES & SUPPLEMENTS
- RELIEVING SYMPTOMS

III. INFERTILITY & REPRODUCTIVE THERAPY
- ALTERNATIVE THERAPIES
- CAUSES & PRECURSORS

IV. OLDER MOTHERS

V. PREGNANCY COMPLICATIONS
- BIRTH DEFECTS
- CESAREAN SECTION
- ECTOPIC PREGNANCY
- LOW BIRTH WEIGHT
- MISCARRIAGE
- PRE-ECLAMPSIA
- PREMATURE BIRTH
- STILLBIRTH

VI. HEALTHIER BABIES
- ASTHMA & ALLERGIC DISEASES
- BEHAVIORAL PROBLEMS
- BONE DENSITY & BONE HEALTH
- CHILDHOOD CANCERS
- DIABETES
- DRUG DEPENDENCY
- HEART DISEASE & HEART DEFECTS
- MEMORY & COGNITIVE FUNCTION

VII. MOMS WITH PRE-EXISTING HEALTH PROBLEMS
- AIDS
- ASTHMA
- CELIAC DISEASE
- DIABETES
- HYPOTHYROIDISM

VIII. BREASTFEEDING & FORMULAS
- BREASTFEEDING BENEFITS
- BREASTFEEDING CAVEATS

I. STAYING HEALTHY THROUGH YOUR PREGNANCY

823. MOM'S NUTRIENT NEEDS ARE HIGHER

Since a woman's nutrient needs increase during pregnancy and lactation (to support fetal growth and milk synthesis), make sure you are eating well and supplementing with essential vitamins and minerals. Adjustments made by the body to meet these needs alter the amount of ingested nutrients retained. Calcium absorption, for example, increases twofold during pregnancy but drops to values for non-pregnant women during the lactation period. In women chronically consuming a low calcium diet, calcium absorption increases to more than *80 percent* during reproduction.

Zinc absorption also tends to increase during pregnancy and lactation, and selenium absorption is high (80 percent of intake) in both pregnant and non-pregnant women. Pregnant women conserve selenium by decreasing urinary selenium excretion.

Source: *Journal of Nutrition* 2001;131:1355S-1358S.

824. EARLY SCREENING FOR PREGNANCY DIABETES

If you are pregnant, having your blood screened early on for the onset of pregnancy-induced diabetes is a smart idea. Earlier testing (at 16 weeks rather than the standard third trimester) for gestational diabetes should become standard practice, as it can identify more than half of the women who will become diabetic during their pregnancies. Early glucose screening may help reduce the morbidity and mortality rates associated with gestational diabetes to even lower levels than current ones – by permitting appropriate counseling, monitoring, and treatment at the earliest possible time.

Source: *Journal of Reproductive Medicine* 2002;67.

825. LIGHT THERAPY FOR PREGNANCY DEPRESSION

If you are suffering from depression during your pregnancy, bright-light therapy may be an effective treatment. Around five percent of pregnant women meet the criteria for major depression, but doctors are reluctant to prescribe antidepressant medications for fear of their effect on the fetus. But exposure to bright light (phototherapy), a technique used to treat those suffering from seasonal affective disorder (SAD), also works on women suffering from depression during pregnancy. This therapy is nontoxic and inexpensive.

Pregnant women suffering from depression who expose themselves to an hour a day of bright ultraviolet light from a light box within 10 minutes of waking up show moderate improvements after just three weeks. After five weeks of light therapy, depression decreases by 59 percent. (And when the light therapy is discontinued, signs of depression begin to increase.)

Source: *American Journal of Psychiatry* 2002;159:666-669.

WANT TO KNOW MORE?
Light therapy may advance the timing of the daily biological clock, which may bring about the antidepressant effect.

II. MORNING SICKNESS & NAUSEA

MORNING SICKNESS: ALTERNATIVE THERAPIES

826. ACUPUNCTURE AGAINST PREGNANCY NAUSEA

If you are suffering from unpleasant feelings of nausea due to your pregnancy, acupuncture may be able to relieve your symptoms. Pregnant women who experience severe vomiting appear to recover more quickly when they receive acupuncture in addition to more standard treatments. The severity of nausea and the frequency of vomiting both decrease *significantly* and more quickly with active acupuncture than with placebo administration, regardless of when standard medical treatment is received. The beneficial effects of acupuncture are often seen within minutes of the treatment.

Source: *Journal of Pain Symptom Management* 2000;20:273-279.

827. WRIST ACUPRESSURE AGAINST NAUSEA

Learning how to self-administer simple acupressure may help to relieve your symptoms of pregnancy-related nausea quickly and safely, any time you are feeling ill. Try this: Look at your wrist on the palm side. Locate the crease farthest from your hand between your hand and wrist. Measure two thumb widths up from this crease, and press in the middle of your wrist at this spot. There is an acupressure point here, which if stimulated for several seconds, relieves nausea and motion sickness in most people. If you have the point, you should feel a distinct twinge when you stimulate it. (This treatment can be administered several times a day.)

Source: *Journal of Obstetrics & Gynecology; Neonatal Nursing* 2001;30(1):61-70.

MORNING SICKNESS: NATURAL REMEDIES & SUPPLEMENTS

828. VITAMIN B6 & ZINC AGAINST NAUSEA

Taking vitamin B6 (in the pyridoxal form) helps to relieve pregnancy nausea, especially if taken with zinc. Approximately 70 percent of women experience some degree of nausea and vomiting during their pregnancies, but the good news is that these symptoms almost always end by the fourth month. In fact, pregnancies in which nausea and vomiting occur are more likely to have favorable outcomes.

(As I wrote in my book on nutrition and pregnancy over 20 years ago, pregnancy nausea is the body's way of detoxifying to protect the baby. This information has recently been released in a new study, as though it has just been discovered!)

The amount of B6 to be taken should be at least 10 mg (but not exceeding 20 or 30 mg) and should be taken both before and after conception.

Sources: 68th Annual Meeting of The Royal College of Physicians and Surgeons of Canada, 1999; B. Kamen, *The Kamen Plan for Total Nutrition During Pregnancy* (available only online through www.publishingonline.com).

WANT TO KNOW MORE?
Low magnesium levels have also been associated with nausea and vomiting. Consuming magnesium-rich foods (kelp, almonds, greens, and whole grains) could be therapeutic.

829. GINGER HELPS REDUCE PREGNANCY NAUSEA

If you are experiencing nausea and vomiting due to pregnancy, taking ginger may help to relieve symptoms. One gram of ginger a day *significantly* reduces the severity of pregnancy-related nausea and vomiting. In a group of pregnant women given 250 mg of ginger daily, only 37.5 percent had vomited after four days, and 87.5 percent reported their symptoms had improved after one week compared to a control group.

Adverse effects were minor and did not prevent the mothers-to-be from continuing the treatment regimen. No significant differences were observed in spontaneous abortions (miscarriages), term deliveries, or cesarean deliveries, and there were no cases of congenital anomalies.

Source: *Obstetrics & Gynecology* 2001;97:577-582.

MORNING SICKNESS: RELIEVING SYMPTOMS

830. SIMPLE MORNING-SICKNESS RELIEF TIPS

If you are feeling nauseous due to pregnancy, some of these simple tips may bring relief, a list compiled by pregnant women:

- Eat small meals frequently, high in carbohydrates and protein (but avoid fatty or spicy foods).

- Avoid cooking, eating, or smelling spicy or greasy foods.

- When symptoms appear, lie down and rest.

- Try eating dry toast or crackers when you first wake up.

- Eat something every one to two hours while awake (and keep a snack by the bed).

- Salty foods or lemony smells may help settle your stomach. Ask yourself what will make you feel better: something crunchy, salty, sour, fruity, or sweet? Eat it, and don't worry about perfect nutrition right now.

- Avoid getting overtired.

- Keep track of situations and factors that trigger your nausea so that you can avoid those things. Odors, sudden motion, or even looking at busy patterns can serve as triggers.

- Drink peppermint or spearmint tea first thing in the morning. And sipping teas containing mint, raspberry leaf, ginger root, anise, or fennel may help. (In fact, drink plenty of raspberry-leaf tea, as it supplies B vitamins and needed minerals. You can drink one cup of tea daily throughout your pregnancy to tone and prepare your uterus along with relieving your nausea.)

- Try sucking on candied ginger.

- Tincture of wild yam (one dropperful) may be added to a glass of water or mint tea twice a day.

- Homeopathic remedies such as Ipecac 30x, Nux vomica 6x, and Cannibus 30x have been used by some women with success.

- Relaxation, visualization, or self-hypnosis may help.

- Increase B-complex vitamins in your diet. (Try 50 to 100 mg of vitamin B6 twice a day.)

III. INFERTILITY & REPRODUCTIVE THERAPY

INFERTILITY: ALTERNATIVE THERAPIES

831. ACUPUNCTURE & PREGNANCY SUCCESS

If you are considering reproductive therapy, you should know that acupuncture may greatly improve your chances of getting pregnant. Among women undergoing assisted reproductive therapy, acupuncture given before and after embryo transfer *significantly* improves pregnancy rates.

Acupuncture is performed 25 minutes before and after the embryos are transferred. Needles are placed along the spleen and colon meridians (to improve blood flow and energy to the uterus) and at other points to influence the uterus and to stabilize the endocrine system.

The needles are left in place for 25 minutes, and further acupuncture treatment is given after embryo transfer.

Source: *Fertility & Sterility* **2002;77:721-724.**

WANT TO KNOW MORE?
[Acupuncture may also be helpful in reducing the symptoms of pregnancy-induced nausea. See Hint #814 earlier in this section for more details.]

832. THERAPY GROUPS HELP INFERTILE WOMEN

Infertile women, take note: Group support and group therapy can *significantly* increase pregnancy rates. Group psychological intervention could prove to be a cost-effective first step for women who have tried for a while to get pregnant, and could spare women the cost and discomfort of medical interventions.

Fifty-five percent of women in a cognitive-behavioral group and 54 percent in a support group developed viable pregnancies, compared with only 20 percent of women in a control group.

Psychological interventions may affect pregnancy rates at an earlier point than entry into an in vitro fertility program can, and should perhaps be implemented in conjunction with initial medical treatment.

Source: *Fertility & Sterility* **2000;73:805-811.**

INFERTILITY: CAUSES & PRECURSORS

833. PESTICIDES & IN VITRO FERTILIZATION

If you are a couple seeking in vitro fertilization, be aware that fertilization rates are *significantly* impaired when the male partner has had occupational exposure to pesticides. Because most individuals are exposed to multiple pesticides with various active ingredients, it is impossible to draw conclusions as to which specific chemical may be responsible.

Source: *Lancet* 1999;354:484-485.

834. DOES MERCURY LEAD TO INFERTILITY?

Reducing your intake of seafood may help to protect against elevated levels of mercury, which may be an important contributor to infertility in both women and men. Infertile couples have significantly higher blood-mercury levels than do their fertile counterparts, and these mercury levels may be directly related to the amount of seafood consumed.

[Although tuna is the most commonly consumed fish in the US, it is suspected to contain dangerously high levels of mercury due to environmental pollution.]

Mercury gets deposited in the pituitary gland and testicular tissues. Exposure to such endocrine disrupters in the womb and during adulthood is one possible explanation for impaired reproductive health.

Sources: *British Journal of Obstetrics & Gynecology* 2002;109:1121-1125; *Nederlands Militair Geneeskundig Tijdschrift* 2000;107(12):495-498; *Journal of Dentistry* 1999;27(4):239-256; *Occupational & Environmental Medicine* Mar 1995;52(3):214.

WANT TO KNOW MORE?
Women with high occupational exposure to mercury, such as those who work with amalgam in dental offices, are also less fertile than unexposed women.

[Endocrine disrupters are compounds cooked up in test tubes (or byproducts of these compounds), produced for daily industrial, agricultural, or domestic purposes. Endocrine disrupters are new to human existence. *Xenoestrogen* is the name for an endocrine disrupter that is or emits a synthetic estrogen. (*Xeno* meaning "foreign.")

To learn more about: where endocrine disrupters come from, and how they affect fertility, sexual health, and even serious disease, see chapter four of my book, *She's Gotta Have It!*. The chapter also explains where these disrupters come from and what you can do to protect yourself from their harmful effects.]

IV. OLDER MOTHERS

835. AMNIOCENTESIS DANGER FOR OLDER MOTHERS

Older moms, take heed: Women over 40 are nearly *twice* as likely as younger women to lose their babies following a second-trimester amniocentesis. Of course it doesn't have to happen! but if you are an older mom-to-be, you should be especially careful about your diet and risks.

Source: *British Journal of Obstetrics & Gynecology* 2001;108:1053-1056.

V. PREGNANCY COMPLICATIONS

BIRTH DEFECTS: CAUSES

836. ACNE DRUG CAUSES SEVERE BIRTH DEFECTS

If you are pregnant or even considering pregnancy, stay away from the acne drug, Accutane (isotretinoin), which may contribute to severe birth defects, depression, or even suicide. Before taking this medication, you should have two negative pregnancy tests — including one on the second day of your next normal menstrual period. Additionally, if you are taking Accutane, you should use two forms of birth control, have repeat pregnancy tests every month, and register with a survey that monitors the experiences of women taking the drug.

Pregnancies affected by exposure to Accutane continue to occur in the US despite package warnings and a manufacturer pregnancy prevention program (PPP) initiated in 1988. Don't confuse the teratogen warning symbol — a pregnant woman depicted in a circle with a slash through it — with that of a birth-control symbol.

Sources: *Journal of the American Academy of Dermatology* 2002;46:505-509; US Centers for Disease Control and Prevention (CDC), reports released Feb 2000, Aug 2001.

WANT TO KNOW MORE?
The number of Americans using Accutane has soared over the past decade: retail pharmacies filled nearly 20 million prescriptions for the drug between 1982 and 2000. Accutane is used to treat individuals with mild to moderate acne, but too many women taking it become pregnant despite efforts to warn them that the product is known to cause *severe* birth defects.

837. AMNIOCENTESIS & RISK OF CLUBFOOT

If you are pregnant and considering amniocentesis, be warned that the procedure done too early may increase your baby's risk of being born with a clubfoot. No one knows why amniocentesis might lead to clubfoot deformities, but the relationship between early administration of this test (performed between gestational week 11 and week 12 plus 6 days) and congenital foot abnormalities is well documented.

However, the risk declines *significantly* if the procedure is performed later (between week 13 and week 14 plus 6 days.)

After early amniocentesis, 1.1 percent of children are born with a foot abnormality. This figure is significantly higher than the 0.4 percent of children who show a foot abnormality when the test is performed during week 13 but before week 15.

And when amniocentesis is performed even later (between week 15 and week 19 plus 6 days) the rate of clubfoot declines even further, to 0.1 percent. But the difference between this group and a group that undergoes the test between week 13 and week 14 plus 6 days is not statistically significant.

Source: University of Calgary Study, reported in *Reuter's Medical News* Oct 2000.

WANT TO KNOW MORE?
Maternal smoking is also associated with the occurrence of clubfoot. Source: *American Journal of Epidemiology* 2000;152:658-665.

838. BOTTLED WATER & SHORTER SHOWERS SMART

Pregnant women: Avoid drinking tap water and take shorter showers or baths to reduce your risk of miscarriage or having a baby born with birth defects. Exposure to dangerous chlorination byproducts (CBPs) in tap water can be reduced by using carbon filters or by switching to non-chlorinated bottled water. And taking shorter showers and baths also helps to minimize your exposure to CBPs, which can be inhaled or absorbed through the skin.

Source: Report by the Environmental Working Group (EWG) and the US Public Interest Research Group (PIRG).

WANT TO KNOW MORE?
Montgomery County, Maryland, has the most pregnant women at risk in an individual community or water system, while Texas is worst on a statewide basis.

839. CHLORINE DANGER FROM SWIMMING POOLS

A chlorine byproduct found in swimming pools may lead to serious health problems, including spontaneous abortion (miscarriage), stillbirths, and congenital malformations – so pregnant women should be especially careful. Chlorination has been the major disinfectant process for domestic drinking water for many years, but recent studies associate chlorine with numerous adverse reproductive outcomes, including central nervous system problems, cardiac defects, oral cleft (cleft palate), and respiratory and neural-tube defects.

Studies done on tap water indicate these negative consequences at even lower levels of this chlorine byproduct, which is formed when chlorine reacts with organic matter such as skin or hair, or even dust. (Filtering the water can help to keep organic matter at low levels.) Swimmers could be absorbing the chemicals through the skin, inhaling them as they evaporate, or swallowing water.

In studies done in London swimming pools, it was found that although the amount of the byproduct varied according to the water temperature and the number of people in the pool, it was higher than levels found in tap water.

Source: *Chemosphere* 2002;46(1):123-130; *Journal of Occupational & Environmental Medicine* 2002;59(4):243-247.

840. PREGNANT? STOP EATING TUNA

Pregnant women should limit their consumption of fish such as tuna because of high levels of mercury contamination (a sad result of today's polluted oceans), which could potentially result in birth defects. The Food and Drug Administration (FDA) is urging pregnant women and all women of childbearing age to limit their intake of tuna (the mostly commonly consumed fish in the US), swordfish, king mackerel, shark, and tilefish, because of suspicions of danger to developing fetuses. Instead, the FDA urges people to eat a "variety of fish" to ensure against potentially high mercury intake.

The FDA is considering a study on the effects of mercury intake from fish in children.

Source: Food and Drug Administration, Sep 2002.

841. DEFECTS ORGANIC SOLVENTS LEAD TO BIRTH

Pregnant women exposed in the workplace to organic solvents (as in healthcare professions and in the clothing and textile industries) are at *substantially* increased risk of major fetal malformations. Occupational exposure to organic solvents during pregnancy increases the risk of major congenital malformations *13 times*! Malformations occur among women who have symptoms related to exposure, such as irritation of the eyes or respiratory tract, breathing difficulties, or headaches.

Women whose jobs expose them to organic solvents during previous pregnancies also have a higher incidence of miscarriages. Symptomatic exposure appears to confer an unacceptable level of fetal exposure and should be avoided by appropriate protection and ventilation.

Source: *Journal of the American Medical Association* **1999;281:1106-1109.**

842. HAMSTERS, MICE & BIRTH DEFECTS

If you are pregnant, avoid contact with pet hamsters, mice, and other rodents because of the risk of infection that can result in serious birth defects. Many cases of birth defects linked to a rodent-borne pathogen may go undiagnosed as physicians ascribe them to other causes. The disease is spread when humans handle infected rodents or breathe in the virus via dust-sized fecal particles floating in the air. The illness usually produces flu-like symptoms, although infection occurs without symptoms in about a third of cases.

While adults almost always recover without permanent damage, infants who contract the virus in utero can suffer lifelong neurological damage including cerebral palsy, mental retardation, seizures, and (most commonly) blindness or impaired vision. Women working in research laboratories should always wear gloves whenever handling rodents or cleaning their cages.

Source: *Clinical Infectious Diseases* **2001;33:370-374.**

843. HEART MALFORMATIONS FROM URBAN SMOG

Pregnant moms living in cities, be warned: High exposure to urban smog in early pregnancy may raise a woman's odds of having an infant with certain heart defects. The babies of women living in areas with the highest carbon monoxide levels have a *three times higher* risk of particular heart defects than those from areas with the lowest levels. Women with moderately high exposure have smaller increases in this risk.

A similar dose-response pattern emerges when researchers look at maternal ozone exposure and aortic artery and valve defects, and pulmonary artery and valve anomalies.

The second gestational month is a critical time for normal migration and differentiation of *neural crest cells* in terms of cardiac development. (Neural crest cells are notorious for their sensitivity to toxins because of their lack of antioxidative-stress proteins.)

Source: *American Journal of Epidemiology* **2002;155:17-25.**

BIRTH DEFECTS: NATURAL & SUPPLEMENTAL PROTECTION

844. TAKE FOLIC ACID AGAINST BIRTH DEFECTS

All women capable of childbearing should consume 400 micrograms of folic acid per day to decrease their risk of having a baby born with birth defects. Evidence for the protective effects of folic acid (also known as folate) on developing embryos is overwhelming: 400 micrograms daily can reduce the incidence of neural-tube defects such as spina bifida by as much as 85 percent.

Women with prior affected pregnancies may need a larger dose to be effective.

Three strategies are available to women to achieve this goal: use of dietary supplements; use of fortified foods; and/or increased intake of naturally occurring folic acid from foods. [Some good dietary sources of this nutrient include spinach, kale, beet greens, chard, asparagus, broccoli, liver, and brewer's yeast.]

Sources: *New England Journal of Medicine* 1999;341:1485-1490; *Journal of the American College of Nutrition* 1998;17(6):625-630; Annual Meeting of the American Academy of Cerebral Palsy and Developmental Medicine, Washington, DC, 1999.

WANT TO KNOW MORE?
More than 65 percent of new mothers recently surveyed were unaware of the role that folic acid plays in the prevention of birth defects. Seventy-five percent of those who were aware of its benefits did also know that folic acid supplementation is linked to the prevention of spina bifida – but only 16 percent took vitamins within the first three to four weeks of pregnancy.

845. FORTIFIED CEREAL NOT ENOUGH

Be warned: Getting your folic acid just from fortified cereal may not be sufficient to prevent birth defects in your child – so you should be supplementing with a daily multivitamin as well. Women of childbearing age cannot on fortified cereal intake alone for the necessary folic acid needed to prevent neural-tube defects, and so they should be taking 400 micrograms in supplemental form on a daily basis, preferably in a daily multivitamin.

Researchers investigated whether or not cereal fortification of folic acid was enough to prevent neural-tube defect problems. Very few women who do not take supplements get the needed 400 micrograms daily, despite cereal intake. Women of childbearing age need a daily multivitamin that provides 400 micrograms of folic acid.

Source: *American Journal of Public Health* 1999;89:1637-1640.

846. SUPPLEMENT WITH ZINC AS WELL

Women, take note: In addition to folic acid, zinc supplementation during pregnancy may also be helpful in avoiding neural-tube defects in your unborn child. Although folic acid supplementation (and the entire complex of B vitamins) has been widely proposed for pregnant women, trace elements have been neglected. The fact that zinc deficiency produces congenital abnormalities in animals prompted studies to link zinc and neural-tube defects in humans, and a correlation between low zinc levels in the hair of mothers and newborns and neural-tube defects was observed. The role of zinc as a cofactor of various enzymes involved in nucleic-acid metabolism could possibly explain the link with birth defects.

Zinc is found in significant quantities in most animal foods. Oysters have 10 times as much as other sources, but it is also found in fish (especially herring), poultry, and egg yolks. Vegetarian moms should consider consuming more whole grains and nuts.

Source: *Indian Journal of Pediatrics* **2001;68:519-522.**

CESAREAN SECTION

847. RECOVERING FASTER FROM C-SECTIONS

If you have had a cesarean section, resuming a regular diet soon after may help you to shorten your hospital stay. Traditional feeding entails a clear-liquid diet on the day after surgery, with a regular diet the next day if the patient reports bowel function. But those who eat solid food shortly after surgery have a significantly shorter hospital stay: 49.5 hours versus 75 hours. [More than a full day less.] Symptoms of mild ileus (obstruction of the bowels) do not occur significantly more often among those women fed early than among those fed in the traditional pattern.

Source: *Obstetrics & Gynecology* **2001;98:113-116.**

ECTOPIC PREGNANCY

848. IUD & THE RISK OF ECTOPIC PREGNANCY

Women using an IUD should be aware that it could play a role in the development of ectopic pregnancies. The use of an IUD *significantly* increases the risk of ectopic pregnancy (the abnormal positioning of the fetus). In addition, the use of a progesterone IUD at the time of conception and a history of miscarriage and tubal damage can also increase this risk.

However, factors associated with a *decreased* risk include a history of treated lower genital tract infections as well as displacement of the IUD.

Source: *Fertility & Sterility* **2000;74:899-908.**

WANT TO KNOW MORE?
A new study of federal census and health data shows that suburban women are increasingly having low-birth-weight babies, a phenomenon that used to be seen only in inner cities. From 1990 to 1999, low-birth-weight rates in the suburbs of America's 100 largest cities increased by *14 percent* (compared to an only five-percent increase in the cities). These cities and their suburbs represent more than half the US population. Northeastern cities had the highest rate of low birth weights (10.4 percent), while the South had the highest suburban rate (7.8 percent). (***Reuter's Medical News* Aug 2002**)

LOW BIRTH WEIGHT: CAUSES & PRECURSORS

849. SMOKING LOWERS INFANT BIRTH WEIGHT

Pregnant women who *cut down* their smoking instead of completely quitting need to reach low levels of exposure in order to improve the birth weight of their babies. Infant birth weight initially declines sharply as cigarette use during the third-trimester increases. However, this decline levels off at more than eight cigarettes per day.

Women with medium levels of exposure who reduce their cigarette use may not experience improvements in infant birth weight unless they achieve levels that are less than eight cigarettes per day.

Source: *American Journal of Epidemiology* **2001;154:694-701.**

WANT TO KNOW MORE?
[Quitting smoking while pregnant, however, is crucial to the health of your baby — not to mention your own! See the "Smoking & Nicotine Addiction" section for helpful quitting strategies.]

850. AVOID EXPOSURE TO PCE WHEN PREGNANT

If you are pregnant, buy a filter for your showerhead and avoid handling dry-cleaned clothes to avoid exposure to percholorethylene (PCE), a dangerous chemical toxin that can result in low-birth-weight babies. Women who are 35 or older and who are exposed to contaminated drinking water are *twice* as likely to give birth to a small-for-gestational-age (SGA) infant than are women of the same age who are not exposed. Drinking bottled water is only part of the solution: since inhaling PCE is such an efficient way of getting it into the body, showering with contaminated water results in as much exposure as drinking it!

PCE is a common dry-cleaning chemical, so pregnant women should also avoid handling dry-cleaned clothes [and the clothes should be removed from the plastic bags and aired out for several hours in a well-ventilated room]. Women over 35 who have had past miscarriages and who are exposed to PCE are at greater risk of having a small-for-gestational-age infant.

Source: *American Journal of Epidemiology* **2001;154:902-908.**

WANT TO KNOW MORE?

People working in the chemical, metal-degreasing, or dry-cleaning industries, or in scientific laboratories (or even those who live with people who work in these industries) may be exposed to higher levels of PCE. Workers may bring the PCE home on their clothes, or expose others by exhaling their own contaminated breath. Health effects of this chemical may exist at a level below which a health advisory would be issued.

851. GUM DISEASE LINKED TO LOW BIRTH WEIGHT

Need another reason to visit the dentist? Be advised that pregnant women with moderate to severe periodontal disease may be more likely to deliver a low-birth-weight infant. Periodontal disease alone, without the presence of other risk factors, can increase the risk of restricted fetal growth. In fact, it's a risk factor as significant as smoking or alcohol use! Mothers with periodontal disease have about a *twofold* increased risk of impaired fetal growth, and this risk can be *six to 10 times higher* if the periodontal disease progresses during pregnancy and is severe from the start.

While *mild* periodontal disease in the mother does increase the risk of fetal growth restriction and low birth weight, the risk is most significant when periodontal disease is moderate or severe.

Source: International Association for Dental Research, San Diego, CA, Mar 2002.

WANT TO KNOW MORE?

[Periodontal disease in mothers may also result in a premature delivery. See Hint #885 later in this section for more details. And see Hint #526 in the *Heart & Cardiovascular Disease* section for information on the link between periodontal disease and coronary artery disease and stroke.]

852. PRE-ECLAMPSIA TREATMENT & LOW WEIGHT

If you are pregnant and receiving treatment for pregnancy-induced hypertension, be warned that it could have a negative effect on the birth weight of your baby. Treatment of mild-to-moderate hypertension related to pregnancy (known as pre-eclampsia) can adversely affect a fetus's growth. A greater difference in a mother's arterial pressure between the beginning of the therapy and delivery [that is, a desired drop in her blood pressure] is associated with a significantly higher proportion of infants born who are small for their gestational age.

Studies strengthen the argument (albeit weakly) for caution in the use of anti-hypertensive therapy for mild-to-moderate pre-eclampsia.

Source: *Lancet* **2000;355:81-82,87-92.**

WANT TO KNOW MORE?
[For more detailed information on pregnancy-induced hypertension, see the extensive *Pre-eclampsia* segment later in this section.]

853. MOMS: A WARNING ABOUT FLAXSEED

Because flaxseed can affect a baby's reproductive development, use caution when consuming it during both your pregnancy and lactation period. Flaxseed has been shown to affect both pregnancy outcome and reproductive development in test animals. If consumed in large quantities, it can decrease birth weight, among other problems.

Source: *Journal of Nutrition* **Nov 1998;128(11):1861-1868.**

LOW BIRTH WEIGHT: REDUCING RISK
854. HELPFUL TIPS TO AVOID LOW BIRTH WEIGHT

Reduce your risk of having a low-birth-weight baby by:

- Eating a balanced diet high in fiber and low in fat.

- Consuming sufficient calories, vitamins, and minerals — including at least 400 micrograms of the B vitamin folic acid every day.

- Gaining a healthful amount of weight during your pregnancy (the recommended amount is at least 25 to 35 pounds).

- Quitting smoking and staying away from tobacco smoke during your pregnancy.

- Not using alcohol or other drugs, including herbal preparations, unless prescribed by your doctor.

Source: *Journal of the American Medical Association* **2002;287(2).**

855. MODERATE EXERCISE EARLY ON HELPFUL

If you are pregnant, starting a moderate-intensity regimen of weight-bearing exercises may be preventive against having a low-birth-weight baby. Women who start a moderate weight-bearing exercise program during early pregnancy have improved fetoplacental growth rates, and infants born to exercising women are *significantly* heavier and longer, with differences seen in both lean body mass and fat mass, compared to babies born to mothers who do not exercise.

In addition, the mid-trimester growth rate of the placenta is significantly faster in women who exercise than in women who are sedentary.

Source: *American Journal of Obstetrics & Gynecology* **2000;183:1484-1488.**

WANT TO KNOW MORE?
[Be warned, however, that *intense* exercise throughout your pregnancy can have just the opposite effect – babies born at a lower birth weight (but not necessarily at a dangerously low weight). See Hint #856 that follows for more details.]

856. BUT DON'T OVERDO PREGNANCY EXERCISE

Don't overdo it: Although women who exercise *moderately* throughout their pregnancies have larger placentas, a more intense exercise regimen may result in babies who weigh less at birth. Women who exercise at the same rate throughout their pregnancy, or boost the intensity of their exercise regimen later in their pregnancy, give birth to infants who are lighter and have less body fat than women who slow down in the final trimester.

However, none of the babies born to women who exercise moderately or intensely through the ninth month are considered "low-birth-weight babies." These infants are significantly lighter and have less body fat, but are not small enough to be at risk for medical or developmental problems.

Women who exercise vigorously early on and then reduce the intensity of their exercise program as they approach their due dates weigh more and have heavier placentas. (The volume of the placenta is a general marker of the structure's ability to transport oxygen and nutrients to the fetus.) While a heavier placenta can be protective in some cases, heavy exercisers do *not* have dangerously light placentas.

Source: *American Journal of Obstetrics & Gynecology* **2002; 186:142-147.**

WANT TO KNOW MORE?
Regular weight-bearing exercise is beneficial for both mother and baby and the amount of benefit varies with the timing and amount of exercise. If the woman is healthy and the pregnancy normal, regular exercise can do nothing but improve the situation.

857. ZINC FOR LOW=BIRTH-WEIGHT BABIES

If your infant was a low-birth-weight baby, giving him/her zinc supplements may be protective. Zinc supplementation is linked to a substantial reduction in deaths from infectious disease in those infants who were born small for their gestational age. In these children, supplementing with zinc results in reduced rates of severe diarrhea, possibly related to enhanced immune system health.

Source: *Pediatrics* **2001;108:1280-1286.**

LOW BIRTH WEIGHT: LATER PROBLEMS

858. ASTHMA LOW BIRTH WEIGHT NOW, LATER?

If you have had a low-birth-weight-baby, be warned: He/she may be at increased risk of developing asthma down the road. Very low birth weight infants may be at risk for respiratory problems during their elementary-school years, even if they had no respiratory symptoms when newborns. Respiratory symptoms (such as asthma) are *twice* as common in very low birth weight children.

All very low birth weights babies should be followed for respiratory health as they grow — even those with few or no respiratory symptoms.

Source: *American Journal of Epidemiology* **2001;154:521-529.**

WANT TO KNOW MORE?
[If you have had a low-birth-weight baby, read the extensive "Childhood Asthma" section to learn about how to prevent and treat asthma in kids.]

859. LOW BIRTH WEIGHT = LOW IQ IN BOYS?

Pregnant women should be aware that a low birth weight can have an adverse effect on the intelligence of your child, especially for boys — all the more reason to take steps now to prevent it. For reasons that remain unclear, a significant direct association between birth weight and IQ is seen in male babies. It may be because boys are larger than girls at birth and also grow more in the latter part of the pregnancy, so they may be more sensitive to aspects of the uterine environment that restrict fetal growth. It may also have to do with differences in prenatal brain development that are known to exist between boys and girls.

However, this doesn't mean that birth weight is not important for girls – it is simply more significant for male development.

Source: *British Medical Journal* **2001;323:310-314.**

WANT TO KNOW MORE?
IQ is directly linked to birth weight even among children with *normal* birth weights. (In other words, this relationship continues into the normal birth-weight range.)

860. LOW WEIGHT & LATER BEHAVIORAL PROBLEMS

Children born at low birth weights are more likely to have behavioral problems and psychiatric disorders than those born at normal weights. Forty percent of low-birth-weight children are reported to have behavioral problems (this is true of even "heavier" low-birth-weight babies, such as those weighing up to 2,000 grams at birth). The most common problems seen in this group are attention-deficit/hyperactivity disorder (10 percent) and phobia (seven percent). Other problems can include depression, separation anxiety, enuresis (bed-wetting), oppositional defiant disorder, conduct disorder, distractibility, impulsivity, lack of adaptability or social skills, and difficulties in relating to peers. Of all of these, inattention may be the primary issue for the low-birth-weight child.

Source: *Archives of Disease in Childhood: Fetal & Neonatal Edition* **2002;87:F128-F132.**

861. LOW WEIGHT & LATER DEPRESSION IN MEN

Pregnancy is no time to be counting calories: Fetal malnourishment can predispose men to depression later in their adult life. Male infants weighing less than 6.5 pounds at birth may be nearly *four times* more likely to develop depression in old age than their peers who are heavier at birth. But the likelihood of depression at age 68 declines with increasing birth weight among men. (For instance, those weighing less than 6.5 pounds at birth are three to four times more likely to be depressed than male infants weighing more than 8.5 pounds at birth. Those who weigh 6.5 to 7.5 pounds are slightly more than three times as likely to develop depression, while those who weigh 7.5 to 8.5 pounds are 2.8 times as likely to be depressed.)

Males may be more vulnerable than females to poor fetal nutrition because they have faster growth trajectories.

Source: *British Journal of Psychiatry* **2001;179:450-455.**

WANT TO KNOW MORE?
[If you are suffering from depression (from any cause), see the *Depression* section of this book for helpful information.]

862. LOW BIRTH WEIGHT & DIABETES 2 RISK

If you have had a baby born at a low birth weight, he/she may be at increased risk for diabetes later on and should be screened for the disease. Low birth weight is associated with later development of type 2 diabetes and glucose intolerance in men – particularly those with a family history of diabetes. Men who weigh 3,000 grams or less at birth are four times more likely to develop type 2 diabetes than those with a higher birth weight, regardless of family history. (Add a family history of the disease and that risk is 10 times higher!) And low-birth-weight men are about twice as likely to have impaired glucose tolerance and impaired fasting glucose.

Infants weighing less than 5.5 pounds at birth may be more likely to develop insulin resistance, a precursor to type 2 diabetes (as well as heart disease). Insulin resistance syndrome is more common among low-birth-weight infants by the time they reach the ages of eight to 14. Hyperinsulinemia, decreased beta-cell function, elevated blood fats, and central obesity (which are associated with low birth weight) might be the first components of insulin resistance during childhood.

Screening for type 2 diabetes is important for children and adolescents, especially if they are overweight, have a positive family history of type 2 diabetes and are African American, Native American, or Hispanic. On top of these risk factors we can now add low birth weight.

Sources: *Diabetes Care* **1999;22:1043-1047;2001;24:2035-2042;** *Annals of Internal Medicine* **2000;132:253-260;** *American Journal of Clinical Nutrition* **2002;76(2):399-403.**

863. LOW-BIRTH-WEIGHT MOMS & DIABETES

If you yourself were a low-birth-weight baby, you are at increased risk of developing pregnancy-related diabetes – so be sure to get screened early for it. Low birth weight is related to insulin resistance and the development of type 2 diabetes in adults (mainly due to a delay in organ maturation caused by the smaller neonatal size). Pregnancy itself is known to create insulin resistance, and many women develop a condition known as *gestational diabetes mellitus* (GDM), which generally clears up after the baby is born.

A pregnant woman's own weight when she was born could be helpful in determining whether or not she is at especially high risk of developing GDM, as women who were classified as "low birth weight" when they were born are more likely to develop pregnancy-related diabetes. (This link is especially strong for low-birth-weight women who give birth to larger babies.)

Source: *Diabetes Care* **2002;25:1761-1765.**

WANT TO KNOW MORE?
[See Hint #824 earlier in this section for more information on the benefits of early screening for pregnancy-related diabetes.]

864. LOW BIRTH WEIGHT & HEART DISEASE

Death from coronary heart disease is associated with low birth weight, so moms – – please – no dieting during pregnancy! Body mass index in childhood is strongly related to the mother's body mass index, which in turn is related to coronary heart disease. The highest death rates from coronary heart disease occur in boys who were thin at birth but whose weight caught up to them, so that from age seven on they had an average or above average body mass.

Death from coronary heart disease may be a consequence of poor prenatal nutrition.

Source: *British Medical Journal* **Feb 1999;318(7181):427-431.**

865. LOW BIRTH WEIGHT KIDS & HYPERTENSION

Yet another health concern for low-birth-weight kids: An increased risk for hypertension, both in childhood and adulthood. Poor maternal nutrition during pregnancy reduces the baby's birth weight and influences (through a process known as "programming") blood pressure control. There is an inverse association seen between birth weight and blood pressure in both childhood and adulthood (so *lower* weight means *higher* pressure, unfortunately).

Early fetal-placental mechanisms may be critical to the later development of high blood pressure.

Sources: *American Journal of Epidemiology* **2001;153(8):779;** *British Medical Journal* **1999;319:1325-1333.**

WANT TO KNOW MORE?
[See the extensive *Hypertension* section to learn about this condition, as well as helpful information on how to prevent and treat it.]

866. LOW-BIRTH-WEIGHT *MOMS* & HYPERTENSION

Just as women who were themselves low-birth-weight babies have an increased risk of developing pregnancy-related diabetes, they also have an increased risk of pregnancy-related hypertension – so protect your own baby by not dieting during your pregnancy. Women who were born preterm or small for their gestational age have an increased risk of subsequently developing pregnancy-induced hypertension (known as pre-eclampsia) compared with those women born at a normal size and gestational age.

Such findings provide further evidence that the origins of many of the diseases of adulthood (such as hypertension) are at least in some cases occurring very early in life, perhaps even before birth. An important goal of such research is to determine whether these factors are modifiable, and, if so, to what extent. [I believe they are.]

Source: *Archives of Internal Medicine* 1999;159:1607-1612.

WANT TO KNOW MORE?
[For more detailed information on pregnancy-induced hypertension, see the extensive *Pre-eclampsia* segment later in this section.]

867. HIGHER RISK FOR RESPIRATORY PROBLEMS

Pregnant moms, be warned: If you yourself were a low-birth-weight infant, you are approximately *three times* more likely to have baby with respiratory distress syndrome. Women who deliver infants with respiratory distress syndrome had *significantly* lower birth weights when they were born compared to their counterparts giving birth to infants who do not develop respiratory distress syndrome.

Source: *Obstetrics & Gynecology* 2000;95:174-179.

MISCARRIAGE: CAUSES & PRECURSORS

868. PREGNANT? STOP DRINKING COFFEE!

If you are pregnant, stop drinking coffee *immediately* to avoid the risk of having an early miscarriage Consuming high amounts of caffeine daily could increase your risk of having a spontaneous abortion (miscarriage) or a low-birth-weight infant, especially if you experience pregnancy-related nausea. Women who consume at least 20 mg of caffeine daily during the first trimester have a greater risk of miscarriage, and there is an obvious dose-dependent relationship after the occurrence of nausea (which means the greater your caffeine consumption, the greater your risk).

Caffeine may cause a decrease in estrogen levels, which could allay discomfort of pregnancy, decrease the severity and duration of nausea – but subsequently increase the risk of spontaneous abortion. Pregnant women should also monitor their intake of other foods and drinks that contain caffeine, such as tea, soft drinks, and chocolate. (For example, one bar of chocolate, three cups of tea, one can of cola, and one cup of instant coffee would add up to 300 mg of caffeine a day!) And don't forget that caffeine can also be found in many cold and flu medicines.

Sources: *New England Journal of Medicine* 2000;343:1839-1845; *Epidemiology* 2001;12:38-42; **Committee on Toxicity of Chemicals in Food, Consumer Products, and the Environment, UK, Oct 2001.**

WANT TO KNOW MORE?
How much caffeine is in there?
- Average cup of instant coffee: 75 mg
- Average cup of brewed coffee: 100 mg
- Average cup of tea: 50 mg
- Regular cola drink: up to 40 mg
- Regular energy drink: up to 80 mg
- Normal bar of chocolate: up to 50 mg

869.   DON'T FLY UNLESS ABSOLUTELY NECESSARY

Pregnant women at risk for preterm labor or with placental abnormalities should avoid air travel, and it is not generally advisable to fly once gestational age of 32 to 38 weeks is reached. Because air turbulence cannot be predicted and the risk for trauma is significant, pregnant women should be instructed to continuously use their seat belts while seated, as should all air travelers. Pregnant air travelers with medical problems that may be exacerbated by a hypoxic environment, but who must travel by air, should be prescribed supplemental oxygen during air travel. See Hint #763 for information about the risk of flight attendants and miscarriages.

Source: *International Journal of Gynecology & Obstetrics* 2002 ;76(3):338-9; *Obstetrics & Gynecology* 2001;98(6):1187; *Aviation Space & Environmental Medicine* 2000;71(8):839-42.

WANT TO KNOW MORE?
Other potential on-the-job hazards for both female and male flight attendants include increased gravitational forces and radiation exposure.

870.   PREGNANT MOMS: WATCH OUT FOR LEAD

Pregnant moms, be warned: Levels of lead in the blood once considered moderate may increase a woman's risk of having a miscarriage. Lead may be an important contributor to pregnancy loss. Miscarriage in a group of Mexican women associated with lead exposure increased steadily as blood lead levels increased. The lead levels observed in these women were actually *lower* than acceptable standards for occupational exposure in the US and Mexico.

This risk appears to be dose-dependent, as spontaneous-abortion risk associated with lead exposure increases steadily in women as blood lead levels increase.

Source: *American Journal of Epidemiology* 1999;150:590-597.

WANT TO KNOW MORE?
[One potential source of lead exposure could be imported ceramic dinnerware. See Hint #1,079 in the *Environmental Toxins* section for more details.]

MISCARRIAGE: DIETARY TACTICS

871. FOLATE REDUCES MISCARRIAGE RISK

Eat your greens, moms! The risk of having an early miscarriage is *significantly* reduced in women with adequate or even high blood folate levels. In addition to being protective against birth defects, *adequate* folate (folic acid) levels in the mother protect against miscarriage — and *high* folate levels do not increase the risk. In fact, there may even be a protective effect associated with high folate levels. A high folate status, as increasingly seen in the US and many other Western countries because of food fortification and supplement use, is not associated with an increased risk of spontaneous abortion (as was previously believed). However, *low* folate levels are associated with an increased risk.

In addition to low blood folate levels, women with elevated homocysteine concentrations are also at greater risk for early miscarriages – so adding vitamins B6 and B12 to your supplement regime (which in conjunction with folate helps to lower homocysteine) may also be protective. [Folate can be found in leafy greens, which include spinach, kale, beet greens, beets, chard, asparagus, and broccoli, as well as brewer's yeast. Bean sprouts such as lentil and mung are also good. But keep in mind that this nutrient is only available from unprocessed, fresh food.]

Source: *Journal of the American Medical Association* **2002;288:1867-1873;** *Obstetrics & Gynecology* **2000;95:519-524.**

WANT TO KNOW MORE?
[Homocysteine is an amino acid produced naturally in your body, but high levels in the blood are associated with many health problems, including Alzheimer's and heart disease. See Hints #73 and #550 for more details.]

PRE-ECLAMPSIA: CAUSES & PRECURSORS

872.. HIGHER PULSE PRESSURE & PRE-ECLAMPSIA

If you are a pregnant woman whose pulse pressure is elevated early in your pregnancy, you may be at risk for developing a condition known as *pre-eclampsia*. Pre-eclampsia is a pregnancy complication marked by high blood pressure and swelling in the legs that affects as many as one in 10 women pregnant for the first time. If left untreated, pre-eclampsia can develop into *eclampsia*, a life-threatening condition in which a woman has convulsive seizures in late pregnancy or during the first week after her delivery.

Among women who develop pre-eclampsia, pulse pressure at week seven through 15 of their pregnancy is *significantly* higher (45 mm Hg) compared with women who develop gestational hypertension (41 mm Hg) or women with normal blood pressure (normotensive) women. [Gestational hypertension is an elevated blood pressure induced by pregnancy, but unlike pre-eclampsia, pressure does not reach such a dangerously high level.]

A 1-mm Hg increase in pulse pressure during early pregnancy increases the risk of developing pre-eclampsia by six percent, but does not increase the risk of gestational hypertension.

Source: *Obstetrics & Gynecology* 2001;97:515-520; *Journal of Epidemiology* 2002;13:409-416.

WANT TO KNOW MORE?
An estimated 50,000 women worldwide die from pre-eclampsia each year.

873.. THE "BIOMARKERS" OF PRE-ECLAMPSIA

When you are pregnant, early signs in your body – "biomarkers" – can indicate whether or not you may be at risk for developing pre-eclampsia. Compared with low-risk women, women with pre-eclampsia have decreased concentrations of ascorbic acid (vitamin C) in the blood, which may lead to oxidative stress in the mother due to damaging free radicals. [Vitamin C, a powerful antioxidant, normally helps to protect us from free-radical damage.]

Early signs of oxidative stress in the body, along with endothelial dysfunction and placental insufficiency, are all associated with the development of this dangerous form of pregnancy-induced hypertension. These abnormalities appear several weeks before the onset of the condition.

Source: *American Journal of Obstetrics & Gynecology* 2002;187:127-136.

874. LOW BIRTH WEIGHT & PRE-ECLAMPSIA

If you have already given birth to a low-birth-weight baby, be warned that your risk for pre-eclampsia may be higher during your next pregnancy. Women who deliver low-birth-weight infants have a *threefold* increased risk of developing pre-eclampsia during a future pregnancy. This increase in risk is independent of other known risk factors for pre-eclampsia, such as age, the time between pregnancies, education, diabetes, and hypertension.

Low birth weight also predicts a substantial proportion (as high as 34 percent) of pre-eclampsia cases during second pregnancies.

Source: *Obstetrics and Gynecology* 2000;96:696-700.

WANT TO KNOW MORE?
[See the *Low Birth Weight* segment earlier in this section for helpful information on helping your baby reach a healthy birth weight.]

875.   SNORING MOMS MAY MEAN HIGH PRESSURE

If you are a pregnant woman who snores during her sleep – especially if you did not snore before – you may be at risk for pregnancy-induced hypertension and pre-eclampsia.   Snoring during pregnancy is a sign of pregnancy-induced hypertension. Upper-airway obstruction during the night may contribute to the development of both pregnancy-induced hypertension and pre-eclampsia (pregnancy hypertension that has reached a dangerous level of 45 mm Hg or higher).

Only four percent of women report snoring habitually before becoming pregnant, but during the last week of pregnancy as many as 23 percent of them snore habitually and 25 percent snore occasionally. Hypertension occurs in 14 percent of women who snore compared with only six percent of non-snorers, while pre-eclampsia develops in 10 percent of snorers compared with four percent of non-snorers. Both of these differences are statistically significant.

Pregnant women may be especially vulnerable to increases in upper-airway resistance, as breathing may also be restricted by an increase in the abdominal pressure affecting the diaphragm.

Source: *Chest* 2000;117:137-141.

WANT TO KNOW MORE?
Snoring during pregnancy can also indicate a greater risk of fetal-growth retardation.

PRE-ECLAMPSIA: DIETARY TACTICS
876.   AVOIDING PRE-ECLAMPSIA THROUGH DIET

As high levels of certain nutrients can increase your risk for pre-eclampsia, watch your diet carefully when you are pregnant – especially your consumption of protein and sodium. Dietary intake during the first half of your pregnancy may affect your risk of developing pre-eclampsia. A connection is seen between the onset of pre-eclampsia and an excess of certain nutrients: too many calories, proteins, lipids, simple sugars, polyunsaturated fatty acids, or sodium (or a combination of any of these).

A reduction in the amount of these nutrients, *especially* proteins and sodium, when applied during the early stage of pre-eclampsia symptoms, may aid in the disappearance of clinical signs of the disease.

Sources: *Acta Biomed Ateneo Parmense* 1997;68 Suppl1:95-98; *American Journal of Obstetrics & Gynecology* 2001;185:451-458.

PRE-ECLAMPSIA: NATURAL REMEDIES & SUPPLEMENTS

877. RIBOFLAVIN DEFICIENCY & PRE-ECLAMPSIA

If you are pregnant, reduce your risk of developing pre-eclampsia by consuming sufficient levels of vitamin B2 (riboflavin). In pregnant women already at high risk of developing this condition, riboflavin deficiency can increase the risk of pre-eclampsia by nearly fivefold. So expectant mothers should make sure they are getting an adequate supply of this nutrient. [Good dietary sources of riboflavin include egg yolks, cheese, fish, milk, spinach, yogurt, and whole grains.]

Source: *Obstetrics & Gynecology* **2000;96:38-44.**

878. VITAMIN C AGAINST PRE-ECLAMPSIA

If you are pregnant, consuming foods rich in vitamin C may help to lower your risk of developing pre-eclampsia. Low levels of vitamin C can adversely affect vascular function during pregnancy, thereby contributing to the development of pre-eclampsia, a toxic condition of late pregnancy. Women with pre-eclampsia have lower levels of vitamin C compared with normal pregnant women, or with non-pregnant healthy women.

Women who eat less than the recommended five servings of fruits and vegetables daily (up to a year before delivery) are nearly twice as likely to develop pre-eclampsia. And women who consume less than 85 mg of vitamin C daily are twice as likely to be diagnosed with the condition. The recommended daily intake for vitamin C is 85 mg for adults and more for pregnant women.

Women with the lowest levels of vitamin C in their blood during labor are nearly *four times* more likely to be diagnosed with pre-eclampsia, compared with women who have the highest levels – regardless of their age, calorie intake, and whether or not they are overweight before pregnancy.

[Vitamin C is one of the least stable vitamins, and cooking can destroy much of it. Some good dietary sources of vitamin C are citrus fruits, strawberries, green peppers, broccoli, dark leafy greens, and tomatoes.]

Source: 13th World Congress of the International Society for the Study of Hypertension in Pregnancy, Toronto, 2002; *Hypertension in Pregnancy* **2002;21(1):39-49;** *Journal of Epidemiology* **2002;13:409-416.**

WANT TO KNOW MORE?
Low levels of vitamin C cause the arteries to overreact, and so they are more prone to vasoconstriction. Vitamin C prevents nitric oxide from being destroyed, and nitric oxide is an important vasodilator.

879. ADD VITAMIN E FOR MORE PROTECTION

In addition to vitamin C, supplementing with vitamin E as well may further reduce your risk of developing pre-eclampsia while pregnant. Prenatal supplementation with vitamins C and E can help prevent the onset of pre-eclampsia in women at high risk for this complication. Only eight percent of women given vitamin C (1,000 mg/day) and vitamin E (400 IU/day) developed pre-eclampsia compared to 17 percent not given these vitamins who *did* develop the condition. (The vitamins were given between weeks 16 and 22 of gestation and continued until delivery.) When only women who completed the study were included in the final analysis, the risk was reduced even more.

Oxidative stress may contribute to the development of pre-eclampsia, and antioxidant therapy may have an important role to play in its prevention. [Vitamin E can be found in butter, egg yolks, liver, oils such as palm oil and rice bran oil, wheat germ, barley, saw palmetto, and some nuts and grains.]

Source: *Lancet* 1999;354:788-789,810-816.

880. MAGNESIUM PROTECTION AGAINST ECLAMPSIA

If you *do* have pre-eclampsia, taking magnesium sulfate may be protective against your condition progressing to life-threatening *eclampsia*. In pregnant women with pre-eclampsia, magnesium sulfate cuts the risk of eclampsia and possible maternal death *in half*. [Eclampsia, a result of untreated pre-eclampsia, is a life-threatening condition that can bring about convulsive seizures in pregnant women.] But magnesium sulfate can prevent as well as control the convulsions brought on by eclampsia.

Magnesium sulfate reduces the relative risk of eclampsia by 58 percent and the risk of maternal death by 45 percent. Magnesium sulfate is an inexpensive drug.

Source: *Lancet* 2002;359:1877-1890,1872-1873.

PRE-ECLAMPSIA: REDUCING RISK

881. WORKING MOMS & PRE-ECLAMPSIA RISK

Working moms-to-be: Reduce your risk of pregnancy-induced hypertension and pre-eclampsia by taking it easy when you are expecting. Working during your pregnancy *significantly* increases your risk of developing pregnancy hypertension and pre-eclampsia. Women who work through pregnancy are *five times* more likely to develop pre-eclampsia than are nonworking moms.

This link between working and pre-eclampsia is significant. It is possible that the stress of work may lead to an increased release of stress hormones, which in turn can cause blood pressure to rise.

Sources: *Journal of Epidemiology and Community Health* **2002;56:389-393;** *British Press Digest*, **as reported in** *Reuter's* **Apr 2002.**

882. STAY AWAY FROM IRON SUPPLEMENTS!

If you are pregnant and already at risk for pre-eclampsia, be sure to avoid taking iron supplements, which may actually contribute to this condition. Women with pre-eclampsia have *significantly* higher levels of iron concentration in their blood. Therefore, it is inadvisable, in the absence of evidence of iron deficiency, for pregnant women at high risk for pre-eclampsia to take iron supplements.

Source: *American Journal of Obstetrics and Gynecology* **2002;187:412-418.**

883. MODERATE EXERCISE HELPS PRE-ECLAMPSIA

If you are a pregnant woman at risk for hypertension, a program of moderate exercise (such as walking) is an effective way to lower your diastolic blood pressure. After 10 weeks of walking, systolic pressure in women with a history of pregnancy hypertension does not change significantly but *diastolic* pressure does. (The women in this study did not lose weight, and researchers believe that walking was the only cause of the decrease in diastolic blood pressure.)

Hypertension can lead to pre-eclampsia, a leading cause of maternal death that can also have a negative effect on the baby and necessitate a premature delivery. Women at risk can exercise safely if they are supervised properly.

Source: *Journal of Reproductive Medicine* **2000;45:293-301.**

PREMATURE BIRTH: CAUSES & PRECURSORS

884. MOMS: MAKE SURE TO EAT REGULARLY

Pregnant moms, make sure you are eating right, as skipping meals regularly during your pregnancy can induce stress on the body that could lead to a premature delivery. Women who are expecting are advised to eat three meals daily, as well as to consume at least two nutritious snacks during the day to prevent going for long periods without any food. Women who fall short of these guidelines have a 30 percent increased risk of delivering their babies prematurely.

Skipping meals can result in elevated levels of stress hormones that have been implicated in the events leading to a preterm delivery. Skipping meals becomes a "stressor" to the body, and stress during your pregnancy may lead to a preterm birth.

Source: *American Journal of Epidemiology* **2001;153:647-652.**

885. GUM DISEASE LINKED TO PRETERM BIRTH

If you are considering having children, see your dentist! Pregnant women with periodontitis have an increased risk of premature delivery. Women should have a periodontal examination and have any periodontal disease treated early on – ideally before pregnancy.

Source: *Journal of the American Dental Association* **2001;132:875-880.**

WANT TO KNOW MORE?
[Periodontal disease is also a significant factor for delivery of a low-birth-weight baby. See Hint #851 earlier in this section for more information.]

886. PREVIOUS ABORTIONS & PRETERM RISK

If you are a pregnant woman who has had induced abortions in the past, you have an increased risk of having a prematurely delivered baby. Women who have had one or more induced abortions have a significantly increased risk of having a preterm delivery in subsequent pregnancies. This increased risk is associated with the number of previous induced abortions a woman has had.

This association is the same for very preterm, moderately preterm, as well as spontaneous or induced deliveries. However, there is no significant link between previous induced abortions and a woman's risk of giving birth to a small-for-gestational-age (SGA) or low-birth-weight (LBW) infant.

Source: *British Journal of Obstetrical Gynecology* **2001;108:1036-1042.**

887.. DOUCHING COULD LEAD TO PRETERM BIRTH

If you are pregnant, avoid vaginal douching, as it may increase your likelihood of having a preterm delivery. Women should have a periodontal examination and have any periodontal disease treated early on – ideally before pregnancy.

Source: *Journal of the American Dental Association* **2001;132:875-880.**

PREMATURE BIRTH: DIETARY TACTICS

888. FISHY METHOD TO AVOID PRETERM BIRTH

Go fish! Eating lots of seafood during the early part of your pregnancy helps to reduce your risk of having a preterm birth or a low-birth-weight baby. Low consumption of seafood during early pregnancy is a risk factor for preterm delivery and low birth weight. (Especially in women eating less than 15 grams of fish daily). However, the risk of low birth weight, preterm birth, and intrauterine growth retardation all decrease with increasing fish consumption. The risk of preterm birth falls progressively from 7.1 percent in women who never eat fish, to 1.9 percent in those who eat fish at least once a week. In women with zero or low intake of fish, small amounts of n-3 fatty acids – from fish or fish oil – may offer some protection against both preterm delivery and low birth weight.

Preterm birth is a strong predictor of an infant's later health and survival. Intake of seafood rich in fatty acids can increase birth weight by prolonging gestation or by increasing the growth rate of the fetus.

Source: *British Medical Journal* **2002;324:447.**

WANT TO KNOW MORE?
[However, not all fish is safe to consume during your pregnancy! Tuna – as well as fish like swordfish, king mackerel, shark, and tilefish — may contain high levels of mercury due to environmental pollution, and should be avoided by pregnant moms because of potential dangers to developing fetuses. In fact, the FDA urges *everyone* to eat a variety of fish to ensure against a potentially high mercury intake.]

PREMATURE BIRTH: NATURAL REMEDIES & SUPPLEMENTS

889. VITAMIN A AGAINST PRETERM-BIRTH RISK

If you are pregnant, be sure you are getting enough vitamin A to reduce your risk of premature delivery. A deficiency in vitamin A during the third trimester is *significantly* associated with an increased risk of preterm delivery (as well as moderate to severe maternal anemia). No significant association is seen, however, between a vitamin A deficiency and pregnancy-induced hypertension (pre-eclampsia).

[Vitamin A can be found in liver, fish liver oil, and green and yellow vegetables and fruits.]

Source: *British Journal of Obstetrics and Gynecology* **2002;109:689-693.**

PREMATURE BIRTH: LATER PROBLEMS

890. PREMATURE GIRLS & ANOREXIA NERVOSA

Premature delivery and birth trauma may increase a girl's risk of developing anorexia nervosa later on – on more reason for moms-to-be to watch their diets during pregnancy. Anorexia nervosa is associated with preterm birth and birth trauma, which may cause subtle brain damage.

In conjunction with other individual or environmental factors, this may result in the inability to correctly identify hunger and satiety sensations.

Source: *Archives of General Psychiatry* 1999;56:634-638.

STILLBIRTH: CAUSES & PRECURSORS

891. OBESE MOMS & HIGHER STILLBIRTH RISK

Obese pregnant women, be warned: You are more likely to have an unexplained stillbirth than a leaner mother. Of all unexplained stillbirths, more than half (51 percent) occur in women with a body mass index over 30. Obese pregnant women usually have other known risk factors for stillbirth, such as diabetes or high blood pressure.

These women may also be in a "prediabetic" state with insulin resistance, which causes metabolic disturbances in the developing fetus.

Another potential explanation is that when obese women sleep on their backs, the pressure from their thicker abdominal walls can restrict blood flow from the placenta to the fetus.

Source: Annual meeting of the American College of Obstetricians and Gynecologists, Los Angeles, May 2002.

WANT TO KNOW MORE?
Important note: At the same time, women should avoid dieting during their pregnancies. One approach is for the expectant mother to keep a "kick-count" sheet to record how often the fetus is moving about – a sign of good health.

VI. HEALTHIER BABIES

HEALTHIER BABIES: ASTHMA & ALLERGIC DISEASES

892. AVOID ANTIBIOTICS DURING PREGNANCY

Avoid taking antibiotics during your pregnancy, as they may increase your child's risk of later allergic diseases such as asthma, hay fever, or eczema. Because much of the immune system develops in utero, factors that modify microbial exposure during this time may have a long-term impact on a baby's risk of developing allergic diseases.

Children exposed to antibiotics in utero have a 68 percent increased risk of developing asthma, a 56 percent increased risk for hay fever, and a 17 percent increased risk for eczema.

This adverse result does not depend on the type of antibiotic or the trimester in which the antibiotics are prescribed, but there is a dose-response effect, especially for asthma.

Source: *American Journal of Respiratory & Critical Care Medicine* 2002;166:827-832.

893. BUTT OUT OR FACE ASTHMATIC KIDS

If you are pregnant, stop smoking immediately to protect your child from asthma and other respiratory problems down the road. Exposure in utero to maternal smoking – with or without subsequent exposure to environmental tobacco smoke – occurs in 18.8 percent of children, and is associated with later physician-diagnosed asthma and a lifetime history of wheezing. Kids exposed in utero to maternal smoking are more likely to have asthma than children exposed to environmental smoke after birth.

Because the airway structures of the lung are largely complete at birth, exposure in utero may increase the occurrence of asthma by altering critical developmental pathways, leading to poorer lung function.

Sources: *British Medical Journal* 2001;322:450; *Archives of Diseases of Childhood* 2000;83:307-312.

WANT TO KNOW MORE?
Other factors that increase a child's risk of early wheeze include a maternal history of asthma and premature delivery.

HEALTHIER BABIES: BEHAVIORAL PROBLEMS

894. MOMS, ALCOHOL & KIDS WITH ADHD

Steer clear of alcohol during your pregnancy: It may lead to attention and hyperactivity problems in your child. Attention-deficit/hyperactivity disorder (ADHD) may be the result of damage to the fetal midbrain caused by the mother's alcohol intake during pregnancy. In test animals given alcohol when pregnant, the electrical activity of dopamine neurons is reduced in their offspring.

These neurons normally generate a certain amount of spontaneous electrical activity resulting in dopamine release in the areas of the brain responsible for attention. Attention and hyperactivity problems may be caused by the reduced activity in these dopamine neurons.

Substances such as cocaine and certain psychiatric medications can also reduce dopamine-neuron activity, and any events that disrupt dopamine neurons during fetal development (including stress) could lead to dysfunction of these neurons and ADHD.

Source: *Alcohol Clinical Experimental Research* **1999;23:1801-1807.**

895. ALCOHOL & LATER DELINQUENCY IN KIDS

Pregnant women: Avoid *any* amount of alcohol (even a few sips of wine), as children whose mothers consume even small amounts of alcohol while pregnant have an increased risk of behavioral problems later in life. Maternal alcohol consumption during pregnancy is linked to problems in children such as aggression, delinquent behavior, and attention problems. Children with low levels of prenatal alcohol exposure (equivalent to an average of one cocktail per week throughout the mother's pregnancy) are *three times* as likely to exhibit later delinquent behavior.

Source: *Pediatrics* Aug 2001..

896. SMOKING & NEGATIVE TODDLER BEHAVIOR

In addition to the risk of later asthma, smoking during your pregnancy may lead to having children with negative behavior. Women who smoke during pregnancy are more likely than those who do not to have children who display negative behavior as they approach the age of two. The levels of this negative behavior are directly related to the mother's level of smoking during her pregnancy.

Overall, toddlers whose mothers smoke during pregnancy are *four times* likelier to exhibit negative behavior than are toddlers with mom who did not smoke.

Source: *Archives of Pediatrics & Adolescent Medicine* **2000;154:381-385.**

WANT TO KNOW MORE?
Birth complications from cigarette smoking during pregnancy may even be linked to later *criminal* behavior in children. [See Hint #897 that follows for more details.]

897. SMOKING & LATER CRIMINAL BEHAVIOR

It's not just the risk of temper tantrums: Smoking during your pregnancy may lead to children who grow up to exhibit *criminal* behavior. Adult men whose mothers smoked during pregnancy are more likely than others to become violent criminals. There is a dose-dependent relationship between the amount of maternal prenatal smoking and arrests for nonviolent and violent crimes.

The association appears to be strongest for persistent criminal behavior. These findings confirm and extend a previously reported association between prenatal maternal smoking and *adolescent* criminal activity.

Source: *Archives of General Psychiatry* **1999;56:215-219.**

HEALTHIER BABIES: BONE DENSITY & BONE HEALTH

898. MINERALS & BABY'S BONE DENSITY

If you are pregnant, make sure you are getting sufficient dietary phosphorous, magnesium, and potassium to ensure healthy bones in your baby. The bone-mineral density of young children is associated with the mother's diets during her pregnancy. Phosphorus and magnesium are both associated with significantly higher femoral neck density in children. A child's lumbar (lower) spine density is also significantly higher when born to mothers with the highest intake of phosphorus, magnesium, and potassium – and significantly lower in those born to moms with high fat intakes.

[These minerals are found in many foods, but some sources that contain all three include dairy products, nuts, fish, whole grains, and brewer's yeast.]

Source: *European Journal of Clinical Nutrition* **2000;54:749-756.**

HEALTHIER BABIES: CHILDHOOD CANCER

899. TAKE FOLATE FOR LEUKEMIA PROTECTION

Taking supplemental folate during your pregnancy may help to protect your child from developing leukemia. n are advised to take folate (folic acid) before conception to protect against serious birth defects. And now we know that continuing to take folate during pregnancy has a protective association against the risk of acute lymphoblastic leukemia.

Additional analysis indicates that the protective effect of folate varies very little according to the time the supplement is first taken or the duration of use.

[Low blood levels of folate are present in at least 25 percent of normal pregnancies. High concentrations are found in spinach, brewer's yeast, and lentils. Moderate amounts are found in dark green leafy veggies, carrots, eggs, and avocadoes.]

Source: *Lancet* **2001;358:1935-1940.**

900. MOMS: AVOID ACRYLAMIDE-LADEN FOODS!

Pregnant women and nursing mothers, be warned: You should sharply limit, or even cease, consumption of french fries, potato chips, or other foods that contain the cancer-causing chemical *acrylamide*. This chemical first received global attention in April 2002 when Swedish researchers reported finding acrylamide in fried and oven-baked foods, especially in potato chips and french fries. These findings were at first greeted with skepticism, but scientists in other nations have since produced similar results.

High levels of acrylamide have been found to cause cancer in test animals. Last September the FDA announced a plan to reduce or eliminate concentrations of acrylamide in potato and cereal products. Acrylamide is a neurotoxic agent that is believed to also cause cancer in humans.

The danger of pregnant and breastfeeding mothers ingesting acrylamide has now been positively confirmed. Fetuses and newborn babies are *particularly* susceptible to the potential harmful effects of this chemical, and are at greater risk because of their generally higher body water levels. Furthermore, blood-brain barriers in fetuses and newborn infants are not fully developed.

Source: Institute for Biomedical and Pharmaceutical Research in Nuremberg, Germany, Jan 2003, reported in *Reuter's Medical News* Jan 2003.

901. MULTIVITAMINS AGAINST NEUROBLASTOMA

Pregnant moms: Reduce your baby's risk of developing a specific childhood cancer by taking multivitamins supplements – both before and during your pregnancy.
Women who take multivitamins before or during their pregnancies *significantly* reduce the risk of their babies developing *neuroblastoma*, a malignant tumor occurring chiefly in infants and young children. Women who use a vitamin and mineral supplement in any trimester, or even the month before becoming pregnant, reduce the risk of this childhood cancer by 30 to 40 percent.

The specific vitamin(s) potentially responsible for the reduced risk remains unknown. But the reduced incidence of several birth defects with vitamin supplementation as well suggests that a mother's vitamin use before and during pregnancy may be very beneficial to a baby's health.

Source: *Epidemiology* **2002;13:575-580.**

HEALTHIER BABIES: DIABETES

902. SMOKING MOMS, DIABETIC KIDS

In addition to putting your child at risk for future asthma and behavioral problems, smoking during your pregnancy also increases his/her risk of developing diabetes.
Maternal smoking during pregnancy increases both the risk of early-onset type 2 diabetes and non-diabetic obesity in children. In utero exposure to smoking may increase the risk of both diabetes and obesity through "programming" – resulting in lifelong metabolic problems due possibly to fetal malnutrition or toxicity.

Source: *British Medical Journal* **2002;324:26-27.**

WANT TO KNOW MORE?
Cigarette smoking as a young adult is also independently associated with an increased risk of subsequent diabetes. [See the extensive *Diabetes Type 2* section for many tips on preventing and treating this disease.]

In a representative sample of pregnant women across a number of obstetrics clinics in Michigan, it was discovered that at least 15 percent of pregnant women used alcohol. (***Alcoholism, Clinical & Experimental Research*** **2003;27(1):81-7**)

Premature births have now reached near-epidemic proportions in the US. More than 475,000 infants were born prematurely in 2001, up 27 percent from two decades before. (**National Center for Health Statistics, Jan 2003**)

903. PREGNANCY NUTRITION & DIABETES

Pregnant women: Reduce your baby's risk of developing type 2 diabetes later on by making sure to eat well during your pregnancy. Poor nutrition while in the womb is implicated in the later development of type 2 diabetes. Undernourishment in utero has been shown to produce insulin resistance in genetically normal, second-generation test animals.

Source: Journal of Nutrition 2000;130:741-744.

WANT TO KNOW MORE?
[Want to eat better but don't know where to start? See the *Better Nutrition* section in the *Healthier Living* appendix of this book for many helpful tips.]

HEALTHIER BABIES: DRUG DEPENDENCY

904. PROTECT KIDS BY FOREGOING LABOR DRUGS

Reduce your child's risk of future drug abuse and dependency by deciding to forego some of your own drug use during labor and delivery. Drug abuse and/or dependence on cocaine, hallucinogens, narcotics, or other drugs were compared with the mother's use of drugs during labor. Twenty-three percent of drug abusers were found to have had mothers who took multiple doses of strong pain medication during labor, compared to only six percent of controls.

Other potential factors such as prolonged labor, asphyxia, birth order, and low birth weight were similar in both groups.

Source: Epidemiology 2000;11:715-716.

HEALTHIER BABIES: HEART DISEASE & HEART DEFECTS

905. CARDIAC DISEASE & MATERNAL NUTRITION

If you are pregnant, eating well and being serious about nutrition will help protect your unborn child from cardiovascular problems later in life. Undernourished fetuses and low-birth-weight infants have an increased risk of developing cardiovascular diseases in adulthood, including hypertension, coronary heart disease, and stroke.

Adequate protein intake is as important as total caloric intake. (Amino-acid metabolism in the fetus appears to have a key influence on the development of organs.) In addition, early nutrition may also affect cell number, among other factors that stay with us into adulthood.

Sources: *American Journal of Clinical Nutrition* Feb 1999;69(2):179-197; *Journal of Physiology* Feb 1999;514(3):617-627; *Heart* 2000;84:595-598.

906. OBESE MOMS & HEART DEFECTS IN KIDS

Overweight moms, be warned: You have an increased risk of giving birth to a child with a heart defect. Women who are overweight before conception appear to have an increased risk of giving birth to infants with isolated heart defects. And compared with infants of average-weight women, infants of underweight women are less likely to have a major isolated heart defect.

Source: *Epidemiology* 2001;11:439-446.

WANT TO KNOW MORE?
[However, pregnant women are advised never to diet, as this can lead to low-birth-weight babies. But see Hints #855 and #856 earlier in this section for important information on exercising safely during your pregnancy.]

907. MULTIVITAMINS & FEWER HEART DEFECTS

Taking multivitamins *before* you conceive, rather than during your pregnancy, reduces the risk of congenital heart defects in your baby. A mother's multivitamin use prior to conception is associated with a 24 percent lower risk of all heart defects in her baby, while no reduced risk is detected in those women who start taking vitamins during the second or third month of pregnancy. By this time the heart structures are already formed in the embryo.

It cannot be ruled out, however, that the diet of women who take multivitamins might differ from the diet of women who do not.

Source: *American Journal of Epidemiology* 2000;151:878-884.

WANT TO KNOW MORE?
Infections during pregnancy are a major cause of premature delivery. Nearly 12 percent of all births are now premature, occurring before 37 completed weeks of pregnancy.

Premature births are also the leading cause of mortality among US infants, causing more than 4,000 deaths each year, according to figures from the National Center for Health Statistics.

HEALTHIER BABIES: MEMORY & COGNITIVE FUNCTION

908. CHOLINE FOR BETTER BABY BRAINS

Moms, be advised: Getting enough of the little-known nutrient choline during your pregnancy may play a vital role in the formation of your baby's brain and memory function. Choline intake during pregnancy affects the memory center of the baby's brain and has long-lasting effects on his/her cognitive function and visual-spatial memory. The critical time in which choline is needed is in the last trimester of pregnancy. If test animals are not given enough choline at that time, their babies suffer memory problems throughout their lives and are more likely to become senile.

Choline is a naturally occurring amino acid and an essential building block for a memory forming brain chemical called *acetylcholine*. It plays a major role in the formation of cell membranes throughout the body. [Foods rich in choline include egg yolks, milk, nuts, meat, liver, and soybeans. Breast milk contains much more of this nutrient than many infant formulas.]

Sources: *Developmental Brain Research* **1999;** *Journal of the American College of Nutrition Oct 2000.*

WANT TO KNOW MORE?
If a mother consumes extra choline during her pregnancy (about three times what she'd normally take in from food) her babies will be born with enhanced memory that will last their entire lives. In the adult brain, dietary choline is also associated with learning and memory processes.

909. LATE DHA & BABY BRAIN DEVELOPMENT

Moms-to-be: Supplementing with the fatty acid DHA at the end of your pregnancy may have a very beneficial effect on your baby's cognitive development. This strongly suggests the importance of DHA levels during the last trimester. Infants born to mothers with high DHA levels are more likely to demonstrate mature sleeping patterns than infants born to mothers with lower levels. And infants who receive DHA-rich breast milk also exhibit more mature brain development than their formula-fed peers.

In addition, early DHA levels may influence the risk of heart disease later in life. In animal studies, low DHA levels have been associated with the development of high blood pressure. [Fish such as mackerel, sardines, herring, and salmon are all good sources of DHA.]

Source: *American Journal of Clinical Nutrition* **2002;76:608-613.**

910.   MEMORY-BOOSTING INFANT FORMULAS

If you are not breastfeeding your infant, be sure to use a formula that contains essential fatty acids, because these nutrients can boost your baby's brain development and improve vision. Infant formulas containing two fatty acids believed to aid in neurological and visual development are now available. The added compounds, docosahexaenoic acid (DHA) and arachidonic acid (ARA), are present in breast milk, and infants fed these supplemented formulas for at least 17 weeks show long-term cognitive advantages. (DHA and ARA have already been added to formulas in some European countries for some time now.)

Since rapid infant brain development occurs in the early months of life, a number of researchers believe that a direct dietary source of DHA and ARA at that time can be beneficial for both brain and retinal development. Infants who are fed formula supplemented with DHA and ARA score better at 10 months of age on a test assessing problem-solving skills than do infants fed regular formula.

Sources: *Developmental Medicine in Child Neurology* **2000;42:174-181;** *Reuter's Medical Report* **Jan 2002.**

WANT TO KNOW MORE?
[I wrote about this potential over 20 years ago in my book, *Total Nutrition for Breastfeeding Mothers*, now available only online. (For availability, check out www.publishingonline.com.)

DHA supplementation may also help improve adult cognitive function as well. See Hint #699 in the *Memory & Cognitive Problems* section for more details. In addition, it may also be protective against diseases such as asthma (see Hint #118), type 2 diabetes (Hint #403), and lupus (Hint #670).]

VII. MOMS WITH PRE-EXISTING HEALTH PROBLEMS

PRE-EXISTING PROBLEMS: AIDS

911.   PROTECTING KIDS BORN TO HIV+ MOMS

If you are a pregnant woman who is also HIV-positive, supplementing with specific vitamins may help protect the health of your baby. Vitamins B, C, and E provided to HIV-positive women during pregnancy and lactation are likely to reduce the risks of mortality and other adverse effects among children born to these women. In mothers who are immunologically or nutritionally compromised, multivitamin supplementation – *excluding vitamin A* – reduces the risk of HIV transmission through breastfeeding, which has been associated with poor maternal micronutrient status. (Supplementation with vitamin A, however, is associated with a *higher* risk of HIV-1 transmission through breastfeeding.)

Multivitamin use has no effect on the overall HIV-1 transmission rate, but total child mortality is lower among mothers taking multivitamins than among those not taking multivitamins.

Source: *AIDS* **2002;16:1935-1944.**

PRE-EXISTING PROBLEMS: ASTHMA

912.   UNDER-TREATED ASTHMA & PRETERM BIRTH

Asthmatic moms: Don't let your asthma go untreated, as women with under-treated asthma during their pregnancies are at risk of having a premature delivery, and one possibility is learning about self-management. This risk of preterm birth is increased in women with untreated asthma. (Women with *severe* asthma actually have a lower risk of preterm birth because they are more likely to have their disease controlled with drugs). The theory is that women who have hyper-responsivity of smooth muscle in the bronchi also have it in the uterus.

The same drugs used to control preterm labor are the same that are used to treat asthma (although they are given in larger doses for preterm labor). The smaller doses used by a woman with asthma give her substantial protection against preterm delivery.

On the other hand, those with asthma who are directly involved in management of their asthma do "at least" as well as those given the usual care. Self-management of asthma has been demonstrated to be an efficient patient-centered approach to asthma management. Self-managed asthmatics show an improvement in quality of life with improvement in emotion [which has to benefit the baby]. These patients feel less worried or insecure about the influence of their asthma in daily life.

Researchers conclude that a lower burden of asthma can be achieved with more patient autonomy, making this approach an interesting one.

Source: *Thorax* **2003;58:30-36; 98th International Conference of the American Thoracic Society, 2002.**

WANT TO KNOW MORE?
[See the *Premature Birth* segment earlier in this section for more advice on how to avoid a premature delivery.]

PRE-EXISTING PROBLEMS: CELIAC DISEASE

913. CELIAC DISEASE & POOR BIRTH OUTCOME

If you are a woman who has been diagnosed with celiac disease, be sure to maintain a gluten-free diet before becoming pregnant to reduce your risk of having a low-birth-weight baby. Birth outcomes are worse in women with *untreated* celiac disease compared to women without the disease – as well as compared to women with celiac disease but who have been hospitalized for it.

[Celiac disease is an inflammation of the intestinal lining in response to the ingestion of a protein known as gluten, which is present in many grains including wheat, rye, oats, barley, and triticale.]

Women with untreated celiac disease have a 2.6 times higher risk of having a low-birth-weight baby, and a 3.4 times higher risk of experiencing retarded intrauterine growth when compared to non-sufferers. (But again, these risks are not increased in women who have been hospitalized for celiac disease.)

Source: *American Journal of Gastroenterology* 1999;94:2435-2440.

PRE-EXISTING PROBLEMS: DIABETES

914. DIABETIC MOMS & LARGER BABIES

Diabetic moms: Be careful to control your glucose levels during your pregnancy to reduce your risk of having a *high*-birth-weight baby. Insulin-dependent diabetic women with poor glycemic control during their pregnancies are more likely than other diabetic women to deliver infants who are large for their gestational age (LGA). But if strict blood glucose control is maintained during the first and second trimesters, it might reduce the incidence of LGA infants.

Growth acceleration in the fetus begins at 20 weeks in insulin-dependent diabetic pregnancies, but this acceleration is determined by elevations in the mother's glucose concentration that starts weeks earlier. Maternal hyperglycemia causes fetal hyperglycemia – and can result in pancreatic problems in the fetus that can lead to the birth of an LGA baby.

[See the *Diabetes* section for food and supplement suggestions for the diabetic.

Source: *Obstetrics & Gynecology* 2000;95:190-194.

915. GUM DISEASE & TYPE 1 DIABETIC MOMS

Diabetic moms-to-be, see your dentist! You are at higher risk for serious gum disease, which can affect your glucose control as well as increase your risk of having a low-birth-weight child. Problems related to periodontal disease are more severe in pregnant women with type 1 diabetes than in non-diabetic pregnant women, such as significantly higher levels of plaque and gum inflammation.

Like other bacterial infections, periodontitis in pregnant diabetics may affect blood-glucose control. And periodontal disease may be an independent risk factor for preterm, low-birth-weight infants.

Source: *Journal of Periodontology* **2001;72:1485-1490.**

PRE-EXISTING PROBLEMS: HYPOTHYROIDISM

916. HYPOTHYROIDISM & MISCARRIAGE RISK

If you are a pregnant woman with a low thyroid hormone levels, be warned that you have an increased risk of having a miscarriage. Pregnant women with low thyroid levels have nearly *four times* the risk of miscarriage in the second trimester than do other women. Expectant mothers with elevated levels of thyroid stimulating hormone (which translates to low thyroid levels) have a 3.8 percent risk of late miscarriage. (Pregnant women without the problem have only a 0.9 percent miscarriage risk.)

Six out of every 100 late miscarriages may be attributed to hypothyroidism.

Source: *Journal of Medical Screening* **2000;7:127-130.**

WANT TO KNOW MORE?
Even if you are in the best of health, this is the time to throw your can opener away and put a lock on the freezer door. When will you ever again be in such complete and total control of your child's diet? This is the time to eat unprocessed foods, particularly complex carbohydrates, take the supplements recommended by your alternative physician, exercise moderately (walking is best), and enjoy the power you have to influence the outcome of your pregnancy.

Once upon a time, in the Fiji Islands, the mayor of each town assigned two men to a woman as soon as she became pregnant. Their mission was to obtain from the sea – daily – a particular kind of crab. This variety of seafood is extraordinarily rich in nutrients. It is unlikely that two men will appear to do the same for you, but seeking the best, most nutritious food should not be difficult in today's world, wherever you live.

VIII. BREASTFEEDING

BREASTFEEDING: BENEFITS

917. BREASTFED KIDS ARE SMARTER KIDS

Breastfeeding your baby for at least six months may help to give him/her a higher IQ. Mothers should breastfeed their babies *exclusively* for the first 24 weeks of life, in order to enhance their child's cognitive development. Children who are breastfed for the first six months demonstrate improved cognitive function. Unfortunately, supplemental foods are often introduced by three months of age. The improvement in IQ associated with breastfeeding is even more dramatic for children who are born small for their gestational age. The duration of exclusive breastfeeding has a significant impact on cognitive development in these small-for-gestational-age babies, without compromising their growth.

Source: *Acta Pediatrician* 2002;91:267-274.

WANT TO KNOW MORE?
[Low-birth-weight babies are at risk for numerous health and behavioral problems later in life. See the *Low Birth Weight* segment earlier in this section for advice on how to reduce your baby's risk of being born too small.]

918. BREASTFEEDING AGAINST CHILD CANCERS

Breastfeeding your child for at least six months may also help to protect him/her from certain childhood cancers, such as leukemia and lymphoma. The risk for contracting childhood acute leukemia and a lymphoid malignancy is higher among those children who are breastfed for less than six months, compared to kids breastfed for at least six months or more.

Source: *European Journal of Cancer* 2001;37:234-238.

WANT TO KNOW MORE?
[Did you know that substances in hot dogs have also been linked to leukemia in children? See Hint #212 in the *Cancer, Leukemia* section for more information.]

919. BREASTFEEDING LOWERS MOM'S CANCER RISK

In addition to protecting your baby from childhood cancers, breastfeeding may protect *you* from breast cancer! Women who breastfeed their babies for at least two years have *half* the risk of developing breast cancer compared with women who breastfeed for less than six months. This protective effect applies to risk even after menopause. Women who have breastfed for at least 73 months (just over six years) over the course of their lives have an even lower risk of breast cancer. The researchers speculate that reproductive-cycle hormones linked to some forms of breast cancer are suppressed during breastfeeding, while protective compounds may be released.

Source: *American Journal of Epidemiology* **2000;152:1129-1135;2001;154:37-42.**

WANT TO KNOW MORE?
Unfortunately, American women rarely breastfeed for more than four months – which is why the protective association was not made until studies were done in other countries. Other factors that also lower a woman's risk of breast cancer include a later age of menstruation and a younger age of first pregnancy.

[See the extensive *Cancer, Breast* section for many hints about protecting yourself from this disease.]

920. BREASTFEEDING LOWERS BLOOD PRESSURE

In addition to reducing your risk of breast cancer, breastfeeding your baby can also help lower blood pressure – for both of you! Breastfeeding can help to lower a mother's blood pressure for a sustained period of time. Infant holding is also thought to be a reliever of stress. In fact, infant cuddling – even without breastfeeding – has a positive effect on stress reduction. And in children born prematurely, breast-milk consumption is associated with lower blood pressure later on. Blood pressure is lower in children ages 13 to 16 given banked breast milk as babies (alone or in addition to mother's milk) compared to those given formula.

[See the *Hypertension* section for many hints on preventing and treating high blood pressure.]

Sources: American Psychosomatic Society Annual Meeting; *International Journal of Epidemiology* **1999;28:396-402;** *Lancet* **Feb 2001;357(9254):413-419.**

921. BREASTFEEDING: FOR HOW LONG?

When should you stop breastfeeding your baby? Researchers suggest that modern humans should actually be breastfed for between two and a half to seven years. Humans have slightly longer durations of all stages of the life span than our nearest relatives, chimpanzees. We have a slightly longer gestation period, later dental eruption, later sexual maturity, and therefore would expect slightly later ages of weaning. Chimpanzee mothers breastfeed their babies for four to five years. Around the world, many children are breastfed for two and a half to seven years. A healthy start in life from several years of breastfeeding should be followed by a lifelong diet low in animal protein and fat and high in physical exercise, to maximize heart health in adulthood.

Source: *British Medical Journal* **2001;323:689.**

RESPIRATORY ILLNESS & INFECTION

Inappropriate antibiotic therapy is still being used for viral respiratory tract infections. Physicians are slowly improving their prescribing patterns, but almost half of patients with such infections still receive antibiotics. (*Archives of Pediatric Adolescent Medicine* **2002;156(11):1114-9**) Despite advances in nutrition and critical care, limitations of currently available treatment for severe respiratory infection are paramount. (*Respiratory Research* **2000;1(1):9-11;** *Clinical Microbiology & Infection* **2002;8 Suppl 2:1-11**)

Prevention of recurrent wheezing and good control of allergic rhinoconjunctivitis is critical for preventing subsequent development of bronchial asthma. (*Journal of Miecrobiology, Immunology & Infection* (China) **2001;34(4):259-64**)

IN THIS SECTION:
- CAUSES & PRECURSORS
- DIETARY TACTICS

- NATURAL REMEDIES & SUPPLEMENTS
- REDUCING RISK

RESPIRATORY ILLNESS: CAUSES & PRECURSORS

922. GAS STOVES & YOUR RESPIRATORY HEALTH

Cooking with gas stoves can increase respiratory symptoms and lead to chronic airway inflammation – despite no sign of an acute respiratory infection. The use of gas stoves is associated with respiratory symptoms of chronic airway inflammation and higher rates of respiratory infections. And now researchers have also found increases for the respiratory symptoms of "cough without cold" and "morning cough."

The strongest effect for chronic inflammation (reflected by an increase in white blood cell counts) is found for those likely to have been exposed at higher levels: those exposed to stoves without fans, stoves in smaller homes, or those people who spend more time indoors. (Although these studies were done on children, other evidence suggests similar results with adults.)

Source: *International Journal of Hygiene & Environmental Health* **2000;203(1):29.**

923. TOO MUCH GIRTH & AIRWAY OBSTRUCTION

Is your belt buckle at the last hole? Be warned: Too much around the middle can lead to respiratory ills, but vitamin C and beta-carotene could help. Airway obstruction is found to increase *significantly* with increased waist circumference. The cause of the inverse association between girth and pulmonary function is not clear, but one possible explanation is that a large waist circumference may affect the movement of the diaphragm and the chest wall.

However, obstruction decreases with the intake of vitamin C, which is directly associated with good lung function. And a positive association is also seen with beta-carotene.

Source: *American Journal of Epidemiology* **2001;153:157-163.**

RESPIRATORY ILLNESS: DIETARY TACTICS

924. FRUITS THAT IMPROVE RESPIRATION

Eating more whole apples, pears, bananas, and tomatoes can help to improve your respiratory health. In a study done on over 13,500 healthy adults, a high intake of apples and pears (fruits rich in flavonoids) was found to be protective against chronic cough and breathlessness, or chronic obstructive pulmonary disease.

Consumption of more than five apples per week and more than three tomatoes a week shows a strong association with increased respiratory control. In addition, wheezing is less common among those who frequently consume apples, tomatoes, and bananas. These fruits have high levels of antioxidants, which researchers suspect are the reason for their benefits. Could any health program be easier?

Intake of solid fruit – but *not* tea – is tied to these beneficial effects, despite the fact that tea also contains some of the ingredients believed to be responsible for these benefits (including catechins, flavonols, and flavones).

Source: *American Journal of Respiratory & Critical Care Medicine* **2001;164:61-64; 97th Annual Meeting of the American Thoracic Society, San Francisco, May 22, 2001.**

925. THE POWER OF CHICKEN SOUP

Traditional chicken soup with matzoh balls has the ability to inhibit metabolic responses that promote inflammation – making it a wonderful home remedy for respiratory problems. Samples taken from traditionally prepared chicken soup with matzoh balls at nearly each step of the preparation showed inhibitory properties against the processes that promote inflammation. In fact, all the individual ingredients showed inhibitory properties, including the boiled chicken extract. The inhibitory activity observed in the study is likely achievable by consuming one 350 ml (12 fluid ounces) bowl of soup, and the effect appears to be dose-dependent. [So drink up!]

Source: *Chest* **2000;118:1150-1157.**

WANT TO KNOW MORE?
Chicken soup has been recommended for treating respiratory symptoms as long ago as the 12th century, promoted by Maimonides.

RESPIRATORY ILLNESS: NATURAL REMEDIES & SUPPLEMENTS

926. PROBIOTIC MILK & RESPIRATORY INFECTION

Parents, take note: Giving children probiotic milk may help to reduce the rate and severity of respiratory infections. In a seven-month trial, kids receiving milk with added *Lactobacillus* GG had 11 percent fewer absences due to illness, 17 percent fewer respiratory infections (both upper and lower), and a 19 percent reduction in antibiotic use compared to children in a control group who did not receive the milk.

The administration of probiotic milk products is an easy and acceptable method, with no adverse effects. More and more studies suggest that these health-promoting organisms may help prevent both respiratory and diarrhea-related diseases in children at increased risk of such infections, such as those kids in daycare facilities. {Viable yogurt, now available, can accomplish the same goal.]

Source: *British Medical Journal* 2001;322:1318-1319,1327-1329.

WANT TO KNOW MORE?
[The use of daily doses of liquid *acidophilus* (available in most health food stores) for both adults and children is something I have been advocating for decades.]

927. ACIDOPHILUS, PNEUMONIA & BRONCHITIS

More good news about probiotics and respiratory health: Supplementing with *Lactobacillus acidophilus* can help to suppress pneumonia and decrease bronchitis in children 6 to 24 months old. Children who are undernourished suffer twice the severities, but the *lactobacillus* proves to be beneficial for both undernourished and normal children.

Source: *Archivos Latinoamericanos de Nutricion* 2002;52(1):29-34.

WANT TO KNOW MORE?
[Probiotics are helpful against a host of maladies. I have been recommending the use of large amounts of *Lactobacillus acidophilus* for years to teenagers suffering with acne, and have endless reports of great success. See Hint #352 in the *Dermatological Conditions* section for more information.]

928. RUNNERS: TAKE VITAMIN C BEFORE RACES

Runners, take note: Supplementing with vitamin C before running a marathon can reduce the effects of upper respiratory tract infections – a common problem following marathon participation. The incidence of symptoms of upper respiratory tract infections during the two weeks following a marathon is reduced by more than half in runners who consume 600 mg of vitamin C for three weeks before the race compared with runners consuming a placebo.

Intense prolonged exercise can wreak havoc on your immune system. Vitamin C has attracted interest in the sports community as a supplement that might reduce the risk of overtraining. [I follow the same regimen before flying.]

Source: *Exercise Immunology Review* **1997;3:32.**

RESPIRATORY ILLNESS: REDUCING RISK

929. DID YOU WASH YOUR HANDS?

Want to avoid respiratory illness? Make sure to wash your hands. A three-year study of a hand-washing program on a military base, involving over a million healthy young adults, was associated with a 45 percent reduction of respiratory illness. Frequent hand-washers reported fewer respiratory illness episodes when compared to infrequent hand-washers.

Although surveys reveal challenges with hand-washing compliance, this should be added to our list of techniques for preventive medicine.

Source: *American Journal of Preventive Medicine* **21:2:79-83.**

930. IS THERE SOMETHING "GOING AROUND"?

If you're wondering if your respiratory symptoms are caused by something that might be "going around," click on www.rtialert.com to see a report of infections in your area, and whether or not your neighborhood will be hit hard. After you enter your zip code, you will get a local report. You will also be informed if levels in your area are expected to peak soon. Bronchitis, sinusitis, and pneumonia are three common respiratory tract infections that this site monitors.

SHINGLES

Varicella zoster virus is a herpes virus that can cause two distinct clinical diseases, chickenpox and shingles. Primary infection of varicella, often called chickenpox, results in a generalized eruption of a rash which is usually seen in children and is highly contagious. This virus can then become latent and later reactivate causing herpes zoster, commonly known as shingles.

931. PEPPERMINT OIL FOR SHINGLES PAIN

If you are suffering from the painful effects of shingles, peppermint oil may offer some relief. Postherpetic neuralgia, an outcome of shingles, may be relieved with peppermint oil (containing 10 percent menthol) applied directly to the skin at the area of pain. Postherpetic neuralgia remains a difficult problem to treat. But applying peppermint oil topically may result in an almost immediate improvement.

Source: *Clinical Journal of Pain* **2002;18(3):200-202.**

SLEEP APNEA

Sleep apnea refers to a serious condition in which there is intermittent cessation of breathing during sleep, which forces the individual to repeatedly wake up to take breaths of air.

932. PROGESTERONE AGAINST SLEEP APNEA

Sleep apnea (temporary stopping of breathing during sleep, resulting in daytime sleepiness) afflicts as many as half of all women over the age of 45 or 50, but it can be alleviated with the use of progesterone. Sleep apnea is twice as likely to occur in postmenopausal women as it is in women who are still premenopausal, and is more severe when it does occur. As many as 17 respiratory events can occur per hour, compared to nine in premenopausal women.

It has been known for some time that progesterone is a breathing stimulant, and therefore may protect against sleep apnea.

Source: 96th International Conference of the American Thoracic Society, May 2000.

WANT TO KNOW MORE?
For additional benefits of progesterone, see my book, ***Hormone Replacement Therapy: Yes or No? How to Make an Informed Decision.*** The application of a progesterone cream, applied topically, could be an easy solution.]

SLEEP DISORDERS & DEPRIVATION

The last four decades have seen the emergence of a new medical specialty, sleep medicine. In response to an unfulfilled clinical need, sleep medicine developed medical solutions for age-old problems with sleep and wakefulness. (***Dental Clinics of North American*** **2001;45(4):631-42)** The drug solution, however, is not without side effects.

933. COFFEE & YOUR SLEEP PATTERN

If you are having trouble sleeping at night, avoid those late afternoon coffee breaks. Coffee after lunch can wreak havoc with sleep patterns because (in addition to being a stimulant) caffeine interrupts the flow of melatonin, the hormone that sends us to sleep at night. Secreted by the pineal gland, melatonin controls body rhythms and helps our body know when to sleep and when to wake. People who drink coffee after lunch sleep on average 5.5 hours a night compared with seven hours if they drink decaffeinated coffee.

Melatonin secretion is reduced not only by caffeine, but also by alcohol and some commonly prescribed drugs.

Sources: *British Press Digest* reported in *Reuter's* 2002; *Nurse Practitioner* 1997;22(2):66-67,71-72,77.

WANT TO KNOW MORE?
Reductions in melatonin secretion have also been associated with many disorders, including cardiovascular disease, Alzheimer's disease, diabetes, SIDS (Sudden Infant Death Syndrome), as well as aging.

934. SEVEN HOURS OF SLEEP IS BEST

If you tend to sleep for a long period of time each night, you should be aware that seven hours of sleep per night appears to be ideal, while an hour or more in excess of seven hours results in an increased risk of mortality. Those who sleep an average of 8.5 hours nightly, or less than 3.5 or 4.5 hours, have an increase mortality risk that exceeds 15 percent. In those who sleep 10 or more hours per night, the increased risk is primarily due to cerebrovascular deaths.

The risk associated with the use of prescription sleeping pills is greater than any risk associated with insomnia.

Source: *Archives of General Psychiatry* 2002;59:131-138.

935. MODERATE SLEEP DEPRIVATION IS HARMFUL

Make sure you are getting enough sleep – even moderate sleep deprivation can be harmful to your health. While *severe* sleep deprivation has been repeatedly shown to have harmful effects on mental and physical functioning, we now know that restricting normal sleep by only two hours a day can also be disastrous.

Even modest sleep restriction impairs daily functioning, increases inflammatory markers, and adversely affects hormone levels.

After one week of mild sleep deprivation, study participants fall asleep faster and sleep more deeply, a sign of the body's attempt to adapt to sleep loss. And during the daytime, these sleep-deprived individuals show more signs of sleepiness and perform worse on vigilance tests.

Sleep deprivation is also shown to affect hormonal levels, and both men and women have a 40 to 60 percent average increase in important inflammatory markers. [inflammation is elevated in many disease conditions].

It is interesting to note that women seem to fare better; they are more resilient and able to sleep more soundly than men.

Source: Annual Meeting of the Endocrine Society, San Francisco, CA, Jun 2002.

WANT TO KNOW MORE?
Short-term sleep restriction results in impaired glucose tolerance. Sleep restriction may be an independent risk factor for developing symptomatic diabetes. (***Diabetes Care*** **2003;26(2):380-384)**

936. HERBS FOR FORTY WINKS

Natural herbs used for sleep disorders include chamomile, gotu kola, hops, l-tryptophan, lavender, passionflower, skullcap, and valerian. These are generally safer and offer a more natural alternative to the drugs. [When starting to use these herbs, begin slowly and build to the recommended doses gradually. Many of these herbs are available in tea form. This avoids the need for tablets or capsules, binders and fillers. Credible tea companies use techniques to maintain the integrity of the herbs they are processing.]

For those who are on drug therapy, note that clinical studies comparing dietary supplements with low-dose anti-depressants or high-dose anti-depressants find no sgnificant difference between treatments.

Source: *Lippincotts Primary Care Practice* 1999;3(3):290-304

937. BRIGHT LIGHT FOR NIGHT SHIFT WORKERS

Short-term bright light treatment may help the adaptation to an extended night-work period, and especially the subsequent re-adaptation to day life. Night workers complain of sleepiness, reduced performance and disturbed sleep due to lack of adjustment of the circadian rhythm. Bright light treatment of 30 minutes per exposure was applied during the first four nights of the night-shift period and the first four days at home following the shift period.

The bright light exposure was scheduled individually to phase delay the circadian rhythm. Bright light treatment modestly facilitated the subjective adaptation to night work, but the positive effect of bright light was especially pronounced during the re-adaptation back to day life following the return home. Sleepiness was reduced and the quality of day was rated better after exposure to bright light.

Source: *Journal of Sleep Research* **1999;8(2):105-12.**

938. YAWNING? TRY SIBERIAN GINSENG

Siberian ginseng can be a prophylactic for fatigue. Short term treatment with ginseng significantly prolongs aerobic endurance. Japanese students wouldn't think of entering the exam room without having taken their supplemental ginseng. (Far better than the bar of chocolate my mother gave me!)

Many controlled studies demonstrate the effectiveness of Siberian ginseng for relieving stress, acting as a stimulant tonic, and boosting the immune system.

[An ancient Chinese herbalist is quoted as saying, "Person would rather take handful of ginseng than cartload of gold and jewels.]

Sources: *Planta Medica* **1998;64(2):130-3; B Kamen,** *Siberian Ginseng: Up-to-Date Research On The Fabled Oriental Tonic Herb.*

WANT TO KNOW MORE:
Many people have a temporary spell, often in early afternoon, when they feel drowsy. This passing desire for a quick nap is completely different from excessive daytime sleepiness, which is a much more significant problem.

Excessive daytime sleepiness is a serious concern in the workplace with respect to errors, accidents, absenteeism, reduced productivity and impaired personal or professional life. More women than men appear to be affected. (*Social Science Medicine* **2003 Feb;56(4):883-94**)

SMOKING & NICOTINE ADDICTION

Researchers are telling us that the consequence of chronic smoking have been underestimated. For example, the scientists have just learned that smoking one cigarette, whether by a smoker or nonsmoker, causes an acute increase in arterial stiffnes.. (*Hypertension* **2003;41:183-187**) Sadly, smoking by young people is on the increae.

The good news is that those who stopped smoking at least ten years ago have a lower risk of cancer than current smokers and those who stopped more recently. (*American Journal of Epidemiology* **2002;156:1011-1020**) There doesn't seem to be much point in telling all this to smokers. They know how detrimental the habit is. At best, smokers need to be aware of nutritional help to mitigate the dire consequences.

N THIS SECTION:
- DIETARY PROTECTION
- HEALTH RISKS
- NATURAL & SUPPLEMENTAL PROTECTION

- QUITTING STRATEGIES
- SECOND-HAND SMOKE PROTECTION

SMOKING: DIETARY PROTECTION

939. SMOKERS: BALANCE ANTI- & PRO-OXIDANTS

If you are a smoker, altering your diet to balance dietary antioxidants and pro-oxidants can be protective against smoking-related damage. Smokers may benefit from more fresh fruits and vegetables and less meat, and/or combined supplements of vitamin C, beta-carotene, and iron. The point is to balance the antioxidants and the pro-oxidants. (Vitamins C and beta-carotene are antioxidants, while iron is a pro-oxidant.) The findings of a 10-year Belgian study done on over 2,800 male smokers were consistent with the hypothesis that the oxidative balance of the diet is associated with subsequent mortality.

Source: *Journal of Nutrition* **2002;132:756-761.**

SMOKING: HEALTH RISKS

940. QUIT SOON OR "FACE" THE CONSEQUENCES

Young women should know that after many years of smoking, the skin of a 40-year-old woman has aged an additional 20 years. If the desire to be beautiful is a more powerful weapon than fear of lung cancer, the high risk of wrinkles should be a significant deterrent for smoking.

The wrinkle effects are reversible if women quit smoking early enough. But the damage done to skin and the subsequent formation of wrinkles are irreversible if smoking continues for decades.

Source: *European Week Against Cancer* **2001.**

WANT TO KNOW MORE?
Lung cancer is rising more rapidly among women than among men in the European Union, and in some countries lung cancer among women under 45 years of age is more common than among men in the same age group.

941. FEWER CIGARETTES NOT THE ANSWER

A reduction in the number of cigarettes smoked each day, short of completely quitting, does NOT appear to reduce the risk of tobacco-related diseases. (15 or more cigarettes a day) who reduce their cigarette intake by half experience no reduction in serious risk from any cause. Quitters, however, have a 35 percent lower risk of disease from all causes compared with heavy smokers.

There is also no difference seen in respiratory disease or death from cardiovascular disease between people who reduce their smoking and those who continue to smoke heavily.

Source: *American Journal of Epidemiology* **2002;156:994-1001.**

SMOKING: NATURAL & SUPPLEMENTAL PROTECTION
942. VITAMIN PROTECTION FOR SMOKERS

Smokers: A combination of beta-carotene, vitamin C, and vitamin E can be protective by increasing your levels of antioxidant enzymes (which are depleted by smoking). Smoking tobacco products reduces the body's levels of many nutrients, including antioxidants. At the same time, the liver needs higher levels of some of these nutrients to promote the detoxification (breakdown) of hazardous compounds found in tobacco smoke.

When male smokers are given a combination of antioxidant supplements daily for six weeks, blood levels of several key antioxidant enzymes — catalase, glutathione peroxidase, and superoxide dismutase — increase *significantly*. At the same time, decreases are seen in both oxidized (free-radical damaged) fats in cholesterol as well as iron levels, which can promote free-radical reactions. (Benefits are seen even in those taking a moderate daily dose of 15 mg of beta-carotene, 500 mg of vitamin C, and 400 IU of vitamin E.)

Sources: *Biochemistry* **2002;13:427-434;** *Journal of the National Cancer Institute* **1999;91:1738.**

WANT TO KNOW MORE?
If you are a male smoker, you should know that high serum levels of alpha-tocopherol (vitamin E) are associated with a decreased incidence of lung cancer.

943. AGED GARLIC EXTRACT FOR PROTECTION

Dietary supplementation with aged garlic extract may be protective against smoking-related damage. Some components of garlic are known to possess antioxidant properties, and supplementation with aged garlic extract may help to reduce the oxidative stress resulting from smoking or other toxic exposures. [Aged garlic extract is available in most health food stores, and doesn't irritate the gastrointestinal lining the way raw fresh garlic can.]

In a study done on both smokers and nonsmokers, significant beneficial effects were observed for both groups after supplementation with aged garlic extract. However, two weeks after discontinuing the garlic, the parameters went back to what they were before – indicating that aged garlic extract should be continually taken.

Source: *Journal of Nutrition* **2002;132(2):168-171.**

WANT TO KNOW MORE?
[Aged garlic extract is also helpful against atherosclerosis (see Hint #522) as well as poor circulation (Hint #822).]

944. TAURINE PROTECTION FOR SMOKERS

Supplementing with taurine, an amino acid, can help younger smokers reverse damage to their blood and lymph vessels. Taurine is shown to have a protective effect on endothelial structure and function, which refers to the thin layers of flat cells that line the blood vessel and lymphatic membranes. In fact, in young adult smokers, taurine supplementation largely reverses this endothelial dysfunction, restoring it to that of nonsmokers. (The benefits appear to stem from taurine's effect on nitric oxide metabolism.)

Although beneficial for young smokers, it is not yet known if taurine could help the dysfunction that commonly occurs with chronic cigarette smoking. [Some good dietary sources of taurine include eggs, milk, meat, and fish. It is not found in vegetable proteins.]

Source: *Circulation* **2003;107.**

WANT TO KNOW MORE?
Although pretreatment with vitamin C also significantly improves this problem in smokers, it's not enough to match that of nonsmokers.

945. *FORMER SMOKERS NEED PROTECTION TOO*

FORMER smokers, be advised: Compared with those who have never smoked, former smokers still tend to have lower antioxidant levels — so it's a good idea to go heavy on antioxidant supplementation. Cigarette smoke is a significant source of oxidative stress, one reason for its unhealthful effects. Compared with nonsmokers, active smokers have more than 25 percent lower circulating concentrations of ascorbic acid (vitamin C) and alpha- and beta-carotenes.

But even after you stop smoking, you still have less circulating amounts of these antioxidants than someone who has never smoked. (Smoking is less strongly associated with circulating concentrations of vitamin E and the carotenoids lutein, zeaxanthin, and lycopene.)

But there's good news: Since dietary micronutrient intake is associated with blood micronutrient concentrations, you can boost your antioxidant levels through supplementation and diet.

Source: *Toxicology* 2002;180(2):121.

WANT TO KNOW MORE?
The same associations hold true for passive smoking, so even low-dose exposures to tobacco smoke can result in lower circulating antioxidant concentrations. [See later in this section for hints specifically on protection from *second-hand* smoke.]

SMOKING: QUITTING STRATEGIES
946. *LAUGHING GAS CAN HELP YOU QUIT*

A dose of "laughing gas" (nitrous oxide) seems to help smokers kick the habit. It is believed that nitrous oxide helps smokers quit because it replenishes stores of dopamine, which become depleted during drug and alcohol withdrawal. Nitrous oxide decreases withdrawal symptoms, and the procedure is extremely safe.

When smokers were given the gas, an 85 percent reduction in the number of cigarette smoked per day was seen for three days following treatment. Nicotine cravings were greatly helped, and many remained cigarette-free for as long as six months. (None of the smokers used any other kind of smoking cessation therapy.)

Source: 2001 Annual Scientific Assembly of the American Association of Family Practitioners, Atlanta, GA, Oct 2001.

947. ACUPUNCTURE TO HELP QUIT SMOKING

If you are a smoker who needs some extra help in quitting, consider acupuncture, which is shown to be effective. Acupuncture treatment (five days a week, for four weeks) can help smokers decrease the number of cigarettes they smoke, as well as help them give up smoking altogether. (It is the most addicted smokers who show the largest benefit with this method.) When acupuncture is combined with education about the dangers of smoking, the greatest effect is seen.

Source: *American Journal of Public Health* **2002;92:1642-1647.**

SMOKING: SECOND-HAND SMOKE PROTECTION
948. CAROTENOIDS LOWER IN PASSIVE SMOKERS

If you live or work with a smoker, be sure to add carotenoids to your supplement regimen because you most likely have low levels of these beneficial substances. [Carotenoids are compounds related to vitamin A, of which beta-carotene is the most well known. Others include alpha-carotene, lycopene, and lutein.] Among nonsmokers, exposure to passive smoking tends to be associated with lower blood concentrations of carotenoids, as second-hand smoke may result in decreased circulating concentrations of selected micronutrients.

[Palm oil tocotrienols are an excellent source of carotenoids. They are also found in foods such as spinach, broccoli, kale, asparagus, lettuce, carrots, sweet potatoes, winter squash, pumpkin, red cabbage, apricots, peaches, mango, cantaloupe, papaya, cherries, and watermelon.]

Source: *American Journal of Clinical Nutrition* **2000;72(6):1576-1582.**

949. ANTIOXIDANTS & SECOND-HAND SMOKE

In addition to carotenoids such as beta-carotene, supplementing with natural vitamin E, vitamin C, bioflavonoids, and other antioxidant nutrients can protect those exposed to second-hand smoke. Cigarette smoke contains more than 4,000 chemicals, many of which are hazardous free radicals. In addition to their direct damage, free radicals can also initiate an inflammatory response, which further injures tissues. [Inflammation is elevated in many disease conditions.] Test animals exposed to cigarette smoke have higher levels of free radicals in the liver, the organ that breaks down hazardous chemicals. If they receive an antioxidant-nutrient combination, they maintain normal levels of free radicals.

Source: *Environmental Health Perspectives* **2001;109:1007-1009.**

950. VITAMIN C FOR KIDS EXPOSED TO SMOKE

If children are exposed to even *minimal* amounts of second-hand smoke at home, both their dietary and supplemental sources of vitamin C should be significantly increased. Previous research has shown that adults exposed to second-hand smoke have increased dietary vitamin C requirements, and this exposure can also lower vitamin C levels in children. Even very low exposure can result in lower levels of vitamin C, and for reason not yet fully understood, a greater difference is found in girls.

Source: *American Journal of Clinical Nutrition* 2003;77:167-172.

WANT TO KNOW MORE?
[Some good dietary sources of vitamin C include citrus fruits, "tart"-tasting fruits, green leafy veggies, and sauerkraut. Grains and beans have little vitamin C until they are sprouted (sprouts have been known since the 18th century to cure scurvy, a disease that results from severe vitamin C deficiency). Green peppers contain more vitamin C than an orange. As for supplements, there are newer, better sources than the allergenic corn-extracted vitamin C.]

STOMACHACHES

Although stomachaches and headaches are often considered characteristic of children with anxiety disorders, there is converging evidence that a broader range of somatic symptoms may be associated with these expressions of anxiety. (***Journal of Abnormal Child Psychology* 1991;19(6):659-70**) As for adults, we've all had them, and very often we know why. It's when we can't identify the cause that we need to pay more attention..

951. ACIDOPHILUS AGAINST STOMACH UPSET

Every household should have a bottle of liquid *acidophilus* in the fridge. Very few natural products work as fast to alleviate stomachaches, abdominal cramps, or even vomiting. Even if you suspect mild food poisoning as the cause of stomach upset, start with the *acidophilus*. Take two tablespoons, and if symptoms aren't relieved after the first dose, repeat in a half hour. Probiotics such as *acidophilus* should be taken regularly by everyone, anyway, but at times of stomach distress, the liquid is usually fast acting.

Acidophilus does not have a medicinal taste, and you'll find that even children won't offer resistance. [Liquid *acidophilus* is readily available at most health food stores.]

Source: Betty Kamen's decades of experience.

STRESS

Stress has a major impact on degenerative diseases and mental disorders. It plays a significant role in susceptibility, progress, and actual outcome of these diseases. Also, subjective or individual differences have to be taken into account. And not all stress is bad. Stress that is not overwhelming may even improve performance/biological functions and be beneficial in certain cases. (*Neuroendocrinology Letters* **2002 Jun;23(3):199-208**)

IN THIS SECTION:
- NATURAL REMEDIES & SUPPLEMENTS
- REDUCTION STRATEGIES

STRESS: NATURAL REMEDIES & SUPPLEMENTS

952. VITAMIN C: A STRESS BUSTER?

Supplementing with a specific form of vitamin C may help you to better deal with stress. Subjects given 1,000 mg of vitamin C were shown to deal with stress better: Their average increase in blood pressure was only 23 mm Hg compared to the 31 mm Hg increase seen in those given a placebo. In addition, their blood pressure and cortisol (the stress hormone) levels returned to normal more quickly.

It was concluded that people may feel less stressed when they are saturated with vitamin C. (Important note: The researchers caution that the vitamin C in this study was different from the vitamin C found in oranges – the same results may not be seen when taking natural vitamin C.)

Source: *Psychopharmacology* 2002:159:319-324.

953. AGED GARLIC EXTRACT IN TIMES OF STRESS

If you are under a great deal of psychological stress, protect your health by supplementing with aged garlic extract. Psychological stress can have deleterious effects on your immune system and overall health, but aged garlic extract (AGE) is shown to be helpful in preventing this stress-induced damage. When given to psychologically stressed test animals, AGE helped to *significantly* prevent a number of factors (such as decreased spleen weight) used to determine the ill effects of stress on the body.

[Aged garlic is a remarkable supplement. It protects the body against liver toxicity caused by industrial chemicals and the damage done by acetaminophen (Tylenol). Evidence shows that aged garlic can also protect against damage from aging, radiation, and chemical exposure, as well as reduce the risk of cardiovascular disease, stroke, and the brain cell damage related to Alzheimer's disease. Aged garlic is available in most health food stores.]

Sources: *Phytomedicine* Nov 1999;6(5)325-330; B. Kamen, *Everything I Know About Nutrition I Learned from Barley*.

954. STRESSED OUT? CHLORELLA CAN HELP

Supplementing with chlorella can help your body protect itself against the unhealthful effects of psychological stress. Many people who take the supplement chlorella report beneficial results against stress. [Chlorella is a green algae, grown in fresh mineral water pools and supercharged with nutrients.] When given to psychologically stressed test animals, chlorella has a protective effect against tumors and reduced cortisone levels, indicating that it can prevent psychological stress and help to maintain homeostasis in the face of external environmental changes. Chlorella has also been shown to reduce the demise of certain immune cells normally caused by psychological stress.

[Chlorella is available in health food stores, where you will notice it is referred to as "cracked-cell" or "broken-cell" chlorella. As the algae cell wall cannot normally be broken down in the human digestive system, a special process is required to safely "crack" the algae cell open without harming the beneficial enzymes within.]

Source: *International Journal of Immunopharmacology* 2000;22(11):877-885.

955. VELVET ANTLER FOR STRESS & FATIGUE

In addition to enhancing your immune system, the supplement velvet antler may be very helpful against stress and fatigue. Extracts of velvet antler are found to exhibit *significant* immuno-stimulating activity, as well as having an anti-fatigue effect. In addition, these extracts show a significant anti-stress effect when given to test animals. (Velvet antler extracts have even shown some anti-thrombotic activity.)

These findings are indicative of the adaptogenic properties of antlers during stressful conditions. [An adaptogen is something that normalizes a physiological process or condition, unlike drugs, which tend to influence a process or condition in the same predictable direction.] The extracts also have a beneficial effect on the neuromuscular and endocrine systems.

Sources: Antler Science & Product Technology 2001, Alberta, Canada; "Immuno-Stimulating, Anti-Stress and Anti-Thrombotic Effects of Unossified Velvet Antlers," K.H. Shin, et al., pp 236-249.

WANT TO KNOW MORE?

[To learn about how velvet antler can also help with diseases such as osteoporosis and arthritis (and how it is better than isolated chondroitin and glucosamine sulfate), see my book, *The Remarkable Healing Power of Velvet Antler*.]

956. FAMILY FEUDS? SERVE ANTI-STRESS TEA

At your next family get-together, promote a sense of calm and tranquility by serving anti-stress tea. When families get together (such as on holidays) emotions and tempers can often run high, resulting in high stress all around – but serving anti-stress tea may help. Just sipping a hot liquid imbues a feeling of calmness, and when that beverage contains anti-stress herbs such as St. John's wort, balm leaves, and valerian root, so much the better. The synergy of these herbs — used only in very small amounts – helps to promote a feeling of peace and serenity.

So think of serving such a tea to your mother-in-law, or to the rambunctious cousins who act out noisily when they see each other only once a year.

WANT TO KNOW MORE?

Tea is more popular than ever in America today. Currently, there is a reawakening of interest in tea as many seek a more positive, healthful lifestyle. As I travel about, I have noticed that many hotels are restoring the tradition of the afternoon tea service. Makes sense!

It's interesting to note that experiences of early life stress are more prevalent among depressed patients than healthy controls. (*Nueropsychopharmacology* 2002;27(6):756-64)

And chronic unpredictable stress exacerbates the vascular and cellular inflammatory responses. (*Integrative Physiological and Behavioral Science* 2002;77(1):79-83)

957. PHOSPHATIDYLSERINE, A MOOD ENCHANCER

Taking 300 mg of phosphatidylserine each day for a month is associated with feeling less stressed and having a better mood. This study for the first time reports an improvement in mood following phosphatidylserine supplementation in a group of young healthy adults.

It accomplishes this effect on mood because it blunts the release of cortisol. Cortisol has a long list of adverse effects when in excess, and is now considered a major cause of insomnia and memory loss due to brain damage.

Source: *Nutritional Neuroscience* 2001;4(3):169-78.

STRESS: REDUCTION STRATEGIES

958. SIMPLE TIPS FOR STRESS RELIEF

To help cope with any kind of stress (especially during these stressful times), consider some of these helpful stress-relieving practices:

- Try to exercise aerobically one-half hour daily; it's a good release for anxiety.

- Practice deep breathing exercises or other relaxation techniques (meditation, yoga, etc.).

- Avoid watching the news while eating; listen to soothing music during that time instead.

- Have long talks with close friends about your fears and frustrations. (But not at mealtime.)

- Fortify with specific supplements demonstrated to improve coping capacity, such as antioxidants like vitamin C (the single most important anti-stress nutrient), and vitamins A and E.

- Add supplements containing nutrients that stress can deplete, such as calcium and zinc.

- Include a probiotic to minimize the digestive problems that can be induced by stress.

- Include enzymes to increase nutrient absorption.

- Drink lots of water to help circulate nutrients.

- Take a short walk before retiring to encourage better sleep. B vitamins and calcium may be as effective for sleep as Grandma's glass of warm milk.

- Consider one or more anti-stress herbs, such as licorice root, fennel, or gotu kola leaf.

- Since stress upsets hormone metabolism, this is a good time for both men and women to become familiar with the low-dose progesterone creams, particularly those containing Siberian ginseng and other beneficial "feel-good" and hormone-balancing herbs. (There are specific formulas for men and women.)

STROKE

Stroke is one of the oldest but least understood diseases, and it is one of the major public health problems facing our seniors. Investigations have found that the incidence of stroke has been underestimated by about 50 percent. Recent clinical and basic research indicates that stroke is neither unpredictable nor irreversible. Many risk factors for stroke are readily identifiable, and evidence-based treatment may be used to reduce the likelihood of stroke among those at risk. (*Mt Sinai Journal of Medicine* 2003 Jan;70(1):27-37)

IN THIS SECTION:
- ALTERNATIVE THERAPIES
- CAUSES & PRECURSORS
- DIETARY TACTICS

- NATURAL REMEDIES & SUPPLEMENTS
- RECOVERY STRATEGIES
- REDUCING RISK

959. TAKING STROKES SERIOUSLY

Public awareness continues to falter with respect to strokes. Textbook symptoms include tingling, paralysis, or loss of vision, particularly on one side of the body, and other symptoms that are less frequently identified include headache, nausea and vomiting, and vertigo. According to a survey of 1,000 adults, when asked which health threat they feared the most, 33 percent reported cancer, 13 percent heart disease, and a dismal ONE percent feared stroke (even though 35 percent of those surveyed reported having had a stroke themselves or knowing someone with a recent stroke!)

Another discouraging survey involving 4,000 Americans aged 18-30 years pointed to the fact that although they possessed the knowledge that a family member suffered a stroke, young adults are still unlikely to change their own risky lifestyle behaviors. [The issue of why we don't change our lifestyle in spite of a proliferation of serious messages is addressed extensively in my new book, *Everything I Know About Nutrition I Learned from Barley*. The book also offers a few simple solutions.]

Source: *Medscape Cardiology* 2002;6(2),PAGE.

STROKE: ALTERNATIVE THERAPIES
960. BOTOX INJECTIONS FOR STROKE PATIENTS?

If you have had a stroke and are experiencing weak or spastic muscles in the hands, Botox injections may be helpful. Injections of Botox can help reduce the weakness or spasticity of wrist and finger muscles and associated disability in men and women who have had strokes. [Botox, derived from the bacteria that causes botulism, has been gaining more and more popularity these days as an anti-wrinkle treatment.]

Botox can improve the quality of life in those with post-stroke spasms. It may be an effective treatment for many of the over four million patients in the US who have had a stroke (and it is an extremely safe treatment for stroke patients).

Source: *New England Journal of Medicine* **2002;347:382-383,395-400.**

STROKE: CAUSES & PRECURSORS

961. BEWARE HIGH DOSES OF ASPIRIN!

Beware taking high doses of aspirin, which could raise your odds of having a hemorrhagic stroke. Women taking 15 or more tablets of aspirin per week *double* their risk of hemorrhagic stroke compared with women not taking aspirin. Among older women and those with hypertension, the risk of hemorrhage is actually *tripled* with a high weekly dose of aspirin.

Long term therapy with aspirin is also associated with a significant increase in the incidence of gastrointestinal hemorrhage. No evidence exists that reducing the dose or using modified release formulations would reduce the incidence of gastrointestinal hemorrhage.

Sources: *Stroke* **1999;30:1764-1771;** *British Medical Journal* **2000 11;321(7270):1183-7.**

962. SLEEP PATTERNS & YOUR RISK OF STROKE

If you sleep more than eight hours a night, snore frequently, or fall asleep during the day, you should be especially careful of your lifestyle and food and supplement intake because you may be at high risk for a stroke. The frequency of stroke is found to be higher among those who sleep for more than eight hours per night (14 percent), compared with those who sleep only six to eight hours (5.4 percent) and those who sleep less than six hours (also 5.4 percent). In addition, those with daytime sleepiness also have a higher frequency of stroke (12 percent) compared with those without (4 percent). This increased stroke risk is independent of cardiovascular risk factors.

The reason for the link between sleep and stroke risk remains unclear.

Source: 26th International Stroke Association Conference of the American Heart Association, Feb 2001.

963. BLOOD-CLOT RISK IN OVERWEIGHT PEOPLE

Taking steps now to reduce excess weight can help you to lower your production of a specific hormone that puts you at increased risk for dangerous blood clots and stroke. People who are overweight have a higher risk of developing blood clots than people who are not overweight because of a hormone produced by fat cells. Overweight people develop more and larger fat cells that produce this hormone (called leptin), which makes them more susceptible to blood clotting. The more leptin in blood plasma, the higher the risk of forming clots.

Researchers conclude the best way to prevent blood clots and the subsequent strokes and heart attacks caused by them is the same message we keep hearing, again and again: *Eat right and exercise.* Losing weight helps to lower the amount of leptin in the blood.

Source: *Journal of the American Medical Association* 2002;287:1706-1709.

964. MODERATELY HIGH HOMOCYSTEINE & STROKE

Beware even moderately high levels of homocysteine, which can put you at increased risk for a stroke, as well as many other health problems. There is an association seen between moderately elevated blood levels of homocysteine and these three conditions: stroke, cerebrovascular dementia, and Alzheimer's disease. Since B vitamins can reduce homocysteine levels, B vitamin supplementation may be a good idea for most adults.

[My suggestion for increasing B vitamins with supplementation is to use food-type supplements such as sprouted young barley leaf, brewer's yeast, bee pollen, and chlorella. If your homocysteine levels are *extremely* high, use isolated vitamins B12, B6, and folic acid.]

Source: *Stroke* 2002;33:2351-2356.

WANT TO KNOW MORE?
[Homocysteine is an amino acid produced naturally in your body, but high levels in the blood are associated with many health problems, including Alzheimer's and heart disease. See Hints #73 and #550 for more details.]

965. GUM DISEASE & THE RISK OF STROKES

Periodontal disease and tooth loss can increase your risk of having an ischemic stroke (most likely because of inflammation) – so if you have these problems, check out anti-inflammation regimens such as the herb cat's claw and green tea. Men who have no more than 24 teeth are 57 percent more likely to experience an ischemic stroke than are men with more teeth. An ischemic stroke is caused by a decrease in the blood supply caused by constriction or obstruction of blood vessels.

Periodontal disease is known to cause inflammation and inflammation is known to play an important role in the development of coronary artery disease as well as stroke.

Sources: *Stroke* **2002;34;** *Journal of Periodontal Research* **2002;37(6):433-438.**

WANT TO KNOW MORE?
[Poor dental health, especially gum disease, has been linked to many serious diseases and health problems, such as rheumatoid arthritis (see Hint #103), heart disease (see Hint #526), and low birth weight (see Hint #851).]

STROKE: DIETARY TACTICS
966. VEGGIES PROTECTIVE AGAINST STROKES

Eat your vegetables! Eating fresh veggies several times a week can *significantly* reduce your risk of both ischemic AND hemorrhagic strokes. The risk of stroke can be as much as *58 percent* lower among those who consume vegetables six to seven days per week compared to those who only consume them up to two days per week. High concentrations of dietary vitamin C appear to reduce the risk of both *ischemic* and *hemorrhagic* stroke, independent of other stroke risk factors such as hypertension, total cholesterol, body mass index, physical activity, smoking, alcohol drinking, antihypertensive medication, atrial fibrillation, and a history of ischemic heart disease.

During a 20-year follow-up period of a large number of men and women, researchers found strong inverse associations between vitamin C concentration and all strokes. The risk of stroke was *70 percent* higher among those with the lowest vitamin C levels compared to those with the highest.

[Vitamin C is one of the least stable vitamins, and cooking can destroy much of it. Some good dietary sources of vitamin C are citrus fruits, strawberries, green peppers, broccoli, dark leafy greens, and tomatoes.]

Source: *Stroke* **2000;31:2287-2294.**

WANT TO KNOW MORE?
[See Hint #970 for information on the protective effects of vitamin C *supplements* against strokes.]

967. REDUCE STROKE RISK BY EATING FISH

Adding fish or other seafood to your diet at least a couple of times per month can greatly reduce your risk of having an ischemic stroke. Men who eat fish once or twice a month often have a *significantly* lower risk of *ischemic* stroke compared with those who eat fish less frequently.

The word ischemia refers to "holding back." An ischemic stroke is caused by a blockage or decrease in the blood supply. (Fish consumption is not associated with the prevention of a *hemorrhagic* stroke, caused by bleeding.)

Eating fish two to four times per week is associated with a nearly 50 percent reduction in the risk of *thrombotic* stroke (a blood clot inside the brain's arteries, blocking the blood flow). The beneficial effect of fish intake on the risk of ischemic stroke may approach a maximum at a relatively low level of consumption. More fish intake (up to five or more times per week) does not appear to provide further benefit.

Sources: *Journal of the American Medical Association* **2001;285:304-312;2002;288:3130-3136.**

WANT TO KNOW MORE?

Strokes usually occur because the artery has become narrowed by a condition where fatty deposits (plaques) build up along the walls of blood vessels. However, it may also happen when a blood clot forms in some distant part of the body, breaks loose and travels in the bloodstream to the brain.

Researchers have also found that fish consumption reduces lacunar stroke (blockage of the smaller of the brain's arteries). They hypothesize that the beneficial effect of fish is due to the omega-3 fatty acids, but they caution that not all fish are created equal from the standpoint of pollutants or omega-3 fatty acids.

968. USE GRAPESEED OIL TO LOWER STROKE RISK

Start using grapeseed oil for your cooking and your salad dressings, as it contains high amounts of linoleic acid, which is shown to be protective against the risk of strokes. Several studies show that a lower proportion of linoleic acid (omega-6 fatty acid) is associated with an increased risk of total stroke or ischemic stroke. In fact, linoleic acid is inversely related to stroke risk in a dose-response fashion (so the more linoleic acid you consume, the lower your risk.) Dietary intake of linoleic acid may also lower blood pressure, and it may even improve glucose tolerance! (And it is well known that higher levels of linoleic acid may also lower cholesterol.)

For every five percent increase in the level of linoleic acid, there is a 28 percent reduction in the risk of either type of stroke, a 34 percent drop in the risk of clot-related strokes, and a 19 percent decline in hemorrhagic strokes.

Grapeseed oil has a mild flavor and a high smoke point (485 degrees), so it's great for frying and baking. Other attributes make it ideal for use right out of the refrigerator. It also has a high content of vitamin E (probably one of the reasons it is such a stable oil). You may want the cold-pressed oil for cooking, and the garlic- or basil-flavored oil for your salads.

Source: *Stroke* Aug 2002;33(8):2086-2093.

WANT TO KNOW MORE?

[Linoleic acids are essential acids, which means your body doesn't make them – you must *eat* them. Even though we are consuming 40 percent more fats today than we did about a hundred years ago, we are not getting enough of this essential fatty acid. In therapeutic doses, essential fatty acids can lessen the pain of arthritis, prevent abnormal heart rhythms, and help treat conditions such as eczema and PMS.]

Linoleic acid can also be found in black currant, borage, and evening primrose oils.

969. SWEET NEWS ABOUT CHOCOLATE & STROKES

This may be the best-received hint of all time: The bioflavonoids in a small amount of semisweet chocolate chips prolong clotting time and have a blood-thinning effect – protecting you from strokes! The amount the researchers are talking about is 25 grams. (One ounce is about 32 grams, so the serving size studied was one-sixteenth of a pound.) That doesn't mean more is better. With more chocolate, we get more sugar, and more of other substances that are not necessarily in our best health interest – to say nothing of adversely perpetuating the sweet tooth.

Furthermore, the people who participated in this research project had no heart disease or other chronic diseases [so any other disadvantages may not have been as deleterious as for those who do have medical problems.] The fact remains, however, that a small amount of chocolate consumption causes a *significant* increase in flavonol concentrations in the blood, and an antithrombotic response after two hours.

Small amounts of foods rich in flavonoids – such as chocolate – can beneficially affect platelet function for a limited period. [But I think we all know that there are better choices out there, albeit perhaps not as appealing to the taste buds!]

Source: *Journal of the American Medical Association* **2002.**

WANT TO KNOW MORE?

[If you must have chocolate, indulge in the purest chocolate you can find (or afford). The caveat is to avoid cheap chocolates to which too much sugar and modified fat has been added. See Hint #1,062 in the *Healthier Living* section for more interesting information about chocolate.]

STROKE: NATURAL REMEDIES & SUPPLEMENTS

970. SUPPLEMENTAL VITAMIN C AGAINST STROKES

In addition to consuming lots of vitamin C-rich fruits and vegetable, taking supplemental vitamin C may also help to reduce your risk of having a stroke. Low levels of vitamin C in the blood are associated with an increased risk of stroke in middle-aged men, especially among hypertensive and overweight men. Vitamin C may exert protective effects against strokes by enhancing endothelial function. [These are the layers of cells that line the cavities of the heart, the blood and lymph vessels, and the serous cavities of the body.] The link could also be that people who take vitamin supplements or eat vitamin-rich fruits and vegetables may be more health-conscious than those who don't.

Source: *Stroke* 2002;33:1568.

971. GINKGO AGAINST STROKE-RELATED DAMAGE

Small doses of the herb ginkgo (as in Ginkgo biloba) may help limit the brain damage caused by a stroke. While a low dose of ginkgo appears to offer protection against stroke — reducing the area of the brain affected by 30 percent – a larger dose does not seem to have a beneficial effect. Warning: Because ginkgo is also a mild blood thinner, it may be risky to use it in patients already on blood-thinning medications commonly prescribed for people at risk for stroke.

Source: 52nd Annual Meeting of the American Academy of Neurology, San Diego, CA, May 2000.

WANT TO KNOW MORE?
[Ginkgo has a beneficial effect on many other health problems, including Alzheimer's disease (see Hint #77), dementia (Hint #335), and lagging libidos caused by anti-depressants (Hint #346).]

972. VITAMINS PROTECTIVE AGAINST STROKES

Supplementing with multivitamins combined with antioxidant vitamins (such as vitamin E) can help reduce your risk of having a stroke. Mortality risk from stroke (and heart disease) is *15 percent* lower in those who take a combination of multivitamins and antioxidants. (The antioxidants used in the study were vitamins A and E. Vitamin E has been found to effective in preventing a wide variety of diseases.)

Source: *Annals of Internal Medicine* 1999;130(12):963-70.

973. POTASSIUM AGAINST STROKES

Increasing your intake of the mineral potassium may help you to reduce your risk of stroke. An increased potassium intake may help reduce the risk of stroke among nonusers of diuretics (and aggressive potassium supplementation should be considered for diuretic users). Among those who do not use diuretics, potassium intake below 2.4 grams a day is associated with an increased risk of stroke. A particularly high risk of stroke is noted among diuretic users with low potassium levels and atrial fibrillation.

[Bananas are famous for being a great source of potassium. But other dietary sources of this mineral include brewer's yeast, dairy foods, fish, garlic, nuts, spinach, whole grains, and meat and poultry.]

Sources: *Neurology* 2002;59:302-303,314-320; B. Kamen, *Everything You Always Wanted to Know About Potassium But Were Too Tired to Ask.*

WANT TO KNOW MORE?
[Once again, those of us involved in nutrition research have been ahead of the curve. My book, *Everything You Always Wanted to Know About Potassium But Were Too Tired to Ask*, published in 1992, points to the fact that the risk of stroke decreases as your level of potassium increases, a process entirely unrelated to blood pressure. The book also explores the reasons for low levels of potassium, and specifically defines in detail the kind of supplementation to look for.]

974. NATURAL ANTICOAGULANTS AGAINST STROKES

VERY IMPORTANT FOR ALL STROKE VICTIMS OR THOSE AT RISK FOR STROKE: Protect yourself from the risk of blood clots and stroke by using natural anticoagulants, which are less harmful to the body and do not cause bleeding as many anticoagulant drugs can. Two new natural anticoagulant products have recently appeared in the marketplace. One, nattokinase, is an enzyme derived from the traditional Japanese food called natto [made from fermented soybeans].

The other is a group of enzymes from China, called lumbrokinase, extracted from a specific species of earthworm. Lumbrokinase also decreases fibrinogen significantly.

Among other advantages, these natural products do not cause the risk of excessive bleeding or other side effects that result from the usual anticoagulant drugs. It is also used in valves to decrease clot formation in artificial hearts.

Source: *Arteriosclerosis, Thrombosis, & Vascular Biology* 2002;22:1354-1359; *Clinical Hemorheology Microcirculation* 2000;23(2-4):213-8; *Artificial Organs* 1999;23(2):210-4.

975. MAGNESIUM, TO CONTROL HOMOCYSTEINE

Since magnesium regulates the effects of vitamin B6, B12, and folate on homocysteinemia, this mineral should be added to your stroke-prevention program.
High homocysteine levels cause dose-dependent loss of magnesium [which means, the higher the homocysteine, the greater the magnesium loss.] Adding the B vitamins alone does not affect the magnesium loss. The increased homocysteine, by causing abnormal metabolism of magnesium in vascular smooth muscle cells, primes these cells for atherogenesis, cerebral vasospasm, and stroke.

Source: *Neuroscience Letters* 1999;274(2):83-6.

STROKE: RECOVERY STRATEGIES

976. POSITIVE THOUGHTS & STROKE RECOVERY

Attitude really *can* make a difference: A positive outlook after having suffered a stroke can greatly improve both your mental and physical health. Whether it's faith, laughter, or acceptance, stroke patients who cope better after a stroke live longer. Those who use humor and positive reinterpretation are more outgoing, active, and positive a year after their stroke. However, stroke patients who avoid talking or thinking about their stroke are *more* depressed after a year. These patients may also refuse to change their diet and exercise patterns to prevent future strokes.

Support from family and friends can also play a large role in a stroke patient's recovery, and this includes transportation to doctor visits, medication pick-up, and listening without judgment.

Source: The American Stroke Association's 27th International Stroke Conference, San Antonio, TX, Feb 2002.

977. HYPERBARIC OXYGEN QUICKLY FOR STROKES

Find out NOW where the nearest center for hyperbaric oxygen treatment is located, as it can prevent stroke-related damage if administered quickly. Hyperbaric oxygen treatment, when given within the first *three hours* following the onset of an ischemic stroke, can reduce damage and help functional recovery. Hyperbaric oxygen treatment supplies oxygen to the brain, salvaging structurally intact brain tissue at risk of irreversible damage following a stroke. All hyperbaric oxygen sessions are well tolerated.

This treatment has positive effects on tissue oxygenation. Studies show that hyperbaric oxygen treatment following a stroke helps to reduce ischemic brain damage and behavioral dysfunctions.

Source: Regional Stroke Meeting of the International Stroke Society, Buenos Aires, Argentina, Jun 2002; *Singapore Medical Journal* 2001;42(5):220-3; *Experimental Neurology* 2000;166(2):298=306..

STROKE: REDUCING RISK

978. WALK AWAY FROM THE RISK OF STROKES

Regular, moderate physical activity, such as going for a nice brisk walk, can greatly reduce your risk of suffering a stroke. In women, greater leisure-time physical activity *substantially* reduces the risk of all strokes. Results from the famous Nurses' Study show that the most active women are approximately *50 percent* less likely to have any kind of stroke than the least active women. Simple walking is associated with a reduced risk, and *brisk* walking reduces both the overall stroke risk and the risk of ischemic stroke when compared with casually paced walking. And it's never too late! Even those women who become active for the first time in middle age lower their stroke risk compared to those women who remain sedentary.

Source: *Journal of the American Medical Association* 2000;283:2961-2967.

979. KEEPING FIT KEEPS STROKES AWAY

Guys, are you keeping fit? The more heart and lung fitness you have, the less your chance of suffering a stroke – *at any age*. A definite inverse relationship is seen between cardiorespiratory fitness and the risk of death from stroke, even after adjusting for factors such as smoking, alcohol consumption, weight, hypertension, and diabetes. Between the ages of 40 to 87, highly fit men have a 68 percent lower risk of stroke, and moderately fit men a 63 percent lower risk, when compared to men who are the least fit.

Source: *Medical Science & Sports Exercise* 2002;34(4):592-595.

980. LECITHIN: THE BRAIN-INJURY PROTECTOR

The nutrient lecithin, if administered soon after a person has suffered a stroke, may be very helpful in minimizing more serious brain injury. Choline precursors (such as lecithin) may offer substantial beneficial effects in the treatment of strokes, including reductions in the rate of death and disability. Choline precursors are transformed into substances in the brain that may improve ischemic brain injury through nerve protection and enhanced nerve repair. The protective lecithin *must* be given within the first few hours following the stroke, however. [In addition to lecithin, administering magnesium sulfate en route to the hospital in patients who have suffered an acute stroke is also feasible, safe, and well tolerated by stroke patients.] There's lots of good data indicating that these neuroprotectants can make a big difference in stroke patients.

Source: *Journal of the American Medical Association* 2001;285:1719-1728.

981. STROKE PATIENTS & HIP-FRACTURE RISK

If you have had a stroke, start getting involved in bone-health therapies NOW, as you may also have an increased risk of hip fracture. Hip fracture is *two to four times* more likely to occur in stroke patients than in the general population. Since most fractures in stroke patients occur on the side paralyzed by the stroke, fractures are most often caused by accidental falls – usually about six months following the stroke. Stroke patients tend to fall to the side of the paralysis and are less able to cushion their own falls.

In addition, those with visual impairments are also more likely to fall. [Carpeted floors, rather than wooden floors, can help to cushion falls.]

Source: *Stroke* 2002;33:1432-1436.

982. AVOID THE HIP FRACTURE RISK WITH D3

If you have had a stroke, there's a good chance you are deficient in vitamin D3, especially if you are older. A group of stroke patients were checked for vitamin D status, and then followed for two years. Those who were deficient in D3 had a high hip fracture rate, unlike those in the group who had sufficient D3.

Source: *Stroke* 2001;32(7):1673-7.

WANT TO KNOW MORE?
[See the extensive *Osteoporosis & Other Skeletal Problems* section for lots of hints on how to both prevent and improve this condition.]

Caveat: Long-term oral anticoagulation reduces bone mass. Warfarin therapy inhibits vitamin K-dependent blood-clotting. Although this could reduce the risk of stroke, it increases the risk of severely lowered bone mineral density. Both warfarin-induced reduction of vitamin K function and lowered vitamin K concentrations are probable causes of osteopenia. (*Stroke* 1997;28(12):2390-4)

Antioxidant vitamins play a role in the prevention of stroke because they scavenge free radicals and prevent LDL oxidation.

Antioxidant enzymes such as superoxide dismutase (SOD) and glutathione peroxidase (GPx) provide a defense system that plays a critical role in protecting the cell from free radical damage, particularly lipid peroxidation. (*Journal of Medical Investigation* 2002;49(3-4):172-81)

TRAVEL STRESS & HEALTH CONCERNS

"There's no place like home," yet international travel by American families and their children is increasingly more common. The ease of access to air travel and its increased popularity over the last thirty years have led to a significant incidence of imported infectious diseases and potential infectious hazards. (*Journal of the Royal Society of Health* 2002;122(2):86-8) For example, nine million tourists annually arrive in countries where yellow fever is endemic. (*Clinical Infectious Diseases* 2002 Jul 1;35(1):110) And even on short flights, the change of air pressure takes its toll.

983. REDUCE EAR PAIN WITH A DECONGESTANT

If you suffer from middle-ear pain when flying, a timed-release oral decongestant taken before the trip can help. Since the greatest problem for middle-ear trauma occurs during takeoff and landing, a timed-release decongestant is advisable. If it's not timed release, the effect may wear off if your flight is delayed. (If you feel extra nervous or sweaty, not to worry — it may just be a reaction to the decongestant.) Taking ginger is also a good idea, because it acts as a partial decongestant and also relieves motion sickness.

Source: *Clinical Evidence.* 2002;(7):466-8.

984. HOW I SURVIVE AIR TRAVEL

The next time you travel by plane, you may want to follow these tips that I use to protect my own health and stress levels while in the air:

- When I fly, I get up every half hour and go into the lavatory, where I jump up and down for a few minutes. The jumping helps to compensate for the absence of muscular activity in the calves from sitting so long, which severely slows the rate of blood flow in your lower limbs.
- I carry extra bottles of water, and drink as much as I can to keep hydrated.
- I also take a washcloth with me, which I douse with water periodically and apply to my face to compensate for the dry air. Dry air, even for a short period of time, leads to fine wrinkles. This humid cloth on your face also helps respiration! (See Hint #999 for more information on dry air and wrinkles.)
- I take vitamin C galore before and after the trip, in addition to extra zinc (which gets zapped by the adrenaline increase caused by stress). Doubling the usual intake of nutrients helps to counter the physiological stresses of pressure change, reduced level of oxygen, dry air, immobility due to cramped seating, noise, vibration, and turbulence.
- I call 24 hours in advance to order a hot seafood or vegan meal, and I pack a special treat (either fruit or a CC Pollen energy bar) so I will not feel deprived when I refuse the mixed salted nuts or chemical-laced pretzels.

WANT TO KNOW MORE?
Catecholamines (adrenaline and noradrenaline) increase significantly with noise exposure, such as the kind we hear in a plane. Another reason to increase your vitamin C for adrenal-gland nourishment!

985. STAY DRY WHEN YOU FLY

Avoid drinking alcohol while flying, as it can cause dehydration, impaired mental function, and may even put you at risk for a heart attack One study shows that the effects of alcohol, when added to the specific toxic effects of flying, quickly and readily lead to a drop in overall psychophysical efficiency. (And who wants to arrive at the in-laws with curtailed performance of any kind!) And more seriously: A correlation has also been seen between the ingestion of alcohol on long flights and heart attacks in men.

Source: *Aviakosm Ekolog Medicine* 2001;35(3):6-14; *Aviation Space & Environmental Medicine* 2002;73(5):481-4.

986. FREQUENT FLYERS & RADIATION EXPOSURE

Frequent flyers: Before and after you fly, reduce your cancer risk by increasing those supplements that counteract radiation exposure, such as chlorella or any powerful antioxidants. Frequent flyers are at risk of developing cancer, due to repeated exposure to cosmic radiation, which peaks at 50,000 to 60,000 feet. (The atmosphere protects the earth from this potentially harmful radiation.) Passengers are flying more frequently and planes are flying higher as air traffic increases – and frequent flyers may be at higher risk than cabin crew, who have very regulated shifts. Cosmic radiation contains very energetic particles, and when there is a solar flare, the radiation released can be 1,000 times the dose.

Source: *Reuter's Medical Report* Oct 2000.

987. PREVENTING "ECONOMY CLASS SYNDROME"

Protect yourself from "Economy Class Syndrome": When you fly, be sure to avoid alcohol, drink plenty of fluids, wear loose clothing, and exercise your legs during the flight. "Economy Class Syndrome" refers to blood clots formed during air travel. A new study reveals clinically relevant increases for several clotting factors during exposure to an environment similar to a pressurized cabin, contradicting recent assertions that there is no link between venous thrombosis (blood clotting) and air travel. After only two hours, some clotting factors increase 2.5 times, while others increase by more than *eightfold*!

Always make sure to drink plenty of nonalcoholic beverages while flying to prevent dehydration. [I take my own teabags and ask for hot water, so I get antioxidants in addition to liquids.]

Sources: *Lancet* **2000;356:1657-1658;2001;357(9267):1461-1462; World Health Organization Report, Aug 2001;** *Angiology* **Jun 2001;52(6):369-374.**

WANT TO KNOW MORE?
The association of blood clots with air travel may make this problem an occupational health risk to otherwise healthy business travelers. Passengers who remain seated for the bulk of a flight are at risk, particularly important for larger people crammed into economy-class seats.

988. COMPRESSION STOCKINGS FOR LONG FLIGHTS

Wearing elastic compression stockings when flying is another way to help reduce your risk of deep-vein thrombosis (blood clots). Deep-vein thrombosis occurs in as many as 10 percent of travelers during long airplane voyages, and varicose veins can make you more susceptible to blood clots. But wearing below-knee graduated elastic compression stockings during long flights can be protective.

Source: *Lancet* **2001;357:1461-1462,1485-1489.**

989. THROMBOSIS CAUSED BY FEAR OF FLYING?

In addition to cramped conditions and long periods of immobility on airplanes, new theories indicate that a fear of flying may actually be one of the main causes of deep-vein thrombosis. A fear of flying is often exacerbated by the stress of departure deadlines, crowded terminals, and excessive waiting, followed by cramped seating (which causes the blood supply to pool into your legs). All of this leads to a high secretion of adrenaline resulting in the constriction of the blood supply, which can result in the formation of blood clots in the legs of vulnerable passengers. Clots can form without symptoms and sudden death may occur several days later as a result of a pulmonary embolism.

Source: *Reuter's Medical News* **Jan 2002.**

WANT TO KNOW MORE?
[See the "Stress" section for helpful hints on how to control and reduce the negative effects of stress. You might also want to try learning stress-control techniques such as self-meditation, to help yourself relax while flying.]

990. MORE AIRPLANE-RELATED ILLS

In addition to blood clots, air travelers are at increased risk of infection and pressure-related health stress – all the more reason to increase your intake of protective supplements before and after plane trips. The absence of smoking on modern planes has encouraged designers to cut back on the rate of cabin ventilation, hence introducing filtered recirculated air back into the cabin. A lower ventilation rate may lead to a lower air quality in some parts of the plane and an increased risk of possible cross-infection from other passengers. [Remember you are in close proximity to strangers from all over the world.]

Technological advances in jet-engine design have permitted larger passenger planes to fly longer distances and at greater altitudes than ever before. Higher altitudes mean lower cabin pressure, which can lead to acute altitudinal hypoxemia (below normal oxygenation of the arterial blood), especially bad for the very young, seniors, or those who are less fit.

Source: *Journal of Social Health* Mar 2001;121(1):29-37.

WANT TO KNOW MORE?
Air travel should always be delayed after scuba diving to minimize the chance of developing decompression sickness.

ULCERS

Although ulcers have been associated with stress, we now know that there are correlations with allergies, nutrition status, infection, immune integrity, and drug intake. Symptoms include stomach pain or upset, feelings of acute hunger and pain after eating or lying down, and burning sensations in the stomach. The incidence of ulcers is very common.

IN THIS SECTION:
- CAUSES & PRECURSORS
- DIETARY TACTICS

- NATURAL REMEDIES & SUPPLEMENTS

ULCERS: CAUSES & PRECURSORS

991. PAIN KILLERS CAN LEAD TO PEPTIC ULCERS

Be careful when taking acetaminophen, as high doses may lead to peptic ulcers. Those who take acetaminophen (Tylenol, Excedrin, etc.) at doses exceeding two grams per day are at nearly *four times* the risk of peptic ulcer compared with non-users, and the risk skyrockets when nonsteroidal anti-inflammatory drugs (NSAIDs, such as Advil, Motrin, Aleve, Bayer) and high-dose acetaminophen are taken together.

These studies were conducted in Spain and at the Harvard School of Public Health in Boston, MA. The researchers also reported that the risks associated with the newer NSAIDs etodolac, meloxicam, and nabumetone are comparable to those of "the average NSAID effect." Dosage is the most significant factor associated with risk due to NSAIDs.

Source: *Epidemiology* 2001;12:570-576.

ULCERS: DIETARY TACTICS

992.. BROCCOLI SPROUTS FOR PEPTIC ULCERS

A single ounce of broccoli *sprouts* offers as much protection against peptic ulcers (as well as cancer) as a pound and a quarter of cooked broccoli. We have known about broccoli's protective benefits against cancer for some time, and now we can add peptic ulcers to that list. Infections known to cause gastritis and peptic ulcers dramatically enhance the risk of developing gastric cancer. Eradication of these infections is complicated by resistance to conventional antimicrobial agents and by the persistence of a low-level reservoir of *H. pylori* infection within our gastric epithelial cells. Eating broccoli sprouts is a simple –- and less flatulent! –- way to protect yourself.

[I have been enthusiastically sprouting for decades. It's easy, cheap, and requires only a few minutes each day. Or you can supplement instead with a nutraceutical prepared from young sprouted leaves, such as young barley leaf powder.]

Source: *Proceedings of the National Academy of Sciences* 2002:28;99(11):7610-7615; 1997;94(19):10357-10372.

ULCERS: NATURAL REMEDIES & SUPPLEMENTS

993. ULCERS? PROBIOTICS TO THE RESCUE

Probiotics (specifically, *Lactobacillus acidophilus* and *Lactobacillus casei*) can help to inhibit the organism that causes duodenal and gastric ulcers (*H. pylori*). Clinical studies show a persistent reduction with the administration of these lactobacilli. The lactobacilli decrease the density of *H. Pylori* in the stomach and also enhance the antibiotic therapy that helps get rid of the *H. Pylori*.

[I recommend liquid *acidophilus* or the powerful Bio-K yogurt, sold in the refrigerated supplement section of health food stores.]

Sources: *Journal of the Thai Medical Association 2002;85(Suppl1):S79-84,739-742; Digestive Liver Diseases 2002;34(Suppl2):S81-83; Archives of Latin-American Nutrition 2002;52(1):29-34; European Journal of Gastroenterology & Hepatology 2002;14:663-669*

WANT TO KNOW MORE?
These probiotics may also suppress pneumonia, decrease bronchitis in children, and prevent antibiotic-associated diarrhea.

It should also be noted that *H. pylori* infection is also associated with an increased risk of reduced fertility and coronary heart disease.

URINARY TRACT INFECTIONS

It's no fun! Frequent urges to urinate; burning sensations, sometimes stinging pain. The problem can start slowly, or, without warning — there it is! But it doesn't happen for no reason! After clearing the infection, it's time to think about what you can do to prevent future events

994. CRANBERRY JUICE FOR URINARY INFECTIONS

Regular drinking of cranberry juice reduces the recurrence of urinary tract infections, thereby reducing the need for anti-microbials. Up to 60 percent of women have a urinary tract infection at some point during their life, and at least a third experience a recurrence in the following year. Both cranberries and blueberries contain condensed tannins called *proanthocyanidins*, which inhibit bacterial action. *E. coli* is the most common bacterium causing urinary tract infection, but these compounds are also protective against *H. pylori*.

[Pure, unsweetened cranberry juice is available at health food stores.] One note of warning: The juice is better than the concentrated supplements, which have been shown to cause kidney stone formation in susceptible women.

Sources: *FEMS Immunology Medicine & Microbiology Dec 2000;29(4):295-301; Urology Jan 2001;57(1):26-29; British Medical Journal 2001;322:1571.*

WANT TO KNOW MORE?
Every year in the US, anti-microbials are given to over 11 million women with urinary tract infections, and this has resulted in an alarming increased resistance to these medications. This emerging resistance underlines the need for better and more natural alternatives.

VARICOSE VEINS

Varicose veins have a thickening wall. An imbalance in the two types of collagen protein could explain the lack of elasticity causing varicose veins. (*Journal of Vascular Research* **2001;38(6):560-8**)

995. HORSE CHESTNUTS FOR VARICOSE VEINS

An extract from the seed of the horse chestnut may be an effective natural remedy against varicose veins. Horse chestnut seed extract is a natural substance with *venotonic* properties. [A venotonic is any substance that improves venous tone by improving the elasticity of the vein wall. Relaxation of the vein wall contributes to varicose vein development.] Components found in horse chestnut help to improve both venous tone and vein elasticity.

In addition, horse chestnut is vascular protective and has anti-inflammatory effects. It is also a free radical scavenger, removing harmful particles in the body caused by oxidative stress. Horse chestnut seed extract corrects capillary hyper-permeability, which can lead to edema.

Source: *Archives of Dermatology* **1998;134(11)1356-1360.**

VERTIGO

Feeling like you're on a roller coaster, but you aren't? Dizzy or faint? Perhaps nauseous, too? That swimming or swirling sensation in your head or lack of equilibrium is vertigo! The hallucination of motion is most unpleasant, but often just temporary. If you do feel dizzy but haven't just disembarked from a ten-day sailing cruise, or even if you have, here's what you can do.

996. HOMEOPATHY FOR VERTIGO

The homeopathic remedy, Vertigoheel, was compared with a commonly used drug in the treatment of patients with vertigo of various origins, and both treatments showed a clinically relevant reduction in the frequency, duration, and intensity of the vertigo attacks during a six-week treatment period. Vertigo-specific complaints were significantly reduced in both treatment groups.

Source: *Archives of Otolaryngology, Head & Neck Surgery* **1998;124(8):879-85.**

WARTS

Common warts (referred to medically as verruca vulgaris) are caused by infection and are very resistant to treatment. Many, largely ineffective modalities for cure have been tried in the past – almost always unsuccessfully.

997. DUCT TAPE TO COMBAT WARTS

If you are suffering from warts, you should know that simple duct tape is significantly more effective in treating common warts than any other method. It is also the most promising, safest, and most nonthreatening treatment for children.

Here's the process:
1. Cover the wart with a piece of duct tape and leave in place for six days.
2. Remove the tape after six days and soak the area in water.
3. Debride [gently scrape] the wart with an emery board or pumice stone.
4. Twelve hours later, recover the wart with duct tape, and repeat the process.

The cycle may have to be repeated a few times, but usually works within two months, although most warts will respond to this treatment within the first month.

Source: *Archives of Pediatric & Adolescent Medicine* **2002;156:971-977.**

WRINKLES

IN THIS SECTION:
- DIETARY TACTICS
- NATURAL REMEDIES & SUPPLEMENTS

Human skin, like all other organs, undergoes chronological aging. In addition, unlike other organs, skin is in direct contact with the environment and therefore undergoes aging as a consequence of environmental damage. The primary environmental factor that causes human skin aging is UV irradiation from the sun. This sun-induced skin aging (photoaging), like chronological aging, is cumulative.

But the sun is good for you! The secret is to take supplements (preferably nutraceuticals) that contain anti-oxidants to chase away those damaging free radicals.

Chronological aging and photoaging share fundamental molecular pathways. These new insights provide exciting new opportunities for the development of new anti-aging therapies. (*Archives of Dermatology* **2002;138(11):1462-70**) Certain lifestyle habits known to have effects on skin aging are identified as phototype, body mass index, menopausal status, degree of lifetime sun exposure, and number of years of cigarette smoking. (*Archives of Dermatology* **2002;138(11):1454-60**)

A short exposure of skin to a low-humidity environment induces changes in the moisture contents in the stratum corneum and skin surface pattern, which means that a dry environment in our daily life makes fine wrinkles related to lack of water in the stratum corneum. (*Skin Research Technology* **2002 Nov;8(4):212-8**)

That's why I use the wet-cloth procedure when I fly. (See Hint #984 for details.)

WRINKLES: DIETARY TACTICS
998. WRINKLES & FOOD

If you are concerned about wrinkles, you should be aware that the types of food you consume *do* influence the look of your skin. There is less skin wrinkling in those with higher intakes of vegetables, olive oil, fish, and legumes. There is more skin damage with the consumption of butter, margarine, milk products, and sugar, and high intakes of meat, dairy, and butter actually appear to have adverse effects on your skin. Prunes, apples, and tea have varied results. (Antioxidants, in general, are of benefit to your skin.) And put out those cigarettes! Smokers look older than their non-smoking peers.

Source: *Journal of the American College of Nutrition* **Feb 2001;20(1):71-80.**

WRINKLES: NATURAL REMEDIES & SUPPLEMENTS
999. VITAMIN C REVITALIZES SKIN COLLAGEN

Vitamin C cream has an anti-aging effect on skin collagen, and can reduce wrinkles after six months of use. Five-percent vitamin C cream, topically applied, can increase the quantity of collagen in the skin and improve the way the collagen is aligned, replacing larger and deeper wrinkles after just six months of use. Vitamin C not only rearranges collagen, but increases the production of collagen and matures it by stimulating enzymes to create cross-linkages between collagen molecules, all of which can alleviate the signs of aging.

Vitamin C compounds are as effective as retinols, but with fewer side effects.

Source: **2nd World Congress in Cosmetic Dermatology, Rio de Janeiro, Brazil (as reported in *Reuter's Health* Nov 2000).**

1000. "LISTEN" TO YOUR BLOOD

Preventive blood testing is an important tool that can help you recognize potential health problems long before they arrive – giving you the chance to do something NOW to avoid them.

There is almost always an avoidable cause for all disease. Just because you "feel" good does not mean you are in excellent health. Yearly *preventive* blood testing (as opposed to the more common *symptom-driven* testing) can provide the evidence that you not only feel well, but that your blood cells *prove* you are.

Having a HealthPrint® done by Ellie Cullen's scientific laboratory can be invaluable in recognizing an "out-of-order" situation in the body long before the standard blood test can. Please read *Normal Blood Test Scores Aren't Good Enough!* by Ellie Cullen, RN, which can be purchased on Amazon.com or by calling YFH Press toll free at 877-468-6934. It's a story so important that I believe it should be shouted from every rooftop.

1001. BETTY KAMEN'S HALF CENTURY SUMMARY

What you eat every day of your life affects the length and quality of your entire life.

PART TWO:

HEALTHIER LIVING

Oh no! 1,001 already! But there's so much more important stuff to tell you...so much information about nutrition, exercise, supplements...protecting yourself from the harmful effects of toxins in our environment.

I can't resist! So here are some more...

BETTER NUTRITION

1,002. COLOR YOUR FOOD BRIGHT!

For optimum health (and protection against diseases such as cancer) make sure your dinner plate looks like a rainbow!

Consuming 400 to 600 grams of fruits and vegetables a day can help reduce the incidence of many common forms of cancer. The phytochemicals found in these foods inhibit cancer in many ways. You can identify the cancer-preventing phytochemicals in your fruits and vegetables by their color:

- Red foods contain lycopene, the pigment in tomatoes, which is localized in the prostate gland and may be involved in maintaining prostate health.

- Yellow-green vegetables, such as corn and leafy greens, contain lutein and zeaxanthin, which are localized in the retina where age-related macular degeneration occurs.

- Red-purple foods contain anthocyanins, which are powerful antioxidants found in red apples, grapes, berries, and wine.

- Orange foods, including carrots, mangos, apricots, pumpkin, and winter squash, contain beta-carotene, helping to prevent cancer, heart disease, and boosts immunity.

- Orange-yellow foods, including oranges, tangerines, and lemons, contain citrus flavonoids, which help to protect against coronary heart disease.

- Green foods, including broccoli, Brussels sprouts, and kale, contain glucosinolates, which possibly produce plant growth hormones and anti-carcinogenic factors.

- White-green foods in the onion family contain allyl sulfides, which help to decrease cholesterol.

You should be eating one serving of each of the above groups daily. (The National Cancer Institute and the American Institute for Cancer Research recommend five to nine servings of vegetables and fruit per day.) Since this may be an unrealistic goal for many people, consider supplements derived from these foods, often available in dehydrated powders.

Source: *Journal of Nutrition* 2001;131:3078S-3081S.

1,003. ARE YOU EATING THE "RIGHT" VEGGIES?

Dump your nutritionally lacking iceberg lettuce and start eating "better" veggies, especially dark green and cruciferous vegetables, which can protect you from cancer. Although more Americans may be eating five portions of vegetables daily, intakes of those that are cancer-protective (dark green and cruciferous veggies, which include bok choy, collards, kale, broccoli, cabbage, cauliflower, mustard greens, Brussels sprouts, radishes, and turnips) remain low – very low!

Iceberg lettuce, tomatoes, fried potatoes, bananas, and orange juice are the most commonly consumed fruits and vegetables, accounting for nearly 30 percent of all fruits and vegetables consumed. The average person consumes between 2.3 and 3.6 servings of vegetables and between 1.6 and 2.0 servings of fruit daily. (The most popular items, lettuce and tomatoes, are consumed by 39 to 42 percent of Americans.)

Only a lowly three percent consume broccoli. White potato averages 1.1 servings daily, with french-fried potatoes representing 0.4 serving. Tomato product consumption averages 0.5 serving daily, dark green vegetable consumption averages 0.2 serving daily, and citrus, berries, or melon consumption amounts to nearly 0.8 serving daily. This indicates that Americans are consuming more fruits and vegetables but that dark green and cruciferous vegetable intake are lagging behind.

Source: *Journal of Nutrition* **2000;130(12):3063-3067.**

1,004. ORGANIC FOODS REALLY ARE BETTER

It's not just hype – organic foods really are better for you. If you are among those wondering if it really pays to buy organic, at least two studies show that organic crops contain significantly more vitamin C, iron, magnesium, and phosphorus – and significantly less nitrates – than conventional crops do. They also appear to have less protein but protein of a better quality, and a higher content of nutritionally significant minerals with lower amounts of some heavy metals.

(One reason for the differences may be due the higher water content of conventional crops, which causes nutrient dilution.)

Few studies have examined the effects of herbicides or other pesticides on nutrient content. But animal studies show better growth and reproduction in animals fed organically grown feed compared with those fed conventionally grown feed.

Sources: *Journal of Alternative & Complementary Medicine* **2001;7(2):161-173;** *Alternative Therapy & Health Medicine* **1998;4(1):58-69.**

1,005. MORE BENEFITS OF ORGANIC VEGGIES

More good reasons to buy organic: Organically cultivated vegetables have a much longer shelf life, a better taste, and better mutagen protection than do generally cultivated vegetables. Research conducted at the Department of Food Science and Technology at Tokyo University found that organic vegetables show 30 to 57 percent anti-mutagenicity, while the generically cultivated ones demonstrate only 5 to 30 percent protection.

Source: *Mutation Research* **2001;496(1-2):83-88.**

1,006. GET YOUR FOLATE FROM FOOD

Increasing your intake of folate (folic acid) helps to decrease harmful homocysteine levels, but there are advantages to getting your folate from food rather than from supplements: you will also be getting more fiber and more bioavailable vitamins and minerals. Increased intake of vegetables, legumes, cereals, orange juice, fruit, and nuts and seeds increases folate in general. Apples, peaches, and plums have a low folate content; oranges and bananas have a high folate content.

Source: *American Journal of Clinical Nutrition* **2002;76(4):758-765.**

WANT TO KNOW MORE?
[Homocysteine is an amino acid produced naturally in your body, but high levels in the blood are associated with many health problems, including heart disease. Increasing your intake of folate, along with vitamins B6 and B12, can help reduce these levels.]

The association between vascular disease and elevated homocysteine is caused, in part, by inadequate intake of dietary folate. But adding folate can reduce your risk of vascular disease.

1,007. WHERE ARE THOSE NUTRIENTS HIDING?

You are being good and healthy and eating lots of fruits and vegetables – just make sure you aren't missing the best parts! For most fruits and vegetables, the greatest concentration of nutrients is found in the peel or just under the peel, rather than in the pulp. (Carrots are one exception.)
Many nutrients (such as carotenoids) are found in higher concentrations in foods grown in hot climates. In fact, indigenous foods have greater quantities of most nutrients than introduced crops do. And many nutrients also increase greatly during ripening. Finally, when seeds and grains are *sprouted*, their nutrient value also greatly increases.

Source: *Archives of Latinoamerican Nutrition* **1999;49(3Suppl1):74S-84S.**

1,008. PHYTOESTROGENS & DISEASE PROTECTION

Help protect yourself against many chronic diseases by increasing your intake of phytoestrogens, consumed in whole-food form. [Phytoestrogens, also called plant estrogens, are substances found in plants that have an estrogen-enhancing or estrogen-like effect.] Higher consumption of phytoestrogens may be protective against certain chronic diseases, but our consumption of such foods in Western culture is extremely low. (Included in these phytoestrogens are certain lignins, isoflavones, and coumesterols). Some good sources of phytoestrogens are peas and beans, vegetables, nuts, grain products, tea, fruit, and soy products. [Please note that it is important to obtain phytoestrogens from whole, unprocessed foods. Once they are isolated from food, their value diminishes.]

Source: *Journal of Nutrition* 2002;132:1319-1328.

1,009. BANANAS CONTAIN POTENT ANTIOXIDANT

Monkeys have the right idea: Bananas contain an important substance that can protect you from free-radical damage. Dopamine, a powerful water-soluble antioxidant found in popular commercial bananas, has a greater potency for scavenging certain free radicals (such as the food additives BHA and BHT) than does glutathione. Dopamine is a *catecholamine*, and has a similar potency to strong antioxidants like ascorbic acid (vitamin C). Bananas contain dopamine at high levels in both the peel and pulp, making them an important antioxidative food.

Source: *Journal of Agriculture and Food Chemistry* 2000;48(3):844-848.

WANT TO KNOW MORE?
[Keep in mind, however, that bananas are high in carbohydrates. Remember the adage for optimal health: For every fruit, consume three portions of vegetables.]

1,010. BROCCOLI: THE CANCER FIGHTER

Boys *and* girls: Eat your broccoli and other cruciferous veggies, which protect you against a host of cancers. Cruciferous vegetables (such as broccoli and cauliflower) have been shown to have a dose-dependent effect on the death and growth arrest of prostate cancer cells (so the more you eat, the more protection you will have). Scientists have finally identified the phytochemicals in cruciferous vegetables that are responsible for this protection.

In test animals, selenium-enriched broccoli decreases intestinal tumor growth, and has been shown to be protective against chemically induced mammary and colon cancer.

Sources: *International Journal of Oncology* 2002;20(3):631-636; *Journal of Nutrition* Feb 2002;132(2):307-309.

1,011. BROWN RICE NOT SO NICE

Because of the oil content in brown rice, this grain becomes rancid within hours of hull removal, and should not be consumed. The rice grain is not edible as is. The modern two-step rice milling process includes the removal of the hull, a component of little value, which comprises 20 percent of the original grain. The grain that remains after removal of the outer husk is brown rice. The second step is polishing of the kernel. The process of polishing removes the bran and germ of the kernel. Brown rice is polished several times to get white rice, and the polishes put together (known as rice bran) accounts for eight percent of white rice. The bran, or brown rice (because it contains the germ with its high oil content), becomes rancid within hours of husking, and, unfortunately, rancidity is not always detected by smell or taste.

You may be aware that wheat germ (the germ of the wheat) becomes rancid unless vacuum packed or frozen. The same is true of the germ of the rice. This makes sense, because it is the germ of these grains that contains the valuable oil. This news may fly in the face of the commonly held belief that brown rice is good for you, but it turns out that this food is not in your best health interest because of this rancidity problem. (White rice, of course, is a nutrient-poor food, but safer than brown rice in terms of rancidity.)

Source: R. Cheruvanky, "Bioactives In Rice Bran and Rice Bran Oil," *Phytochemicals as Bioactive Agents* **2000, Technomic Publishing Co, Lancaster, PA.**

WANT TO KNOW MORE?
[The bran removed from rice, however, is a powerhouse of nutrients. Stabilized rice bran, a supplement found in most health food stores, is an excellent nutritional supplement that may also be protective against diseases such as diabetes and atherosclerosis.]

1,012. WHOLE CARROTS BETTER THAN JUICE

Carotenoids in carrots help prevent lipid peroxidation (very important for your health), but carrot juice offers no such benefit – so munch your carrots, don't drink them. Carotenoids are protective pigments found in red, orange, and yellow plants. They help protect the chlorophyll of the plant from oxidation, and offer you a similar kind of protection. But carotenoids degrade with the breakdown of the cellular structure (as in juicing).

Because carotenoids are highly unsaturated, they are susceptible to oxidation during processing and storage. Carrots that have been dehydrated are not in your best health interest either, as carotenoids can give rise to volatile compounds in dehydrated carrots.

Source: *Journal of Nutrition* **2000;130(9):2200-2206.**

1,013. A COLD CEREAL THAT'S GOOD FOR YOU

If you and your children are still locked into the tradition of eating cold cereal for breakfast, at least consume one that offers some decent nutrition. Have you ever wondered why you can leave a box of cold cereal on a pantry shelf without refrigeration? No self-respecting bug would ever think of attacking this non-food, usually devoid of enzymes or anything else resembling substances of nutritional value.

Because I go around the world advising people against the use of cold cereals, I have come to be known as the most notorious "Cereal Killer."

Source: Common sense.

1,014. CITRUS *PULP* WHERE THE GOOD STUFF IS

The white pulp on the inner side of grapefruit and orange rind is chock-full of nutrients, so it's a good idea to scrape it out and eat it too. When manufacturers started to can fruit juices extensively about 40 or 50 years ago, they hired scientists to see if the mountains of rind left over had any use. That's when bioflavonoids were discovered, which we now know are a group of chemical substances found in many plants. Bioflavonoids help to keep the cell walls of small blood vessels permeable, and have also been shown to suppress prostate tumor proliferation.

The pectin contained in the white pulp is also extremely beneficial. In fact, it's extracted and sold as modified citrus pectin because it is rich in residues that help to prevent metastasis of certain cancers, including melanomas, prostate, and breast cancers.

Sources: *Journal of Agricultural Food Chemistry* **2000;48(10):4918-4923;** *Alternative Medicine Review* **2000;5(6):573-575;** *Nutrition & Cancer* **2000;38(1):116-122.**

1,015. EGGS: GO AHEAD & EAT THEM!

Eat your eggs – they are an important source of essential nutrients and do NOT raise your cholesterol levels. It is now known that there is little if any connection between dietary cholesterol and blood cholesterol levels, nor does consuming up to one or more eggs per day adversely affect blood cholesterol levels. [It is gratifying to researchers like myself to see scientific validation from the traditional medical community for concepts we have had for decades.]

Functional foods are foods that provide health benefits beyond basic nutrition and include whole, fortified, enriched or enhanced foods, which have a potentially beneficial effect on health. An excellent example is the egg, nature's original functional food. Eggs are an excellent dietary source of many essential components that may promote optimal health, such as: excellent quality protein, choline (the memory and good-brain-function nutrient), and lutein and zeaxanthin (nutrients that help prevent cataracts).

Source: *Journal of the American College of Nutrition* **2000;19(5Suppl):499S-506S;556S-562S.**

WANT TO KNOW MORE?

One study showed that the daily nutrient intake of egg eaters was *significantly* greater than that of non-egg eaters for all nutrients studied. Eggs contributed 20 to 30 percent of vitamins A, E, and B12. Non-egg eaters had inadequate intake of vitamin B12, vitamin A, vitamin E, and vitamin C. After adjusting for demographic (age, gender, and ethnicity) and lifestyle variables (smoking and physical activity), dietary cholesterol was not related to serum cholesterol concentration.

[See *Dietary Misconceptions* in the *Heart & Cardiovascular Disease* section for more information on this topic.]

1,016. WINTERTIME? EAT FISH FOR VITAMIN D

Eating fish, especially in the dark winter months, can help keep you from becoming vitamin-D deficient. If you live in a climate where the sun doesn't shine much in the winter, high consumption of fish will help supply vitamin D, a nutrient available basically only from the sun and from very few foods (and *essential* for preventing osteoporosis).

In a study done on Japanese women during the winter months, only 4.6 percent of them showed vitamin D insufficiencies – a value lower than that found in Western populations. The concentrations of vitamin D in those who consumed fish frequently (about four times or more a week) were *significantly* higher than levels of those with a moderate consumption of fish (one to three times a week).

The nutritional status of vitamin D in Japanese populations seems to be better than that in most Western populations. Frequent fish consumption is believed to help maintain adequate concentrations during the winter.

Eating eggs may also have a similar effect: Those who did not consume eggs have significantly lower vitamin D levels.

[Caveat: Beware farmed fish. Farmed fish may not be properly fed, and may be devoid of the right fatty acid profiles.]

Source: *American Journal of Clinical Nutrition* **2000;71:5;1161-1165.**

WANT TO KNOW MORE?

[To understand why vitamin D is so essential for good bone health, see my booklet, *Startling New Facts About Osteoporosis*, as well as the *Osteoporosis & Other Skeletal Problems* section of this book.]

1,017. FLAXSEED: HEART PROTECTION & MORE

Start adding flaxseed to your diet, as it is a rich source of essential fatty acids and other important substances that may be cancer-preventive and heart-protective. Flaxseed contains the phytoestrogen *lignan*, which is similar to the sex hormones produced in the body. It can protect your heart, inhibit mammary tumor development, and even reduce inflammation. Lignans are preventive against the lower aortic stiffness and degeneration associated with atherosclerosis (with the benefits most pronounced in postmenopausal women). In addition, flaxseed supplementation can also lower both total cholesterol and LDL (the unfavorable cholesterol).

[Most physicians recommend one to two tablespoons of ground flaxseed daily. Since flaxseed oil goes rancid easily (even in capsules and in dark glass bottles), it's best to simply grind it daily – easily done with an inexpensive small coffee bean grinder. Ground flaxseed has a light, nutty taste and can be sprinkled over vegetables or salads.]

Sources: *Arteriosclerosis, Thrombosis, & Vascular Biology* 2002;22:1316-1322; *Journal of Clinical Endocrinology Metabolism* 2002;87(4):1527-1532; *Cancer Letters* 2000;161(1):47-55.

WANT TO KNOW MORE?
It was once commonplace to have fresh flaxseed oil delivered to your doorstep, just as milk was delivered several decades ago, or water today.

1,018. IMPORTANT SUBSTANCE IN GRAPE SKIN

Eating grapes may be protective against hypertension, stroke-related damage, and harmful oxidative stress – among many other health benefits. *Resveratrol*, a substance found in the skin of most grapes, helps to prevent the damage that occurs to DNA as a result of oxidative stress (free radicals), which is deeply involved in many disease states.

A powerful phytoestrogen, resveratrol is both an antioxidant and an anti-mutagen, potentially useful against vascular diseases involving hypertension. Findings suggest that resveratrol might also be useful in treating ischemic-induced inflammatory processes occurring from a stroke.

Sources: *Life Science* 2000;67(25):3103-3112; *Clinical Experimental Pharmacology & Physiology* 2001;28(1-2):55-59.

WANT TO KNOW MORE?
[Just make sure the grapes you buy are *organic*, as grapes (as well as green beans, peaches, and spinach) are often sprayed with diazinon – one of the most toxic pesticides. See Hint #1076 in the *Environmental Toxins* section for more details.]

1,019. THE HEALTH BENEFITS OF NUTS

Just some of the many remarkable health benefits of nuts: Walnuts help to reduce both total and low-density lipoprotein (LDL) cholesterol levels in those whose cholesterol levels are too high. Walnuts may also beneficially alter fat distribution, which may be one way in which they are heart-protective.

- Walnuts are among the few foods that are high in potassium and low in sodium, reducing your risk of high blood pressure and stroke.

- The polyunsaturated fatty acid omega-3 improves the biochemical alterations that occur with ulcerative colitis, and walnuts are among the foods that have significant quantities.

- Risk factors for coronary heart disease are *significantly* reduced when whole almonds are added to the diet, especially for those with high blood fat (high cholesterol, triglycerides, etc.).

- Macadamia nuts help to improve cholesterol levels.

- Frequent consumption of pecans is associated with a decreased risk of cardiovascular disease.

- Women who eat more than five ounces of nuts a week have a *significantly* lower risk of total coronary heart disease than women who never eat nuts or who eat less than one ounce a month.

- Nut consumption is inversely associated with risk of type 2 diabetes in women (so the more you eat, the lower your risk).

- Men who consume a diet high in nuts have a reduced risk of developing prostate cancer.

- Nuts and seeds are also great sources of calcium.

Sources: *Circulation* **1999;2002;106;** *Annals of Internal Medicine* **2000;132:538-546;** *Archives of Internal Medicine* **2000;** *American Journal of Clinical Nutrition* **2000;71(5)1166-1169;2001;74(1):72-79;** Experimental Biology Meeting, Orlando, FL, 2001; *Journal of Agricultural Food Chemistry* **2002;50(8):2459-2463;** *Journal of Nutrition* **2002;132(4):703-707;2002;132(5):11-19;1062S-1101S;** *Journal of the American Medical Association* **2002;288:2554-2560;** Department of Nutrition, Harvard School of Public Health, Boston, MA; B. Kamen, *Everything You Always Wanted to Know About Potassium But Were Too Tired to Ask.*

WANT TO KNOW MORE?
[A great gift idea: A bowl of mixed organic nuts in the shell and a couple of nutcrackers. It's fun – and healthful – for family, friends, and kids of all ages to sit around and crack and eat the nuts. (The shells protect against rancidity.)]

1,020. THE PROBLEMS WITH POTATOES

Some potato tips: Make sure to buy only organic varieties, be careful not to overcook them, and discard potatoes that have grown eyes or have turned greenish.
Non-organic potatoes are usually treated with a dangerous additive to prevent the growth of sprouts (or eyes). In fact, in today's world, only organic potatoes *will* grow sprouts – and once they do, the entire potato should be discarded. Green discoloration is also something to look for, caused by the development of a toxic substance occurring when potatoes are exposed to sunlight or artificial light. (This explains the traditional way of harvesting potatoes in Ireland, with a coat of earth kept intact on the potato.)

Also, don't cook your spuds for too long! When overcooked, potatoes can raise blood sugar levels almost as rapidly as pure glucose can, because high or prolonged cooking temperatures break down the complex carbohydrates found in potatoes into simple sugars.

Keep in mind that cooking also destroys vitamin C, and even more of this vitamin is lost if cooked potatoes are kept for later use, especially at room temperature. (And by the way, dehydrated instant potatoes contain almost no vitamin C – the more processed food is, the greater the nutrient destruction.)

Source: R.K. Bernstein, *Diabetes: The Glucograf Method For Normalizing Blood Sugar*, (Crown Publishing, 1981).

WANT TO KNOW MORE?
Here's a simple health tip: When eating in restaurants, ask for double vegetables to replace the rice or potatoes. Or settle for plain white rice (nutrient deficient but safe).

1,021. PRUNES: NOT JUST FOR OLD FOLKS

Eating prunes may be preventive against a host of maladies, including osteoporosis, heart disease, and cancer. Dried prunes are an important source of boron, which plays a role in the prevention of osteoporosis. And despite their sweet taste, prunes do not cause a rapid rise in blood sugar concentration, possibly because of their high fiber content. (Dried prunes contain approximately 6.1 grams of dietary fiber per 100 grams, while prune juice is devoid of fiber due to filtration before bottling.)

Prunes are a good source of energy in the form of simple sugars. They contain large amounts of phenolic compounds, which may aid in the laxative action and delay glucose absorption. The phenolic compounds in prunes have been found to be preventive against chronic diseases such as heart disease and cancer. Additionally, the high potassium content of prunes might be beneficial for your cardiovascular health.

[To learn more about fiber (and why it is so important for optimum health) read my book, *New Facts About Fiber*.]

Source: *Clinical & Pharmacology Therapy* 2002;71(1):21-29.

1,022. SOYMILK NOT A BETTER CALCIUM SOURCE

Soymilk drinkers, take note: The calcium in fortified soymilk is not as easily used by the body as the calcium in cow's milk. In a study comparing the bioavailability of the calcium in fortified soymilk with that of calcium in cow's milk, it was concluded that calcium-fortified soymilk does *not* constitute a calcium source comparable to cow's milk.

[There are better ways to get calcium than from soy or cow's milk. Factors that support calcium metabolism are: Consumption of leafy greens, whole grains, alfalfa sprouts, and nuts and seeds, moderate exercise, and food-type supplements (such as colostrum or velvet antler).]

Source: *American Journal of Clinical Nutrition* 2000;71(5)1166-1169.

1,023. EAT WATERMELON FOR LYCOPENE

Eating watermelon may be protective against heart disease, prostate cancer, and dangerous free-radical damage in the body. Lycopene, the phytochemical associated with reduced prostate cancer risk and lower rates of heart disease, is the red pigment that gives watermelons their color. It is also a powerful antioxidant, scavenging aggressive chemicals that react with cell components and cause damage and loss of proper cell function.

The Women's Health Study suggests that lycopene may reduce the risk of heart disease in middle-aged and older women by as much as 33 percent. Another study found that men with the highest concentrations of lycopene in their fat tissue have a 48 percent reduced risk of developing cardiovascular disease when compared to men with the lowest levels.

Watermelon contains about 40 percent more lycopene than tomatoes (even when compared to heated tomato juice). Although lycopene levels vary among different types of melons, the seedless ones tend to have more, depending on both variety and growing conditions. Watermelon also contains the vitamins A, B6, C, and thiamin. A cup and a half of watermelon contains about nine to 13 mg of lycopene. Red, ripe flesh is the best indicator of the sweetest and most nutritious watermelon.

[Other good sources of lycopene include tomatoes, red and pink grapefruit, red-fleshed papaya, and guava.]

Sources: *Agricultural Magazine* 2002; *Journal of the National Cancer Institute* 2002;94:391-398; *International Journal of Food Science and Nutrition* 2001;52(2):143-149.

WANT TO KNOW MORE?
Lycopene is the most efficient free-radical quencher, devouring over 10 times more oxygenated free radicals than vitamin E can.

1,024. TASTES LIKE ZINC DEFIENCY

If you are a vegetarian family, consider zinc supplementation (especially for the children) to protect your sense of *taste*. A deficiency of zinc can result in changes in the number and size of taste buds and fine structure changes in taste bud cells, occurring especially during a child's accelerated growth stage following weaning – making zinc supplementation all the more important for children being raised as vegetarians.

In addition to taste disturbances, zinc deficiency is also associated with multiple clinical complications, including skin changes.

Reductions in red meat and increases in cereals in the diet may compromise the intake and bioavailability of this mineral. Cereals increase phytate intake, which can interfere with your body's zinc status.

Sources: *Journal of Formosa Medical Association* **2001;100(5):326-335;** *British Journal of Nutrition* **2001;86(1):71-80.**

1,025. VEGETARIAN DIETS & COPPER ABSORPTION

Copper is not absorbed as efficiently in vegetarians as in meat eaters, but because of increased levels of copper in vegetarian foods, vegetarians *actually* have increased copper absorption. Copper is an essential element for life and health. While copper levels appear to be lower in vegetarians, it is not due specifically to their diet. The lower absorption levels may be due to dietary inhibitors that reduce the copper availability in those diets. So while copper is less efficiently absorbed by vegetarians, they actually have higher overall copper absorption due to increased levels of this nutrient in their diet.

[Copper is typically present in mineral-rich foods such as potatoes, beans and peas, nuts, grains, and fruits.]

Source: *American Journal of Clinical Nutrition* **2001;74:803-807.**

1,026. GOOD NEWS: MY KID'S A VEGETARIAN!

If you're the parent of an adolescent who has decided to "become a vegetarian," rather than viewing as a fad or a phase, you should be aware that it's actually a great alternative to the less-than-healthful typical American diet. In fact, adolescent vegetarians are more likely than their meat-eating peers to meet the "Healthy People 2010 Dietary Objectives." The objective of limiting calories per day from fat to 30 percent or less is met by 69.5 percent of vegetarians compared with 47.5 percent of non-vegetarians. Likewise, 26.4 percent of vegetarians consume three or more servings of vegetables per day compared with 13.9 percent of non-vegetarians.

In addition, vegetarian adolescents are also less likely than non-vegetarians to eat fast food or drink regular soda and fruit drinks.

Source: *Archives of Pediatric & Adolescent Medicine* 2002;156:426-427,431-437.

WANT TO KNOW MORE?
For most vegetarian adolescents, the choice to forego meat is not based on a concern for animal welfare or improving the quality of their diet, but to control their weight.

HEALTHIER COOKING

1,027. START USING REMARKABLE GRAPESEED OIL

When cooking with oil, choose grapeseed oil – a highly stable oil that can raise HDL cholesterol (the "good-guy" kind), lower LDL cholesterol (the harmful variety), and help to prevent hypertension caused by excessive sodium. Linoleic acid is one of two essential fatty acids we cannot manufacture ourselves, and the good news is that grapeseed oil is *76 percent* linoleic acid! Research shows that just one ounce of grapeseed oil daily is all that is necessary for the positive HDL effect.

(And as a bonus, triglyceride levels also decrease.) The oil also has lots of vitamin E (another nutrient sadly lacking in the American diet).

More good news is that grapeseed oil is highly stable, so it's the best possible oil for deep-frying. The recommended regular or deep-frying temperature is 360 degrees. At this temperature, there is no smoking, splattering, or burnt taste because the smoke-point of grapeseed oil is unusually high (over 485 degrees) – unlike the much lower smoke-point temperatures of other oils. Keeping the temperature at the normal range prevents conversion to harmful trans fatty acids.

Grapeseed oil is ideal for salad dressings and mayonnaise. It has no fatty aftertaste and enhances the flavor of food, so it can be used for anything from a tuna salad to delicate party appetizers. It has a non-greasy, slightly nutty flavor and will not cloud when chilled. It takes one ton of grape seeds just to make eight ounces of extra-virgin grapeseed oil.

Sources: *Journal of the American College of Cardiology* 1993; *Journal of Arteriosclerosis* 1990;10:5; **Interviews with chefs.**

1,028. LIGHT COOKING FOR BETTER VEGGIES

When preparing meals, be sure to cook your green veggies *lightly* to increase the bioavailability of beta-carotene. Although green vegetables may increase in value with light cooking, keep in mind that extended heating destroys the carotenoids – and may even transform them into substances with lower provitamin A activity.

Source: *Journal of the National Cancer Institute*, **quoted in** *Lancet* **1996;347:249.**

1,029. COOKING INCREASES IRON VALUE

Boiling, steaming, or stir-frying many vegetables can help increase the bioavailability of the iron they contain. Cooking increases the bioavailable iron in cabbage from about 5 percent to 15 percent, and in broccoli flowerets from 6 percent to more than *30 percent*! Cooking even enhances the iron bioavailability of some vegetables that have high available iron content when raw, such as red and green peppers and tomatoes.

Researchers have found that most vegetables are more nutritious if cooked for approximately 15 minutes. Some vegetables, such as spinach, are equally nutritious whether raw or cooked. But storing cooked vegetables overnight, even in the refrigerator, results in dramatic losses in the available iron content.

Source: *Plant Foods in Human Nutrition 1997;51(1):1-16.*

1,030. BOIL, ROAST OR STIR-FRY?

The more protein you eat, the more riboflavin (vitamin B2) you require, but roasting and frying can cause *significant* losses of this important nutrient. (Boiling, however, does not.) So stir-frying leafy greens is not in your best health interest. Storing of foods also causes the loss of B2. A large amount is lost in milk when it is irradiated to create vitamin D.

Tongue inflammation is a common sign of riboflavin deficiency in older people. A riboflavin deficiency has also been implicated as a cause of cataracts. It may also be a cause of Meniere's syndrome, an ear disorder that leads to recurrent attacks of dizziness and ringing of the ears (often accompanied by nausea and vomiting).

Riboflavin is also found in yogurt (real yogurt, not the supermarket varieties), liver, fish, and eggs. Because riboflavin is light sensitive, milk (if you are still drinking it) should only be purchased in opaque containers, not in glass bottles.

Source: *International Journal of Food Science & Nutrition 2002'53(3):197-208.*

1,031. IODINE LOST IN SALT WHEN HEATED

For those using iodized salt to compensate for iodine deficiency, note that iodine is lost when subjected to high temperatures, as in cooking or food processing. Iodine deficiency is a problem for almost all countries of the world. Goiter is its most obvious consequence, but other consequences do more damage, particularly on the developing brain.

The iodine content of iodized salt was calculated in cooked food, and the results indicated a gradual loss of iodine content from the iodized salt samples when subjected to high temperature.

Sources: *Indian Journal of Pediatrics* 1997;64(6):883; *Journal of Clinical Endocrinology & Metabolism* 1996;81(4):1332-1335.

1,032. DON'T SOAK SLICED FOODS

If you are slicing foods (like apples or potatoes) in advance of cooking, do not soak them in water, but place in a tightly sealed container and keep the food dry in the refrigerator to preserve nutrients. Nutrients that dissolve in water pass quickly from food into water during soaking. Sugars, minerals, ascorbic acid, and the B vitamins readily dissolve in water.

When fruits and vegetables are soaked before and during cooking, the fact that the sugars dissolve into the water causes losses in both flavor and sweetness. Try cooking carrots and other vegetables without water and taste the sweetness difference! If you need to crisp salad vegetables, sprinkle with water, but do not soak them. Refrigerate your salads if prepared in advance. And keep in mind that carotene is destroyed by light!

Source: *Nahrung* 2002;46(2):92-5.

1,033. SOME SURPRISING FACTS ABOUT SOUP

Because overcooking vegetables may increase their sugar content, you may want to try blending (instead of cooking) your vegetables for soup preparation, and then add hot water and seasonings just before consuming. Most packaged and restaurant soups contain considerable amounts of simple sugars, and even soups prepared at home from fresh vegetables may contain high glucose levels if cooked for several hours.

Labels of packaged or canned products may use dextrose, fructose, corn syrup solids, etc., to designate the addition of sugars. Don't take label listings for granted.

Source: Common sense.

1,034. A SAFER WAY TO SAUTÉ & STIR-FRY

To prevent oil from exceeding safe temperatures when you sauté or stir-fry, add equal parts of water and oil (preferably grapeseed or red palm oil). If the mixture boils and "spits," your pan is too hot. High heat creates trans fats, which elevate cholesterol, in addition to other negative effects on blood lipids. Different degrees of deterioration of dietary frying oils have been found to negatively affect immune responses in those with autoimmune diseases.

Two of the most stable oils are grapeseed oil and red palm oil. (Vitamin C, by the way, reduces the harmful effects of oxidized frying oil.)

Sources: *Journal of Nutritional Science Vitaminol* (Tokyo) 2000;46(3):137-140; *Prostaglandins Leukot Essent Chung Hua Min Kuo Wei Sheng Wu Chi Mien I Hsueh Tsa Chih 1996;29(3):123-133; Fatty Acids Oct 1997;57(4-5):399-402; Indian Journal of Experimental Biology 1999;37(10):1042-1045.*

1,035. TURN BURGERS OFTEN WHEN FRYING

The safest way to fry hamburgers is to turn them every sixty seconds, rather than once halfway through cooking, to eliminate the formation of carcinogens. Thorough cooking of ground beef is necessary to eliminate potentially dangerous bacteria, but this process can promote the formation of carcinogenic *heterocyclic amines*.

Turning patties every 60 seconds during frying will cook burgers completely in eight minutes at 160 degrees Celsius (300F) or seven minutes at 180 degrees Celsius (324 F), whereas flipping the burgers just once after five minutes results in 16- and 9-minute cooking times, respectively.

Turning the patties every 60 seconds produces lower levels of heterocyclic amines. Use of this cooking method could help to ensure a safer food product and might, therefore, lower human cancer incidence. [You can also make your hamburger patties safer to consume by adding vitamin E to them. See the next Hint for more details.]

Source: *Journal of the National Cancer Institute* 2000;92:1773-1778.

1,036. VITAMIN E PROTECTS BEEF PATTIES

You can inhibit the production of adverse substances formed when frying beef patties by adding vitamin E to the meat before frying. Patties were fried at three temperatures: 175C (347F); 200C (392F); and 225C (445F) for six and 10 minutes each side to determine the conditions for formation of several harmful substances. Vitamin E, when used at two concentrations (1 percent and 10 percent based on fat content) and added directly to the ground-beef patties, *significantly* reduced the harmful substances, the average ranging from 45 to 75 percent reduction.

Comparable inhibition was achieved by the direct addition of vitamin E (1 percent based on fat content) to the surface of the patties before frying. The greatest amount of some of the harmful substances was generated when the patties were cooked at the highest temperatures for the longest time.

Source: Department of Food Science and Human Nutrition, Michigan State University.

1,037. ADDED VITAMIN E STABILIZES OLIVE OIL

Another good vitamin E tip: Breaking open a capsule of vitamin E into refined olive oil increases the stability of the oil under pro-oxidant conditions, and its consumption decreases oxidative (free-radical) damage. Researchers investigated whether or not vitamin E affects the refined olive oil response to oxidation regarding the stability of the oil and the protection against lipid peroxidation in comparison with other edible oils. After frying, refined olive oil supplemented with vitamin E compared with non-supplemented refined olive oil had a higher concentration of alpha-tocopherol and more resistance against oxidation.

Source: *Free Radical Research* 1999;31(Suppl):S129-135.

1,038. BE SURE TO COOK SAUSAGES THOROUGHLY

Sausages cooked too quickly can seem done but may not have reached thetemperature needed to kill bacteria, so be sure you cook sausages for at least 12 minutes at a medium heat when frying, and at least 10 minutes on the barbecue. Researchers injected Salmonella into frozen sausages, and then barbecued or pan-fried them and tested for the presence of surviving bacteria. Although the sausages seemed thoroughly cooked, barbecuing and frying sometimes allowed Salmonella cells to survive.

Source: Public Health Laboratory Service, Bristol, England, Sep 2002.

1,039. KEEP RAW & COOKED FOODS SEPARATE

In the kitchen, keep the raw stuff (steaks, roasts, turkey, chickens, seafood) separate from the ready-to-eat foods. You may start out keeping raw and prepared meats separated, but chances are you will use the same platter on which to place the food once it's cooked. Not a good idea! When juices from raw meats touch cooked or ready-to-eat foods, cross-contamination can occur.

Source: *Health Care Food & Nutrition Focus* 2002;18(7):6-7.

1,040. ANTIMICROBIAL PROPERTIES OF SPICES

Spices help cleanse foods of pathogens and thereby contribute to the health, longevity, and reproductive success of those who find their flavors enjoyable. The reason spices are used obviously is to enhance food palatability. But spices also inhibit or kill food-spoilage microorganisms, and can also serve as powerful antimicrobial (antibacterial and antifungal) agents.

It's interesting to note, however, that researchers discovered that as the annual temperatures (an indicator of relative spoilage rates of unrefrigerated foods) of an area increased, the proportion of recipes containing spices, number of spices per recipe, total number of spices used, and use of the most potent antibacterial spices all *increased* – both within and among countries.

Source: *Neurobiology & Behavior*, Cornell University, NY, reported in *Biology Review* 1998;73(1):3-49.

WANT TO KNOW MORE?
[A component of the common curry spice turmeric may be protective against such diseases and health problems as Alzheimer's (see Hint #76), cancer (Hint #153), and edema (Hint #422).]

1,041. FOOD POISONING: THE PARTY CRASHER

Social functions such as barbecues and dinner parties are the most common source of food poisoning in the home – and the most common foods implicated are poultry, desserts containing raw eggs, and egg-based dishes. The results of a study of food poisoning show that although outbreaks of gastrointestinal infection in the home continue to decline, food remains the major transmitter of infectious intestinal disease. And those infected in home outbreaks are more likely to need hospital treatment than those attending functions outside of the home.

Contamination usually occurs through inappropriate storage, inadequate cooking, and the accidental transfer of bacteria in the kitchen.

Source: *British Medical Journal* 2001;323:1097-1098.

1,042. POST-TURKEY DAY FOOD SAFETY

If you have lots of food left over the day after Thanksgiving, or any holiday when a large amount of food has been prepared, following some basic food-safety rules can protect you and your family from potential food poisoning. Unlike bacteria that cause food to spoil, microorganisms are spread through improper food handling, so be sure that you refrigerate or freeze your leftovers within two hours or less after room-temperature exposure, and that your leftover turkey is then stored in your fridge between 37 to 39 degrees F, or zero degrees in your freezer. Food left out for more than two hours should be discarded. Meat, poultry, fish, eggs, and dairy foods are all potentially hazardous foods. *One bacterium can grow to over 2 million in seven hours*! And bacteria do NOT die in the refrigerator.

Bacteria will also grow on foods as they are thawing at room temperature, making them unsafe. Dangerous microorganisms can grow on the surface of food even if the center is still frozen. Thaw your frozen leftover turkey in the refrigerator or in constantly running drinking water.

If you are taking turkey sandwiches to work on Monday, pack them with a frozen jell pack or a frozen bottle of spring water or juice. (When the water or juice thaws, there's your lunch drink!) Bacteria grow rapidly when the temperature is between 40F and 140F.

Last tip: Don't overcrowd the fridge. If there is no space for air circulation inside the refrigerator, food may not stay at 40 degrees F or less.

Source: Food Safety Education Staff, USDA Meat and Poultry Hotline; North Carolina Cooperative Extension Service.

1,043. DON'T MICROWAVE FOODS IN PLASTIC!

Do not heat food containing fat in a microwave using plastic containers because the combination of fat, high heat, and plastics releases dioxins and other toxins into the food and ultimately into your cells. (Dioxins are carcinogens and *highly* toxic.) After studying several commercial plastic containers, compounds such as methylbenzene, ethylbenzene, 1-octene, xylene, styrene, and 1,4-dichlorobenzene were found in all of them.

Although the cooking of raw foods in a microwave oven can result in an acceptable end product in terms of touch, taste, and smell, the process does *not* address the microbiological safety of the cooked food. Microwave ovens from various commercial suppliers were used to cook naturally contaminated whole raw broiler and roaster chickens according to manufacturers' instructions. Even after microwave cooking, many of the roasters yielded viable *Listeria* bacteria.

Factors such as wattage, cavity size, and the presence or absence of a turntable did not play a significant role in the survival of this contaminant.

Sources: *Food Additive Contamination* 2002;19(6):594-601; *Emergency Medicine* (Fremantle) 2001;13(2):181-185; *Journal of Food Protection* 1998;61(11):1465-1469.

WANT TO KNOW MORE?
[For a good introduction to dioxins and other endocrine disrupters, how they negatively affect your health and what you can do to protect yourself, see my recent book, *She's Gotta Have It!*]

1,044. THE DANGERS OF "BROWNED" FOODS

Boiling and steaming foods is better than waterless cooking (as in baking, roasting, and broiling), because the waterless cooking creates browned foods and contributes to heart attacks, strokes, and nerve damage. Scientists have known for years that cooking proteins with sugars in the absence of water forms products that can damage body tissues. Cooking with water prevents sugars from binding to proteins and forming these poisonous chemicals. So, baking, roasting, and broiling cause the poisonous products to form, while boiling and steaming prevent them.

Brown foods, such as brown cookies, brown bread crust, brown basted meats and brown beans, and even brown coffee beans may increase nerve damage (especially in diabetics who are overly susceptible to nerve damage). On the other hand, since steamed and boiled vegetables, whole grains, beans, and fruits are made with water, they do not contain significant amounts of these dangerous products. Another reason why you should eat your fruits, vegetables, whole grains, and beans fresh, boiled, or steamed.

Source: Annual meeting of the Diabetes Association, San Francisco, CA.

SUPPLEMENTS

1,045. VARIETY'S THE SPICE OF.SUPPLEMENTS

If you are taking large quantities of any supplement, such as vitamin C for example, be sure to mix the brands you purchase. Different manufacturers use different sources and different formulas for their products. *Variety* is a key word in nutrition, even in your choice of dietary supplements. Needless to say, the more natural and the more "whole" the original source, the better.

Source: Common sense!

1,046. AGED GARLIC: A TRUE APHRODISIAC

Aged garlic extract increases the production of an enzyme in the body that validates its reputation as an aphrodisiac. The enzyme nitric oxide synthase increases with the use of garlic. This enzyme is responsible for the production of nitric oxide, which helps to increase blood flow. Nitric oxide plays a critical role in sexual function. (How this all works is a fairly recent discovery that led to a Nobel Prize for Medicine in 1998.)So from a medical point of view, garlic's reputation as an aphrodisiac is scientifically validated.

Source: B. Kamen, *She's Gotta Have It!*

WANT TO KNOW MORE?

[Aged garlic may also be helpful for treating atherosclerosis (see Hint #522) and poor circulation (Hint #822), as well as protecting you against the harmful effects of smoking (Hint #943) and stress (Hint #953).]

1,047. BEET CRYSTALS PACKED WITH NUTRIENTS

Add a teaspoon or more of beet crystals to any powdered nutrient mix to make it more palatable, or add it to cereals or other foods for the recalcitrant who won't take supplements. Beet crystals dissolve easily in any liquid, and are naturally sweet tasting. Beets contain a wizard's brew of important nutrients, and are even reported to normalize high blood pressure.

One of the problems with beets is that they require a lot of cooking, and most of the nutrients go down the drain. Not so with the crystallized variety. Beet crystals are made from organic beets, and available in most health food store.

Source: B. Kamen, *Everything I Know About Nutrition I Learned From Barley***.**

1,048. RECOVER FROM DESSERT WITH FIBER

How do I recover from dessert? With fiber! Because anything sweet disturbs blood sugar levels, which in turn disturbs the production of growth hormone – among other important metabolic processes – make sure you are including a good fiber mix in your supplement regimen. It is difficult to get enough fiber without supplementation from even the most exemplary diet in this country. Five whole heads of lettuce contain only six grams of fiber, and fruits are very low in fiber, too. For optimal health, the recommended amount is 35 to 60 grams.

Fiber improves glycemic control, lowers cholesterol and triglyceride values, and can even promote weight loss. It can increase fecal mass and stool frequency, two health-promoting attributes.

Fiber supplements should contain naturally occurring plant fibers. Health-store fiber formulas are usually derived from old-fashioned foods like fruits or grains, cloaked in modern technology. Since fibers vary in function, and many cause beneficial synergistic reactions with other fibers, it's a good idea to select a fiber product with multi-fiber sources.

It's easy to get a heterogeneous selection of fiber in supplemental form at your local health store. The blend should be palatable, but not sweet (we don't want to undermine the benefits). My favorites are assembled from a mix of organic sprouted seeds, in powder form. You'd have to swallow too many tablets or capsules to get the amount needed for protection. And taking the supplement in powder form assures the intake of lots of water, *a necessity when taking fiber supplements*.

Psyllium seed taken alone (as in Metamucil) actually destroys the villi of the digestive tract if taken regularly over a few years. Again, it's very important to take mixed forms of fiber, so you don't overload on only one kind (unless it's in a whole-food form, as in oatmeal).

For more information on fiber and how it can help many health conditions, including breast cancer, high cholesterol levels, colitis, hiatus hernia, irritable bowel syndrome, and more, see my easy-to-read book, *New Facts About Fiber.*

1,049. FIBER & SUFFICIENT WATER INTAKE

If you use wheat bran as your fiber supplement, be sure to soak the bran overnight. If you don't soak it, the bran will absorb moisture from *you*, and could exacerbate a constipation problem, rather than help it. Fiber is not broken down in your digestive tract the same way that whole foods are broken down. In fact, it's a good idea to drink at least eight ounces of water with any fiber supplement.

Source: B. Kamen, *New Facts About Fiber.*

1,050. THE BENEFITS OF SIBERIAN GINSENG

Long used in traditional Oriental medicine, Siberian ginseng is a remarkable supplement that is protective against a myriad of health problems. Siberian ginseng has been shown to help modulate arrhythmia (irregular heart beat), alleviate allergic symptoms, increase fat utilization, lower cholesterol, moderate insulin levels, and reduce pain. And it also exhibits antioxidant and anti-cancer properties!

The Chinese never regarded ginseng as "curative," but rather as "adjustive." It is able to keep your body in line despite environmental influences. A drug stimulant affects behavior in most situations, but Siberian ginseng acts predominantly when you are faced with a challenge.

[Although American and Korean ginseng are of some value, they are not as powerful and are usually commercially cultivated: grown in artificial environments, often with chemically enhanced fertilizers. Siberian ginseng grows wild in the mountain forests of Hokkaido, Japan. In the area I visited, the Siberian ginseng plants have been growing undisturbed for more than a century. Unhindered in a native environment, the root is more potent. Plants in the wild are often stronger in order to survive the harsh natural conditions.]

Sources: *Immunopharmacology & Immunotoxicology* 2001;23(1):107-17; *Eksp Klin Farmakol* Jul-2000;63(4):29-31; *International Journal of Sport, Nutrition, & Exercise Metabolism* 2000;10(4):444-451; Journal of Ethnopharmacology 2000;72(3):345-393.

An in-depth report on four *super* nutraceuticals appears at the end of *Healthier Living*. These are stabilized rice bran, whole crushed barley leaf, colostrum, and velvet antler.

EXERCISE & FITNESS

1,051. CURRENT EXERCISE MORE IMPORTANT

The incredible benefits of exercise are associated with *recent* activity rather than your collegiate athletic endeavors, or any other exercise programs you practiced in the past – so get moving! It's never too late to begin exercising. Endless studies in recent years show that people who are more active tend to live longer. Exercise has proven beneficial in conditions ranging from osteoporosis to depression to cerebrovascular disease. So it doesn't matter so much that you were an athlete in college: it's recent and current physical activity that will decrease your risk of heart disease and premature death.

Source: *American Heart Journal* 1999;138(5):900-907.

1,052. ARE *YOUR* KIDS EXERCISING ENOUGH?

Current guidelines from the US Centers for Disease Control and Prevention and the American College of Sports Medicine suggest that *all Americans* should strive for at least 30 minutes of moderate exercise daily — with even longer periods of time recommended for children. The rising level of obesity in American kids is a major cause of concern, and the current guidelines for children may not be tough enough. Researchers advise one to two hours of physical activity a day.

Source: *Pediatrics online* 2001;e108.

1,053. EXERCISE AFTER LONG-TERM INACTIVITY

Even substantial decreases in cardiovascular fitness resulting from decades of inactivity can be *significantly* reversed with modest endurance training (such as walking, cycling, or jogging) – at *any* age. The encouraging results of one study showed that men, after a relatively modest six-month endurance-training program, were able to get back to an aerobic-power level consistent with their 20-year-old baseline. So they were able to reverse a substantial portion of the aerobic power that had been lost over the years. Decrease in cardiovascular fitness after age 50 occurs as a result of loss of the ability to take up and use oxygen. But it is never too late to start exercising.

Source: *Circulation* 2001;104:1350-1357.

1,054. AEROBICS EXERCISE BENEFITS FOR MEN

Regular physical exercise can help to reduce abdominal fat and glucose-stimulated insulin responses in middle-aged and older men. A nine-month, moderate-intensity exercise training program with men walking, jogging, or cycling three times a week for 30 to 45 minutes increases aerobic power by 15 percent and reduces body fat and waist circumference.

In addition, insulin responses during glucose-tolerance tests decrease by 16 percent. Regular physical exercise may prevent or improve conditions associated with hyperinsulinemia — including hypertension and atherosclerosis.

Source: *Journal of the American Geriatric Society* **2000;48:1055-1061.**

1,055. LONGER PERIODS OF MODERATE EXERCISE

Those who exercise moderately for longer periods (such as walking or bicycling) use more energy than those who participate in short periods of high-intensity physical activity. Exercisers who spend relatively more time on *moderate*-intensity activity than low-intensity activity have a higher physical activity level than more sedentary people, but time spent on high-intensity activities alone does not affect the physical activity level.

In the normal population, short periods of high-intensity activity are usually followed by extended periods of low-intensity activity. The proportion of time distributed to activities of low and moderate intensity is what influences the total energy expenditure.

Source: *Nature* **2001;410:539.**

1,056. EXERCISE: GET A STEADY "DOSE" DAILY

Walking briskly for half an hour burns more calories than three 10-minute walks spaced throughout the day. Ideally, daily exercise should be done in one steady dose, instead of 10 minutes here and there. The calorie difference could amount to losing roughly five pounds per year. Investigators found that continuous walking burned about 60 more calories per day than shorter intermittent walks.

The National Institutes of Health tells healthy adults to accumulate at least 30 minutes of moderate exercise on most days. Other experts advocate moderate-to-intense activity for 20 to 60 minutes straight, three to five days per week. Some exercise is better than none. Brief periods of activity help to reduce your risk of cardiovascular disease.

Source: *Medicine & Science in Sports & Exercise* **2001;33:163-170.**

1,057.   SIBERIAN GINSENG FOR MUSCLE & ENERGY

With news of the dangers of creatine as a supplement, athletes should know about tried-and-true Siberian ginseng – which is reported to enhance physical performance, improve muscular strength, and maximize oxygen uptake and reaction times. Controlled studies of Asian ginsengs found improvements in overall exercise. Ginseng treatment was shown to shorten reaction time at rest and during exercise. Researchers conclude that ginseng extract improves psychomotor performance during exercise without affecting exercise capacity.

Studies with animals show that ginseng or its active components may prolong survival to physical or chemical stress. Although not everyone is an athlete, everyone can gain from reaching a higher level of effectiveness of motor activity. Siberian ginseng's stimulative effect begins as soon as half an hour to an hour after ingestion. Ginseng also helps to subdue or even eliminate menopausal symptoms.

Sources: *International Journal of Sports Nutrition* 1999;9(4):371-377; *Sports Medicine* 1994;18(4): 229-248; B. Kamen, *Siberian Ginseng: Fabled Tonic Herb* (Keats Publishers).

NATURAL MEDICINES

1,058.   LIQUID ACIDOPHILUS AGAINST MANY ILLS

A tablespoon or two of liquid acidophilus can help relieve over-eating indigestion, with only positive side effects. In fact, no household should be without a bottle of liquid acidophilus in the fridge at any time. Here are just a few ways it can be of benefit:

- Acidophilus can confer protection against pH levels that are too acid.
- It helps prevent the occurrence of antibiotic-associated diarrhea.
- It can suppress pneumonia and decrease bronchitis in children.
- Long-term consumption increases concentrations of HDL cholesterol (the "good-guy" cholesterol), leading to improvement of the LDL/HDL cholesterol ratio.
- It decreases *H. pylori* bacteria (the bacteria responsible for ulcers) in your stomach and helps to enhance any therapy for *H. pylori* eradication.

But even if you haven't been taking acidophilus on a daily basis, you'll find it incredibly effective for relieving acute stomach upset.

Sources: *Journal of Molecular Microbiology & Biotechnology* 2002;4(6):525-532; *Journal of the Thai Medical Association* 2002;85(Suppl1):S79-84;2002;85(Suppl2):S739-742; *Archives of Latinoamerican Nutrition* 2002;52(1):29-34; *European Journal of Clinical Nutrition* 2002;56(9):843.

1,059   THE MANY HEALTH BENEFITS OF ALOE

Aloe vera, long known as an effective treatment for burns, has properties that may be helpful against many other conditions, including skin disorders, diabetes, and ulcers. Aloes have long been used all over the world for various medicinal properties. Aloe vera gel is well known as an effective treatment for treating burns and for aiding wound healing.

It has a protective effect when added to soap regimens for skin reaction treatment. [See Hint #362 in the *Dermatological Conditions* section for information about the use of Aloe vera gel for the treatment of psoriasis.]

In addition, it is believed that the pulp of the Aloe vera plant may help in the treatment of diabetes. In the past 15 years, there have been controversial reports on the hypoglycemic activity of Aloe species, probably due to differences in the parts of the plant used. But researchers conclude that the *pulp* of Aloe vera leaves (devoid of the gel) could be useful in the treatment of non-insulin dependent diabetes.

Aloe gel is also included among those compounds with anti-ulcer activity.

Sources: *Archives of Facial Plastic Surgery* 2001;3(2):127-132; *Oncology of Nursing Forum* 2001;28(3):543-547; *Phytotherapy Research* 2001;15(2):157-161.

1,060.   ALA AGAINST DIABETES & MORE

Alpha-lipoic acid has been shown to improve nerve function in toes, and is also used in Europe to treat diabetes and diabetic complications. Alpha-lipoic acid (ALA) is a naturally occurring antioxidant found in spinach and beef. It is used to treat diabetics and diabetic complications in Europe because it helps in the process in which glucose (blood sugar) is broken down and burned for energy.

American diabetes journals are publishing more studies on alpha-lipoic acid and nerve disorders, reflecting a growing appreciation of this nutrient's health benefits.

Alpha-lipoic acid's antioxidant properties could possibly account for its beneficial effect on nerve function.

Source: *Diabetes* 2000;49:1006-1015.

WANT TO KNOW MORE?
[To learn more about ALA and diabetes, see Hint #404 in the *Diabetes Type 2* section. Alpha-lipoic acid may also be protective against hypertension (Hint #625), as well as play a beneficial role in memory enhancement (Hint #698).]

1,061. NATURAL ANTI-INFLAMMATORY HERBS

Natural anti-inflammatory compounds abound in the herbal world and are found in green tea, the spices turmeric and rosemary, and feverfew. The use of herbs for medical benefit has played an important role in nearly every culture on earth. Herbal medicine was practiced by ancient cultures in Asia, Africa, Europe, and the Americas.

Herbs provide benefit over and above allopathic medicine by allowing users to feel that they have some control in their choice of medications. Herbal products may have benefits similar to pharmaceuticals yet without the side effects of standard drugs. Natural non-steroidal anti-inflammatory products are currently being explored for possible use as cancer preventives.

Source: *Journal of Nutrition* 2001;131:3034S-3036S.

1,062. CHOCOLATE: A HEALTH FOOD?

Here's the Hint you've all been waiting for: *Chocolate* **may prevent the oxidation of LDL cholesterol, be useful as a bronchitis treatment and cough medicine alternative, and has a long history as a natural remedy for hemorrhoids, gout, and digestive problems, among other health problems.** Chocolate has been described as "awesome, calming, dangerous, delectable, erotic, heavenly, intoxicating, irresistible, mysterious, non-nutritious, satiating, sexy, sinful, sticky, and tranquilizing...to taste chocolate is to share in a common connection through history, from a time over 3,000 years ago to the present, from the frothy cacao beverages prepared at the court of King Montezuma, to the era of the modern chocolate bar."

When researchers at the USDA fed cocoa powder and dark chocolate to a group of people for four weeks, they found that LDL oxidation ("bad-guy" cholesterol) was inhibited. This favorable effect was attributed to flavonoids (antioxidants) and copper. Milk chocolate and cocoa powder are among foods having the highest amount of copper, a mineral that most Americans are deficient in (because of soil depletion). By eating chocolate, the daily intake of copper might be three times the daily requirement, or twice the RDA for adults.

[Of course, we could also get our copper from oysters, shrimp, buckwheat, nuts and seeds, and beans.] Dark chocolate contains more of this mineral than light chocolate does. Researchers also theorize that perhaps chocolate enhances the absorbability of copper.

Researchers at the National Heart and Lung Institute in London report that *theobromine*, a chemical found in cocoa and chocolate, is more effective than codeine as a cough medication.

The medicinal use of cacao and chocolate as a primary remedy goes back several centuries. It has been used to help emaciated patients gain weight, to improve digestion and elimination, and even to help lactation and the pain of gout. It also has a long history as a cure for hemorrhoids throughout the centuries.

In the twentieth century, it has been recommended as a skin lubricant, a healing treatment for cracked lips, and as an emollient to treat bronchitis. However, it is also noted that it is difficult to digest if prepared with milk, and that it could "overexcite."

[If you must have chocolate, indulge in the purest chocolate you can find (or afford). The caveat is to avoid cheap chocolates to which too much sugar and modified fat, etc., have been added.]

Sources: *American Journal of Clinical Nutrition* 2002;76(3):687-688; *Journal of Nutrition* 2000;130:2057S-2072S.

1,063. THE MANY HEALTH BENEFITS OF PAPAYA

Papain (an enzyme found in papaya) can accelerate burn healing, produce a therapeutic effect in those with inflammatory disorders in the genitals, intestine, liver, and eyes identical to those of a commercial drug product, and the unripened juice can even lower blood pressure. Most of us are aware of papaya's benefit for digestion. But this amazing fruit can do so much more.

The juice of the unripened papaya fruit can lower blood pressure. Researchers concluded that the fruit juice of papaya probably contains antihypertensive agents, as yet not completely identified. In the West Indies, topical application of papaya is used successfully by nurses in chronic skin ulcer therapy.

Sources: *Phytotherapy Research* 2000;14(4):235-239; *West Indian Medical Journal* 2000;49(1):32-33; *Eksp Klin Farmakol* 2000;63(3):55-57.

1,064. IN PRAISE OF PHYTOESTROGENS

Clover sprouts, alfalfa sprouts, and oilseeds (such as flaxseed) are significant dietary sources of *phytoestrogens*, which help to prevent menopausal symptoms, osteoporosis, cancer, and heart disease. Phytoestrogens extracted from red clover are associated with an increase in high-density lipoprotein cholesterol (the "good-guy" stuff) and a significant increase in bone health after six months of consumption.

Phytoestrogens can exert estrogenic and anti-estrogenic activities *at the same time*, indicating an adaptogenic effect (that is, they adapt to your needs, unlike synthetic estrogen).

Dietary phytoestrogens significantly reduce aortic cholesterol content with a potency comparable to that of hormone therapy. [It's very easy and inexpensive to sprout clover and alfalfa seeds at home.]

Sources: *Annual Review of Nutrition* 1997;17:353-381; *Menopause* 2001;8(4):259-265; *Climacteric* 2001;4(2):151-159.

WANT TO KNOW MORE?
[See my book, *Hormone Replacement Therapy: Yes or No? How to Make an Informed Decision*, for more detailed information of phytoestrogens and the concept of adaptogens.]

1,065. HEALTH BENEFITS OF POMEGRANATE JUICE

Pomegranate juice has been shown to inhibit the production of free radicals, lessen cholesterol accumulation, and destroy several viruses on contact. Pomegranate juice can contribute to the reduction of oxidative stress and hardening of the arteries. In test animals with advanced hardening of the arteries (atherosclerosis), lesions were actually reduced by 17 percent compared with placebo-treated animals.

A substance isolated from pomegranate juice (a tannin-fraction) has a significant anti-atherosclerotic effect. The active constituent that appears to be responsible for pomegranate's multiple health benefits (including its anti-viral properties) is *ellagic acid*. Ellagic acid is a potent inhibitor of a molecule (tyrosine protein kinase) whose activity has been associated with the ability of certain viruses to transform normal cells into cancerous cells.

Sources: *Journal of Nutrition* 2001;131:2082-2089; *Journal of Cell Biochemistry.* 1995;220(Suppl):169.

1,066. ANTIBIOTICS FROM A POTATO PEEL?

An extract made from potato peel prevents adhesion of bacteria to cells – working as a *natural* antibiotic. Although most antimicrobials are chemicals that inhibit growth or annihilate "the enemy," plant components can actually prevent microorganisms from adhering to healthy tissue. Research shows resistance to E. coli and a strep strain with the use of the potato skin extract. (Adhesion is a necessary first step in order to cause disease.)

Using this technique avoids the use of antibiotics, which, after killing bacteria, may cause release of toxic substances that can cause damaging inflammatory responses.

[But beware of non-organic potato peel, which is usually treated with an additive to prevent "eyes" from forming on the potato. Any potato that has "eyes" should be discarded.]

Source: Annual Meeting of the American Society for Microbiology, May 2000.

1,067. ANTIOXIDANT PROPERTIES OF SPICES

In descending order of effectiveness, these spices inhibit lipid peroxidation (rancidity and/or instability that can lead to the formation of free radicals): rosemary, oregano, annatto, sweet paprika, cumin, hot paprika, and saffron. The effect of these Mediterranean food spices on the oxidative stability of refined olive oil was compared with common food additives during storage at room temperature for 72 hours, two months, four months, and six months. The results showed that extracts of these spices have significant stabilizing effects and prove to be superior to commonly used food additives. In addition, the chemopreventive potency of extracts like rosemary on the development of cancer in test animal is very promising.

The substance that gives the curry spice turmeric its yellow color, called curcumin, may help fight cancer, Alzheimer's disease, and may also hasten wound healing.

Sources: *Journal of Food Protection* Sep 2001;64(9):1412-1419; *Food & Chemical Toxicology* Sep 2001;39(9):907-918; Annual Meeting of the American Association for Cancer Research, San Francisco, CA, Apr 2002.

1,068. THE ANTI-DISEASE PROPERTIES OF TEA

Tea has been shown to help curtail the start and development of cardiovascular disease and nutritionally linked cancers, including those in the stomach, colon, breast, prostate, ovary, and endometrium. Tea is one of the most commonly consumed beverages in the world and is rich in polyphenolic compounds collectively known as tea flavonoids. Tea flavonoids possess antioxidant properties and have been proposed as key protective dietary components, reducing the risk of coronary heart disease and some cancers. One aspect involved in these diseases is the abnormal oxidative stress leading to the formation of free radicals, but tea flavonoids can powerfully inhibit these reactions.

Both green and black teas release significant levels of antioxidants into hot water within two minutes of infusion, but green tea possesses the greater antioxidant capacity.

Sources: *Proceedings of the Society of Experimental Biological Medicine* 1998;218(2):140-143; *International Journal of Food Science & Nutrition* 2000;51(3):181-188.

1,069. TEA TREE OIL: THE MICROBE KILLER

If you are visiting a relative or friend in the hospital, tea tree oil is the best possible present because it is effective in killing a variety of resistant microorganisms commonly found in hospitals. Tea tree oil rapidly kills most microorganisms in less than 60 minutes. Observing that resistant microorganisms in hospitals cause problems for both the treatment of patients and infection control, researchers recommend the use of tea tree oil in topical and hand-washing applications to reduce the transmission of many microorganisms associated with "hospital-caused infections."

Source: *Journal of Antimicrobial Chemistry* **2000;45:639-643.**

1,070. WILLOW BARK, THE "NATURAL ASPIRIN"

Excitement, stress, family issues, jet lag, overeating, etc., have too many of us automatically reaching for headache and/or pain relief drugs, but willow bark extract can do the same job as aspirin with none of the adverse stomach side effects. Willow bark is the natural form of salicylic acid (aspirin), and it has comparable anti-inflammatory activities as higher doses of aspirin. Just like aspirin, it reduces pain and can lower fever. In contrast to aspirin, it does not affect the stomach mucosa.

A daily dose of 1,572 mg of willow bark extract has been shown to be helpful for those with osteoarthritis of the hip and the knee and for those with exacerbations of chronic lower back pain. Willow bark extract also has advantages over a routinely prescribed treatment of orthopedic specialists based on nonsteroidal anti-rheumatic drugs.

It may also play a protective role against the formation of blood clots (although the activity here is weaker).

Source: *Wiener medizinische Wochenschrift* **(German) 2002;152(15-16):354-359.**

ENVIRONMENTAL TOXINS

1,071. AVOID FOODS SPRAYED WITH DIAZINON

Avoid eating grapes, green beans, peaches, and spinach, unless *organic*, because these foods are sprayed with one of the most toxic pesticides. Diazinon, a neurotoxicant that can affect key developmental processes, is considered the most toxic pesticide registered for widespread use.

Not only is it in foods that we eat on a regular basis, but it is also commonly found in drinking water and on lawns and in parks. Consumers Union has recommended to the US Environmental Protection Agency that this organophosphate pesticide be phased out of use within four years.

Source: Consumers Union, reported in *Reuter's Medical News* Jul 2000.

1,072. STEER CLEAR OF IRRADIATED FOODS

Avoiding eating foods that have been irradiated, as there is concern that this process may pose many health risks to consumers. The Cancer Prevention Coalition and Public Citizen Group claim overwhelming evidence that: radiation cuts the nutritional value of food by a third; once cooked the food has no nutritional value at all; irradiated food poses a threat to human fertility and reproductive viability; and its byproducts are carcinogenic.

Joined by other groups and several environmental protection organizations, the group claims there are numerous public health threats posed by applying ionizing radiation to food, including dangers from its byproducts. (For example, these groups report that benzene, a known carcinogen, is a byproduct that appears in large quantities in irradiated beef.)

Radiation was first approved as a bactericide for spices in 1983. Since that time, the FDA has approved irradiation of pork, fruit, vegetables, red meat, poultry, and fresh eggs. [But until more information is in place, better safe than sorry.]

Source: *Reuter's Health Medical News* **Oct 2000.**

1,073. THE DANGERS OF FLUORIDE

Take steps to reduce your exposure to fluoride, which has been linked to many health problems, including osteoporosis and fluorosis. Belgium has banned fluoride in its water supply because of the increased risk of osteoporosis it poses, as well as concerns it could damage the nervous system. Despite discontinuation of water fluoridation, no increase was observed in the frequency of dental caries (cavities) in one town over a three-year period.

In another study, it was shown that the prevalence of fluorosis (mottling of the teeth) was 54 percent in a fluoridated area and only 23 percent in a fluoride-deficient area.

[I advocate non-fluoridated toothpaste for *everyone*, which can be easily found in most health food stores.]

Both reverse osmosis and distillation water filters can remove fluoride at a high rate. [To learn more about fluorosis, including the very serious *crippling skeletal fluorosis*, see Hints #770 and #785 in the *Osteoporosis & Other Skeletal Problems* section.]

Sources: *Nutrition Business Journal* **2002; ASDC** *Journal of Dentition for Children* **2000;67(5):302;304;350-354;** *British Dental Journal* **2000;189(4):216-220.**

1,074. SUGAR CAN INCREASE TOXIC EFFECTS

Yet *another* reason to cut out sugar from your diet: Excessive dietary intake of sugars could increase the toxicity of numerous toxic substances. In tests conducted on the effects of glucose on the neurotoxicity of the pesticide *parathion*, it was observed that the toxicity associated with exposure to this chemical increased.

It is postulated that excessive glucose consumption decreases the intake of other dietary components, in particular amino acids. Individuals who get a large proportion of their calories from sugars may therefore be at a higher risk of acute toxicity from such organophosphorus pesticides.

Source: *Journal of Toxicology & Environmental Health* 2001;63(4):253-271.

WANT TO KNOW MORE?

Exposure to methyl parathion is most likely for those people living or working near or on a farm where it is sprayed on crops. It is a powerful poison that affects the central nervous system, and exposure to high levels for even a short time in the air or water can be very serious. Methyl parathion has been detected at low levels in food.

There is no evidence that sugars naturally incorporated in the cellular structure of foods have adverse effects on health. But the intake of extrinsic sugar (from an outside source) does a lot more than cause cavities. (***Public Health Nutrition* 2001;4(2B):569-91**)

An interesting article in the ***British Medical Journal*** (**2002**), discusses the fact that we need more than just labelling changes. We need fundamental changes to food production. Too many foods thought to be "healthy" contain hidden sugars. Among these foods are: breakfast cereals, fruit juices, salad dressings, yogurt, baby foods, and a variety of drinks. As we all know, the sugar conditioning starts with baby foods and drinks, and once the child has acquired a sweet tooth, non-sweetened foods are not so attractive. Until the food industry takes more responsibility, we have to be *personally* responsible.

Fortified foods are often sweetened with added sugars, counteracting the nutrient benefit of the added supplement. (***Journal of Nutrition* 2002;132:2785-2791**)

The largest source of added sugars in the US diet is nondiet soft drinks, accounting for one third of total intake. As we all knw, diets high in sugars have been associated with various health problems. In addition to the familiar dental caries and obesity, there are also correlations with bone loss and fractures. (***Journal of Nutrition* 2001;131:2766S-2771S**)

1,075. FAREWELL TO MERCURY THERMOMETERS

If you still have a mercury thermometer in your medicine cabinet, it should be discarded. The American Academy of Pediatrics is calling for the eradication of mercury thermometers, citing the possible danger of mercury poisoning. The technology is outmoded, and safer and more accurate digital thermometers are widely available. (Besides, mercury thermometers are difficult to use and read.) Among the alternatives are digital, strip, and ear thermometers. Digital thermometers are safe and very easy to read, and ear thermometers are increasingly popular for young children.

As far as accuracy is concerned, the electronic rectal temperature measurements are the most accurate – and the closest to rectal mercury readings. Electronic tympanic (ear), oral, or axillary (armpit) measurements are not recommended.

Eliminating mercury thermometers could also help to reduce the occurrence of mercury dermatitis, which can be caused by broken thermometers. If you are still using a mercury thermometer, be aware that there is no clinical advantage to using a measurement time longer than three minutes.

[Important note: Mercury is an *extremely* hazardous waste product. Mercury thermometers should NEVER be discarded with the household trash – instead bring your old thermometers to your doctor's office where they can be discarded off properly.]

Sources: *Pediatrics* 2001;108:197-205; *European Journal of Surgery* 2000;166(11):848-851.

1,076. WHAT ARE ENDOCRINE DISRUPTERS?

Endocrine disrupters – chemical pollutants in the environment created for industrial, agricultural, or domestic purposes – are now being linked to many serious health problems. The effect on human health of environmental chemicals that are mediated through the endocrine system (called endocrine disrupters) has generated huge interest and investment. Endocrine disrupters are new to human existence, and the idea that trends for prostate cancer, cystic ovaries, endometriosis, breast cancer, increased sexuality problems, and reduced fertility are all connected with environmental pollution is gaining credence internationally.

Synthetic chemicals in the environment are the prime source of the excessive estrogenic stimulation, with exposure through food and water being the primary route. Phthalates (used to make plastics soft or bendable) and bisphenol A (used in lining food cans) both have a high potential for endocrine disruption.

Source: *British Medical Journal* 2001;323:1317-1318.

WANT TO KNOW MORE?
[My book, *She's Gotta Have It! explains* explains why this situation exists today. The book also suggests a course of action to protect your own health from this serious environmental problem.]

1,077. CARBON MONOXIDE RISK FROM FURNACES

Before turning your furnace on for the winter season, have it inspected in order to avoid deadly carbon monoxide poisoning (and check appliances, too, while you're at it). Carbon monoxide poisoning associated with fuel-burning appliances kills more than 200 people each year and sends more than 10,000 to hospital emergency rooms! Carbon monoxide is a colorless, odorless gas produced by burning any fuel. Initial symptoms of carbon monoxide poisoning are similar to flu and can include headache, fatigue, shortness of breath, nausea, and dizziness.

For your own safety, have a professional inspection done on all fuel-burning appliances (this includes furnaces, stoves, fireplaces, clothes dryers, and space heaters) to detect dangerous carbon monoxide leaks. These appliances burn fuels such as gas, kerosene, oil, coal, and wood. Signs of possible carbon monoxide leaks include black stains on the outside of the chimney, flue, or vents. These stains could mean that pollutants are leaking into the house.

The short-term cure for low-level exposure is fresh air, but the long-term solution is to have your furnace checked; not only the burner itself, but also the heat exchanger, piping, and chimney. And don't neglect the appliances!

Source: CPSC's website at www.cpsc.gov.

1,078. NITRATES IN TAP WATER & CANCER RISK

Make sure to always drink filtered and bottled water, and ask your favorite restaurant to do the same, as nitrate found in tap water can increase your risk of several cancers. Nitrate levels in water are rising, and are linked to an increased risk of bladder and ovarian cancer, especially in older women. In one study done on over 16,500 women between the ages of 55 and 69 who had used municipal water supplies for more than 10 years, 3,150 later developed cancer. Although you may be careful about your water supply at home, keep in mind that the coffee, tea, soft drinks, fruit drinks, table water, and soups you order in restaurants are almost exclusively prepared with tap water.

[You might try bringing your own bottled water to your table at your favorite restaurant until they begin to get the idea.]

Source: *Epidemiology* 2001;11:327-338.

WANT TO KNOW MORE?
[See the *Cancer, Bladder* and *Cancer, Ovarian* sections for more information on both of these diseases.]

1,079. AVOID IMPORTED CERAMIC DINNERWARE

Be warned: Imported dishes may contain toxic metals in excessive amounts, and decorative ceramic plates may be improperly labeled regarding permissible use with food. About one-third of imported ceramic dinnerware checked was found to release lead in levels exceeding California Proposition 65 (CA 65) limits – which are *more strict* than FDA rulings. One imported ceramic dish also released cadmium in excess of FDA limits. Some imported decorative ceramic plates may release lead in high concentrations, yet are not permanently labeled as hazardous (which is in noncompliance with FDA regulations).

However, melamine (plastic) dinnerware is proven to be safe.

Source: *Science: Total Environment* 1999;234(1-3):233-237.

1,080. BEWARE CHLORINE GAS IN BATH WATER

Let your bath water fill the tub completely before you enter the room, to allow the chlorine gas to escape in your absence. Chlorine is used to purify tap water. Unfortunately, this becomes a debatable risk-benefit issue. Among the disadvantages of chlorine is the fact that it encourages calcium excretion [putting your bone health at risk]. But simply allowing the water to "gas out" while the tub is filling, but not in your presence, can help to mitigate the problem.

1,081. VENTILATE HOMES AT NIGHT

Because the carcinogen benzene enters homes and gets trapped in carpets, linoleum, and wood surfaces (but not in tiling, marble, or bare walls), houses in city environments should be ventilated at night, when traffic is the least dense. The environmental level of benzene (a known carcinogen) is not an accurate indicator of personal exposure to the pollutant because adsorbent products in the home can trap it.

The population exposure is usually higher indoors than outdoors. Since benzene levels in outside air peak during the day, when more cars are on the road, ventilating at night is recommended, when levels are lower.

Source: *Nature* 2000;404:141-142.

EVERYDAY HEALTH HINTS

1,082. CHECK YOUR "TRANSIT TIME"

To check your "transit time" (the time elapsed from ingesting food to the time you eliminate it), swallow a spoonful or two of corn kernels without chewing them, and examine stools in the next few days. The transit time of someone in Africa consuming a high-fiber diet may be about 18 hours. A healthy American should display a transit time of 24 to 36 hours. Seniors in this country have an average transit time of two weeks.

Transit time is dependent on the fiber in your diet, and is an excellent gauge for determining your diet status. A decreased transit time indicates that there is less time for toxins to be in contact with your intestinal mucosa. Increased bulk also dilutes potential carcinogens. Plus there is less constipation and therefore less straining. A faster transit time can help you to avoid many serious diseases, including colon cancer. To learn more about transit time and fiber foods, see my book, *New Facts About Fiber*.

1,083. THE RISKS OF YELLOW FOOD DYES

Beware FD & C Yellow #5 and #6, dyes shown to be cross-reactive with aspirin and acetaminophen. Yellow #5 can also cause excessive elimination of zinc. Exposure to even small amounts of these synthetic substances can provoke serious reactions. Yellow #5 and #6 have been associated with hives, belching, vomiting, edema, and abdominal pain. Many antibiotics contain these dyes.

Source: Schmidt, et al, *Beyond Antibiotics* (North Atlantic Books).

1,084. WATER: HOW MUCH SHOULD YOU DRINK?

Drinking water equal to half your weight in ounces is in your best health interest. (Example: If you weigh 150 pounds, you should be consuming 75 ounces of water daily.) We all know we can live longer without food than without water. Water helps to keep our skin elastic and it increases urine volume (which helps to flush away end products of metabolism). It is the vehicle for food materials absorbed from the digestive canal. Water is essential for the regulation of body temperature and it is important in lubrication of joint surfaces. It is the medium in which chemical changes take place that underlie most of our obvious activities. The list of metabolic functions involving water is almost endless. Try increasing your water volume and enjoy the benefits.

Source: Wisdom of the Ages.

1,085. HOUSEHOLD SOAPS & DRUG RESISTANCE

Be sure to check the list of ingredients the next time you purchase soap, as dangerous multi-drug resistance may develop from the widespread use of soaps containing antibacterial substances. Antibacterial agents (such as triclosan and triclocarban) are present in about 75 percent of all household liquid soaps and in about 30 percent of bar soaps, *even if not so labeled*, and even though there is no evidence that they prevent infection.

Source: **Meeting of the Infectious Diseases Society of America, as reported in** *Reuter's Medical Report* **Sep 2000.**

1,086. THE DANGERS OF "SUPERCLEAN MANIA"

Beware antibacterial cleaning products as well: hospital-based antibacterial resistance has spread to homes, schools, and workplaces because of the extensive use of these products. The wide use of germicidal household products (and products like ciprofloxacin after last year's anthrax scare) is a major responsible factor. Our medical community is also helping the evolution of drug-resistant bacteria by administering antibiotics indiscriminately. Antibiotics fed to livestock also pose dangers.

As surface antimicrobials seep into sinks and toilets, they wash through sewage systems and into water supplies. Bacterial strains that carry genes for tiny internal pumps eliminate the antimicrobial compounds, recycling them back to the environment unchanged.

Sources: *Journal of the American Medical Association* **2002;288:947-948;** *Morbidity & Mortality Weekly Report* **2002:51;565-567.**

1,087. THE MANY HEALTH RISKS OF FASHION

Protecting your health is *always* in style: Fashion and style trends can cause infections, damage the musculoskeletal system, and impact fertility Fashion health risk summary: *Thong underwear* can cause vaginal and urinary tract infections; *tight pants*, low sperm count, rash, infection; *body piercing* and *tattooing*, hepatitis C transmission and other infections, and these procedures are allergy triggers; *high-heel shoes*, foot, knee and back problems; *big shoulder bags*, shoulder and back problems; *corsets*, atrophy of the back muscles; and, finally, *fashion magazines*, poor body image, eating disorders.

Gynecologists report anecdotally that they are seeing an increasing number of women with recurrent urinary tract and vaginal infection connected with thong underwear. The bacteria go from the rectum to the vagina and to the bladder. Normal healthy people, however, shouldn't really be impacted by this, but anyone who is predisposed may have an increased incidence.

Tight jeans in the 1970s and early 1980s – so tight the zipper had to be pulled up with pliers – were blamed for genital irritation and low sperm counts in men.

Marilyn Monroe deliberately had the stiletto heels of her shoes adjusted. One heel was made shorter than the other so that she swayed and sashayed as she walked. Fashions do change, however, and Marilyn would be considered too heavy by today's standards.

Source: *American Medical News* **Aug 2002.**

1,088. LONG NAILS & DISEASE TRANSMISSION

If your fingernails are long and/or artificial, they could play a role in serious disease transmission, especially for the young children you come in contact with. The disease that may be transmitted via long or artificial fingernails is *Pseudomonas aeruginosa* (a bacteria), and may have caused the death of eleven newborn infants in a hospital setting. Although there is no conclusive evidence yet, it is recommended that neonatal ICU healthcare workers be restricted from having long or artificial fingernails. Positive *P. aeruginosa* cultures were found among healthcare workers with long natural or artificial fingernails, and not among those with short- or medium-length natural nails.
If you care for young children at home, take the same precautions.

Sources: *Infectious Control Hospital Epidemiology* **2000;21:77-85;** *American Journal of Infection Control* **2002;30:252-254.**

1,089. THE RISKS OF "HIGH" PIERCING

Avoid multiple piercing of the ear ("high" piercing), which involves repeated puncture through ear cartilage that often results in serious inflammation – and could lead to a loss of cartilage and "cauliflower ear." Antibiotic resistance to the inflammation caused by ear piercing is increasing. The vast majority of piercings are performed by non-medical practitioners, such as jewelers, hairdressers, or tattooists. These practitioners may not fully appreciate the implications of cartilage damage resulting from high piercing. Abscesses are frequent and cosmetic deformity has proved difficult to avoid.

Children as young as six are having piercings in navels, ears, and noses. The potential complications of the inflammation are serious. Infections involving the cartilage progress rapidly. The long-term cosmetic problems arise from destruction of cartilage. As the inflammation progresses, the abscess peels off layers of the cartilage. The body-piercing phenomenon is poorly regulated, and there is little promotion about its adverse effects.

Source: *British Medical Journal* **2001;322:906-907,936.**

1,090. DON'T WASH YOUR SKIN BEFORE SUNNING

Don't take a bath or shower before you go to the beach or the pool – you'll avoid washing away the fatty oil just under the top layer of your skin that aids in the conversion of ultra violet rays to vitamin D. The connection between vitamin D and the sun was made 2,500 years ago! Unfortunately, no natural food contains vitamin D in anything but trace amounts; not even mother's milk.

For those whose lifestyle shuts them off entirely from sunlight (30 minutes a day can actually help to prevent cancer), fish liver oil is the richest source. You get very small amounts in butter, eggs, herring, liver, salmon, tuna, and mackerel.

Vitamin D deficiency affects your teeth and your bones because this nutrient influences the supply and deposition of calcium.

1,091. HELP YOUR DOG RECOVER FROM ARTHRITIS

If your dog suffers from arthritis, try giving Rover some velvet antler. Many success stories have crossed our desk about crippled dogs regaining their joint flexibility with velvet antler. Since the FDA agrees that the chondroitin sulfate and type II collagen in velvet antler have been scientifically substantiated by research and clinical studies, in compliance with FDA regulations, "to support healthy joint structure and function," why not try this therapy on your canine pet?

To learn more about how velvet antler works for regaining healthy joint function, see my book, *The Remarkable Healing Power of Velvet Antler.*

1,092. NOT THE WINE...IT'S THE *LIFESTYLE*

The often touted health benefits of wine may be a result of dietary habits and other lifestyle factors, and not the wine itself. Those who prefer wine have healthier diets than do those who prefer beer or hard liquor or those who have no preference. Wine drinkers report eating more servings of fruit and vegetables and fewer servings of red or fried meats.

The diets of wine drinkers contain less cholesterol, saturated fat, and (non-wine) alcohol, and more fiber.

Wine drinkers are also less likely to smoke.

Sources: *Archives of Internal Medicine* **2001;161:1844-1848;** *American Journal of Clinical Nutrition* **2002;76(2):466-472.**

1,093. BLUE-LENSES BAD FOR YOUR EYES

Blue-tinted sunglasses, intended to enhance performance when playing tennis, are ineffective and allow transmission of short wavelength light – a potential hazard to the lens of the eye. There is much literature on theoretical risks and additional literature on the potential clinical risks of blue light.

Both the American Academy of Ophthalmology and the American Optometric Association recommend that when individuals are out in bright sunlight, they should wear lenses that absorb *all* ultraviolet and deep blue visible light.

Blue lenses, marketed to increase the color contrast of optic-yellow tennis balls, actually make the balls less visible against a greenish court surface. Also, while blocking most UV light, the lenses block very little "blue light." And by making the world appear subjectively darker, a person wearing the lenses might spend extra time in the sun or have a relatively dilated pupil.

According to researchers, blue is the wrong end of the spectrum if you want to block most harmful rays. The manufacturers of these lenses disagree.

Source: *Archives of Ophthalmology* **2000;119:1064-1066.**

1,094. DON'T EAT THAT GINGERBREAD HOUSE!

If gingerbread houses are traditional in your family, let the children know that they are for decoration only because gingerbread contains *seven times* the amount of acrylamide found in fried potatoes. Acrylamide is linked with cancer, neurological damage, and infertility The potential problem first came to light in April 2002, when the Swedish National Food Administration and Stockholm University reported they had found the chemical in fried and oven-baked foods, especially potato chips and french fries.

Many initially doubted the findings, but scientists in Norway, the UK and Switzerland later reported similar results. Chips, fried potatoes, cakes, and now gingerbread have all been found to contain high levels of acrylamide. The levels depend on the way the foods are prepared and how they are stored.

Gingerbread is among the worst foods for acrylamide levels. The substance is probably formed as the result of a natural chemical reaction while preparing food at high temperatures.

Source: German Consumer, Nutrition & Agriculture Ministry, reported in *Reuter's Health* **Dec 2002.**

DRUGS WARNINGS: OVER-THE-COUNTER

1,095. PROTECT AGAINST ACETAMINOPHEN DAMAGE

The damaging effects of acetaminophen (as in aspirin-free Tylenol, Actamin, Anacin, Bayer Headache Relief, St. Joseph Children's Aspirin-Free analgesic, etc.) can be reduced with grapeseed extract. Well-known over-the-counter analgesics can cause *serious* damage to liver cells and tissues when too much is taken or when used in combination with alcohol. In 1996 alone, 74,000 cases of acetaminophen toxicity were reported in the United States.

Acetaminophen causes cell death in the liver by affecting the DNA of the cells, contributing both to programmed cell death that occurs during cell renewal and the aging process, and death of cells in response to exposure to toxic substances.

Researchers conclude that proanthocyanidin (as found in grapeseed extract) is a natural chemoprotectant and may be useful in defending cells against various environmental toxins.

Source: Experimental Biology Meeting, San Francisco, CA, Apr 1998.

1,096. UK RESTRICTS ACETAMINOPHEN

Acetaminophen poisoning (through the overuse of Tylenol and even aspirin-free Anacin and aspirin-free Excedrin) is the most common type of intentional drug overdose in the United Kingdom, comprising 40 percent of all cases. ("Aspirin-free" almost always means acetaminophen.) Placing restrictions on the sale and packaging of these medications in the UK has reduced the incidence of overdosing. In fact, the national referral rate for liver transplants due to acetaminophen overdose dropped from 3.5 a month to two a month.

The experts conclude that measures for limiting availability seem well founded and are not an unduly harsh restriction on the availability of these widely used drugs.

Parent, take note: Acetaminophen does not alleviate symptoms in children with chicken pox, and may even prolong the illness.

Sources: *Journal of Pediatrics* 1989;114(6):1045-1048; *Lancet* 2000;355:2009-2010,2047-2049.

1,097. ANTIHISTAMINES & IMPAIRED DRIVING

Be warned: Antihistamines can impair your driving ability more than alcohol can, even if you do not feel drowsy. Drowsiness is a poor indicator of driving impairment, and researchers caution that people should *not* drive when taking antihistamines. (Non-sedating antihistamines are preferable to sedating antihistamines, but they are available by prescription only.)

Source: *Annals of Internal Medicine* 2000;132:354-363.

1,098. THE RISKS OF DAILY ASPIRIN USE

Don't be influenced by the Bayer aspirin ads proposing that daily use of aspirin is beneficial for all adults: the US FTC and the US Department of Justice have ordered Bayer to tone down their ads. Bayer's aggressive aspirin marketing campaigns were cited as being misleading and could lead to medical complications. Officials were concerned about its unsubstantiated claims that regular intake of aspirin could prevent heart attacks and ischemic strokes in healthy adults.

Aspirin intake can worsen renal failure and hypertension as well as aggravate asthma in some patients. Bayer has been ordered to add the following to its ads: "For healthy people without any symptoms of heart disease, the risks of aspirin therapy may outweigh the benefits."

Source: *British Medical Journal* 2000;320:208.

1,099. ASPIRIN LEADS TO SERIOUS BLEEDING

Use of low-dose aspirin increases by *threefold* your risk of an upper gastrointestinal (GI) bleed requiring hospital admission, and enteric coating of the aspirin does not reduce this risk. Researchers identified a large number of individuals who regularly used 100 mg or 150 mg aspirin tablets between 1991 and 1995. Among a significant number of first-time hospitalizations for upper GI bleeding during this period, 12 percent involved current users of low-dose aspirin. The problem increased when low-dose aspirin was combined with nonsteroidal anti-inflammatory drugs (NSAIDs). The risk was similar for 100-mg and 150-mg tablets, and for both enteric-coated and non-coated tablets.

The risk remained elevated during the year after treatment, even when aspirin use was discontinued.

Sources: *American Journal of Gastroenterology* 2000;95:2218-2224; *British Medical Journal* 2000; 321:1183-1187,1170-1171.

1,100. PYCNOGENOL AS ASPIRIN ALTERNATIVE

Pycnogenol, an extract from the bark of the French maritime pine tree, is as effective as aspirin in preventing the increase in platelet aggregation that occurs with smoking, with the added advantage that it does not increase bleeding time (as aspirin does).

Source: *Thrombosis Research* **1999;95:155-161.**

1,101. ASPIRIN USE & PLANTAIN PROTECTION

A natural flavonoid found in plantain pulp helps to protect the gastric mucosa from aspirin-induced erosions. The anti-ulcer properties of plantain banana have been well established even though the active ingredient has only recently been identified (the flavonoid *leucocyanidin*). Leucocyanidin significantly increases mucus thickness, and definitely has a protective effect, although the mechanism involved is still not fully understood.

By the way, the leaves of the plantain plant have been used for skin healing for centuries all over the world.

Source: *Journal of Nutritional Biochemistry* **2001;12(2):95-100.**

DRUGS WARNINGS: PRESCRIPTION

1,102. TAKE PROBIOTICS AFTER ANTIBIOTICS

When antibiotics are prescribed in the countries of continental Europe, probiotics (regarded as medicines) are prescribed alongside them, partly because they help to prevent the diarrhea that often accompanies antibiotic treatment. Probiotics are microbes that can protect you against disease. They are immune-modulating bacteria that have very low virulence compared with the more pathogenic gut flora (such as *Escherichia coli* and clostridia).

Lactobacilli and bifidobacteria are examples of probiotics found in the large intestine. In the US, probiotics are marketed as supplements and are sold over the counter.

Lactobacillus GG can prevent diarrhea and allergies in children. Lactobacilli also produce compounds that act as local antibiotics against more toxic organisms.

Sources: *Lancet* **1999;354:1884;** *British Medical Journal* **2002;324:1364.**

1,103. VITAMIN C REDUCES ANTIBIOTIC NEED

If you MUST take an antibiotic, vitamin C given with tetracycline has been shown to reduce the amount of the antibiotic required, and to shorten the course of the antibiotic therapy — thereby minimizing its side effects. 500 mg of vitamin C given with every 250 mg of tetracycline increases the blood level of the antibiotic *15 times* compared with tetracycline alone. And any reduction in antibiotics is a health advantage.

Source: A. Gaby, Townsend Letter for Doctors 1990.

1,104. VITAMIN E & ANTIPSYCHOTIC DRUGS

Twenty-five percent of patients who take antipsychotic drugs develop *tardive dyskinesia*, but 1,200 to 1,600 IU of vitamin E helps to prevent this side effect. Tardive dyskinesia is a syndrome of potentially irreversible, involuntary, dyskinetic (fragmentary) movements caused by antipsychotic drugs, which may increase free-radical damage to brain cells.

The best responses to the vitamin E supplements occur in those who have had the disease for five years or less.

Source: *Annals of Pharmacotherapy* 1999;33:1195-1202.

1,105. GRAPEFRUIT JUICE AFFECT MEDICATIONS

Grapefruit juice is known to increase the oral bioavailability of some medications, and reduce that of others – so to be on the safe side, delete this juice from your diet if you are on *any* drug. Of all fruit beverages tested for drug interactions, grapefruit juice heads the list. Even a normal dietary amount of grapefruit juice can produce a pronounced, unpredictable, and sustained interaction with drugs used for hypertension.

Certain chemicals have been identified in grapefruit juice that are not detected in beverages from orange, apple, grape, or tangerine.

Grapefruit juice-drug interactions have also been noted for drugs like sildenafil (Viagra), and a long list of others.

Sources: *Clinical Pharmacological Therapy* 2000;68:28-34; *Clinical Pharmacokinetics* Jul 2000;39(1):49-75; *Cancer Epidemiological Biomarkers Prevention* Jul 2000;9(7):733-739; *Med Klin* 2000;95(1SpecNo):18-22.

1,106. FORTIFIED ORANGE JUICE & DRUGS

Just as we have been warned about adverse interactions between grapefruit juice and some prescribed drugs, we now know that calcium-fortified orange juice can also interfere with the action of certain drugs. Drug interactions are a major concern. Foods interacting with drugs may be more far-reaching than we assumed.

(For example, milk should not be taken with certain antibiotics.) Orange juice with added calcium may interfere with the effectiveness of specific germ killers, reducing the effectiveness of these drugs by as much as 40 percent. (The now popular Ciprofloxacin is among the drugs affected this way.)

Labels for these medications already say that they should not be taken with calcium supplements, and some even state they shouldn't be taken with milk.

Sources: *Journal of Clinical Pharmacology* Apr 2002;VOL:PAGE; Interscience Conference on Antimicrobial Agents & Chemotherapy, San Diego, CA, 2002.

WANT TO KNOW MORE?
[We are back to square one: Isolated and/or synthesized supplements should not be added to our diets without careful consideration. Just as whole foods are in our best health interest, so are whole-food types of supplements, as explained in detail in my newest book, *Everything I Know About Nutrition I Learned From Barley*.]

1,107. TAKE THE VITAMIN C "SHUTTLE"

If you are taking medications to treat a neurological disorder, then you should know that these drugs appear to get into the brain more easily when accompanied by ascorbic acid (vitamin C). Ascorbic acid works like a "shuttle," helping any compound get transported through what is known as the blood-brain barrier.

The effect of adding ascorbic acid to drugs known to have difficulty crossing this blood-brain barrier could be very significant in treating such diseases as Alzheimer's, Parkinson's, and epilepsy, as well as viral infections such as AIDS.

Source: Web edition of the *Journal of Medicinal Chemistry* Dec 2001.

SUPER NUTRACEUTICALS

1,108. ANTLER FOR ARTHRITIS, AND MORE!

Elk and deer antlers regenerate every year, and are among the fastest growing animal tissue known. "Velvet" antler is harvested from the deer or elk about halfway through the annual growth cycle. Unlike the inert and calcified tissue of horns or teeth, velvet antler is loaded with growth factors, immune factors, cartilage, collagen, glucosamine sulfate and chondroitin sulfate. These last two substances are currently in widespread use as a remedy for arthritis. When they are naturally packaged in velvet antler along with natural co-factors, the result appears to have a significant performance edge over the isolated chemicals.

Antler is "chondro-protective," meaning that it protects and restores damaged cartilage, the source of arthritic pain.]

Velvet antler is one of a very few natural sources for IGF-I and II, the secondary hormones that do the work for human growth hormone. These are probably the substances responsible for the increased effectiveness of velvet antler over isolated chondroitin sulfate and glucosamine sulfate. The only other natural sources of growth factor hormones are colostrum (the "first milk" produced shortly after a cow or a human mother gives berth) and blue-green algae nucleus (chlorella is the most available source).

[FGF-1, or fibroblast growth factor, is particularly abundant in antler. This may be a link to faster bone repair and protection against osteoporosis. Among the other trace co-factors in antler are stem cell stimulators, immune stimulants, antifungal agents, and antiepileptic agents.] Antler is now being used to treat osteoporosis and enhance athletic performance, and enjoys a well-deserved thousand-year-old reputation as a remedy for male sexual dysfunction.

Small-scale clinical trials have demonstrated that pain-relief from antler-derived products can be comparable to that of NSAIDs (non-steroidal anti-inflammatory drugs) with the important difference that side effects tend to be good rather than bad, and there is no known risk associated with long-term use.

Additional data is available from the veterinary community: One study by the Cedar Animal Medical Center in Gallup, New Mexico, found that 70% of arthritic dogs treated with antler supplements showed a positive response. This trial involved 150 animals over two years.

Veterinary experience suggests that most users are still significantly under-dosing. A dose as high as 10 mg of antler per pound of body weight was proposed - which, on the basis of body weight, would be comparable to 1500 mg per day for a 150 pound human, or six 250 mg capsules.

It has recently been shown that antlers retain an internal circulatory system right up to a few weeks before the antler is naturally shed. Even in the fully "calcified" mature condition, the antler contains a lot of living tissue. An antler shed in the wild will be gnawed on by other animals, who presumably know the value of what they are eating.

Source: Proceedings, Antler Science and Product Technology Conference, Banff, Apr 2000

1,109. HAVE A BARLEY LEAF COCKTAIL

Consumption of leafy green vegetables continues to outperform isolated supplements in a wide variety of clinical trials and population studies. But the constraints of modern living (not to mention our modern, if misguided, taste preferences) often make it difficult or impossible to eat the recommended five portions of vegetables every day. One of the best substitutes is green barley leaf extract. This is not a supplement, but a concentrated whole functional food.

Young, rapidly growing barley sprouts are a rich source of chlorophyll, B vitamins, iron, carotenoids and other antioxidants, and a large assortment of other important phytonutrients. Look for a powdered whole leaf product rather than a juice – there's more good stuff in the whole leaf.

Chlorophyll deserves special mention. This is the green pigment necessary for absorbing solar energy and turning it into chemical energy in the form of food for the plant. In human nutrition, chlorophyll is important because of its similarity to hemoglobin, the oxygen-carrying mechanism of red blood cells.

Both hemoglobin and chlorophyll contain a molecular structure called a porphyrin ring. In hemoglobin, there's an iron atom bonded inside the ring. In chlorophyll, there is magnesium instead. Otherwise the two substances are remarkably similar.

There is speculation that eating chlorophyll-rich plants helps with red blood cell production through an indirect pathway, and may be a viable treatment for anemia and other conditions addressed by red blood cells.

The fastest-growing plants have the most chlorophyll. They also need the highest concentration of antioxidants, because the solar radiation brought into the cells to power the conversion of carbon dioxide and water into carbohydrates for food energy can also trigger the oxidation of delicate proteins.

This is why the fastest growing, greenest, and youngest plants tend to have the highest nutritional value.

I start with my barley drink, then add a probiotic, a little fiber, a tablespoon of stabilized rice bran, some beet crystals for taste, some colostrum powder for immunity enhancement, and that's my afternoon cocktail.

Source: My book, *Everything I Know About Nutrition i Learned from Barley* explores the magic of the green leaf in detail. Hundreds of medical references are included.

1,110.   COLOSTRUM: THE IMMUNITY FOOD

Colostrum is the "first milk" produced by cows and by human mothers during the first day or two after giving birth. Once considered a waste product and fed to barnyard animals, it is rapidly becoming an important functional food. One of the more amazing properties of colostrum is its ability to transfer immune factors from cow to calf. A cow exposed to a particular pathogen will produce the specialized protein custom made to fight that particular bug. This is normal immunity at work. The amazing part is that when the calf drinks the colostrum, that same immune factor can be transferred to the calf – or possibly to the human taking a high quality colostrum supplement.

f the cow lives outside and eats grass, then her colostrum will contain a huge array of specific immune factors, many of which apply directly to human pathogens. The theory is that if you mix colostrum from different sources, the odds are excellent that your immune system will receive some special coding to help with the bug du jour.

Colostrum contains:

~ A full complement of vitamins and minerals.

~ Lactobacillus Bifidus, one of the beneficial organisms that prevents the growth of other more dangerous fauna in the intestines.

~ Lactalbumins, the most common protein in human milk, which has been shown to have anti-cancer action under certain conditions.

~ A high concentration of IgG and other immunoglobulins, which are. very effective broad-spectrum antibodies and a key component of the immune system.

~ Lymphokines and cytokines, chemicals that help attract the right kinds of white blood cells to sites of infection and send other chemical messages between white blood cells.

~ Proline, an amino acid needed by the thymus gland, which in turn plays a vital roll in conditioning white blood cells to become effective parts of the immune system.

~ Growth factors, including growth hormone and IGF-I (anabolic growth hormones that can help to burn fat and build protein); EgF (epithelial growth factor), and TgF A & B (transforming growth factors).

~ Glycoproteins, important constituents of cell membranes that provide binding sites for hormones (one glycoprotein in cow's colostrum is thought to be effective in protecting certain immune factors in the colostrum from destruction by digestive enzymes).

~ The glycoprotein lactoferrin, the second most common protein in human breast milk; which selectively binds and releases iron, and has a wide range of other immunity-enhancing effects.

~ Specialized polypeptides (aka "infopeptides") long chains of amino acids that may transmit immunity iinformation specific to thousands of pathogens.

The most intriguing mode of action – the transfer of specific immunity – is well documented but the mechanism is controversial. The more general pathogen-fighting constituents, such as the high concentration of IGg, are much better understood. Some of the other general beneficial actions, such as those made possible by lactoferrin, cytokines and growth factors, are only now being studied. Other modes of action will probably not be understood for many years.

I always throw a dash of colostrum powder into my afternoon cocktail.

Sources: *Alimentary Pharmacology Therapy* **2002;16(11):1917-22;** *European Journal of Nutrition* **(England), 2002, 56 Suppl 3:S24-8.**

1,111. STABILIZED RICE BRAN

Add stabilized rice bran to your daily health cocktail. Whole rice has a very serious shelf life problem. There is a natural enzyme called lipase in the rice bran that causes the oil to become rancid. When the rice is growing, the lipase and the oil are isolated from each other. But as soon as any mechanical processing occurs - such as when the rice is hulled or when the bran is removed from the kernel - the cell walls are ruptured and lipase meets rice bran oil. From there it only takes a few hours for the fragile rice bran oil to become rancid.

For the last seven thousand years, the solution has been to mill the rice to remove the hull and the bran, leaving only the white kernel underneath. This achieves long shelf life, but also removes most of the nutritional value.

But a new extrusion process makes it possible to expose rice bran to just the right amount of heat for just the right amount of time to deactivate the lipase while leaving most of the rice bran nutrients and natural antioxidant preservatives intact. The result is the availability of nutritionally active rice bran with a long shelf life.

Stabilized rice bran is rapidly being recognized as a very potent neutraceutical, particularly effective against liver dysfunction and diabetes. Among the constituents:

~ *Gamma Oryzanol*, beta sitosteryl ferluate, and five other related compounds. These are potent antioxidants and trace nutrients that play a vital role in so many aspects of human physiology that they suggest a symbiotic relationship between fresh rice and humans. Gamma oryzanol is found only in rice bran.

~ *Tocopherals* and *tocotrienols*, at least eight different varieties. These are all types of Vitamin E, although commercial vitamin E supplements are usually in the form of alpha-tocopheral. The importance of the others is probably at least equal to that of the alpha form.

~ *Polyphenols* including ferulic acid, alpha-lipoic acid, and four others. Lipoic acid is believed to play an important role in sugar metabolism at the cellular level.

~ The *metal chelators* magnesium, calcium, and phosphorous. Also manganese and other trace minerals,

~ *Phytosterols*, including beta sitosterol, campesterol, stigmasterol, and at least eleven more. These are some of the trace nutrients that help explain why fresh vegetables are so good for you. Carotenoids, including beta-carotene, alpha carotene, lycopene, lutein, zeazanthin, and more. Although beta-carotene is commonly sold as a single-ingredient supplement, alpha-carotene may in fact be more important. Lycopene is responsible for some of the recent health claims relating to tomatoes.

~ *Essential amino acids* including tryptophan, histidine, methionine, cystein, cystine, and argenine.

~ *Nine B-vitamins, polysaccharides, and phospholipids.* Phospholipids are vital to maintaining healthy cell membranes.

~ *Lecithin* (phosphatidyl choline and phosphatidyl serine).

~ *Seven identified enzymes*, including coenzyme Q10 and superoxidase dismutase.

Can't we get these same nutrients from brown rice? Brown rice is brown because a layer of rice bran is left in place. But the hulling process causes enough disruption to release lipase into the bran. The result is that virtually all brown rice contains rancid oils to some degree, and the most potent nutrients have been damaged by oxidation. The long-held belief that brown rice is nutritionally superior to white rice is suddenly called into question.

Rice bran has probably been used as a nutraceutical for as long as rice has been gown. Even in modern India, it's not uncommon for the mother of a sick child to collect some fresh bran from rice polishings to use for a therapeutic tea. But the bran has to be very fresh, or it's worthless. Because it's been so hard to stabilize this nutrient-rich food, millions of tons of it are discarded or sold for low-grade animal feed every year.

Stabilized rice bran is now available in several forms, with various ratios of soluble to insolube components and other nutraceutical additives. They all share the surprisingly pleasant nutty taste of fresh rice bran, and the safety of a food that's been used by humans for thousands of years.

Some of the most promising uses are against diabetes, arthritis, peripheral neuropathy, high cholesterol and cardiovascular disease. While the exact modes of action are often unclear, many of these chronic conditions have their origins in oxidative damage. It is likely that the right antioxidant at the right time is what is really responsible for the broad-spectrum efficacy of stabilized rice bran.

This is one of the foods that will help reverse our civilization's 10,000 year decline in nutritional quality. And there are no pills to swallow - just mix in a glass of water, or make it a part of your daily health cocktail drink.

Source: R. Cheruvanky, "Bioactives In Rice Bran and Rice Bran Oil," *Phytochemicals as Bioactive Agents* **2000, Technomic Publishing Co, Lancaster, PA; persosnal interviews with Dr Cheruvanky..**

1,112. 12 STEPS OF CHANGE: MAKING IT ALL WORK!

Because very few can make life-altering transformations fell-swoop, initiating the changes a step at a time can often help, especially if we understand why and how the adjustments will improve our health status. My suggestion is to deal with the following suggestions one at a time, taking a full month to make each change.

But for those of you who know at the start that these modifications will not be realistic (no matter how convincing the science), or for those who have tried and failed, Change Number 12 offers hope with *the least amount of lifestyle resistance for the greatest benefit.* Good luck!

Twelve Steps of Change #1: Give Before You Take Away. The first step for the kitchen in transition is to avoid resistance by *adding* instead of taking away. The master stroke is to lay out healthful snacks – raw vegetable strips in tiny attractive pieces; green peas still adhering to their protective pods for the kids to take apart; sections of fruit on toothpicks; nuts and seeds in the shell to crack open while watching TV – treats that boast nutrition, scattered around the house.

Fiber Feasts. Season yogurt (for good-guy bacteria) with sesame or sunflower seeds (for health-giving polyunsaturated oils). Embellish the dip with tofu (for phytoestrogens, calcium, protein, B vitamins and ease of digestion) and/or mashed avocado (for more polyunsaturated fatty acids and other beneficial nutrients). Place in a small pretty dish; surround with strips of bright-colored cucumbers, zucchini, peppers, mushrooms, carrots (for fiber and minerals).

These suggestions should be in addition to, not in place of, the usual. Substitutions create feelings of deprivation. Flip through recipe books in the health store for more ideas.

Twelve Step of Change #2: No-Salt Insurance: The next step is to transform the simplest fare into a gastronomic treat so that the salt shaker won't be missed. For the diehards who salt before they taste, the following herbs have a salty flavor: summer savory, lovage, and celery. These herbs are easiest to use if dried or powdered. Or, while in transition, you could replace the contents of the salt shaker with this composite: one tablespoon of ground course salt (course salt has more flavor than the over-processed free-flowing variety), 1/4 tablespoon each of ground black peppercorns, ground coriander seeds, ground bay leaves, and dried basil. Slowly reduce the salt content and increase other condiments.

Try cinnamon, yogurt, or apple sauce on oatmeal or other cooked cereals to replace salt and/or milk. Melted sweet butter with oregano can be served over fish. There are no rigid rules, but here's a beginner's herb guide:

Food	Herbs to use
Butter spreads	caraway, chives, garlic, parsley, tarragon
Eggs	basil, coriander, cress, dill, parsley, tarragon, thyme
Fish	basil, chives, dill, fennel, parsley, tarragon, sesame seeds

Meats	basil, dill, marjoram, mint, oregano, rosemary, sage, thyme
Poultry	basil, dill, lemon balm, lovage, rosemary, sage, tarragon, thyme
Salad	basil, chives, cress, dill, garlic, marjoram,
Salad dressing	oregano, parsley, savory, tarragon
Soups	basil, bay leaf, chives, dill, oregano, parsley, tarragon; capsicum, cumin

Most herbs should be added in moderation during the last stages of cooking. If cooked too long, they may give a bitter taste to foods.

12 Steps of Change - #3: Gain with Grains: Recent high-tech research offers an understanding of why patterns of grain eating work so well, and why they endured over the years. More people rely on grains for energy than on any other type of food. Americans, however, eat virtually no whole grains. Grains offer: Low cost, easy storage, and a bundle of nutrients not found in meat or dairy products (i.e. fiber, iron, niacin, and thiamin).

~ Oats. Unlike wheat, the germ and the bran of the oat remain intact, even when commercially processed. Oats, however packaged, are always a whole grain. Oats are high in protein and fiber.

~ Buckwheat: Our country grew up on buckwheat pancakes. Let's make it a favorite again. Kasha is rich in iron and B vitamins, plus the amino acid lysine. The quality of buckwheat can be improved further if combined with sesame flour, which is high in methionine. Lysine and methionine are two amino acids in short supply in most plant foods.

~ Millet. Millet is a grain eaten by millions of people in Asia and Africa daily — perhaps because it is one of the most nutritious of all grains. More nearly a complete protein than any other grain, it's also high in minerals, easily digested, incredibly adaptable, and has a bland, slightly nutty flavor. (It's one of my favorites!)

Beware fast-cooking grains. They have been over-processed, one way or another. Because commercial grains are heavily sprayed, they should be purchased in a natural-food store, where organic varieties are available.

Twelve Steps of Change - #4: Eliminate Simple Sugar to Avoid Complex Disease. No one really understands why we have such a love affair with most things sweet. But eliminating refined sugar is essential if we are to progress on the health continuum.

Not only do we feel deprived when this love-object is banished, but we also suffer very real physical discomfort. A partial solution is education. Every member of the family should understand why refined sugar is so devastating to our health status: everyone should know that more processed a food is, the less nutrient value it has, and refined sugar is just about the most processed food there is. Ninety percent of the original sugar cane or sugar beet is removed at the manufacturer's plant. Not one action of refined sugar can be considered beneficial. Far too many actions of sugar are disastrous. To cite but a few:

~ Beet sugar sensitivity has been reported in medical books. It is not uncommon to have sugar allergies.

~ A dietary regimen which eliminates sugar has proved to be effective in helping hyperactive children. Improvements are seen in the ability to concentrate, in longer attention spans, in less irritability, and in less useless motion.

~ Eating sugar with highly refined starches can promote cavities. Jelly or honey on white bread would be an example. The cavity-promoting effect is worse than eating sugar alone.

~ Sugar in processed cereal is refined sucrose. Sugar in apples is a mixture of fructose, glucose, and sucrose, imbedded in a fibrous matrix together with other nutrients designed to accompany the sugars. The insulin and metabolic responses from eating apples and from eating naked sucrose differ greatly. The consumption of refined sugar has played a major role in the increasing incidence of diabetes.

Evidence incriminating sugars continues to accumulate. What I cited above is barely the tip of the iceberg. Don't be fooled by ingredient listings that specify several different kinds of sugar. The manufacturer is allowed to use as many as twelve or more different sweetening agents, and as long as they are not the same, they may be listed separately. This is a ploy to detract from the fact that so much sugar is present in a particular product. Sugar has a way of hiding. It's highly absorbent, and is found in ketchup, some brands of yogurt, juices, instant breakfasts, chewing gum, cough drops, mouthwash, pickles, and even chewable vitamins.

Use natural sweet foods to help fill the gap felt by the lost love. Try the morning cereal with cinnamon and bananas; sweet potatoes as snacks; pineapple and coconut for dessert; grapes and other fruits in a bowl topped with yogurt and freshly ground nuts or seeds.

12 Steps of Change #5 - Protein: Quality, not Quantity. Surely there is a Nobel Prize waiting for the researcher who can scientifically demonstrate the exact amount of protein required by human beings. Different theories abound regarding the specifics, but we do know, in general, that Americans consume too much protein. We also know that protein *quality* rather than *quantity* is the critical factor.

As you eat, the protein in your food is broken down into component parts, called amino acids. These individual amino acids are then reassembled in the unique pattern of human protein. You are literally taking something else and converting it into you. Your body doesn't care where the amino acids come from as long as they are present and accounted for in quantities necessary for the restructuring of your human cell needs.

A steak may contain protein equal to a quarter of its weight, and an apple may have only a trace of protein. All foods contain some protein, although the amount varies. In addition, the quantities of the individual amino acids differ. When you consume meat, chances are you'll have enough of what you require for the rebuilding. An apple, however, does not supply the necessary amount of each amino acid. If you need an amino acid missing in your lunch today, but happened to eat a food containing that amino acid yesterday, it may be too late. The amino acids that are indispensable for creating your new protein should be consumed at or near the same meal for optimal protein metabolism.

More than any other food, with the exception of breast milk, eggs contain amino acids in a pattern closer to that required by humans. There are almost no amino acids left over after the egg's protein is taken apart and rearranged for your use. It's interesting to note that breast milk contains only one percent protein, but all of this small quantity is utilized, leaving virtually no amino acids for disposal. A food that has a large percentage of protein does not necessarily yield a large percentage of totally usable amino acids for conversion to human protein. High quality complete protein means there are enough amino acids for reassembly with not too many parts left over. It also indicates that other food values in that food are especially healthful. Fish is such a food. Among supplements, Sun Chlorella has an excellent amino acid profile.

Meat, although a high protein food, is not in the same category because of other deleterious aspects. Meat contains high amounts of fat and it has been shown that Americans who avoid meat have higher bone densities than meat eaters. The more protein in your diet, the more calcium excreted. Too much protein is not in your best health interest.

Twelve Steps of Change - #6: "GET FRESH." Before World War II, commercially prepared foods were produced by the same methods used at home. Today, the foods you buy are the result of very sophisticated technology which could only be duplicated in factories. Guess who pays for the high tech? Fresh potatoes cost 2/3rds less than canned and 75 percent less than frozen.

The effects of freeze-preservation on nutrients are deleterious. Substantial amounts of nutrients are lost as a result of many factors, including physical separation (peeling & trimming in preparation for freezing), storage (even at correct temperatures), temperature fluctuation, and thawing.

In addition to the damage incurred in processing, your body reacts negatively when the form of a food is changed. An apple is ingested more than ten times faster in the form of extracted apple juice than when it is contained within the fibrous architecture of the whole apple. In the form of applesauce, it is digested nearly three times faster. These findings confirm that the natural fiber of the whole apple slows the ingestion of nutrients. Since no chewing is required in the consumption of applesauce, the process is speeded up.

Apples are more satisfying than applesauce (in terms of satiety), and the sauce more so than juice. Increased satiety conferred by apples and sauce last at least 2 hours. The satisfying effect of an apple is due as much to fiber content as to carbohydrate content, suggesting that extra satiety is partly dependent on the need to chew fiber. What is surprising is that your body handles the different forms of the apple differently, not only when the fiber is removed (as with apple juice), but also when the fiber has merely been physically disrupted (as with applesauce).

There are other disturbances, too. When ingesting applesauce and apple juice, there is a rebound fall in blood sugar levels that does not occur after consuming whole apples. There is a higher level of insulin in the blood after consuming juice and sauce than after apples, which is responsible for the blood sugar drop.

So step #6 suggests that you discard your can opener, put a lock on your freezer door, and consume foods as close to their primal form as possible. In other words, get it fresh and Whole, and eat it that way.

Twelve Steps of Change - # 7: How to Shop For Your Fat. "Fat" has received bad press, but you cannot survive without fatty acids. Fatty acids are essential. An essential nutrient is anything that your body requires in its daily biochemical activity that it is unable to make by its own chemical processes. Your body can make all the parts of the fat molecules except for polyunsaturated fatty acids, called PUFAs.

PUFAs are found in naturally occurring vegetable & fish oils, and in human milk. All you require is about a tspn a day, but believe it or not, it's hard to find good, unprocessed oil. PUFAs are very chemically reactive. Because they are so reactive, they are affected by improper storage and easily become rancid. Early rancidity is not detectable by smell or taste, but it does interfere with the usefulness of PUFAs in your body.

All processed fats have unhealthful forms of fatty acids. Most, if not all, cooking oils and fats contain excessive quantities of trans fatty acids. One of the most important factors triggering rancidity in fat is exposure to excessive heat. PUFA-rich oils may be used for cooking, but only at low heat and for short cooking times. These oils, once opened, should be kept refrigerated, and used promptly. If not used in four months, they should be discarded and replaced. Typical oils high in PUFAs include grapeseed, safflower, sunflower, and sesame. One of the most stable is grapeseed oil.

Twelve Steps of Change - #8: Good Guy Bacteria. Despite the fact that fermented foods have been used for ages, pioneering work which established the scientific reasons for its benefit weren't noted until 1908. The popularity of such foods has only recently come to the fore. Physicians are now prescribing such foods for many patients and for many reasons.

When a healthy intestinal gut is populated with an assemblage of good-guy bacteria, it crowds out bacteria of "disreputable" lineage. You can resist enemy invasion by entrenching your normal flora with good-guy sentries. Studies show that higher nutritional value of cultured products translate into improved physical performance.

So suggestion #8 is to allow viable bacteria to set up housekeeping in your intestine, creating an ecological system that will help you to absorb nutrients and create new ones, and in general serve to increase your well-being.

Twelve Steps of Change - #9: FROM SEED TO SALAD: SPROUTING. There is an ideal way to beat the establishment. Combine half a dozen sprouts (alfalfa, mung, radish, azuki, sunflower, and lentils are possibilities), add herb seasonings, a dash of apple cider vinegar, a few slices of avocado, and enjoy the medley for lunch with a chunk of sprouted grain bread. Cost? Unbelievably low. You also take giant steps forward on the health continuum.

You can use any wide-mouthed jar to help you get started. Seeds may be consumed at any stage of sprouting, but harvesting at peak offers the most value. Vitamin C is synthesized during germination, and the concentrations of some of the B vitamins is also increased, along with other nutrients. Here's the peak germination time for the most popular seeds: alfalfa, 4 days; mung, 3 days; radish, 4 days; azuki, 2 days; chick-peas, 1 day; lentils, 2 days; sunflower seeds, 1 day; soybeans, 1 or 2 days; wheatberries, 2 or 3 days; buckwheat, 3 or 4 days; clover, 4 days; rye, 2 days; sesame, 1 or 2 days.

Since seeds and environments vary, it is advisable to experiment, using a good sprouting book as a guide. Alfalfa, mung, and garbanzo beans are excellent sprouts for beginners. Before consuming, leave sprouts in indirect sunlight. This will "green" the leaves, adding chlorophyll.

Refrigerated sprouts last up to a week. But since they are growing in your kitchen, the "farm" couldn't be any closer. It is best to "harvest" as needed to optimize nutrient value. Sprouts are so inexpensive that we discard, rather than save, any surplus. (For the novice, harvesting sprouts simply means taking them from the jar.)

Twelve Steps of Change - #10: The Exercise Connection. Regardless of how active you are, exercise encourages better health — fostering a lifetime habit, one of the greatest gifts you can give to yourself and your children. It will improve your overall health and extend your life. The easiest and least expensive exercise is walking. Ideally, the exercise program should be done outdoors.

But you know all that. What you may not know is that just before embarking on your exercise program, swallowing a good supply of nutraceuticals helps to enhance all of the advantages. The aerobics that take place during the exercise venture will distribute beneficial nutrients throughout your body, helping cell absorption.

Twelve Steps of Change - #11. Table Talk Substitution Hints:

~ Use more liquid when substituting whole wheat pastry and other whole grain flours for cake flour or all purpose flour. (Be sure to refrigerate whole grain flour.)

~ Replace whole wheat flour kamut flour.

~ Use low-sodium baking powder to replace regular baking powder.

~ Make your own baking powder by combining 1/4 teaspoon of baking soda with 1/2 teaspoon of cream of tartar.

~ Use sesame flour or arrowroot powder to replace cornstarch.

~ Use cider vinegar to replace distilled vinegar.

~ Use grapeseed oil for salads and cooking. When using unrefined oils (sesame, olive, safflower) to replace hydrogenated fats and shortenings, use more dry ingredients or less liquid.

~ Increase nutritional values with the use of vegetable stock or viable yogurt in place of water whenever possible.

~ Milk, buttermilk, and sour cream can easily be replaced with the use of viable yogurt.

General Hints:

~ Keep a tray of organic soybeans in water in your freezer. These presoaked beans are always at the ready for soups, stews, or casseroles.

~ Freeze any pieces of fruit (bananas, berries, peaches, etc.). Blend. Pour into ice cube tray or freezer container. Freeze again. Blend again. Freeze once more. Serve, topped with viable yogurt, freshly-shelled nuts, unsweetened coconut, and/or mashed organic pineapple. Great dessert!

~ Blend 3 cakes of tofu with 1 1/2 teaspoons vanilla; 2 tablespoons lemon juice; 10 ounces raspberries, 1 banana. Puree and chill, and use as a fruit pudding alternative.

~ Make sugar-free lifesavers by freezing any leftover herb tea or pure juice in mini-ice cube trays. For company, add a sprig of mint or herb leaf before freezing.

~ Blend viable yogurt, bananas, real whipped cream and chopped nuts in any combination of quantities. Freeze and serve in place of ice cream pie.

~ Simmer combinations of dried fruit (apples, apricots, etc.), and blend. Use as cake or pancake topping, or as jelly replacement.

~ Use ground, unsalted popcorn to "lighten" cake flour for baking.

Commercial shredded coconut contains additives and sugar. Shred your own: buy an uncracked, milk-filled coconut. Punch holes in the eyes and drain. (Drink the milk or use it for cooking within 24 hours.) Insert coconut in a bag and drop it from a high place to crack it open. (Out a second story window and onto a sidewalk works.) Cut in pieces and blend. (The brown skin contains nutrients, so leave it on.) Moisten with a bit of coconut milk, and freeze.

Good luck, and remember that *the real power of your household is in your kitchen.*

Twelve Steps of Change - #12: The Need for Supplementation. There is no question that there are multiple unknown, but still essential, cofactors that make food different from and more desirable than nutrient supplements. If we all lived on farms in an unpolluted atmosphere where we could pluck, pick, pull, and chase our food, it would not be necessary to add supplements to our dietary regimen. We all know this is not possible in today's world. In fact, many of you may think that all or even some of the above changes are unrealistic. There is one measure that offers "industrial-strength" protection: *the right kind of supplementation.*

The proclivity of modern medicine (and even our health industry) to take the reductionist approach — isolating nutrients down to a single active ingredient — is at the root of many discrepancies concerning the effectiveness of supplementation. Supplements containing only a small number of known nutrients, whether synthetic or natural, seem to miss the point: *a plethora of unknown or poorly understood cofactors are associated with every recognized nutrient.* Hence the superb statistical performance of whole, natural, nutrient-rich foods, and the sometimes poor performance and often confusing aftereffects of traditional isolated nutrients.

But the inescapable conclusion is that we need to supplement our diets to help return to a food milieu that's close to that of our forbears. If isolated supplemental products prove to be too blunt a tool, what kinds of food concentrates should we consider?

The advantage of a whole-food type of supplement is the unrefined "packaging": *supplements that contain a multiplicity of known and unknown cofactors.* They don't have to mimic the actions of healthful food, because technically they *are* healthful food. And their use requires no compromise of a post-industrial lifestyle that generally rules out obtaining adequate nutrition from "normal" food sources.

Try the super food supplements outlined in Hints #1108 to 1111, one at a time. Talk to shoppers at your local health store and find out what nutraceuticals work for them. (By the way, the best way to find an alternative physician in your neighborhood is to query the shoppers at your local health store.) When you start a new supplement, start slowly in terms of quantity. Give yourself a week or two to work up to the amount designated on the packaging. That way, you may avoidd the discomfort of detoxifying too quickly, a common reaction when we start plying our bodies with nutrients it has been craving.

1,113...wait a minute! There's no more room!

But do you know that there is still SO much more information out there that can help you to safeguard your health and well-being? And new information is available every day. If you would like to be among those who are learning the latest, most up-to-date findings in the world of nutritional and alternative medicine – often before this research is publicly known – simply subscribe to my "Daily Hints" email list. Start learning – it could change your life.

The Daily Table Talk Hints are free, and they are short! Usually just one sentence! (More information on each hint is available at the website for those who want it.)

Sign up by emailing to :
           betty@well.com
and simply write HINT in the subject area.

To see the last ten hints mailed to thousands of subscribers, go to:
           www.bettykamen.com
and click on the HINTS button.

GLOSSARY

AA: arachidonic acid, a 20-carbon polyunsaturated omega 6 fatty acid, used in the production of regulatory molecules such as prostaglandins and thromboxanes. Arachidonic acid can be synthesized from membrane phospholipids and other fatty acids.

acetaldehyde: a chemical used to manufacture perfumes and artificial flavors. It is also an intermediate in the metabolism of alcohol and has a general narcotic action, and can cause irritation of mucous membranes.

acetylcholine: a neurotransmitter derivative of the B vitamin choline. It is released at the ends of nerve fibers in the nervous system and is involved in the transmission of nerve impulses across the synaptic cleft, the space between two nerve cells.

acrylamide: a chemical used to make glues, paper and cosmetics, and in the construction of dam foundations and tunnels. Acrylamide appears to be produced in some foods prepared at high temperatures such as snack chips and French fries. It is known to cause cancer in animals, and is toxic to the nervous system of both animals and humans.

adaptogen: a nutritional or supplemental dietary substance with the ability to activate natural healing or immune responses, but which tends to have a reduced effect when no longer needed. Because adaptogens activate natural physiological control mechanisms, they help biological processes tend to the normal. This is in contrast to most drugs, which generally have a strong effect whether needed or not.

adaptogenic: having the properties of an adaptogen.

ADHD: Attention Deficit Hyperactivity disorder, a common behavioral problem in children.

alpha-lipoic acid: a powerful antioxidant found in liver, yeast, certain vegetables, and stabilized rice bran. Dietary alpha-lipoic acid is easily absorbed and can cross the blood-brain barrier. It promotes the production of glutathione, which aids in liver detoxification, and has been used in the treatment of hepatitis C and other liver disorders.

amenorrhea: the cessation of menstrual periods.

analgesic: a substance which can reduce pain, or having the property of reducing pain.

andropause: male menopause, often associated with fatigue, depression, irritability, and reduced libido and potency.

anthocyanins: any of various water-soluble pigments that impart violet, blue and red colors to flowers and other plant parts. They are also metabolic byproducts in blood and urine.

antioxidant: a substance that prevents another substance from becoming oxidized. Most antioxidants are sacrificial - that is, they themselves become oxidized in the process. Vitamins E, C, and Carotene are familiar examples.

aromatase: an enzyme that converts androgens to estrogens, and

arrhythmia: an irregular or abnormal heartbeat.

arteriosclerosis: the progressive narrowing or hardening of the arteries, usually due to high blood pressure, high cholesterol, smoking or diabetes.

arthralgia: joint pain

asparagine: an amino acid found in many proteins and present in large amounts in certain plants such as asparagus.

asymptomatic: showing no symptoms of disease.

atheroma: fatty deposits in the inner lining of an artery that can obstruct blood flow.

atherosclerosis: the progressive narrowing or hardening of the arteries, usually due to high blood pressure, high cholesterol, smoking or diabetes.

atopic: an allergy caused or promoted by a hereditary predisposition.

bacterial vaginosis: infection resulting from a change in the normal balance of vaginal bacteria.

beta-carotene: a form of carotene that is most widely used as a nutritional supplement. It is an antioxidant, and is converted to vitamin A by the liver. Other components of the "carotene complex" may have equal or greater importance in human nutrition.

bioavailability: the rate and degree at which a substance is absorbed into a living system.

biofeedback: the technique of making unconscious or involuntary bodily processes (such as brain waves) perceptible to the senses, so that they might be controlled consciously.

bronchodilator: a drug that eases constricted breathing by widening the air passages of the lungs.

capsaicin: a compound extract from hot chili peppers that is used medicinally.

carcinogenesis: the generation of cancerous cells from previously normal cells.

cardiovascular disease: disease of the heart and blood vessels.

carotenoids: yellow and red plant pigments including the carotenes and the xanthophylls.

casein: a milk protein.

catechins: phenols found in various plants; first obtained by distillation of gum catechu. Also called catechol and oxyphenol.

celiac disease: a disorder of the small intestine resulting from ingestion of gluten.

cetirizine: an antihistamine

chromium polynicotinate: a niacin-bound form of chromium having high bioavailability. Not to be confused with chromium nicotinate, which is similar but may be less safe as a supplement.

colitis: Inflammation of the colon

convergence insufficiency: inability to maintain proper binocular eye alignment on objects as they approach from distance to near

CoQ10: coenzyme Q10, a vitamin-like compound vital to the production of ATP in the electron transport chain. Dietary CoQ10 is found mainly in fish.

corticosteroids: steroid hormones produced by the adrenal cortex or their synthetic equivalents, such as cortisol and aldosterone.

cortisol: an adrenal-cortex hormone active in carbohydrate and protein metabolism

crippling skeletal fluorosis: a crippling bone disease caused by fluoride. The early stages of skeletal fluorosis can be mistaken for arthritis.

Crohn's disease: progressive inflammation of the colon producing frequent diarrhea, abdominal pain, nausea, fever and weight loss.

cytokines: regulatory proteins, including interleukins and lymphokines, that are released by immune system cells and act as intercellular mediators in the immune response.

cytotoxic: toxic to cells.

DHA: docosahexaenoic acid, a 22-carbon polyunsaturated omega-3 fatty acid found in coldwater fish. DHA is also found in eggs and organ meats, and can be extracted from algae. It is necessary for proper function of nerve cell membranes, and is a primary building block of the retina and brain. DHA is the most plentiful fatty acid in human breast milk. Although it can be synthesized by the body from the essential fatty acid linolenic acid, dietary DHA is considered vital.

diabetes mellitus: 1) insulin-dependent or type 1 diabetes, a form of diabetes caused by insufficient production of insulin resulting in abnormal metabolism of sugars and carbohydrates. It typically appears in childhood or adolescence. 2) non-insulin-dependent or type 2 diabetes, a form of diabetes caused by insulin resistance, where insulin becomes ineffective. It typically appears in adults and is exacerbated by obesity and an inactive lifestyle. Type 2 diabetes often has subtle symptoms and is diagnosed by glucose intolerance.

diastolic: the relaxing phase of the heart's ventricles, during which time they refill with blood. Diastolic blood pressure is the lower of the two blood pressure numbers. Systolic blood pressure is the higher number.

dong quai: a type of angelica root used primarily for its uterine tonic, antispasmodic, and "blood purifying" effects. A mild laxative, herbalists recommend it for almost all gynecological ailments, including menstrual cramps and irregular or retarded menstrual flow. Dong quai should not be used during pregnancy or lactation.

dopamine: a neurotransmitter formed in the brain and essential to the normal functioning of the central nervous system. A reduction in its concentration within the brain is associated with Parkinson's disease. As a drug it is used to treat shock and hypotension

dyspepsia: disturbed digestion or indigestion

ectopic pregnancy: Implantation and subsequent development of a fertilized ovum outside the uterus, typically in a fallopian tube.

edema: a swelling from the accumulation of fluid in the cellular tissue beneath the skin or mucous membrane

endometriosis: the unwanted presence of tissue which resembles endometrium, or uterine mucous membrane, elsewhere than in the lining of the uterus. Endometriosis causes premenstrual pain and dysmenorrhea

endometrium: the tissue lining the uterus. It is sloughed off during the menstrual period, then gradually becomes thicker until the next period.

endotoxin: a toxin produced by some bacteria and released upon destruction of the bacterial cell.

EPA: eicosapentanoic acid, a 20-carbon polyunsaturated omega-3 fatty acid found in coldwater fish. Like DHA, EPA is also found in eggs and organ meats. EPA is required for the production of prostaglandins which control blood clotting and related functions. Although it can be synthesized by the body from the essential fatty acid linolenic acid, dietary EPA is considered vital.

epidemiology: the branch of medical science dealing with the propagation and control of disease.

erythromycin: an antibiotic obtained from *Streptomyces erythreus*.

estrogenic: of, related to, or caused by estrogen.

etiology: the cause or origin of a disease or disorder

fibromyalgia: a condition characterized by chronic pain in muscles and soft tissues surrounding joints, along with fatigue and tenderness at specific sites in the body

fibrosis: development of excess fibrous connective tissue in an organ or tissue.

flavone: precursor of a number of yellow pigments occurring on the leaves or in the stems and seed capsules of many primroses.

flavonoids: a group of plant substances that includes the anthocyanins, water-soluble pigments that impart to flowers and other plant parts colors ranging from violet and blue to most shades of red.

flushing: hot flashes.

folate: a B vitamin necessary for energy production, the formation of red blood cells, immunity, cell division and replication, protein metabolism, and regulation of homocysteine levels.

folic acid: another name for folate (see above).

free radicals: an atom or group of atoms that has at least one unpaired electron and is therefore electrically charged. They are highly reactive and unstable. In animal tissues, free radicals can damage cells and are believed to accelerate the progression of cancer, cardiovascular disease, and age-related diseases.

functional food: a food selected because it provides a concentration of nutrients known to have one or more beneficial physiological effects. Functional foods are sometimes processed in ways that render them more concentrated and more practical to use. (Nutraceuticals are essentially the same as functional foods, although they tend to be more highly processed and more concentrated, more supplement-like than food-like, as the term is commonly applied.)

gallotannin: a type of tannin, also called Chinese tannin. Tannin is a yellow substance obtained from nutgalls having an astringent taste. A large class of similar substances from oak bark, willow, catechu, tea, and coffee are also referred to as tannins. Gallotanin is an antioxidant, antiseptic, flavoring agent for various foods, clarifying agent for beverages, beer and wines, and decolorant for soy sauce.

gastritis: inflammation of the lining of the stomach

GERD: gastroesophageal reflux disease, also known as reflux disease or acid reflux.

germanium: a rare element that resembles tin. The healing properties of certain herbs has been attributed to relatively high levels of germanium: Garlic, aloe, comfrey, chlorella, ginseng, watercress, Shitake mushroom, pearl barley, sanzukon, sushi, waternut, boxthorn seed and wisteria knob contain concentrations from 100 to 2,000 ppm

gestational diabetes: diabetes caused by hormones during pregnancy that reduce the effectiveness of the mother's insulin.

ginkgolides: bioactive terpenes found in the root bark and leaves of *Ginkgo biloba.* It is believed to have anti-inflammatory, anticoagulant, antioxidant and antiseptic properties.

ginsenoside: one of the active compounds in panax ginseng, contributing to ginseng's aphrodisiac, anti-aging and energy-boosting properties.

glucose intolerance: a condition in which dietary sugar produces high blood sugar, but not sufficiently high for a diagnosis of diabetes. However glucose intolerance is often considered an early warning sign for type 2 diabetes:

glutamine: a nonessential amino acid common in plant and animal proteins

glutathione: a tripeptide and a powerful antioxidant produced in the liver. Produced by the amino acids cysteine, glutamic acid, and glycine.

glycation: the uncontrolled reaction of sugar with protein. Glycation damages the tissue of diabetics when blood sugar is above normal, and is one of the causes of the aging of nerve cells.

H. pylori: *Helicobacter pylori*, the organism responsible for ulcers.

HDL: high-density lipoprotein. Lipoproteins, classified according to their densities, are the principal means by which lipids (fats) are transported in the blood. HDL is sometimes thought of as the "good" cholesterol, while LDL, or low density lipoprotein, is the "bad" cholesterol.

homeostasis: a state of equilibrium.

homocysteine: an amino acid produced in the body. High levels of homocysteine in the blood are associated with an increased risk of cardiovascular disease such as atherosclerosis.

hyaluronic acid: a gel-like amino-glycan found in the synovial fluid of joints, and in the eyes. It acts as a binding, lubricating, and protective agent.

hyperglycemia: high blood sugar, a common symptom of diabetes

hyperinsulinemia: excessive insulin, a rare but important cause of hypoglycemia or low blood sugar in infants and children.

hypertension: high blood pressure

hypoglycemia: low blood sugar, often the result of over-stimulation of sugar metabolizing enzymes following consumption of a sweet food.

hypothyroidism: a glandular disorder resulting from insufficient production of thyroid hormones

IGF-1: insulin-like growth factor 1

immunomodulator: a substance that alters, suppresses or strengthens the immune system.

immunomodulators: substances that affect or control immune system function.

insulin resistance: condition in which insulin is not effective, as in type II diabetes.

intermittent claudication: leg pain and weakness while walking, usually due to peripheral arterial disease.

inulin: a nondigestible fiber and prebiotic that helps promote the growth of "good" bacteria in the colon.

inverse association: relationship between experimental parameters whereby the increase of one measured quantity is associated with the decrease of another.

ischemia: a decrease in the blood supply to an organ or tissue caused by constriction or obstruction of the blood vessels.

isoflavone: one of a family of phytoestrogens found chiefly in soybeans

isothiocyanates: a group of naturally occurring compounds that occur as glucosinolates in cruciferous or "cabbage family" vegetables such as broccoli, cauliflower, kale and turnips. They are being investigated as possible chemopreventive agents.

isotretinoin: Accutane, a popular acne medication.

kegel exercises: pelvic floor exercises, performed by repeatedly activating and relaxing the muscle that stops the flow of urine.

lactoferrin: • an iron-binding protein found in milk, saliva and tears, functioning as an iron transport protein. It is anti-viral and antimicrobial. It plays an important role in immune function, and is found in neutrophil leucocytes.

LDL: low-density lipoprotein. Lipoproteins, classified according to their densities, are the principal means by which lipids (fats) are transported in the blood. LDL is sometimes thought of as the "bad" cholesterol, while HDL, or high density lipoprotein, is the "good" cholesterol.

letinan: a polysaccharide found in the fruiting body of shiitake mushrooms. A purified form of lentinan has been used in Japan for the treatment of stomach cancer.

lignans: a type of phytoestrogen, although often thought of as a fiber. The lignans found in plants are converted by intestinal bacteria to two forms of mammalian lignans, enterolactone and enterodial. Lignans, as adaptogens, have either mildly estrogenic or antiestrogenic activity. They can inhibit the binding of estrogen and testosterone, or they can act like estrogens themselves.

linoleic acid: an 18-carbon polyunsaturated omega 6 fatty acid. Linoleic acid is one of the "essential" fatty acids that can only be obtained from food or supplements.

linolenic acid: an 18-carbon polyunsaturated omega 3 fatty acid. Linoleic acid is one of the "essential" fatty acids that can only be obtained from food or supplements.

lutein esters: natural lutein compounds found in vegetable and fruits.

lutein: a carotenoid (like beta-carotene and lycopene) found in many fruits and vegetables, with powerful antioxidant properties.

luteinizing hormone: a hormone produced by the pituitary gland that stimulates ovulation and the development of the corpus luteum in the female, and the production of testosterone by the interstitial cells of the testis in the male.

lysine: an essential amino acid having important structural and chemical roles in all proteins

macronutrient: broad nutritional categories including protein, fat and carbohydrates

metastasis: (plural "metastases") a secondary growth of a malignant tumor.

methionine: an essential amino acid, found especially in red meat. High dietary methionnine, If not properly metabolized by vitamins B6, B12 and folic acid, is thought to lead to excess homocysteine which can increase risk of heart and artery disease.

microalbuminuria: damage to the kidney characterized by release albumin into the urine. Microalbuminuria can be the first sign of diabetic kidney disease.

micronutrient: nutrients required in relatively small quantities, such as vitamins, minerals, food enzymes and phytonutrients.

morbidity: the relative incidence of disease, or the quality of being unhealthful

mutagen: an agent that causes mutation, such as radiation

mutagenic: having the property of causing mutation

myocardial infarction: a heart attack.

myopathy: muscle weakness.

neuropathy: dysfunction, pain or pathological changes in the peripheral nervous system.

nitrophenols: compounds connected with autoimmunity problems.

notrosamines: substance found in red and processed meat that has been implicated in the development of colon cancer.

NSAIDs: nonsteroidal anti-inflammatory drugs, such as Ibuprofen.

nutraceutical: a concentrated food or food component selected because it provides nutrients known to have one or more beneficial physiological effects. Nutraceuticals often undergo a natural process such as fermentation or germination which makes them more effective than the foods from which they are derived. (Functional foods are essentially the same as nutraceuticals, although they tend to be less processed and more food-like than supplement-like, as the term is commonly applied.)

oligofructose: a starch or soluble dietary fiber, consisting of fructose chains, that is not absorbed in the small intestine and passes into the large intestine where it is partly fermented. Oligofructose is a prebiotic, forming a substrate for bifidus bacteria that stimulating its activity

oligosaccharide: a saccharide (a simple sugar) that contains a small number of monosaccharide units, such as a disaccharide.

opioid: possessing properties characteristic of opiate narcotics but not derived from opium.

otitis media: Inflammation of the middle ear, occurring commonly in children as a result of infection

Oxidation: the combination of a substance with oxygen, or more generally, a reaction in which the atoms in an element lose electrons.

oxylate: calcium oxylate, kidney stones, deposits of mineral salts lodging themselves in the urinary tract

Pap test: a method of examining stained cells in a cervical smear for early diagnosis of uterine cancer

pathological: relating to or caused by disease.

pathology: the deviations from the normal that constitute or characterize disease.

PC: phosphatidyl choline, the main constituent of lecithin. Phosphatidyl choline has long been recognized as an emulsifier that can break down fat and lower cholesterol. It is also necessary for the production of acetylcholine, required for proper function of nerve endings.

PCBs: polychlorinated biphenyls, manufactured chemical compounds that build up in the environment and cause harmful effects.

perimenstrual asthma: an increase in asthma symptoms immediately before or after menstrual periods.

periodontitis: gum disease.

peroxidase: any of a group of enzymes that occur in plant cells and cause oxidation by a peroxide.

phosphatidyl choline: the main constituent of lecithin. Phosphatidyl choline has long been recognized as an emulsifier that can break down fat and lower cholesterol. It is also necessary for the production of acetylcholine, required for proper function of nerve endings.

photocarcinogenesis: promoting tumor growth or cancer by exposure to light

phthalates: plastic-softening chemicals widely used in cosmetics and toys.

phytofluene: a carotenoid, precursor of zeta-carotene

plays a dominant role in tumor proliferation.

polycystic ovarian syndrome: a disorder characterized by changes to the ovaries such that multiple follicles accumulate in the ovaries without ovulation. The ovary secretes higher levels of testosterone and estrogens, resulting in irregular or no menses, excess body hair growth, occasionally baldness, and often obesity, diabetes and hypertension.

polyphenol: an antioxidant found in green tea

postherpetic neuralgia: the outcome of shingles.

pre-eclampsia: a condition of hypertension occurring during pregnancy, typically accompanied by edema (water retension) and proteinuria (excessive amounts of protein in the urine). It can lead to eclampsia (coma or convulsions associated with pregnancy).

prenatal: before birth.

proanthocyanidins: tannins found in cranberries and blueberries that inhibit bacterial action.

progesterone: a steroid hormone produced in the ovary. One of the principle female sex hormones, progesterone prepares and maintains the uterus for pregnancy.

progestins: natural or synthetic hormones that mimic some or all of the actions of progesterone.

pro-oxidant: a substance which promotes oxidation.

prostaglandins: a group of potent hormone-like substances, made from arachidonic acid, that mediate a wide range of physiological functions such as blood pressure, inflammation and smooth muscle contraction.

pruritis: itchy skin.

PSA test: "prostate-specific antigen" test, used to screen for prostate cancer.

PUFA: polyunsaturated fatty acids, such as the omega-3 fatty acids DHA and LNA.

pulmonary aspiration: entry of gastric contents or other foreign substances into the respiratory tract. This in turn may produce obstruction of the airways or inflammation of the lung.

pulse: the edible seeds of legumes, such as beans, peas, or lentils.

pyridoxine: vitamin B6.

recombinant: recombined fragments from different sources, as in genetic manipulation by "recombinant DNA."

retinoic acid: a vitamin A derivative that has a role in the growth and development of bone and the maintenance of epithelium. A preparation retonic acid is used topically to treat acne and to modify the appearance of wrinkles, hyperpigmentation, and facial skin roughness.

retinopathy: a pathological (disease-related) disorder of the retina.

rhinitis: inflammation of the nasal mucous membrane.

rickets: a deficiency disease resulting from a lack of vitamin D or calcium, and from insufficient exposure to sunlight.

SAMe: S-adenosyl-L-methionine, a naturally occurring compound which is a major source of methyl groups in the brain. It is required in numerous reactions involving nucleic acids, proteins, phospholipids, amines and other neurotransmitters. SAMe has antidepressant properties and may improve cognitive function.

shingles: herpes zoster, an acute viral infection characterized by painful inflammation and eruptions that spread half way around the body like a girdle.

SIDS: Sudden Infant Death syndrome

sildenafil: Viagra

sleep apnea: temporary cessation of breathing, occurring repeatedly during sleep

SOD: superoxide dismutase, an enzyme that protects against oxidative damage by scavenging free radicals in the body.

spina bifida: a congenital defect in which the spinal column is imperfectly closed so that part of the spinal cord protrudes

SSRI: Selective Serotonin Reuptake Inhibitor, a class of antidepressants that includes Prozac and Paxil.

statins: a class of drugs that reduce serum cholesterol levels by inhibiting an enzyme involved in the synthesis of cholesterol.

steatosis: alcoholic fatty liver disease.

strabismus: "crossed eyes," "walleye"; a condition of abnormal deviation of alignment of one eye in relation to the other.

superoxide dismutase: superoxide dismutase, an enzyme that protects against oxidative damage by scavenging free radicals in the body.

systolic: the contraction phase of the heart and arteries, during which time blood is pumped through the circulatory system. Systolic blood pressure is the higher of the two blood pressure numbers, diastolic blood pressure is the lower of the two numbers.

tamoxifen: a nonsteroidal estrogen antagonist used in the treatment of advanced breast cancer. Also used prophylactically by some women at risk for breast cancer.

tannins: naturally occurring plant polyphenols that bind and precipitate proteins. Tannins are common in grapes, persimmon, blueberry, tea, chocolate, and coffee. They produce the astringent taste in wine or unripe fruits, and the colors in flowers and in autumn leaves.

teratogen: a teratogenic agent.

teratogenic: causing developmental malformations or defects.

thrombosis: the obstruction of a blood vessel by a clot formed at the site of obstruction. This is distinct from an embolism, which is an obstruction produced by a clot or foreign body brought from a distance

tocopherols: a group of fat-soluble alcohols constituting vitamin E and similar compounds. They are important antioxidants and are essential for normal reproduction.

tocotrienols: fat-soluble vitamins related to the family of tocopherols, a form of vitamin E.

triglycerides: a molecule consisting of three fatty acids attached to a glycerol backbone. This is the most common form of dietary fats and oils.

triticale: a hybrid of wheat and rye known for high yield

tryptophan: an amino acid.

UST: Unipedal Stance Time, a simple test to calculate risk of falling by standing on one foot.

vector: an organism, such as a mosquito or tick, that carries disease-causing microorganisms from one host to another

velvet antler: deer or elk antler harvested from the animal while still soft and growing, in the "velvet" phase. Widely used in Asia to treat arthritis and male sexual dysfunction.

venous thromboembolism: economy class syndrome, blockage of a vein by an aggregate of blood factors or blood clot. It can occur in any vein of the body but occurs most commonly in those of the lower extremities, and is associated with long periods of immobility in a seated position, such as during airline travel.

VLDL: very low density lipoprotein.

white-coat normotension: a condition in which blood pressure is measured as normal during an office examination, even though it is usually somewhat elevated at other times. It is more likely to occur in men, especially those who are past smokers, older, or alcohol users.

white-coat syndrome: psychologically-induced blood pressure elevation due to anxiety while being examined by physician or other health care professional.

WHO: the World Health Organization.

wild artichoke: another name for the herb milk thistle.

zeaxanthin: a carotene found in corn, fruits, seeds, and egg yolk

INDEX: HINT NUMBERS

Please note that the numbers following each index entry do not refer to the page number but to the relevant HINT number.

More comments from people all over the world; what they are saying about Betty Kamen's life-changing daily health hints:

"I would like everyone to know that Dr. Kamen's Table Talk has meant so much to me. I have learned so much and always in a clear understanding. She has helped me with answers to hormone questions and also cancer. Many times when she mentioned something, I would be happy to see that I was already doing it and wondering if it was the right thing to do, and there would be my confirmation. I would miss it terribly if she stopped doing this."

~ Pat Bosley, Orlando, FL

"I live in Cape Town, South Africa and find your daily hints very interesting and helpful, since I suffer from a lot of allergies."

~ Hilda van der Merwe, Cape Town, South Africa

"I am very pleased to receive these Daily Health Hints, and often pin them up on the bulletin board at work in attempts to alert colleagues to the possible results of the usual choices in nutrition and related areas. Whether my efforts have any impact or not, I have no way of knowing. But I am grateful to you for offering this valuable service."

~ Avvaiyar Kamari, Bobst Library, New York University, New York, NY

"I very much look forward to my daily hints; you are greatly respected for your dedication, research work, and continuity. My sister is into nutrition in a huge way, she was responsible for my daily hint from you. We take your advice, and we *trust* your advice."

~ Janice Ryan, North Island, New Zealand

"Over the years I have come to rely, not only on Dr. Kamen's extraordinary experience and wisdom in the field of health, but also her passion for educating through her many books, articles and health hints, those of us seeking more ways to be healthy and stay that way. Her contributions are legendary and her advice precious, especially in today's health world of contradictions and sometimes overwhelming information. Who can you trust? I have always trusted Dr. Betty Kamen."

~ Joseph Bentley, President and CEO, The Lifestar Millennium, Inc., Novato, CA

"I love your tips! They are short and to the point — perfect for the working mother who has precious little time on her hands."

~ Sherry Greenfield, Kawasaki, Japan

"Each day I look forward to reading your Daily Health Hints. I have used the hints for my own knowledge and have passed on this valuable information to those that need to have it. Keep up the good work."

~ Jan Goroncy, Health Educator and Practitioner, Sydney, Australia

"Words are not enough to describe how helpful Betty's Daily Health Hints are. As well as all the solid, cutting-edge information, the daily reminder that Betty's on the job gives me hope for the future!"

~ Pat on Salt Spring

"Dr. Betty Kamen's messages are an excellent source of information in the field of alternative medicine. I read them every day and I have gained a tremendous amount of knowledge from these messages."

~ Eugene A. Bratoeff, PhD, Professor of Chemistry, University of Mexico City, Mexico City

"I have enjoyed and utilized many of your hints and Table Talk commentaries. I find that by far you have the most common sense, down-to-earth tips that I have read. I am a talk show host and have been in radio for over 30 years. Your hints are so to the point and easy to understand. I hope that people will recognize you for the health advocate that you are."

~ Nelle Reagan, WRGA, Rome, GA

"I'm an herbalist student now and have been studying vitamins and nutrition for about 30 years. Your Daily Hints are part of my huge collection of tips and usually the ones that I pass along to my three adult children. I would be lost without them."

~ Rita Svoboda, Lake Placid, FL

"I am a practicing psychotherapist and a professor at Adelphi University where I teach nursing. I use Betty's Daily Hints in both my practice and my teaching. These hints are informative and invaluable in helping people learn about complementary medicine and alternative ways of helping them to heal themselves."

~ Dr. Arlene Trolman, Huntington, NY

"I think the hints you offer are timely, accurate, and generally agreed upon by those that follow nutrition and its research."

~ Wanda Ciulla, RN, PA-C, New Life Medical Clinic, Paris, IL

"You are providing a credible source for current information on health and nutrition. I truly look forward to your email hints. Keep up the great work."

~ Richie Gerber, LNC, "The Natural Grocer Show, Fort Lauderdale, FL

"I really appreciate your daily health hints — they are the *first* thing I read each day — they are a daily reminder that health really is the best wealth — I'm 88, in excellent physical & mental health, and your work is a great help in staying that way!"

~ Walter Tabor, San Diego, CA

"Your Daily Table Talk Hints are an excellent and concise source of information and I do consider myself quite lucky being able to receive them."

~ George Stastny, Chartered Herbalist, British Columbia, Canada

"I have been receiving the Daily Health Hints for quite some time. I so look forward to them because it has educated me on many issues, especially the ones that have helped me make changes.... You have been a wonderful source for my healing process."

~ Ymelda De Vargas, Albuquerque, NM

"I am extremely involved in helping others with the education of achieving optimum health, and I absolutely look forward to Dr. Betty Kamen's Health Hints every single day, I actually swear by her word, as I respect her so."

~ Janis D. Van Tine, Sr. PR Specialist, Sun Chlorella USA, Torrance, CA

"I am a Wholistic Kinesiologist and also work in a health food store. I often print out your hints for our clients."

~ Claudia Trewet, Albuquerque, NM

"Thanks for your Daily Hints, I really appreciate keeping up with health news and you and your hints fill in a lot of the blanks. I'm an RN in Telemetry/Cardiology and am very concerned with maintaining my own health and helping other to do the same. Keep up your great work!"

~ Barbara Vickers, RN, Los Angeles, CA

"Thanks so much for the valuable nuggets of advice. You educate in a succinct manner that makes the information stick. And every once in a while one of those gems of knowledge just happens to be the missing piece of the puzzle!"

~ Linda, Ontario, Canada

"I really appreciate your information. I am a holistic dentist and I have picked up a lot of new information from your emails."

~ David Doi

"I so enjoy your early morning Health Hints. They are concise, thorough, and most important accurate. Keep them coming please!"

~ Doreen Nowell, Ontario, Canada

"The daily hints help keep me informed as well as keeping my adult children in the know as they are raising their children."

~ Colleen Brewer, Teacher, California

If you would like the free one-line Table Talk Hints emailed to you daily, email to betty@well.com and write: "Hint" in the subject line.